Basics in NURSING RESEARCH AND BIOSTATISTICS

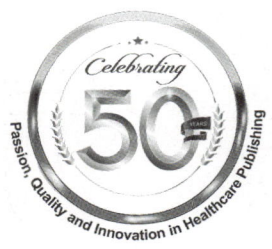

Basics in NURSING RESEARCH AND BIOSTATISTICS

Sreevani Rentala
PhD (Psychiatric Nursing)
Professor and Head
Department of Psychiatric Nursing
Dharwad Institute of Mental Health and Neurosciences (DIMHANS)
Dharwad, Karnataka, India

Foreword

K Reddemma

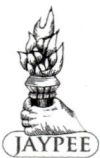

JAYPEE BROTHERS MEDICAL PUBLISHERS
The Health Sciences Publisher
New Delhi | London

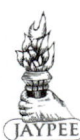 **Jaypee Brothers Medical Publishers (P) Ltd**

Headquarters

Jaypee Brothers Medical Publishers (P) Ltd
4838/24, Ansari Road, Daryaganj
New Delhi 110 002, India
Phone: +91-11-43574357
Fax: +91-11-43574314
Email: jaypee@jaypeebrothers.com

Overseas Office

J.P. Medical Ltd
83 Victoria Street, London
SW1H 0HW (UK)
Phone: +44 20 3170 8910
Fax: +44 (0)20 3008 6180
Email: info@jpmedpub.com

Website: www.jaypeebrothers.com
Website: www.jaypeedigital.com

© 2019, Jaypee Brothers Medical Publishers

The views and opinions expressed in this book are solely those of the original contributor(s)/author(s) and do not necessarily represent those of editor(s) of the book.

All rights reserved. No part of this publication may be reproduced, stored or transmitted in any form or by any means, electronic, mechanical, photocopying, recording or otherwise, without the prior permission in writing of the publishers.

All brand names and product names used in this book are trade names, service marks, trademarks or registered trademarks of their respective owners. the publisher is not associated with any product or vendor mentioned in this book.

Medical knowledge and practice change constantly. This book is designed to provide accurate, authoritative information about the subject matter in question. However, readers are advised to check the most current information available on procedures included and check information from the manufacturer of each product to be administered, to verify the recommended dose, formula, method and duration of administration, adverse effects and contraindications. It is the responsibility of the practitioner to take all appropriate safety precautions. Neither the publisher nor the author(s)/editor(s) assume any liability for any injury and/or damage to persons or property arising from or related to use of material in this book.

This book is sold on the understanding that the publisher is not engaged in providing professional medical services. If such advice or services are required, the services of a competent medical professional should be sought.

Every effort has been made where necessary to contact holders of copyright to obtain permission to reproduce copyright material. If any have been inadvertently overlooked, the publisher will be pleased to make the necessary arrangements at the first opportunity. The **CD/DVD-ROM** (if any) provided in the sealed envelope with this book is complimentary and free of cost. **Not meant for sale.**

Inquiries for bulk sales may be solicited at: jaypee@jaypeebrothers.com

Basics in Nursing Research and Biostatistics

First Edition: 2019

Reprint: **2020**

ISBN: 978-93-5270-580-1

Printed at Nutech Print Services - India

Dedicated to

My loving husband

FOREWORD

It is a matter of great pleasure and pride that after the phenomenal success with her previous two titles "A Guide to Mental Health and Psychiatric Nursing" and "Psychology for Nurses", Dr Sreevani Rentala has embarked on the project *Basics in Nursing Research and Biostatistics*.

Nursing research is an emerging and growing field in which individuals can apply their nursing education to discover new advancements that promote evidence-based care. Though the goal may seem noble, it is easier said than done. Of the many key barriers like lack of time, funding and practical support, a major area of concern is the lack of required skills and confidence to take part in research. This stems from the fact that the nursing community particularly in our country is lacking the resources both in terms of quality teaching and superior reading material to comprehend the basics for carrying out quality research.

It is in this backdrop, I believe that the effort of Dr Sreevani Rentala in coming out with this title will not only bridge the gap but also raise the bar when it comes to publication of similar other titles. Unlike in many other similar titles, the contents of this textbook have been strictly drawn as per the Indian Nursing Council (INC) syllabus. All the listed out topics have been comprehensively covered with elaborations where necessary. A few concepts though may seem abstract or intricate, the author has made a good effort to simplify them by presenting in her own lucid style.

I was particularly impressed with the apt usage of illustrations in the form of figures and tables. Research examples have been used liberally to underline the various concepts and bring home the point. Review questions along with multiple choice questions (MCQs) have been included at the end of each unit.

I am confident that this text on nursing research and biostatistics will serve as a good companion and a one-stop shop for both undergraduate and postgraduate nursing students who are looking to some genuine reference material. This endeavor will not only improve the research prowess among the nursing community but also set a new benchmark. I wish her the very best in all her future assignments.

K Reddemma
PhD (Psychiatric Nursing)
Nodal Officer
National Consortium for PhD in Nursing, INC
Formerly
Dean, Behavioral Sciences
Professor, Department of Nursing
National Institute of Mental Health and Neurosciences (NIMHANS)
Bengaluru, Karnataka, India

PREFACE

Over the past decade, nurses have been the focus of the movement that reflects probably more changes than in the past decades combined. Though nursing established itself as an applied science much early, it was only in 1990s that it became clear that producing new knowledge was not enough. It became evident that the transformation of new knowledge into clinically useful forms and effectively implementing it across the entire care team was required to produce a meaningful impact on performance and patient outcomes. For the nurses to improve delivery systems and care, new competencies in terms of producing research evidence and utilizing knowledge in clinical decision making will have to be developed to transform health care.

Time is now advent for the nurse community to wake up to the fact that it is only research that can legitimize nursing as a profession and provide evidence to support nursing practice. To keep up with the times, even the curricula for nursing education has been radically reformed to reflect a research base, and academic nurses are weaving their careers around it. Though it has all been on the agenda for some time, the outcome in terms of improvement in research base is not commensurate to the all round effort.

As an educator and an author, I have always felt that burgeoning need to address this issue and fill in the gap in my own small way. A close look at the issue revealed that a part of the difficulty is in improving the statistical literacy and developing a positive perception to research among nurses. This can best be done by making available resources in the form of genuine reading material among the student community. This textbook is a legitimate effort to draw the student nurse towards research and meet their intellectual needs. Another matter of concern is that, though most of the textbooks on nursing research dwell upon biostatistics too, due importance is not attached to it as a separate discipline. Biostatistics is dealt in a routine manner resulting in huge knowledge gaps when it comes to application. The students of nursing research are thus confused and compelled to look to teacher's notes or refer books exclusively catering to biostatistics. Though advised to limit the element of biostatistics to a bare minimum, I have gone ahead and given the subject its due. I have put genuine effort in integrating both nursing research and biostatistics, by quoting subject-related examples and employing as many tables and figures as permissible. The goal was to make the central ideas more simple and approachable. This should truly make the book a one-stop purchase so far as the complete subject is concerned.

Sreevani Rentala

ACKNOWLEDGMENTS

I would like to begin by thanking the Almighty God, who bestowed upon me the spiritual strength and perseverance to make it all happen. Without His blessings, this would still have been a dream.

Though I had begun this project much earlier, it kept getting postponed as I was going through some testing times. Every time the goal post kept getting farther away, it only made my resolve much stronger to reach it. I would like to thank the publishers M/s Jaypee Brothers Medical Publishers (P) Ltd, New Delhi, for being very patient all through and especially Shri Jitendar P Vij (Group Chairman), Mr Ankit Vij (Managing Director) and Mr MS Mani (Group President), for reposing faith in me.

I would like to thank Dr K Reddemma (Formerly, Dean, Behavioral Sciences and Professor, Department of Nursing, NIMHANS, Bengaluru), my teacher and mentor, for her timely suggestions and guidance, and for accepting to write the foreword for this book.

I am not only grateful to all those with whom I have had the pleasure to associate while writing this book but also to those who have provided me professional guidance and taught a great deal about both scientific research and life in general.

Nobody has been more important to me in the pursuit of this title than the members of my family. I would like to thank my grandparents, parents and in-laws, whose love and guidance are with me in whatever I pursue. They are the ultimate role models. Most importantly, I wish to thank my loving and supportive husband, Mr Giridhar, who has been a pillar of support, and my two wonderful children, Pranith and Daivik, for their unending inspiration.

It would be inappropriate if I omit to acknowledge the reviewers for their careful reading of the manuscript and their insightful comments and suggested edits. Review done by my dear colleagues Dr Sunanda GT and Ms Rajashree, PhD students Mr Dayananda and Mr Harsha, MSc (N) students particularly Mr Sharanabasappa H and Ms Leemol need a special mention.

I wish to present my special thanks to Mr Venugopal, Associate Director–South (Bengaluru Branch), M/s Jaypee Brothers Medical Publishers (P) Ltd, for his small talks which have been a huge inspiration in over a decade's association with him. Sincere thanks to Dr Madhu Choudhary (Publishing Head–Education), Ms Pooja Bhandari (Production Head), Ms Sunita Katla (Executive Assistant to Group Chairman and Publishing Manager), Mr Rajesh Sharma (Production Coordinator), Dr Astha Sawhney (Development Editor), Ms Seema Dogra (Cover Visualizer), Mr Laxmidhar Padhiary (Proofreader), Mr Nitesh Jain (Graphic Designer), and Ms Uma Adhikari (Typesetter), for the wonderful back office support.

CONTENTS

PART A—NURSING RESEARCH

Unit 1. Introduction to Nursing Research 3
- Methods of Acquiring Knowledge 3
- Problem Solving and Scientific Method 6
- Research 8
- Scope of Nursing Research 23
- Problems in Nursing, Health, and Social Research 24
- Evidence-based Practice 26
- Ethics in Nursing Research 31

Unit 2. Research Process 41
- Quantitative Research Process 41
- Steps in Quantitative Research Process 41
- Advantages and Disadvantages of Quantitative Research 46
- Qualitative Research Process 46
- Steps in Qualitative Research Process 48
- Advantages and Disadvantages of Qualitative Research 52
- Differences Between Qualitative and Quantitative Research 52
- Selecting Quantitative vs Qualitative Research 52

Unit 3. Research Problem and Hypothesis 57
- Meaning 57
- Sources of Research Problem 57
- Criteria for Selecting a Research Problem 59
- Formulation of Research Problem 61
- Components of Problem Statement 63
- Purposes of Research Study 64
- Research Question 64
- Research Objectives 65
- Variables 68
- Types of Variables 68
- Assumptions 74
- Hypothesis 75
- Delimitations 81
- Limitations 82

Unit 4. Review of Literature 88
- Definitions 88
- Importance of Literature Review 88
- Purposes of Literature Review 88
- Elements of a Literature Review 89
- Types of Literature Reviews 91
- Sources of Review of Literature 93
- Criteria for Selection of Sources 96
- Steps in Literature Review Process 96
- General Guidelines for Reviewing the Literature 100

Unit 5. Theory and Conceptual Framework in Nursing Research 105
- Overview of Theories 105
- Theoretical Framework/Conceptual Framework 110
- Conceptual Models 110

Unit 6. Research Approaches and Designs 120
- Meaning and Definition 120
- Purpose of a Research Design 121
- Characteristics of a Quantitative Research Design 121
- Characteristics of a Qualitative Research Design 122
- Key Elements of Research Design 122
- Selection of Research Design 123
- Decision on Selection of Research Design 124
- Types of Research Designs 124

Nonexperimental Designs
- Descriptive or Explorative Designs 127
- Correlational Designs 128
- Cross-sectional Design (Data Collected at One Point in Time) 131
- Longitudinal Designs (Data Collected at Multiples Time Points) 133
- Retrospective Designs 134
- Prospective Designs 135
- Survey Research Designs 136

Experimental Research
- Validity of Experimental Designs 138
- Elements of Experimental Research 142
- True Experimental Designs 143
- Posttest Only Control Group Design (After Only Design) 145
- Pretest-Posttest Control Group Design 146
- Solomon Four-group Design 147
- Cross-over Design 148
- Factorial Design 149
- Randomized Block Design 150
- Randomized Controlled Trials 151
- Clinical Research 151
- Quasi-experimental Designs 153
- Nonequivalent Control Group Pretest Posttest Design 153
- After-Only Nonequivalent Control Group Design 154
- One Group Pretest Posttest Design 155
- Time-Series Design (Repeated Measures Design) 156
- Epidemiological Research Designs 157
- Ethnography 161
- Phenomenological Design 163
- Grounded Theory Approach 163
- Case Study 164
- Developing Research Plan 167

Unit 7. Sample and Sampling Techniques 174
- Sampling Process in Quantitative Studies 178
- Sampling Techniques or Methods 180

- Sample Size 194
- Sampling Bias 200
- Sampling Errors 201
- Sampling Process in Qualitative Research Studies 202

Unit 8. Tools and Methods of Data Collection ... 208
- Purposes of Data Collection 208
- Concepts of Data Collection 208
- Data Sources 209
- Developing a Data Collection Plan 209
- Data Collection Process/Procedure 210
- Selection of Data Collection Method 212
- Types of Data Collection Methods 214
- Survey Method 216
- Questionnaire 217
- Attitude Scale/Attitude Questionnaire 224
- Opinionnaire 225
- Interviews 225
- Observation 234
- Ethics 240
- Biophysiological Measures 240
- Psychological Measures 241
- Records, Documents and Available Data 246
- Validity and Reliability of the Measuring Instrument 247
- Item Analysis 255
- Critiquing Data Collection Methods 257
- Implementing Research Plan 257
- Avoiding Bias—Collecting Reliable Data (Bias in Research) 260
- Pilot Study 260

Unit 9. Plan for Data Analysis and Interpretation ... 265
- Advantages of Planning for Data Analysis 265
- Phases of Quantitative Data Analysis 266
- Types of Quantitative Analysis 270
- Qualitative Data Analysis 280

Unit 10. Dissemination (Communication) and Utilization of Research Findings ... 288
- Meaning of Dissemination 288
- Features of Dissemination 288
- Criteria for Effective Dissemination 290
- Research Report 291
- Dissertation or Thesis 301
- References 305
- Research Critique 311
- Research Utilization 312
- Bridging Gap Between Research and Practice 319
- Barriers in Utilization of Research Findings 322
- Research Utilization Studies 325
- Research Proposal 325
- Role of Computers in Research Process 329

PART B—BIOSTATISTICS

Unit 11. Introduction to Biostatistics 337
- Historical Notes   337
- Definitions   337
- Characteristics of Statistics   338
- Limitations of Statistics   338
- Uses of Biostatistics in Medicine   338
- Significance of Biostatistics in the Field of Nursing   338
- Scope of Biostatistics   338
- Terminology   339
- Commonly Used Symbols in Statistics   339
- Types of Data and its Measurement   339
- Types of Statistics   343
- Organization and Presentation of Data   344

Unit 12. Measures of Central Tendency 364
- Characteristics of a Good Statistical Average   364
- Mean (Arithmetic)   364
- Median   366
- Mode   369
- When to Use the Mean, Median, and Mode   370

Unit 13. Measures of Variability 374
- Dispersion   375
- Measures of Variability (Dispersion)   375

Unit 14. Normal Probability Distribution 393
- Normal (Gaussian) Distribution   394
- Skewness   396
- Kurtosis   396

Unit 15. Measures of Relationship 399
- Correlation   399
- Correlation Coefficient   399
- Types of Correlation   400
- Need for Correlation   403
- Measures of Correlation   403
- Regression Analysis   409
- Regression Line   410
- Regression Equation   410
- Comparison Between Correlation and Regression   411

Unit 16. Inferential Statistics and Hypothesis Testing 414
Inferential Statistics
- Purposes of Inferential Statistics   414
- Types of Inferential Statistics   414

Hypothesis Testing
- Types of Hypothesis   418
- Steps in Hypothesis Testing   419
- Errors in Hypothesis Testing   419
- Parametric and Nonparametric Tests   422
- Parametric Tests Used in Nursing Research   428
- Nonparametric Tests Used in Nursing   440

Contents

Unit 17. Application of Statistics in Health and Use of Computers for Data Analysis ...457
- Definitions   457
- Need for Vital Statistics   457
- Sources of Vital Statistics (Mechanisms for Collection)   457
- Uses of Vital Statistics   459
- Basic Formulae in Vital Statistics   460
- Basic Measurements in Vital Statistics   461
- Statistical Packages   466
- Use of Computers for Data Analysis   467

Glossary 471

Appendices 489
- Appendix 1: Distribution of t-Probability   489
- Appendix 2: Significant Values of F 490
- Appendix 3: Distribution of χ^2 Probability   493
- Appendix 4: Significant Values of the Correlation Coefficient   494
- Appendix 5: Mann-Whitney U Test Table   495
- Appendix 6: Table of Critical Values for the Wilcoxon Test   496
- Appendix 7: Table of Random Numbers   497
- Appendix 8: Model Information Sheet for Research Participants and Consent Form   498
- Appendix 9: Model Letter to Institutional Ethics Committee   501
- Appendix 10: Model Summary Sheet of the Research Project Submitted to the Institutional Ethics Committee   502
- Appendix 11: Model Research Proposal Format   504
- Appendix 12: CONSORT 2010 Checklist of Information to include when Reporting a Randomized Trial   506
- Appendix 13: CONSORT Flow Diagram   508
- Appendix 14: The Strengthening the Reporting of Observational Studies in Epidemiology (STROBE) Statement: Checklist of Items that should be addressed in Reports of Observational Studies   509
- Appendix 15: CARE Checklist (2013) of Information to include when Writing a Case Report   511
- Appendix 16: PRISMA 2009 Checklist for Reporting of Systematic Reviews and Meta-analyses   512
- Appendix 17: PRISMA (2009) Flow Diagram   514
- Appendix 18: TREND Statement Checklist   515
- Appendix 19: TREND Flow Diagram   519

Index 521

PART A—NURSING RESEARCH

- **UNIT 1 :** Introduction to Nursing Research
- **UNIT 2 :** Research Process
- **UNIT 3 :** Research Problem and Hypothesis
- **UNIT 4 :** Review of Literature
- **UNIT 5 :** Theory and Conceptual Framework in Nursing Research
- **UNIT 6 :** Research Approaches and Designs
- **UNIT 7 :** Sample and Sampling Techniques
- **UNIT 8 :** Tools and Methods of Data Collection
- **UNIT 9 :** Plan for Data Analysis and Interpretation
- **UNIT 10 :** Dissemination Communication and Utilization of Research Findings

UNIT 1

Introduction to Nursing Research

Nurses represent the single largest professional group among healthcare providers who for the most part have direct contact with individuals, families, and communities. They provide nursing interventions to patients, their caregivers, and population in general. Their decisions and actions influence the lives of entire populations. Hence, nursing practice should be based on scientific evidence. Research-based practice is essential if the nursing profession is to meet its mandate to the society (American Nurses Association, 2003). To have a research-based practice, the nurse should have adequate knowledge and skill in designing and conducting research in a rigorous manner so as to produce accurate and generalized results.

METHODS OF ACQUIRING KNOWLEDGE

Knowledge is the awareness or perception of reality acquired through insight, learning, or investigation and expressed in a form that can be shared (Chinn and Kramer, 1995).

Knowledge refers to crucial information that should echo reality and provide a direction to the course of action. In nursing, it is the nurse's level of knowledge that directs patient care. Thus, such knowledge should be superior and credible in nature, and lead nurses' actions ranging from providing care to practicing life-saving procedures.

Nurses have relied on numerous sources of knowledge to guide nursing practice. The knowledge can be acquired from highly structured (logical reasoning, scientific, and research approach) as well as unstructured methods (tradition, authority, experience, trial and error, intuition, and role modeling) (Fig. 1.1).

❖ **Tradition**: Tradition passes knowledge from one generation to another and directs the actions. In tradition, knowledge is based on truths and beliefs that develop from customs and trends. Tradition limits the ability to seek new ways of doing things. In nursing, some interventions are based on tradition, customs, and culture rather than on scientific evidence. Traditions have existed over long periods of time

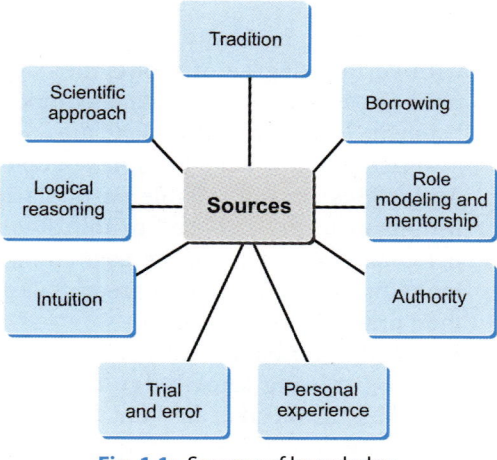

Fig. 1.1: Sources of knowledge

and usually supported by people with power and authority. Hence, it is difficult to change the traditional practices.

- **Borrowing**: Borrowing in nursing refers to utilizing knowledge from other disciplines to guide nursing practice. These disciplines include medicine, sociology, psychology, physiology, and education. Borrowing from another discipline works when the borrowed knowledge is integrated into nursing's body of knowledge. Since disciplines share knowledge, it is sometimes difficult to know where the boundaries exist between that of nursing and other disciplines. Borrowed knowledge has not been adequate for answering many questions generated in nursing practice.

- **Role modeling and mentorship**: Watching and imitating the behavior of an expert nurse is another way nurses' gain knowledge. Many clinical orientation programs for nurses are based on the concept of role modeling. Examples of role models are admired teachers, practitioners, and researchers who inspire students through their roles. An intense form of role modeling is mentorship. Role modeling may result in close personnel relationship between the mentor and the mentee.

- **Authority**: An authority is an individual with certain degree of proficiency and power having the ability to influence others behavior. Experts in a given field are often a source of knowledge for other people. Authorities are not reliable particularly if their expertise is based primarily on personal experience. In the past, nurses looked to physicians for a great deal of their practice knowledge.

- **Personal experience**: Personal experience implies gaining knowledge by being personally involved in an event, situation, or circumstance. For example, when a student nurse gives the first injection she may feel more stressed, but with experience she becomes quite skillful about how to administer the least painful injection. Practice leads to the development of routines that help in building skills. Nurses gain knowledge and experience by seeing and practicing. If experience causes a person to learn something incorrectly, the person uses the knowledge wrongly.

- **Trial and error**: This approach deals with trying out alternatives in succession until an answer to the problem is found. Nurses may engage in certain amount of trial and error when performing interventions involving individuals. This way of acquiring knowledge can be time consuming because multiple interventions are implemented before one is found to be effective. This is an unsystematic and haphazard way of learning.

- **Intuition**: It can be defined as an awareness or perception of a situation or a happening resulting more due to an instinctive feeling rather than conscious reasoning. This is best described as having that "hunch" about something. It is a combination of past experience and knowledge that is unconsciously used to come up with an insight or solution to a problem. It is difficult to develop policies and practices for nurses on the basis of intuition. It is generally considered unscientific and unacceptable for use in research.

- **Logical reasoning**: Logical reasoning as a problem-solving method brings together experience, intellect, and a logical system of thought. There are two types of reasoning: (1) inductive reasoning and (2) deductive reasoning.
    1. *Inductive reasoning* is the process of developing generalizations from specific observations. Theory development is a typical example of inductive reasoning wherein different concepts are put together to form a whole. For

Table 1.1: Differences between inductive and deductive reasoning

Inductive reasoning	Deductive reasoning
Associated with qualitative research	Associated with quantitative research
Moves from specific observations (data) to general (theory) conclusions	Moves from the general conclusions (theory) to specific observations (hypothesis)
Data analysis helps in drawing conclusions which in turn aids the researcher in hypothesis development and framing a possible theory	Theory is either used to develop a hypothesis or is tested
Proceed from data collection and content analysis to the discovery of abstract concepts	Theory is initially reviewed which then leads to evolving systematic procedures for data collection and analysis
Conclusions are developed from specific observations	Conclusions are developed from general observations

example, a nurse may observe the aggressive behavior of a hospitalized schizophrenia patient (specific) and conclude that all schizophrenic patients are aggressive (in general). Inductive reasoning method is usually employed in qualitative research studies.

2. *Deductive reasoning* is the process of developing specific predictions from general principles. Theory testing is a typical example of this type of reasoning wherein the relationship between individual concepts in a theory is examined. For example, if a nurse assumes that aggressive behavior occurs among chronic mentally ill patients (in general), then she might predict that schizophrenia patients in chronic wards (specific) manifest aggressive symptoms. Deductive reasoning is associated with quantitative research or experimental research.

Both the systems of reasoning contribute to enhancing an understanding of the phenomena. However, it is the accuracy of the information that defines the validity of the reasoning. The differences between inductive and deductive reasoning are presented in Table 1.1 and Figure 1.2.

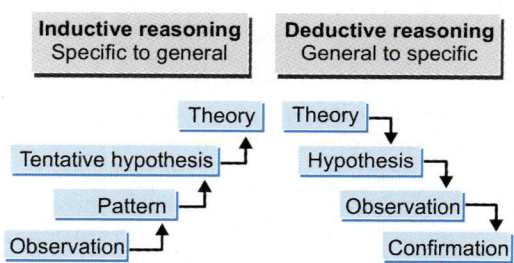

Fig. 1.2: Differences between inductive and deductive reasoning

❖ **Scientific/research approach:** In any discipline, it is the pursuit of research that augments and refines the knowledge. It is the findings from systematic and rigorous research that are placed at the top of evidence hierarchies. The recent emphasis on evidence-based healthcare suggests that the nurses should prominently support their clinical practice with research-based findings and not simply base them on tradition, authority, instinct, or personal experience.

The knowledge needed for nursing practice needs to be precise, holistic as well as outcome, and process oriented. To generate this knowledge, various research methods are required. Nurses need to be taught the way to evaluate various sources of knowledge and must evolve as critical thinkers as this will increase the base for nursing knowledge both in terms of quality and quantity.

PROBLEM SOLVING AND SCIENTIFIC METHOD

Nursing research uses many methods to study clinical problems. Problem solving and application of scientific method are the commonly used methods.

Problem Solving

Problem solving is a systematic approach to seek solution to a problem. In this approach, possible solutions are carefully evaluated and one of them is chosen for implementation.

Steps in Problem Solving (Fig. 1.3)

- *Identification of the problem*: Collect the information from different sources to get a clear interpretation of the problem.
- *Analyzing the problem:* Analyzing means to gather information as to how the problem effects the situation, who are involved in the situation, and find out the factors that are contributing to the problem. This analysis helps in understanding the root causes of the problem.
- *Generating possible solutions:* It is a very innovative step which involves identifying all possible solutions to the problem.
- *Analyzing the solution:* Each solution is evaluated for its strength and weakness, potential risks and benefits, and short- and long-term consequences.
- *Selecting the best solution:* Select the best solution that is most appropriate to fix the problem given the circumstances, resources, and other considerations.
- *Implementing the solution:* Putting into the action of actual solution.
- *Evaluation of outcome of action*: Establish criteria for evaluating effectiveness of solution and review the results.

Scientific Method

Scientific method refers to a set of techniques for investigating phenomena, generating new knowledge, validating previous knowledge, and integrating new knowledge with old knowledge. In this method, the researcher progresses systematically beginning with the definition of the problem and moves through the design of the study and collection of

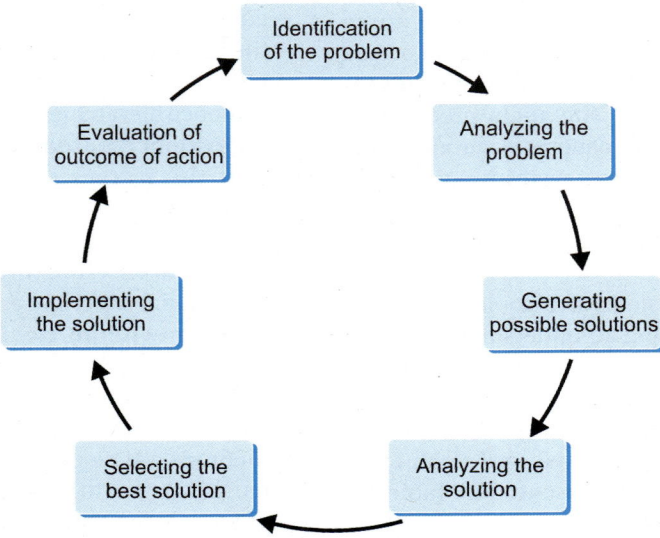

Fig. 1.3: Steps in problem-solving process

information to the solution of the problem. This method is used to understand, explain, predict, or control phenomena.

Characteristics of Scientific Method

- *Orderly and systematic process*: It progresses logically and orderly in a planned series of steps to limit errors or bias.
- *Commitment to objectivity*: Facts are examined without any bias and judgment is based on facts.
- *Based on empirical evidence*: Data are collected using reliable and valid measurements, analyzed scientifically, and conclusions made based on evidence.
- *Ethical neutrality*: Science does not declare whether results are good or bad.
- *Generalizability*: Results can be generalized to other settings.
- *Verifiability*: Outcomes are verifiable.
- *Controls external factors*: Factors which are not under the study are controlled.
- *Replication*: Experiments are repeated to ensure accuracy and conclusions are tested through replication.

Steps in Scientific Method

Scientific method is a systematic process of exploring observations and answering questions. The steps in scientific method are presented in Table 1.2.

Scientific method and problem-solving process are similar in many ways. Both processes begin with identification of a problem area, developing a plan, collecting data, and evaluating the data (Table 1.3).

Though both problem-solving process and scientific method are similar in many ways, problem-solving approach is different from the scientific method. Problem solving targets a single problem related to a patient or an organization whereas a scientific method solves the problems in an organization in a systematic way (Table 1.4).

Table 1.2: Steps in scientific method

Steps	Description
1. State the problem	Understanding the problem.
2. Identify the rationale for the study	Purpose of the study explains why the study is being done.
3. Review the literature	Critical appraisal of research on a given topic which helps to put that topic in context.
4. Define the variables	Specify the variables that are being studied.
5. Formulate the hypothesis	Expected outcome is formulated after gathering information about the problem.
6. Determine ethical consideration	Rights of the subjects should be protected and permission obtained before they are approached to participate in a study.
7. Determine research design and methods of data collection	Research design specifies the methods and procedures for conducting the research study.
8. Define study population and sample	It directs the type of participants needed to be selected for the study and allows the researcher to conduct the study on a sample and apply the results to the entire population.
9. Collect the data	Researcher observes or collects and measures phenomena.
10. Analyze the data	Analyze the data to answer the problem.
11. Draw conclusions	After examining the data from the experiment, conclusions can be drawn. The conclusion will either reject or accept the hypothesis.
12. Communicating findings	Researcher prepares research reports in order to communicate findings to the appropriate audience.

Table 1.3: Comparison between the steps of scientific method and problem-solving process

Scientific method	Problem-solving process
State the problem	Problem identification
Identify the rationale for the study	Problem analysis
Review the literature	Generate possible solutions
Form a hypothesis	Analyze the solution
Determine research design and define study sample	Select the best solution
Collect the data	Implement the solution
Analyze the data	Evaluate and revise
Draw conclusions	
Communicate the findings	

Table 1.4: Differences between problem-solving approach and scientific method

Problem-solving approach	Scientific method
Critical thinking process	Scientific inquiry
Goal is to solve the problem	It validates, predicts, explains, and controls the phenomenon of interest to profession
Replication is not possible	Replication is possible and findings are verified
No statistical analysis is used	Rigorous statistical methods are used to analyze the data
No control is imposed	Controls the extraneous and confounding variables
No informed consent is necessary	Informed consent of participants is necessary
Findings are specific to a particular situation	Findings are generalizable to a larger population
Ethical considerations are minimal	Ethical consideration is a major concept
Report includes how the problem is solved	Report includes systematic description of findings which help to share new knowledge with others

Distinguishing characteristics that set nursing research apart from problem solving is the degree of systematic diligent enquiry and investigation.

RESEARCH

The word "research" is derived from the old French word "cerchier" meaning "to seek" or "to search". The word "research" is composed of two syllables "re" and "search". "Re" means again and "search" means to examine, to test, to try, to investigate, and to probe. Research means to investigate again and again for new knowledge or to find answers to problems.

"Research is a systematic inquiry that uses disciplined methods to answer questions and solve problems". —**Polit and Beck, 2010**

"Research means looking carefully again for new or adapted knowledge".
—**Taylor, Kermode, and Roberts, 2007**

"Research is a systematic investigation to find answers to a problem". —**Burns, 1994**

"Research is a systematic, controlled, empirical, and critical investigation of hypothetical propositions about the presumed relations among natural phenomena".
—**Kerlinger, 1973**

Characteristics of a Good Research

A good research should have the following characteristics:
- *Systematic*: Good research follows orderly and sequential procedures with specified steps.
- *Purposiveness*: Research should be based on specific purpose; it can be conducted in an effective manner if it begins with a clearly defined purpose.
- *Objectivity/impartiality*: Objectivity simply means that truth must be reflected in research. Scientific research must be factual and clear from personal bias, prejudice, feelings, likes, or dislikes.

- *Measurability*: The research variables should be measurable. As various techniques and tools are used to measure the variables in a research study, accurate measurement is required for the researcher to measure the variables adequately.
- *Generalizability*: Research results are generalizable to other settings. It can be defined as application of sample study results to the larger population from which the sample was selected.
- *Accuracy and precision*: Research findings should be accurate and precise. Accuracy is the closeness of a measurement to the true value or the correctness of the data while precision is the degree to which two or more repeated measurements show the same results each time, also termed as consistency or reliability of the data.
- *Verifiability*: The data collected in a research study must be subject to verifiability and testability. For example, the statement, "smoking is injurious to health". This proposition would be regarded as a scientific fact because it verifies the observation that the proportion of health issues are more among smokers compared to nonsmokers.
- *Empirical evidence*: Research should be based on observations and experimentation of theories. A good research always strives to develop empirical evidence which can be used to improve the professional practice.
- *Logical*: Research is guided by rules of logical reasoning. All findings are logically based on empirical evidence.
- *Controlled*: In research, all variables except those being tested or experimented are kept constant so as to find out the true relationship between variables.
- *Analytical*: The collected research data is adequately and appropriately analyzed using standardized method of data analysis to avoid error in data interpretation.
- *Replicable and verifiable*: The research outcome is reproducible in nature and can be verified by replicating the study.
- *Relevant*: Research should be appropriate to what is required, i.e. it is essential that research studies benefit the communities where the research is carried out.
- *Generates new questions*: A good research suggests directions for future studies and generates new questions.
- *Expertise*: A researcher can conduct the study only when he has the necessary personal experience and skill in carrying it out.
- *Centers around existing problems*: Resolving current issues pertaining to any discipline is one of the fundamental purposes of any research. Therefore, a good research must be based on existing professional problems. This enables the particular discipline to be up-to-date with solutions to professional concerns.
- *Recording and reporting*: In research report, every term should be defined and illustrated clearly. The procedure must be described in detail and the report should be written by the researcher to clarify the phenomenon.
- *Original work*: A good research must be an original work and not copied information. Actually research starts from the point where the existing knowledge ends.

According to BW Tuckman (1978), the characteristics of research can be explained using the acronym MOVIE: M—Mathematical precision and accuracy, O—Objectivity, V—Verifiability, I—Impartiality, and E—Expertise.

Criteria for Good Research

Irrespective of type, every research should meet some criteria so that it can be considered as good research. The criteria for a good research are as follows:
- Should address current professional issues

- Should have clear purpose and find a wider acceptance within the research committee
- Emphasize to develop, refine, and expand professional knowledge
- Should be conducted in an orderly and systematic way
- Should clearly state the variables
- Research methods should be described in a comprehensible manner with adequate details which will allow replication of the study
- The research design should be planned methodically so that the results generated are as objective as possible enabling easy understanding of the research findings
- There should be adequate data to investigate the research topic
- The researcher should carefully check the reliability and validity of the data
- The researcher should clearly highlight the limitations and assumptions of the study which will validate and support the findings of the research study
- Research information should be carefully recorded and reported to generate quality empirical evidence
- A good research depends a great deal on the integrity and commitment of the researcher. It also needs lots of time and patience

Purposes of Research

Research involves systematic investigation of phenomena, the purpose of which could be to:
- Explore and better understand the phenomena (exploratory research studies)
- Measure the characteristics of a particular individual, group, or event accurately (descriptive research studies)
- Determine the association and frequency of events (diagnostic research studies)
- Test hypothesis of a cause and effect relationship between variables (hypothesis-testing research studies)

Qualities of a Good Researcher

A researcher is a person who is conducting research and the success of the research work to a great extent depends upon his qualities. The qualities of a good researcher are presented in Figure 1.4.

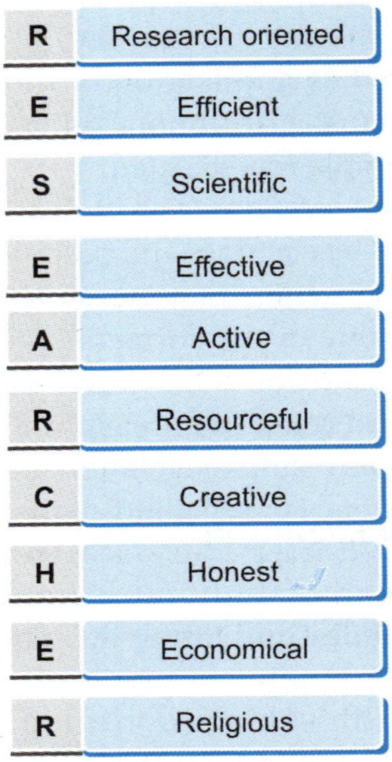

R	Research oriented
E	Efficient
S	Scientific
E	Effective
A	Active
R	Resourceful
C	Creative
H	Honest
E	Economical
R	Religious

Fig. 1.4: Qualities of a good researcher

NURSING RESEARCH

Nursing research is defined as the systematic, objective process of analyzing phenomena important to nursing. It comprises of all studies relating to nursing practice, education, administration, and the nurses themselves.

A systematic approach to gathering information for the purposes of answering questions and solving problems in the pursuit of creating new knowledge about nursing practice, education, and policy (Hek and Moule, 2006).

Nursing research is a formal, systematic, rigorous, and intensive process used for solutions to nursing problems or discovers and interprets new facts and trends in clinical practice, nursing education, and nursing administration (Waltz and Bausell, 2001).

Nursing research is a scientific process that validates and refines existing knowledge and generates new knowledge that directly influences nursing practice (Burns and Grooves, 1993).

Nursing research refers to the use of systematic, controlled, empirical, and critical investigation in attempting to discover or confirm facts that relate to specific problem or question about the practice of nursing (Schotfetdt, 1977).

Nursing research is a systematic study and assessment of nursing problems or phenomena, finding ways to improve nursing practice and patient care through creative studies, initiating and evaluating change, and taking action to make new knowledge useful in nursing (Vreeland, 1963).

Historical Evolution of Research in Nursing

The history of nursing research comprises of many changes and developments. The groundwork for what has flourished was laid late in the 19th century and throughout the 20th century and continues even today. Understanding of how historical issues influenced current nursing research will help to predict future developments in nursing research. The key factors which influenced development of nursing research over the years are presented in Box 1.1.

Box 1.1	Key factors which influenced development of nursing research
• The work of Florence Nightingale • Development of educational programs in nursing • Nursing associations • Trends in health care • Changes in illness orientation • Funding organizations for nursing research	

The Work of Florence Nightingale
❖ Nursing research began when Florence Nightingale (1850s) collected and analyzed information about soldier's morbidity, mortality, and the various factors that influenced these conditions during the Crimean War.
❖ Nightingale mainly focused on a healthy environment and factors influencing physical and mental well-being of the patient. She identified patient problems in practice and undertook a systematic data collection to find answers to those problems and presented the results in tables and pi diagram. Her publication, "Notes in Nursing" described her contribution to nursing research.
❖ In the due course, her research led to a reform in the environment for the sick including hygiene, ventilation, clean water and adequate diet.

Development of Educational Programs in Nursing
❖ Nursing education shifted from hospital training schools to academic settings which helped in development of nursing as a scientific discipline.
❖ As specialized hospitals increased, there was a greater demand for well-educated, specialized, and well-prepared nurses. These changes led to the development of Masters in Nursing.
❖ Nursing organizations gradually developed well-educated faculty and taught how to conduct research. Later, the faculty was involved in conducting research, publishing books, chapters, articles, and clinical studies in patient care.
❖ Research conducted by nurses, nursing faculty, and doctoral nursing students' contributed in the development of nursing interventions for patients, combating serious health problems in the community, influenced the formulation of healthcare policy, and strengthened the professional status of nursing.

- Research initiatives, doctoral dissertations, and scholarly publications continued to advance the nursing science, improve patient care, and promote the health of communities.

Activities of Nursing Associations
- Nursing associations conducted regional, national, and international conferences for nurses and provided an extensive coverage for nursing research at all levels.
- Nursing associations also supported and conducted training activities on clinical research for nurses on health and illness issues to build the scientific basis for clinical practice.
- Most of the organizations/associations provided financial support to research training and research projects related to patient care.
- Several nursing associations developed priorities for nursing research.

Trends in Health Care and Changes in Illness Orientation
Aspects such as increased health problems, comprehensive quality services, and alternative care settings, wanting more holistic orientation in health care demanded for newer interventions that led to the expansion of nursing research.

Funding Organizations for Nursing Research
- Nurse scientists obtain funding from various government and non-government agencies. These funding agencies are essential in maintaining and enhancing the necessary research infrastructure. The federal funding resources provide funding for nursing research and support pre, postdoctoral students, and new investigators.
- The funding organizations contributed towards the advancement of nursing research and enhanced patient care.

Landmarks in Development of Nursing Research

1850–1900
Florence Nightingale (1820–1910) is often seen as the very first nurse researcher. Her "research" eventually led to changes in the environment for sick people including cleanliness, ventilation, clean water, and adequate diet.

1900–1950
- Following Nightingales work, research received minimal attention until the 1950s. During this period, research activities were limited. Most of the studies were concerned with nurse's education.
- Goldmark report identified many inadequacies in the educational backgrounds and concluded that advanced educational preparation is essential. Based on this recommendation, more schools of nursing were established in university settings.
- Published nursing research in the 1900s was concerning problems in nursing education and staffing issues.
- Teachers college Columbia offered the first doctoral program for nurses in 1924.
- The association of collegiate schools of nursing was organized in 1932 to conduct research with a view to improve education and practice.
- The American Journal of Nursing was published in 1900. In 1920s and 1930s, case studies began to appear in this journal. These case studies were the beginning of practice-related research.
- Researches during 1940–1950s focused on nursing services. In 1952, nursing research gained ground with the publication of the first issue of *Nursing Research*, a journal specifically dedicated to reporting nursing research.
- During 1950s, it was mainly sociologists and psychologists who were conducting

research studies on nursing and nurses, while only a few nurses were conducting research on nursing and nurses themselves.

1950–2000

- From 1960s, the value of nursing research gradually increased but only a few nurses had the educational background to conduct studies until the 1970s. Research became a higher priority and many schools began to introduce research steps at baccalaureate level.
- During 1960s, conceptual framework, conceptual models, nursing process, and theoretical base for nursing practice began to appear in the literature to guide nursing practice.
- In 1960s, International Journal of Nursing Studies, a Canadian Journal of Nursing Research was published. During this period, clinical research began to publish studies on nursing care outcomes demonstrating the importance of establishing a scientific basis for nursing practice.
- During 1960s, several professional nursing organizations established research priorities to overcome the dearth of research in nursing practice. This period saw the emergence of practice oriented research on various clinical issues.
- The 1970s saw new growth in the number of masters and doctoral programs for nursing and started research utilization movement. These programs along with the American Nurses Association (ANA), National League for Nurses, Sigma Theta Tau, and Western Interstate Council for Higher Education in Nursing supported nurses not only in learning research process but also producing research that could be used to enhance quality care.
- In 1970s, serious consideration for nursing research in the UK came with the publication of the Brigg's Report that recommended that nursing should become a research-based profession. During this period, there was a marked shift from teaching nursing research to actually utilizing research findings to improve patient care. This is the turning point in the context of nursing research in utilizing research findings in clinical practice.
- During 1976, the Journal of Advanced Nursing and International Journal of Nursing Research began publishing from the United Kingdom.
- In 1980s, computers were widely utilized for collection and analysis of research data.
- In 1983, the first volume of the Annual Review of Nursing Research was published. It incorporated summaries of research evidence on select areas of research practice and supported utilization of research findings.
- The 1980s were exciting and productive for research in nursing. This period saw the extended growth among PhD programs in nursing. Mechanisms for communicating research through journals and reviews also increased. Most nursing organizations have research sections that serve to advance the conduct and use of research. During this period, research became a major force in developing a scientific knowledge base for nursing practice. Outcome research emerged as a significant technique in documenting the effectiveness of healthcare services.
- In 1986, the National Center for Nursing Research (NCNR) was established at the US National Institute of Health. The purpose of NCNR was to promote and financially support research projects and training related to patient care.
- By 1990, nursing science attained maturity in the United States with a focus on outcomes research. The task group on the strategy for research in nursing addressed many deficiencies in nursing

becoming a research-based profession and recommended that all nurses gain research knowledge for effective nursing practice.
- The 1990s brought the promise of reducing the gap between practice and research. The publication "Healthy People 2000" in 1992 by the US Department of Health and Human Services laid the national health agenda for the future.
- Many journals were launched in the 1990s in response to the development in clinically oriented research and interest in evidence-based practice (EBP). Of particular importance is the Cochrane Collaboration. Inaugurated in 1993, this collaboration is an international network of institutions and individuals, maintains and updates systematic reviews of hundreds of clinical interventions to facilitate EBP (www.cochrane.org).

Nursing Research in 21st Century

- In the 21st century, the vision of nursing research is to enable implementation of EBP through development of scientific knowledge base.
- In 2002, the Joint Commission on Accreditation of Healthcare Organization (JCAHO) supported the implementation of evidence-based healthcare.
- In 2004, evidence-based nursing (EBN) was supported with the initiation of world views on EBN journal.
- The Healthy People 2000 and Healthy People 2010 documents published by the US Department of Health and Human Services increased the visibility of health promotion goals and research.
- In 2005, the Sigma Theta Tau International published a paper on nursing research priorities incorporating the priorities of nursing organizations.
- In 2006, the American Association of Colleges of Nursing (AACN) revised position statement on nursing research.
- The National Institute of Nursing Research (2013) provided the most current information on the institute's research funding opportunities and supported studies.

In 21st century, the nurse researchers need to focus on outcome research, biophysiological research, systematic reviews, EBP, cultural and health disparity issues, and develop stronger knowledge base through multiple confirmatory strategies, strengthen multidisciplinary collaboration, and expand the dissemination of research findings to improve the quality care, education, and service.

Evolution of Nursing Research in India (Fig. 1.5)

In *1946*, the Bhore Committee report recommended improvement in various aspects of nursing, including the need for nursing education.

In *1953*, Ms Edith Buchanan of the Rajkumari Amrit Kaur College of Nursing (RAKCON) became the first nurse in India to obtain a doctoral degree in education from Columbia University with the sponsorship of the World Health Organization (WHO).

During *1950–1970s*, many Indian nurses were sponsored by the Rockefeller Foundation to achieve their doctoral degree from Columbia University.

In *1955*, Ms Margaretta Craig attended the International Council of Nurses Meet and presented a paper on the need for nursing research in India.

In *1960*, master degree program in nursing was introduced at RAKCON, New Delhi, which included nursing research as a subject with thesis work on nursing topics. From then on, postgraduate nursing students involved themselves in research activities.

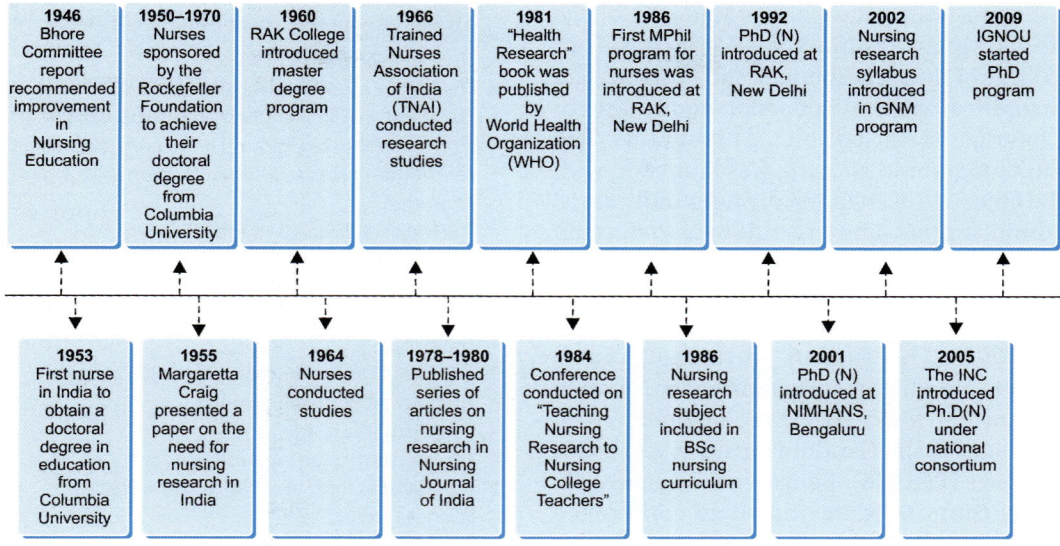

Fig. 1.5: Evolution of nursing research in India

In *1964*, Dr Mary Furguson with other nurses conducted studies on nursing and nonnursing functions of nursing personnel.

In *1966*, the Trained Nurses Association of India (TNAI) conducted research studies under the chairmanship of Ms Margaretta Craig.

From *1978 to 1980*, Dr Aparna Bhaduri and Dr Marie Farrell wrote series of articles on nursing research in Nursing Journal of India, conducted seminars on nursing research to strengthen it further.

In *1981*, Dr Farrell and Dr Bhaduri's book on "Health Research" was published by WHO.

In *1984*, the University Grants Commission sponsored a conference at Bangalore titled "Teaching Nursing Research to Nursing College Teachers".

In *1986*, the first MPhil program for nurses was introduced at RAK, New Delhi followed by Manipal Academy of Higher Education University, Manipal.

In *1986*, the Nursing Research Society of India was established to promote research in India (Box 1.2). Nursing research was included

| Box 1.2 | Aims and objectives of Nursing Research Society of India |

- Support the development of nursing research activities and nursing healthcare institutions to provide nursing care standards
- Provide a platform to nurse scientists to exchange views on nursing research
- Promote and sponsor scientific meets, seminars, and conferences to advance nursing research
- Create public interest in the contribution of nursing in promotive, preventive, and restorative activities contributing to health and family welfare
- Establish a Nursing Research Journal of India and bring out other documents pertaining to innovations in nursing

in BSc (N) curriculum by the Indian Nursing Council.

1992—PhD (N) at RAK College, New Delhi was introduced.

2001—PhD (N) at NIMHANS, Bengaluru was introduced.

2002—The nursing research syllabus was introduced in general nursing and midwifery course and Post Basic BSc (N) curriculum by the Indian Nursing Council.

Some universities such as Manipal College of Nursing, Manipal; Sri Ramachandran College of Nursing, Chennai; and Postgraduate Institute of Medical Education and Research, Chandigarh started PhD(N) programs. The PhD program in Nursing was launched with the objective of enabling the nurse educators, administrators, and practitioners to develop advanced research skills, carry out systematic research, and implement EBN care to patients/clients in various settings.

2005—The Indian Nursing Council introduced PhD (N) program under National Consortium for PhD (N) in collaboration with WHO and Rajiv Gandhi University of Health Sciences (RGUHS), Bengaluru. Presently, six study centers are having video conference facility to impart this program, viz. St. John's College of Nursing, Bengaluru; RAK College of Nursing, New Delhi; CMC College of Nursing, Vellore; Government College of Nursing, Thiruvananthapuram; Government College of Nursing, Hyderabad; and CMC College of Nursing, Ludhiana.

2009—The Indira Gandhi National Open University (IGNOU) started PhD (N) program.

Several nurses and organizations are presently conducting research in various areas with an aim to improve quality nursing care, education, and management. Many research journals have been launched in an effort to further advance research in nursing and transform the areas of practice, education, and management in nursing (Box 1.3).

Box 1.3	List of some nursing journals in India

- The Nursing Journal of India
- The Indian Journal of Nursing Studies
- The Journal of Nursing Research Society of India
- The Kerala Nursing Forum
- The Trends in Nursing Administration and Education
- The Indian Journal of Holistic Nursing
- The Nursing and Midwifery Research Journal
- The Indian Journal of Continuing Nursing Education
- The Nurse
- The International Journal of Nursing Education
- The Journal of Nursing Trendz
- The Prism's Nursing Practice
- The Journal of Nursing Research
- The Manipal Journal of Nursing and Health Sciences, etc.

Current Trends in Nursing Research

The field of nursing research is fast improving and well predicted to widen its scope in the 21st century. The purpose of future nursing research is to promote excellence in nursing science. According to Polit and Beck (2012), the following are the trends anticipated for the earliest 21st century:

- *Evidence-based practice*: The continued focus on EBP will necessitate improvements both in the quality of the studies and in nurses' skills in discovering, understanding, critiquing, and using relevant study results.
- *Translational research*: Translational research is a step beyond EBP and refers to translating research into practice, i.e. ensuring that new treatment measures and research knowledge actually get to the patients or populations for whom they are intended and are implemented correctly. This will encourage the nurses to go for new investigations. The generated new knowledge translates into EBP which in turn will improve patient experience and/or outcome.
- *Use of multiple and confirmatory strategies*: It is crucial to have well-built research designs for development of stronger evidence. Substantiation can be achieved through replication of studies with different clients, settings, and timings.
- *Systematic reviews*: Systematic reviews are the base for EBP. The purpose of a systematic review is to gather and integrate all-inclusive research information on a theme and arrive at a conclusion about the level of evidence.

- *Research in local healthcare settings*: In the current evidence-based environment, there is an increased need to expand small, localized research to find solution to crucial problems. Evidence from such studies can be shared with others in similar situations through communication and collaboration among the nursing faculties.
- *Interdisciplinary collaboration*: Partnership of nurses with researchers and interdisciplinary collaboration among nurse researchers (team research) in the 21st century will address basic problems at the biobehavioral and psychobiologic interface. Such collaboration will facilitate the nurse researcher in playing a more active role in national and international healthcare policies.
- *Dissemination of research findings*: During 21st century, the internet as an information superhighway will have a bigger impact on dissemination of research information, which will in turn promote EBP.
- *Visibility of nursing research*: Most people are ignorant about a nurse's field of work and job categorization. There is an increased need to highlight and publicize the potentialities in the profession through the media. In a bid to promote and gather fresh support for research in nursing, the nurse researchers should showcase their work to professional organizations and Governments.
- *Shared decision making*: The major challenge in the present healthcare system is to appropriate both research evidence and patient preferences into clinical decisions, and structuring research to study the process and the outcomes. This is an emerging trend in health care which is a move towards putting patients at the focal point in their decision making about health care (Barratt, 2008).
- *Cultural issues and health disparities*: The issue of health disparities has emerged as a major concern in nursing and other health disciplines which has in turn raised awareness about the cultural sensitivity of health interventions and the healthcare workers. To address this concern, the nurses' will be required to incorporate cultural needs and beliefs into their practice to provide care appropriate to the client's needs. Thus, nursing research must take into cognizance the health beliefs, behaviors, and values of culturally and linguistically diverse population.

Nursing research helps in implementing new changes in the life-long care of individuals and developing interventions that provide the most optimum level of care. For nursing to continue to uphold its professional status in the health sector, research is imperative.

Need for Nursing Research

The important need for nursing research is to develop a scientific knowledge base for nursing practice. Through a process of systematic scientific enquiry, new facts and effective interventions are discovered. Research not only helps in the discovery of new knowledge but also refines existing knowledge. The generated new knowledge can be used to improve patient care in clinical practice, community health, nursing education, and nursing administration.

Research in nursing practice is needed to:
- Gather data on patient condition about which little knowledge is available.
- Validate nursing actions, develop and evaluate nursing theories, concepts and new nursing interventions.
- Provide accountability to the nursing actions by incorporating research evidence into clinical decision making (EBP).
- Generate new knowledge that will provide scientific base for nursing practice. The generated new information will help to define the unique role of nursing as a

profession, which may facilitate nurses' role in the delivery of healthcare services.
- Define scope of practice which will determine the parameters in nursing and identify its boundaries.
- Document its relevance to the society and efficacy to the public and healthcare providers.
- Predict probable outcomes of nursing decisions in relation to patient care so as to control the occurrence of undesired outcomes.
- Provide knowledge for the purpose of problem solving, decision making, critical thinking, and generating creativity in nursing practice.
- Prevent undesirable patient reactions, answer problems related to health care, and avoid costly unsafe interventions.
- Develop observatory tools for generating knowledge as a basis for predicting and controlling various phenomena.
- Develop advancements that aid patients recovery and help maintain high standards in providing quality care.
- Bridge the gap between nursing education and practice.
- Maintain professional dignity and autonomy in nursing.
- Evaluate the effectiveness of nursing intervention modalities and determine the impact of nursing care on the health of the patients or test out theory.
- Improve quality nursing care by providing care based on scientific knowledge.
- Initiate activities aimed at promoting desired patient outcomes.

Scientific knowledge for nursing practice can be generated through research. Clinical practice without research is practice based on tradition without validation.

Research in community area is needed to:
- Develop knowledge and standards relating to promotion of healthy lifestyles and prevention of diseases and illnesses.
- Develop standards to reduce the number of diseases in the community.
- Facilitate interdisciplinary collaboration in healthcare research.
- Achieve scientific progress and discover more vaccines translating into fewer illnesses and better quality of life for the community as a whole.

Research in nursing education is needed to:
- Provide high quality learning experience to nursing students.
- Develop best methods of teaching and refine existing methods.
- Incorporate research-related content into nursing course.

Research in nursing administration and health services are needed to:
- Improve quality and cost effectiveness of care as studies on nurses and nursing roles can influence work productivity, job satisfaction, and retention in nursing job.
- Know effective ways to recruit individuals into nursing profession and retain them in the profession.
- Evaluate effectiveness of national programs.
- Develop policies relevant to healthcare delivery system.
- Understand the varied dimensions of profession.

With nursing research, new changes in patient care will continue to be implemented and developed into interventions that will ultimately bring more rapid healing and better quality of life to the patients.

Purposes of Nursing Research

The main purpose of research is to find answers to questions through application of scientific procedures (Fig. 1.6).
- *Description*: By conducting research, nurses are able to describe what exists in nursing practice, find out new information, and classify it for use in nursing practice, education, and administration. In

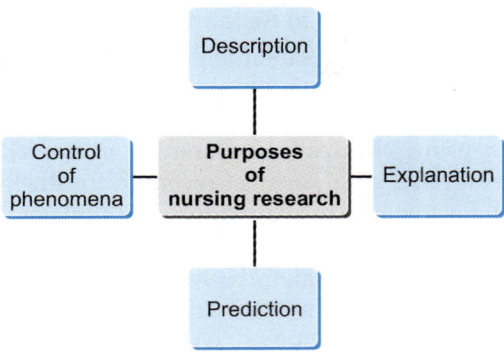

Fig. 1.6: Purposes of nursing research

quantitative studies, description involves the prevalence, incidence, and measurable attributes of a phenomena. Qualitative studies describe attitudes, qualities, habits, customs, etc. Research focused on description is essential for groundwork as it serves the basis for explanation, prediction, and control of nursing phenomena.

* *Explanation*: Through explanatory research, full nature of phenomena, underlying causes for events, relationship among phenomena, and reasons why certain events occur are identified.
* *Prediction*: Through prediction, one can estimate the likelihood of specific outcome in a given situation. With this predictive knowledge, nurses can infer the effects that nursing interventions would have on a patient.
* *Control of phenomena*: Through control, the situation or event can be manipulated or changed to produce the desired outcomes.

According to French (1968), the purposes of research are:

* To uncover new facts about known phenomena.
* To find answers to problems which are partially solved by existing methods and information.
* To improve existing methods and develop new instruments or products.
* To discover previously unrecognized substances or elements.
* To discover pathways of action of known substances and elements.

Importance of Nursing Research

Nurse's primary duty is to give the best possible care to patients. It includes creating and maintaining a safe environment while using interventions that are both appropriate and effective in getting the desired effects. To ensure that nursing practice is efficient and effective, the practice should be based on research. The significance of research in nursing is as under:

* Nursing research generates information which defines the unique role of nursing as a profession.
* It develops and refines nursing knowledge for providing effective patient care and defines the effective strategies in nursing education and administration.
* It ensures credibility of the nursing profession by using research findings to guide clinical actions and take informed decisions.
* It can promote EBP thus, providing accountability for nursing practice.
* It evaluates the efficacy of nursing interventions which will help positive patient outcome.
* Through research, unsafe and trial-and-error interventions are avoided, thus improving quality and cost-effective care.
* It enables the nurses to understand situations about which little is known and explore the factors involved.
* Through research, probable outcomes of certain nursing interventions can be predicted, thus controlling the occurrence of undesirable patient outcomes.

Hence, research is an integral part of nursing profession for continual development of its body of knowledge.

Characteristics of Nursing Research

The following are the characteristics of nursing research:

- *Orderly and systematic process*: It has an order and follows an acceptable procedure for conducting the study. It is carefully and systematically designed, implemented, and analyzed rigorously.
- *Logical*: It attempts to be logical while applying every possible test to validate the procedures so that the researcher is confident of the results.
- *Solving the problem*: It uses systematic method of problem solving that is directed towards the solution of the problem.
- *Empirical*: It is based on direct experience and demands close observation and exact description of what is being studied.
- *Development of knowledge*: Emphasizes on development of principles, theories, and generalizations; refinement and expansion of professional knowledge. It deals with gathering first-hand information and data from various other sources.
- *Analytical*: The data is collected using a carefully designed procedure that is interpreted using a rigorous analysis.
- *Based on purpose*: It can be conducted only with clearly defined purposes.
- *Patient oriented and unhurried activity*: It is an honest exercise that is characterized by patient and unhurried activity.
- *Requires expertise*: The researcher should not only have expertise in the topic being studied but also have writing and reporting skills.
- *Replicable*: It can be replicated to enable the researcher achieve valid and comprehensive results.
- *Innovative approach*: Requires innovative approaches and determination to succeed.
- *Carefully recorded and reported*: Care should be exercised while recording and reporting research information.

Role of a Nurse in Research

The ANA, 1981 has identified various roles for nurses associated with research projects in accordance with their educational level. These are principal investigator, member of research team, evaluator, user of research findings, client advocate during studies, and subjects.

- *Principal investigator*: The individual who is primarily responsible for a research study and is the first author listed on publications or presentations. The nurse actively participates in research activities and is prepared beyond the baccalaureate level to carry out independent research. She keeps herself abreast of current research evidence, engages in ethical conduct of research by generating honest and accurate data, avoids plagiarism in the dissemination of research information, and reports unethical practices to authorities. She disseminates research findings through scientific presentations and journal publications for wider integration of research into current practice.
- *Member of research team*: The nurse can serve as a member of the research team and may collect data or administer the intervention of the study.
- *Evaluator*: The nurse evaluates the research findings.
- *User of research findings*: The nurse uses research findings to improve quality care to individuals, families, and communities. She also uses research to shape health policy in direct care, within an organization, and at the local, state, and national levels. She promotes a workplace environment to support integration of nursing research into practice.
- *Client advocate*: The nurses have the responsibility to act as a client advocate when clients are involved in research. She can explain a study to the potential participants before its commencement and also provide support during the study process.

❖ *Subjects*: The nurse can act as a subject in the research.

TYPES OF RESEARCH

The type of research method is chosen based on the problem to be studied and the current level of knowledge about the phenomena. Research can be classified based on purpose and methodology (Fig. 1.7).

Classification of research by purpose depends on the degree to which findings have direct application and the degree to which they are generalizable to other situations. These are basic research, applied research, action research, and evaluative research.

Classification of research by methodology is based on the approach which is used to conduct the study. These are quantitative, qualitative and mixed.

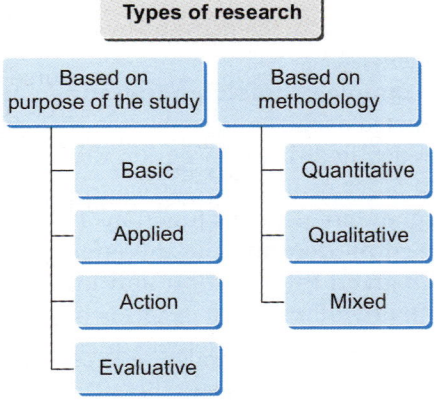

Fig. 1.7: Types of research

Basic Research

Basic research also known as pure or fundamental research is the scientific investigation for the invention of new knowledge and facts. It is appropriate for discovering general principles of human behavior and biophysiologic processes. The basic research includes laboratory investigations with humans or animals to understand physiological functioning, pathological processes, and genetic disorders. This type of research tends not to be directly applicable to the real world, but enhances understanding. Jean Piaget conducted a basic research on intellectual growth of all children wherein he proposed that the children learnt something new in each passing stage.

Purposes
❖ Develop and refine theories
❖ Generate new knowledge
❖ Extend the base of knowledge in the discipline
❖ Establish general scientific principles
❖ Provide a basis for conducting applied research

Example: A study to understand the normal grieving process.

Applied Research

Applied research also known as practical research is a scientific investigation conducted to find a solution to immediate practical problems in the discipline. Basic research generates theory or knowledge that is validated in practice through applied research. This type of research is usually performed in natural (actual) practice setting on subjects who represent the group to which the results will be applied.

Purposes
❖ Tests theory and validates its usefulness in clinical practice.
❖ Solves problems and make decisions in the practice setting.
❖ Evaluates nursing interventions, procedures, processes, and methods.
❖ Findings are useful to policy makers to address health and social problems.

Example: A study to determine the effectiveness of a nursing intervention to ease grieving.

Action Research

Action research is a form of research wherein the researcher and practitioner work together to investigate and evaluate their own work. This form of research is increasingly used in healthcare research. It aids in generating new knowledge and at the same time advance practice.

Action research is cyclical in nature and involves the development, evaluation, and redefining of an action plan using four basic steps: (1) planning (2) action (3) observation and (4) reflection. These cycles of action continue until the researcher's objectives have been met.

Main Features
- Participatory in nature—wherein the researcher and practitioner work together to investigate and evaluate their own work.
- Researcher actively involves in the solution of the problem.
- Democratic impulse—wherein grassroot level practitioners and their managers are allowed to change the context in which they work together.
- Contribution to development of knowledge and change in practice (Rolfe, 1998; Meyer, 1999).
- Findings are evaluated as they are generated for further action and data collection.
- Incorporates both humanistic and natural scientific methods.

Purposes
- Bridges gap between theory, research, and practice.
- Generates new knowledge through systematic study of process and outcomes of change.
- It is quick, service oriented, takes immediate action, and sensitive to time and place.

Example: Glasson J in 2006 conducted a study on "Evaluation of a model of nursing care for older patients using participatory action research in an acute medical ward". The main aim of this study was to improve the quality of nursing care for older acutely ill hospitalized medical patients through developing, implementing, and evaluating a new model of care using a participatory action research process.

Evaluative Research
Evaluative research is a form of research wherein the researcher uses standard social research methods for evaluating a program. Practitioners involved with a policy or program may conduct evaluation research.

Purposes
- To facilitate decision making regarding the relative worth of two or more alternative actions.
- To test the existing solution so as to check if it meets people's needs.
- Used to provide feedback on an event, organization, program, policy, person, activity, etc.
- Measures the effectiveness of a program or policy.
- Used in social sciences and by government agencies.

For example, Neufeld and Strang in 1991 conducted a study to evaluate the structured adult day healthcare program designed to assist older or disabled adults to maintain a level of independent function. This study focused on determining the effectiveness of the given intervention and measuring the quality of a service in terms of patient, professional and management quality.

Quantitative Research
Quantitative research is a formal, objective, and systematic process of explaining phenomena by collecting numerical data that are analyzed using statistical methods. Quantitative methods used in healthcare research are descriptive, correlational, quasi-experimental, and experimental.

Purposes
- Used to describe variables
- Test relationships between variables

❖ Examine cause and effect relationships among variables

Qualitative Research

Qualitative research is a systematic, subjective, and methodological approach used to describe life experiences and situations from the viewpoint of the person in the situation. The main types of qualitative research methods include phenomenology, ethnography, historical research, and grounded theory.

Purposes
❖ Describes and promotes understanding of human experiences related to health.
❖ Used to generate hypotheses.

Mixed Research

Mixed research is the combination of qualitative and quantitative approaches. In this approach representatives and generalizability of quantitative research and in-depth contextual nature of qualitative research are combined in a single research study.

Purposes
❖ Increase the confidence in study data
❖ Expand understanding of the phenomena and integration of theories
❖ Assist the researcher in overcoming the bias that comes from single method

SCOPE OF NURSING RESEARCH

Globally, research in nursing is committed to rigorous scientific inquiry that yields valid and reliable results. It adds significant knowledge to nursing practice and contributes to the well-being of people at large. Nursing research covers a wide range of scientific inquiry ranging from clinical research to research in health administration and education (Fig. 1.8).

Nursing research provides a wide scope for scientific inquiry in clinical trials, health systems research, epidemiological investigations, and qualitative research.

Clinical research involves biological, behavioral, and other types of researches.

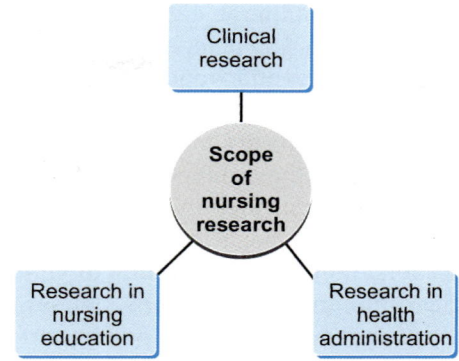

Fig. 1.8: Scope of nursing research

It presents a scientific base for care of individuals across the lifespan. It ranges from acute to chronic care and takes place in a variety of settings across the continuum of care where nursing care is provided either to the individuals, families, or communities, the continuum of care levels spanning from illness to wellness states.

Clinical research emphasizes on health promotion, prevention of illnesses, care and comfort, restoration, and rehabilitation of individuals. In clinical research, the nurse researchers investigate on physical, psychological and social aspects of illness and wellbeing.

Common areas where clinical research is conducted:
❖ Promotion of wellbeing, prevention of illnesses, and care and treatment for patients.
❖ Providing safety and comfort, reduction of disability.
❖ Risk reduction interventions.
❖ Behavioral changes in chronic illnesses, interventions to improve quality of life of chronic patients.
❖ Treatment adherence, side effects or complications associated with drugs, and other treatment modalities.
❖ Interpersonal (social), organizational, or other environmental circumstances and their effects on well-being of individual, family, and community.

- Studies on vulnerable groups—women, infant, youth, and older adults.
- Holistic interventions and also community interventions.

Today the scope of clinical research is not restricted within the confines of biobehavioral studies (studies that identify the relationships among biological, behavioral, psychological, and social factors) but extends to genetic background and cell functions. Nurses are well qualified to lead and participate in interdisciplinary research teams and focus on their integration while providing quality and comprehensive care to patients.

Health administration research examines the ease of access, cost, and quality of health care. It also deals with appropriateness and advancement in care and treatment.

Research studies involving health administration include:
- Issues in organization, financing, quality of care, informatics, cost effectiveness, and staffing pattern.
- Patient satisfaction, performance evaluation, methods to retain staff, and working conditions, etc.
- Effective ways to recruit individuals into nursing profession and retain them.
- Healthcare delivery system, evaluation of national programs.

Increasing healthcare costs, inaccessibility of health services to many people, and efforts to develop comprehensive and quality care increased the demand for nurse researchers to conduct studies in health administration.

Nursing education research deals with making advancements in learning strategies so as to produce better nurses. Qualified and competent nurses are required for improving the nation's health.

Nursing education research centers on:
- Developing, testing, and improving effective educational techniques.
- Finding more effective approaches to enhance learning.
- Assessing teaching and learning process outcomes.
- Refining old evaluation methods and developing new ones to judge the efficiency of the teaching learning process.
- Strategies to motivate students to learn in class room and clinical area.

Nurses conduct research, use research in practice, and teach research. Nursing research is important for the development of scientific knowledge to promote EBN care. A nurse should incorporate research into practice to ensure a solid basis for nursing actions in the clinical area.

PROBLEMS IN NURSING, HEALTH, AND SOCIAL RESEARCH

Researchers in common face numerous problems while conducting research. The problems can be organized under the following headings:
- **Problems in conceptual phase**
  - Faulty reasoning, lack of knowledge, and lack of autonomy to conduct research.
  - Human behavior depends on several factors such as biological, psychological, social, geographical, and cultural factors. It is the complexity in social data that human beings cannot be put to scientific test.
  - As most of the studies are conducted in natural settings, there is minimal possibility of laboratory research.
  - In most of the social science researches, finding the cause and effect relationship is difficult.
  - *Lack of interest among researchers*: Poor knowledge, lack of autonomy, and nonconducive environment lead to lack of interest among researchers.
- **Problems in planning and empirical phase**
  - *Handling multiple variables*: Researchers in nursing attempt to find

factors that are responsible for human behavior. However, as several factors are responsible for human behavior, the researcher finds himself dealing with multiple variables in a single study. This leads to problems in data collection, analysis, and data interpretation.
- *Difficulty in controlling external variables*: As most of the nursing studies are conducted in natural setting, it is difficult to control extraneous or contaminating factors (uncontrolled variables that influence the findings of the research study).
- *Problems in maintaining objectivity*: Natural researchers work in laboratories under controlled conditions whereas nurse researchers work in natural settings which to some extent have the potential for subjectivity to creep in. Subjectivity or bias can result from subjectivity of the researcher, faulty sample selection, faulty methods of data collection, and faulty study design. In any research study, bias cannot be controlled completely as the potential for its occurrence is all pervasive.
- *Unpredictability*: Predictability is an important characteristic of science. In case of physical science, high degree of predictability is possible as the studies are carried out in controlled artificial settings. But it is not so in case of nursing research as human behavior is influenced by various factors that are difficult to predict and also studies are carried out in natural setting.
- Lack of standardized tools specific to a particular population.
- Lack of expertise in conducting qualitative research studies.
- *Difficulty in use of true experimental methods*: Nursing studies cannot be subjected to laboratory test. In most of the experimental studies, the subjects are aware about their artificial conditions and blinding becomes difficult. Their responses are subjected to the awareness of their presence in the artificial setting.
- *Difficulty in replication/verification of inferences*: Replication of study is important for verification of inferences. In nursing studies, repeated experimentation is not possible because of the dynamic and nonrepetitive nature of the human phenomenon.
- *Time and money*: Due to lack of autonomy, the nurses are poorly funded by the agencies. Lack of scientific knowledge and training is a drag on time and financial resources.
- *Ethical issues*: Nursing researches are mostly conducted on human beings. Obtaining ethical clearance and consent from the subjects for participating in research is difficult.

❖ **Problems in analytical phase**
- *Measuring qualitative information through quantitative measures*: In most of the nursing researches, the phenomena are qualitative in nature. This qualitative phenomenon is converted to quantitative phenomena by the use of standardized measures. This leads to alteration of evidence.
- *Dynamic nature of human phenomena*: The human civilization undergoes constant change. What is true today may be not true tomorrow. The techniques used in past may prove inadequate/ineffective for present and future studies. On account of this dynamic nature of human phenomena, the researchers task of analyzing data becomes much complicated and the inferences drawn may be misleading.

❖ **Problems in dissemination phase**
- In the field of nursing, research studies are generally conducted in partial fulfillment for obtaining a particular

degree or meet the criteria for getting regular promotions. Much interest is not exhibited in percolating the findings due to which the knowledge does not reach the target group.
  - In most of the states as continuing nursing education program is not mandatory for renewal of their State Nursing Council Registration, the nurses do not exhibit interest in attending conferences/workshops/seminars.
- **Other problems in nursing research**
  - Though nurse educators are carrying out lot of research, their working in clinical area is not compulsory. Alternately, the nurses working in clinical area are seldom engaged in research.
  - The evidences brought by the nurse educators may not be appreciated by the medical community.
  - The majority of research done by nurse researchers has not been implemented in practice setting.
  - Education, research, and practice are treated as different entities.

Suggestions to Improve Nursing Research

- Nurses should be given more opportunities as a specialty nurse with license to practice independently. This will pave the way for conducting research independently.
- Clocking a minimum number of continuing education hours should be made mandatory for renewal of their licenses. This will facilitate better dissemination of research findings. Nurses who excel should be encouraged and supported.
- Amalgamation of nurse educator and nurse administrator will improve the education, care, and research aspects. It will aid in bridging the gap between education, practice, and research.

Problems Encountered by Nurse Researchers in India

- Overlapping research studies are quite often undertaken for want of adequate information resulting in duplication and wastage of resources which are otherwise scarce.
- There does not exist a clear code of conduct for researchers. Also, interuniversity and interdepartmental rivalries are quite common.
- Level of interaction between nursing education and nursing practice needs to be improved.
- Lack of scientific training in the area of research methodology.
- Lack of resources and support from funding organizations.

EVIDENCE-BASED PRACTICE

Evidence-based practice (EBP) is the meticulous and thoughtful use of current best evidence to guide healthcare decisions. EBN is a process of integrating clinical knowledge, judgment, expertise skills, and individual preferences with the best available clinical evidence (Box 1.4).

Evidence-based nursing involves identifying sound research findings and implementing them in nursing practices, so as to improve quality of patient care. The main goal of EBN is to provide a high quality and cost-efficient nursing care.

Definitions

Evidence-based practice is the conscious, explicit, and judicious use of current best

Box 1.4	The evidence-based nursing (EBN) practice integrates
	• Best evidence available
	• Nursing expertise
	• Values and preferences of the individuals, families, and communities

evidence in making decisions about the care of individual patients. —**Sackett, 1996**

Evidence-based practice is a problem-solving approach to the delivery of health care that integrates the best evidence from studies and patient care data with clinician expertise and patient preferences and values.
—**Fineout-Overholt E, 2010**

Scope of Evidence-based Practice

Evidence-based practice in nursing not only helps in taking decisions about patient care but also extends to:
- Identify knowledge gaps
- Find scientifically evaluated knowledge
- Condense the evidence to assist clinical expertise

Features of Evidence-based Nursing

- Is a problem-solving strategy.
- Discourages decisions based on custom, tradition, authority, intuition, opinion, or ritual.
- Emphasizes on identifying best available research evidence and integrate it with other factors.
- Is based on knowledge evolving from research, quality improvement and risk data, international, national and local standards, cost-effective analysis, benchmarking data, patient preferences, and clinical expertise.
- Incorporates evidence gathered from research, clinical expertise, and patient preferences into decisions about health care.
- Makes an effort to personalize the evidence to suit a specific patient needs and clinical situation.

Components of Evidence-based Nursing

Decision making in EBN involves best available research evidence, needs, values and preferences of population, practitioner expertise in environment, and organizational context (Fig. 1.9).

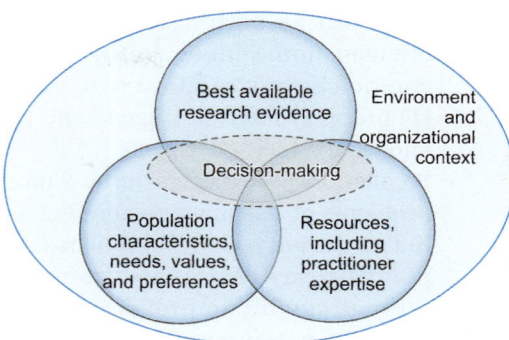

Fig. 1.9: Components of evidence-based practice

Steps in Evidence-based Nursing

To practice EBN, the nurses must not only recognize and appreciate the concept of research but also know how to evaluate the research findings accurately. These skills should be integrated into the nursing curriculum and made a part of their professional training. There are six steps in EBN process (Box 1.5).

Box 1.5	Six steps in evidence-based nursing (EBN) process
	1. Select a research problem
	2. Form a team
	3. Evidence retrieval
	4. Evaluate the evidence
	5. Apply the evidence
	6. Evaluate the efficacy

1. *Select a clinical problem*
   - The EBN process begins with selecting a clinical problem. The following points need to be considered while selecting a problem:
     - Priority and severity of the problem
     - Whether the topic would apply to many or few clinical areas
     - Support of the organization/member of interdisciplinary medical team
     - Availability of solid evidence
   - Members of the interdisciplinary medical team should collectively come up with an agreement regarding selection of clinical problem.

- Ideas for selection of a problem originate from various sources. These can be categorized into two areas: (1) problem-focused triggers and (2) knowledge-focused triggers.
- Problem-focused triggers can be clinical problems or risk management issues. In this category, clinical problems are identified by healthcare members through quality improvement, risk surveillance, recurrent clinical problems, benchmarking data, or financial data. When forming a clinical problem/question, the following information should be included (PICO model):
  - *P*—Patient population (the disease or disorder of patients)
  - *I*— Intervention
  - *C*—Comparison intervention or control group
  - *O*—Desired outcome
- Knowledge-focused triggers are created when nursing staff read research, pay attention to scientific paper presentations at research conferences, or encounter EBP guidelines published by national agencies or organizations. Knowledge-based triggers could be new research findings that further enhance nursing or new practice guidelines.

  It is important that individuals work closely together to reach the optimum outcome for the chosen topic

2. *Form a team*
   - Forming a team is paramount in successful implementation and evaluation of the EBP.
   - Forming a team enhances the chance of EBP being implemented, decrease the rejection, and have an understanding of the project.
   - It is important to have a team comprised of representatives from the highest authority in the organization to the grass-root level members.
   - The EBP team should be aware of the types of patients, setting, interventions, and outcomes.
   - The practitioner should educate the coworkers, clarify their doubts, and clear any misconceptions to improve the outcomes.
3. *Evidence retrieval*
   - Once the clinical problem is finalized, the relevant literature must be extensively reviewed by including electronically and nonelectronically available literature in addition to other relevant literature.
   - In the literature retrieval process, clinical studies, systematic reviews, and EBP guidelines should be accessed (Box 1.6).
4. *Evaluate the evidence*
   - Once the literature is located, the article needs to be classified as either conceptual (theory and clinical articles) or data-based (systematic research reviews).
   - Before reading and critiquing the research, it is useful to read theoretical and clinical articles to have a broad view of the nature of the topic and

---

Box 1.6   Sources of evidence links

- The Cumulative Index to Nursing and the Allied Health Literature (CINAHL) database covers the nursing, allied health, and health sciences literature from 1982 to the present.
- The Medical Literature Analysis and Retrieval System Online (MEDLINE) is the world's most comprehensive source of bibliographic information for health.
- The Cochrane Library covers databases prefiltered for quality of evidence and clinical applicability.
- PsycINFO database covers the online collection of bibliographic references of psychological literature.
- PubMed is a free full-text archive of biomedical and life science journal literature at the US National Library of Medicine.

related concepts. Later, the existing EBP guidelines may be reviewed followed by reading and critiquing the original research article.
- For reviewing, it is better to include higher levels of evidences such as meta-analysis, systematic reviews, and randomized control trials (Fig. 1.10).
- The reviewer must examine the flaws and use rating system to determine the quality, internal and external validity of the research study (Box 1.7).
- Some articles are filled with opinions and biased statements that could lower the credibility of the article. The reviewer should also evaluate for current information.

5. *Apply the evidence*
   - After determining the internal and external validity of the study, decision is taken about appropriateness of the evidence to the present clinical problem/question and also address risk-benefit ratio and any harm involved with implementation of evidence and prognosis.
   - The information gathered should always be shared with fellow nurses and researchers.
   - Develop workplace culture to support implementation of evidence in nursing practice.

6. *Evaluate the efficacy*
   - After application of evidence into practice, undertake clinical audit or a program evaluation, self-reflection, or peer assessment to evaluate the effectiveness.
   - Then translate evidence into practice by developing care pathways to improve clinical efficacy.
   - Evidence-based practice is undertaken to provide safe, effective, and cost appropriate care to the individual.

Benefits of Evidence-based Practice

❖ *For patients*:
   - Provides high quality cost-effective nursing care.
   - Results in better patient outcomes that increases the patient satisfaction.

❖ *For nurses*:
   - By reading all published literature in the specialized area, the nurse can keep herself abreast with latest information.
   - Increases efficiency in providing care to the patients.
   - Provides rationale to all the nursing interventions that help in development of the profession.
   - Nurses can communicate effectively with patients and other healthcare team members about the rationales for decision making and care plan.
   - Provides legal accountability for the practice.
   - Resolves problems in the clinical setting.

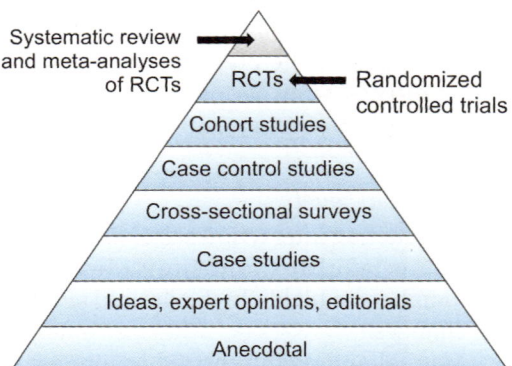

Fig. 1.10: Evidence hierarchy

Box 1.7	Activities important to review the article

- Read article closely
- Examine for flaws
- Use rating system to determine the quality of the research
- Assess for recent or current information
- Assess for credibility and quality of the article
- Determine internal and external validity

- Achieves excellence in care delivery, even exceeding quality assurance standards.
- Introduces innovation.
- Reduces the variations in nursing care.
- Unnecessary practices are eliminated and ineffective practices replaced with effective ones.
- Assists with efficient and effective decision-making that increases confidence.

❖ *For healthcare organization*:
  - Helps the hospital in achieving Magnet status. The Magnet Recognition Program acknowledges quality patient care, nursing excellence, and innovations in nursing practice. Being a magnet facility, patients are assured of excellent nursing service.
  - Since care is delivered based on best evidence, it is less likely to attract litigation and will be able to defend the care.
  - Allows scrutinizing of practice for effectiveness. This process results in significant cost savings.

❖ *For community*:
  - Resources are preserved by not wasting them on implementation of ineffective interventions.
  - Ensures most effective care and limits the amount of disability and suffering of people.

Limitations or Barriers in Implementation of Evidence-based Practice

❖ Resistant to changes in nursing practice.
❖ Time, workload pressures, and competing priorities.
❖ Lack of continuing education programs.
❖ Poor administrative support or lack of support from professional colleagues and lack of confidence in research field.
❖ Lack of knowledge in research methods and critical appraisal skills.
❖ Overwhelming amount of information available in the literature sometimes contradicts findings of research outcome which causes confusion among practitioners.
❖ Shortage of research in some areas.
❖ Lack of autonomy for nurses in implementation of newer interventions.

Strategies to Facilitate Evidence-based Practice in Nursing

At Organizational Level

❖ Providing nurses ample time for activities that promote EBN such as visiting library and conducting electronic searches.
❖ Conducting journal club meetings.
❖ Establishing nurse researcher positions and constituting nursing research committees.
❖ Associating staff nurses with nurse faculty researchers.
❖ Ensuring the facility of print or online subscription to nursing research journals at the healthcare institutions.
❖ Making available preprocessed evidence resources such as clinical evidence, Cochrane library, and abstraction journals.

At Individual Level

❖ Conducting interaction sessions between nurse faculties and individual staff members to highlight the desired practice changes.
❖ Manual and computerized reminders to facilitate behavioral changes.
❖ Promotion should be based on their level of participation in EBP.
❖ Conduct regular educational meetings which allow learners to participate actively.
❖ Audit and feedback in which clinical performance is assessed through chart reviews and direct observation of practice based on which feedback is provided.
❖ Use of more than one strategy is likely to be more effective than a single strategy.

Role of a Nurse in Implementation of EBP in Practice

❖ Read widely and critically
❖ Attend professional conferences
❖ Become involved in a journal club
❖ Pursue and participate in EBP projects

ETHICS IN NURSING RESEARCH

Ethics is that branch of philosophy which deals with dynamics of decision making concerning what is right and wrong. These are norms for conduct that distinguish between acceptable and unacceptable behavior. Thus, ethics can be defined as a method, procedure, or perspective for deciding how to act and for analyzing complex problems and issues. Research involving human subjects or participants raises ethical, legal, social, and political issues that are unique and complex. Research ethics are specifically interested in the analysis of such ethical issues.

The main objectives of research ethics are:
❖ To protect the human participants.
❖ To ensure that research is conducted in a way that serves interests of individuals, groups, and/or society as a whole.
❖ To examine research activities for their ethical soundness—management of risk, protection of confidentiality, and the process of informed consent.

Ethics in nursing research refers to the moral principles the researcher has to adhere to while conducting research so as to ensure the rights and welfare of the subjects under study. As nursing studies primarily deal with human participants, there is a growing concern for protecting individuals from any harmful effects that might result from participation in the study. Thus, ethics have become a keystone to achieve effective and meaningful nursing research.

History of Ethical Codes

❖ In order to prevent scientific abuse of human lives, various professional codes and laws were introduced. The Nuremberg Code was introduced in 1947 to protect human rights in research. This code mainly emphasizes on risk-benefit balance, informed consent, voluntary participation, and protection of participants from physical or mental harm.
❖ In 1964, the Declaration of Helsinki was initiated which asserted that well-being of the individual is more important than scientific interest.
❖ In 1977, the Royal College of Nursing published code for nurses in research.
❖ In 1985, the ANA developed research guidelines.
❖ In 1995, the ANA published ethical guidelines relating to conduct, dissemination, and implementation of nursing research.
❖ These ethical guidelines in research provided strong assistance to professional nurses and a reassurance to patients, public, and society about professional intensions.

Ethical Principles of Research

Ethical principles are used as a framework to guide the research through research process. These principles help to ensure the highest possible standards in every aspect of research process. The Belmont Report is an authentic source about research ethics which was published in 1979. It was commissioned by the US Government in response to ethical failures in medical research, such as Tuskegee Syphilis Study. The Belmont Report proposed three principles that should underlie the ethical conduct of research involving human subjects: (1) Respect for persons (2) Beneficence and (3) Justice. These principles serve as the guiding factor when faced with a research ethics challenge.

Respect for Person (Autonomy)

It refers to the self-determination of a person to participate in a study. The Belmont Report suggests that respect for persons consists of two distinct principles:

i. *Individuals should be treated as autonomous*: Each individual has the worth and freedom to decide whether or not to participate in a research project without risking any punishment or damaging/harmful treatment. It also includes the right of the individual for full disclosure, ask questions, refuse to give information, ask for clarification, or terminate their participation in research.

ii. *Individuals with diminished autonomy should be entitled to additional protections*: Persons unable to take decisions for themselves must be protected from coercion, compulsion, and harmful activities of others. Vulnerable people like children, pregnant women, prisoners, institutionalized people, mentally ill individuals, aged people, terminally ill patients, poor, unconscious patients, etc. are unable to take care of their own welfare and protect their individual rights.
   - Before commencing the research study, the researcher should analyze the potential risks and benefits to participants.
   - Careful approach must be shown while acquiring consent and collecting data from vulnerable people.

The principle of respect for persons suggests that the researcher should receive informed consent from participants.

Informed consent: It refers to a person voluntarily and knowingly giving his/her consent to participate in research. Through informed consent, patient's right to autonomy is protected. The researcher's main task is to ensure that participants have a complete understanding of the study.

The two types of consent are: (1) direct and (2) substitute. In direct consent, an agreement is obtained directly from the participant to be involved in the study. In substitute consent, third party consent is given by someone other than the study participant. Substitute consent is obtained when participant does not have the capacity to take a decision, such as subjects below the age of 18 years, people with cognitive or emotional disabilities.

The four essential parts of informed consent are: (1) disclosure of information, (2) comprehension, (3) competency, and (4) voluntariness.

1. *Disclosure of information*: The participants must be fully informed of all the aspects of the research project (Box 1.8). It also refers to the individual's right to be told the truth and not be deceived about any aspect of the research. The participants should not only be made to understand all the aspects of the research project but also the implications of the study.

2. *Comprehension*: The researcher must ensure that the participants understand the disclosed information accurately. To ensure this, the participants should be explained in a simple and understandable language.

3. *Competency*: It is the person's capability to acquire and retain knowledge. He/she must be competent to understand and be able to arrive at a decision about what is involved. It is determined by age, cognitive, and emotional ability of the participant. Persons below the age of 18 years are considered as legally incapable of taking certain decisions.

Box 1.8	Components of disclosure

- Purpose of the study
- Procedure and selection of the research subjects
- Anticipated physical harm, discomfort, and invasion of privacy
- Compensations in case of any harm
- Expected benefits and alternatives
- Participant's right to withdraw from the research at any time

Also, adults who have cognitive or emotional disability are not competent to take decisions about their welfare.

4. *Voluntariness*: Consent to participate must be given voluntarily, without compulsion, persuasion, or manipulation. Participants should know that participation is voluntary and no punishments are given for refusal.

Documentation for informed consent: The researcher usually documents the informed consent by having participants sign in the consent form. The consent form should contain all the information (Box 1.9). The participants should be provided sufficient time to read the document before signing. The researcher should also sign the document and both parties retain a copy of it. The consent form should be organized coherently, use large font to aid easy reading, and avoid technical terms if possible. The written statement should be at the readable level of study participants.

Box 1.9	Informed consent should contain

- Title of the study and its purpose
- Researcher's credentials
- Duration of participation with number of participants
- Study population, method of selection, and size
- Methods of data collection
- Interventions involved in the study, if any
- Expected time to be spent during each session and total number of sessions with the researcher
- Potential risks, benefits, and compensations
- Policy on compensation, available risk management
- Assured anonymity and confidentiality
- Assurance that participation is voluntary
- Assured the right to refuse to participate or withdraw at any time
- Information on sponsoring agency or academic requirement
- Researcher's contact information
- If test for genetics and human immunodeficiency virus (HIV) is to be done, counseling for consent for test must be given as per national guidelines

Beneficence

It refers to the doing of good to another and positively helps a person. In the Belmont Report, beneficence refers to "do no harm" and "maximize possible benefits and minimize possible harms" to the individual research participant. In nursing research, beneficence suggests that:

❖ No individual is harmed by serving as a participant in the research.
❖ No research study shall be undertaken that shall cause direct harm to research subjects ("do no harm"—nonmaleficence).
❖ Developing new interventions, so also preventive interventions to maximize benefit to the patient and the society alike.
❖ Minimize all types of risks—physical, psychological, social, economic, and other discomforts to participants as much as possible, i.e. participants should not be subjected to any form of suffering, discrimination, or stigmatization as a consequence of having participated in the study.
❖ Establish a risk-benefit ratio to assess the potential benefits and risks of being a participant. If the risks prevail over the benefits, the study should be revised.
❖ The potential harmful effects should be detected early so that study can be terminated if necessary.
❖ The researcher should be concerned about psychological or emotional distress caused from disclosure, fear, personal embarrassment, or humiliation.
❖ Research should be conducted by a qualified expert so as to provide comfort to the study participants.

Justice/Fairness

It refers to the researcher's obligation to treat subjects fairly and equitably before, during, and after the research study. The benefits and risks of research must be distributed fairly.

- In research, participants must be treated fairly and receive what they are allocated or is comparable to other persons in the same situation.
- Ensure reasonable, nonexploitative, and well-considered procedures are administered fairly, i.e. fair distribution of cost and benefit.
- Participants should be chosen based on research requirement and not on convenience, i.e. selected simply because they are easily available or vulnerable or easy to manipulate.
- No harmful treatment should be given or quality treatment withheld to those who refuse to participate or withdraw from the study after agreeing to participate.
- Researcher should be available to participants at any point in the study to seek necessary clarification.

The summary of ethical principles of research and their application in research study are presented in Table 1.5.

Other Ethical Principles

Fidelity: It refers to the researcher's commitment to protect the participants since the participants place trust in researchers.

Privacy and confidentiality: It refers to the researcher's responsibility in ensuring privacy of the participants and confidentiality of the data obtained from them.

- The researcher needs to be aware that invasion of privacy may cause loss of dignity, create guilt, anxiety, and embarrassment.
- As sensitive information like sexual preference, age, weight, personal income, beliefs, attitude, opinion, records, etc. may invade the privacy, it should be minimized to the best extent possible.
- The researcher should be alert in maintaining confidentiality of sensitive information and cannot ignore privacy.
- Subject's privacy is protected if the subject is informed, has consented to participate in the study, and voluntarily shares information with the researcher.

Table 1.5: Application of ethical principles in research study

	Ethical principles of research	*Application of ethical principles in research study*	
Respect for persons	• Individuals should be treated as autonomous • Persons with diminished autonomy are entitled to protection	Person knowingly giving his/her consent to participate in research. The consent process should include: • Disclosure of information • Comprehension • Competency and voluntariness	Informed consent
Beneficence	• Human participants should not be harmed • Research should maximize possible benefits and minimize possible risks	The nature and scope of risks and benefits must be assessed in a systematic way	Assessment of risks and benefits
Justice	• The benefits and risks of research must be distributed fairly	There must be fair procedures and outcomes in the selection of research participants	Selection of participants

- The participants should be assured that the collected data will be held in strict confidence and anonymity protected by not linking the individual identities to responses provided by them.
- Identity and records of the research participants are to be kept confidential. Identification numbers should be assigned to the participants and only those numbers are to be used for analysis rather than the identity data.
- Information should not be disclosed without any valid scientific reason.
- Researcher should sign the confidential pledge if they have access to identification information.
- Research information may be reported in the collective, but if the information of a specific participant needs to reported, fictitious name may be used.

Research Misconduct

Researchers are expected to adhere to ethical, legal, and professional guidelines while conducting a research study. Research misconduct is the violation of standard codes of scholarly conduct and ethical behavior in scientific research. Research misconduct includes fabrication, falsification, or plagiarism in proposing, performing or reviewing research, or in reporting research results.

- *Fabrication* includes completing a questionnaire without assessing or interviewing and creating data without actually conducting the study. It is a type of research misconduct where data or results are made up.
- *Falsification* is manipulating research material, equipment, and accepting subjects into the study who do not meet inclusion criteria, changing, or omitting data. Falsification also includes the selective omission of conflicting data without justification. Adding false statements in the published paper and publishing same research results in multiple papers.
- *Plagiarism* is the use of another person's ideas, processes, and results without giving appropriate credit. A type of research misconduct where ideas, statements, results, or words are not attributed to the author but claimed as one's own work.

Importance of Ethics in Nursing Research

Every researcher has an accountability to protect the participants in an investigation. Nurses who participate in research have to deal with societal values, ethics of caring, and values of scientific research. As nurses engage in various research activities, it is important that the profession operates from sound ethical knowledge base. Reasons that support importance of ethics in nursing are:

- Nursing research usually deals with human beings where implications of ethics become very essential to ensure protection of human rights and welfare, compliance with law, and public health and safety.
- Ethical research is essential for generating sound empirical knowledge for evidenced-based practice.
- Ethical norms help to ensure that researchers funded by public money can be held accountable to the public.
- Adherence to ethical norms helps to build public support for research. Research projects are more likely to receive funding if the quality and integrity of research can be trusted.
- Nursing research usually involves a great deal of collaboration between various disciplines and institutions. Ethical standards promote standards that are crucial for collaborative work, such as trust, accountability, respect, and fairness.

- Ethical norms help in prohibitions against fabricating, falsifying, and plagiarism. This promotes truth and minimizes error.
- Ethical norms ensure protection of vulnerable groups as study participants from harmful effects of experimental interventions.
- Ethics also safeguard the participants from exploitation by the researcher and ensure fullest respect, dignity, privacy, confidentiality of information, and fair treatment for study subjects.

Role of Nurse in Ethical Conduct of Research

The nurse should adhere to strict ethical conduct of research. These include:
- Generating honest and accurate data.
- Obtaining informed consent from all the subjects involved in the study.
- Ensuring fullest respect, dignity, privacy, disclosure of information, and fair treatment for study participants.
- Establishing the risk-benefit ratio for the study participants.
- Taking special precautions when involving vulnerable people.
- Minimize all types of risks to research participants to the best extent possible.
- Avoid plagiarism.
- Report unethical practices in the conduct of research to authorities.

The nurse should play an important role in integrating the research findings into practice.

Guidelines for Critiquing the Ethical Aspects of a Study

- Was the study approved by an Institutional Ethics Committee?
- Was informed consent obtained from all the participants?
- Is there information about provisions for anonymity or confidentiality?
- Is it evident that the benefits of participation in the study outweighed the risks involved?
- Were the subjects provided the opportunity to ask questions about the study?

Institutional Review Board or Institutional Ethics Committee

Research studies that involve human subjects must be reviewed by the Institutional Review Board (IRB). After the researcher has outlined the proposal and data collection methods in detail, the final step before commencing the research is to get the necessary approval from the organizations that will either sponsor the research or give necessary access to the subjects.

Clinical researchers are ethically obligated to protect human participants. The two principal safeties presented to an individual taking part in research are: (1) Written informed consent and (2) Ethics committee (EC) review.

The IRB is a committee having officially selected or nominated members to protect the rights, safety, and well-being of humans involved in a clinical trial by reviewing all aspects of the research study and approving its startup. This committee operates in accordance with national/local regulations as well as clinical practice guidelines.

There are two types of IRBs: (1) local and (2) central. While the functioning of the local IRBs are limited to a substantive and meaningful review of trials conducted by the academic institutions, the central IRBs provide review services for several other entities too.

Purpose
- The IRB reviews the clinical protocol to assess whether the participant's human rights have been violated and evaluates the risks and benefits to the study participants. Through this participant's dignity, rights, safety, and well-being are safeguarded.
- It ensures that clinical trial participants are exposed to minimal risks when compared to benefits likely from research.
- The IRB helps the researcher determine if there is a potential for legal or ethical breach and ensure safeguards are in place to avoid it.
- The IRB is also the organization's assurance that basic quality, ethical, and legal

requirements have been met by the research study as proposed.

Members

- The Institutional Ethics Committee (IEC) members should be multidisciplinary and multisectorial in composition. The number of persons in an ethical committee should be kept fairly small, say from seven to nine members (according to Indian Council of Medical Research, 2016). It is generally accepted that a minimum of five persons are required to compose a quorum. The chairperson of the committee should preferably be from outside the institution. The member secretary who generally belongs to the same institution should arrange meetings of the committee. Other members should be a mixture of medical/nonmedical persons including lay public to reflect the different viewpoint. The members should be competent in reviewing and evaluate the science, medical aspect, and ethics of the proposed research study.
- The composition may be as follows:
  - Chairperson
  - One to two basic medical scientist
  - One to two clinicians from various institutes
  - One legal expert
  - One social scientist
  - One philosopher
  - One lay person from the community
  - Member secretary

Responsibilities of the Principal Investigator

The principal investigator should not deviate from the study protocol without prior approval and must immediately notify the IRB of any removal from the protocol as soon as possible. The IRB holds the principal investigator of the study responsible for ensuring that:

- Individuals are adequately informed of the risks and benefits of research participation and the procedures that will be involved in the research.
- Informed consent will be obtained from each prospective subject in advance in accordance with the institutional and government regulations.
- Routine monitoring of the data collected to ensure the safety of subjects.
- The privacy of research subjects is protected and the confidentiality of data maintained.
- Appropriate additional safeguards are included in the study to protect the vulnerable subjects from coercion or undue influence (e.g. children, prisoners, pregnant women, mentally disabled persons, or economically or educationally disadvantaged persons).

The future of research in nursing should focus on developing sound knowledge base for nursing practice and disseminate research findings through conferences, clinical groups, electronic formats, and publications.

BIBLIOGRAPHY

1. American Nurses Association. (2003). *Nursing's social policy statement* (2nd ed). Silver Spring, MD: Nursesbooks.org.
2. Barratt, A. (2008). Evidence-based medicine and shared decision making: the challenge of getting both evidence and preferences into health care. *Patient education and counseling,* 73, 407- 412.
3. Burns, N., & Grove, S.K. (2005). *The practice of nursing research*: Conduct, critique and utilization (5th ed.). St. Louis, MO: Elsevier Saunders.
4. Burns, N., & Grove, S.K. (1993). *The Practice of Nursing Research*. Sydney: Saunders.
5. Burns, N., & Grove, S.K. (2001). *The Practice of Nursing Research*: conduct, critique & utilization. (4th ed.). Philadelphia: WB Saunders.
6. Chinn. P.L., & Kramer, M.K. (1995). *Theory and nursing*: A systematic approach (4th ed.). St. Louis: Mosby Yearbook.
7. Fineout-Overholt, E. (2010). Evidence-Based Practice, Step by Step: Critical Appraisal of the Evidence Part III. *The American Journal of Nursing,* 110 (11), 43-51.
8. Glasson, J.1., Chang, E., Chenoweth, L., Hancock, K., Hall. T., Hill-Murray, F., & Collier, L. (2006). Evaluation of a model of nursing care

for older patients using participatory action research in an acute medical ward. *Journal of Clinical Nursing*, 15, 588-598.
9. Hek, G., and Moule, P. (2006). *Making Sense of Research: An Introduction for Health and Social Care Practitioners* (3rd ed.). London: Sage Publishers.
10. Houser, J. (2012). *Nursing Research: Reading, Using, and Creating Evidence* (2nd ed.). Sudbury, MA: Jones and Bartlett Learning.
11. Kerlinger, F. (1973). *Foundations of Behavioral Research* (2nd ed.). Holt, Rinehart and Winston.
12. Kerlinger, F. (1986). *Foundations of behavioral research* (3rd ed.). New York: Holt, Rinehart & Winston.
13. Meyer, J., Spilsbury, K., Prieto, J. (1999/2000). Comparison of findings from a single case in relation to those of a systematic review. *Nurse Researcher*, 7, 37–53.
14. Neufeld. A., Strang. V. (1992). Issues in the evaluation of small-scale adult day care programs. *International Journal of Nursing Studies*, 3, 261-273.
15. Nursing Research Society of India Mission: NRSI. Retrieved from www.nrsindia.org.
16. Polit, D.F., & Beck, C.T. (2010). *Essentials of Nursing Research*: Appraising Evidence for Nursing Practice. Philadelphia, PA: Lippincott Williams & Wilkins.
17. Polit, D.F., & Beck, C.T. (2012). *Nursing research*: Generating and assessing evidence for nursing practice (9th ed.). Philadelphia: Lippincott Williams & Wilkins.
18. Polit, D.F., & Beck, C.T. (2004). *Nursing research*: Principles and methods (7th ed.). Philadelphia, PA: Lippincott Williams, & Wilkins.
19. Polit, F.D., & Hungler, B.P. (1997). *Nursing Research* (6th ed.). Philadelphia: Lippincott.
20. Rolfe, G. (1998). The theory practice gap in nursing: from research-based practice to practitioner-based research. *Journal of Advanced Nursing*, 28, 672-679.
21. Sackett, D.L., Rosenberg, W.M., Gray, J.A.M., & Haynes, R.B. (1996). Evidence-based medicine: What is and what it isn't. *British Medical Journal*, 312, 71-72.
22. Schotfetdt, R.M. (1977). Nursing Research: Reflection of value. *Nursing research*, 26(1), 4-8.
23. Taylor, B., Kermode, S., & Roberts, K. (2007). *Research in Nursing and Health Care: Evidence for Practice*, (3rd ed.). Sydney: Thomson.
24. The purposes of research French. (1968). Retrieved from http://www.1stessays.com/services-research-paper.html.
25. Tuckman, B.W. (1978). *Conducting Educational Research*. New York: Harcourt Brace Jovanovick, Inc.
26. Waltz, C., & Bausell, B.R. (1981). *Nursing research: design statistics and computer analysis*. Philadelphia, PA: Davis FA.
27. Welford, C., Murphy, K., & Casey, D. (2012). Demystifying nursing research terminology: Part 2. *Nurse researcher*, 19, 29-35.

REVIEW QUESTIONS

I. Long Essays

1. Define research and explain various types of research with suitable reference to nursing.
2. Enumerate ethical considerations in nursing research.
3. Discuss fundamental ethical principles in research.

II. Short Essays

1. Explain the methods of acquiring knowledge.
2. Enumerate the evolution of nursing research in India.
3. Describe need for nursing research.
4. Explain characteristics of nursing research.
5. Write a brief on evidence-based practice.
6. Narrate problems in nursing research.
7. Describe scope of nursing research.

III. Short Answers

1. Define inductive and deductive reasoning with examples
2. Steps in problem-solving process
3. Define research
4. Define nursing research
5. Logical reasoning
6. Purposes of nursing research
7. Meaning of ethics
8. Define informed consent

IV. Multiple Choice Questions

1. Which of the following is the most sophisticated method of acquiring knowledge?
   a. Trial and error
   b. Intuition
   c. Scientific research
   d. Logical reasoning
2. Following are the core concepts of scientific method *except*
   a. Generalizability
   b. Objectivity
   c. Verifiability
   d. Predictability
3. What type of quantitative research is conducted to generate knowledge that will directly influence clinical practice?
   a. Basic research
   b. Historical research
   c. Phenomenological research
   d. Applied research
4. Deductive reasoning is applied in
   a. Qualitative research
   b. Applied research
   c. Action research
   d. Quantitative research
5. Research means
   a. It is a form of audit
   b. Collecting information on a particular topic
   c. Systematically finding answers to a question
   d. It is an evaluation process
6. Florence Nightingale is most noted for which of the following contributions to nursing research?
   a. Case study approach
   b. Framework and model development
   c. Providing quality care
   d. Data collection and analysis
7. NRSI was established in the year
   a. 1966
   b. 1976
   c. 1986
   d. 1996
8. The characteristics of good research include all, *except*
   a. Orderly and systematic process
   b. Gathering new data
   c. Providing quality data
   d. Conducting study by using large number of samples
9. Which of the following is a research characteristic?
   a. Data are collected systematically
   b. Data are interpreted systematically
   c. There is clear purpose to find out the things
   d. All of the above
10. Which of the following research method is formal and objective?
    a. Phenomenological research
    b. Grounded theory approach
    c. Quantitative research
    d. Qualitative research
11. The following are the components of evidence-based practice *except*
    a. Using best available research evidence
    b. Considering needs and values of population
    c. Practitioner expertise
    d. Cost-efficient nursing care
12. Fundamental or pure research is *called*
    a. Basic research
    b. Applied research
    c. Action research
    d. Interventional research
13. A systematic study directed towards generating knowledge or understanding of the fundamental aspects of phenomena
    a. Basic research
    b. Pure research
    c. Applied research
    d. A and B both
14. Which research refers to scientific study and research that seeks to solve practical problems?
    a. Basic research
    b. Fundamental research
    c. Applied research
    d. Exploratory research

15. The rights of the participants in research include all, *except*
    a. Anonymity
    b. Confidentiality
    c. Voluntary participation
    d. Jurisprudence
16. Following are the purposes of evidence-based practice, *except*
    a. To improve patient care outcome
    b. To eliminate unsound practices
    c. To obtain more research funds
    d. To provide high quality care
17. Following are the barriers of EBP, *except*
    a. Lack of scientific literature
    b. Having autonomy in implementing care
    c. Lack of administrative support
    d. Workload pressure
18. Making patient care decision based on research findings is called
    a. Critical care
    b. Research implication
    c. Applied research
    d. EBP
19. In order to use research in practice, a nurse must
    a. Examine a research study and follow researcher's recommendations
    b. Read many studies in the same area and follow recommendations of the studies with similar findings
    c. Explore strength of evidence available
    d. Replicate studies in their own setting to make sure the recommendations are appropriate
20. In which of the following research questions would qualitative methodology be probably used?
    a. Which pain medication decreases the need of sleep medication in an elderly?
    b. What is the meaning of health for migrant coolie worker woman?
    c. Under what condition does a decubitus ulcer heal most quickly?
    d. How does frequency of medication administration impact in degree of pain experienced following a knee replacement surgery?
21. "Above all, do no harm". This principle encompassed in the ethical dilemma of
    a. Human dignity
    b. Justice
    c. Nonmalfeasance
    d. Anonymity
22. Voluntary agreement by a study subject to participate in a research study is termed as
    a. Informed consent
    b. Agreement
    c. Intervention
    d. Innovation
23. Plagiarism means
    a. Using another person's ideas or results without giving appropriate credit
    b. Creating a data without actually conducting the study
    c. Adding false statements in the published paper
    d. Publishing same research results in multiple papers
24. Informed consent to serve as a subject in research requires signing a document that states
    a. The purpose of the study
    b. That the subject may end participation at any time
    c. The probable risks involved
    d. All of the above

ANSWER KEY

1. c	2. d	3. d	4. d	5. c	6. d
7. c	8. d	9. d	10. c	11. d	12. a
13. d	14. c	15. d	16. c	17. b	18. d
19. c	20. b	21. c	22. a	23. a	24. d

UNIT 2

Research Process

Research process can be defined as a systematic process that deals with identifying, gathering and analyzing data in an objective manner to support research question. This process is used in all forms of research regardless of the research method (scientific method of inquiry, evaluation research, or action research) that enables the researcher to carry out research effectively. It is a multiple-step process where the steps are interlinked with each other in a sequential order.

Nursing research falls within the two broad worldviews, the positivist and naturalistic paradigms. While the positivist paradigm presumes the existence of a single reality that can be measured, the naturalistic paradigm on the contrary believes in the existence of multiple realities that are continuously changing making it difficult to measure. The two main types of research methods viz. qualitative and quantitative research align with these worldviews. While the quantitative research aligns with the positive paradigm which is a formal, objective and deductive approach to problem solving, the qualitative research design aligns with the naturalistic paradigm which is a more informal, subjective and inductive approach to problem solving.

QUANTITATIVE RESEARCH PROCESS

It is a traditional approach to research which involves identifying and measuring the variables in a reliable and valid way. It is a formal, objective, systematic process in which numeric data is used. The main aim of a quantitative study is to conduct a study on small sample and generalize the findings to a larger population using descriptive or inferential statistics.

Characteristics
- Concerned with objectivity and tight control over the research situation.
- Based on concept of manipulation and control of phenomenon.
- Gathers empirical evidence objectively.
- Deals with numbers; findings are presented in numerical or statistical language.
- Verification of results done using statistical analysis.
- Has ability to generalize the findings.

Purposes of Quantitative Research
- Measure concepts or variables objectively.
- Examine relationship between concepts.
- Test hypotheses.
- Develop tools and methods for numerical measurement and assessment.
- Control and manipulation of variables in an experimental setting.

STEPS IN QUANTITATIVE RESEARCH PROCESS

Quantitative research process is a rational, series of actions and goals. The scientific research process progresses in a systematic way and involves a logical flow as every step builds on the previous step. These steps can be classified into five phases: Conceptual phase, design and planning phase, empirical phase, analytic phase and dissemination phase (Flowchart 2.1).

Conceptual Phase

1. Identify the problem
- ❖ Identifying the research problem is the most important step in the research process which is both difficult and time consuming.
- ❖ Generally, a broad area of the topic is selected which is then narrowed down to a specific research problem.
- ❖ The specific research problem should hold the interest of the researcher, be feasible and significant to the nursing profession.
- ❖ Research problems can be sourced from own experiences, literature review and even theories.

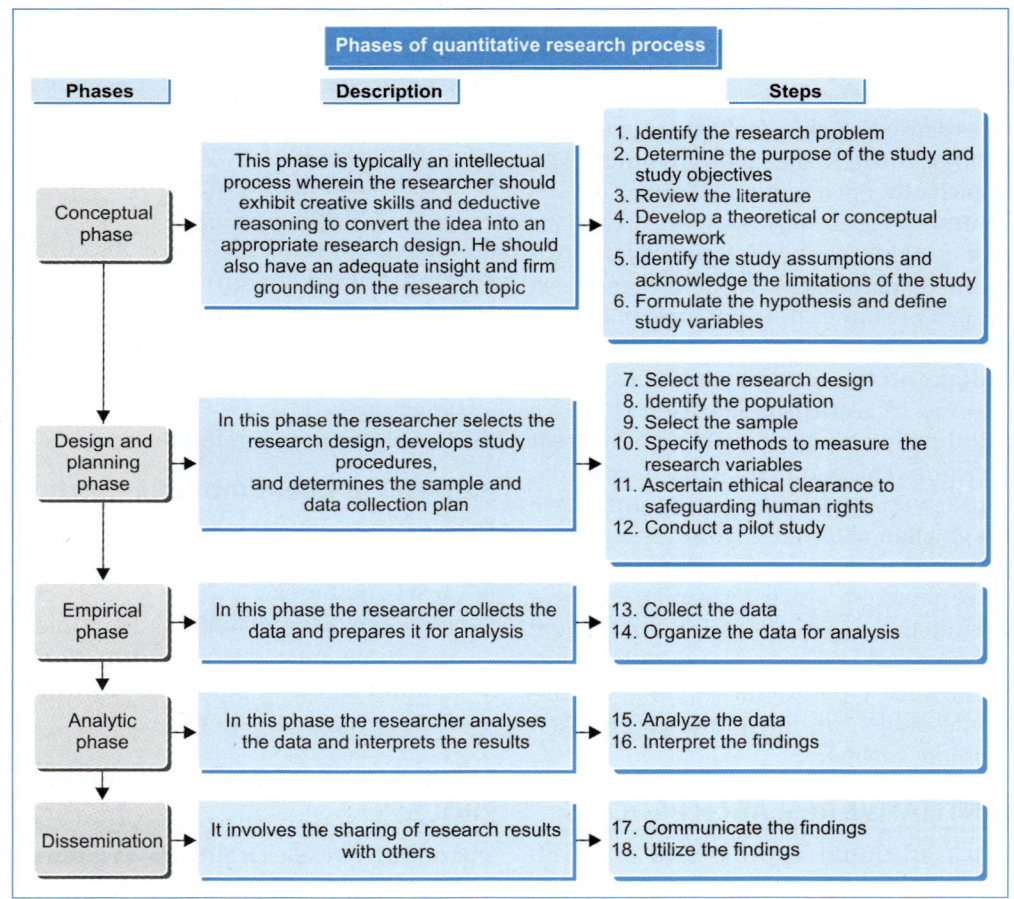

Flowchart 2.1: Phases of quantitative research process

- ❖ The research problem should indicate the sample and the variables being studied.
2. **Determine the purpose of the study and study objectives**
- ❖ The purpose describes why the study is being carried out.
- ❖ Every research project must have a clear rationalization or purpose.
- ❖ If the study purpose is clear and justified, the researcher is likely to receive approval for the study and much more likely to find the necessary subjects for the study.
- ❖ Objectives of the study provide guidelines for the research process.

3. **Review the literature**
- ❖ Literature review is a critical analysis of the relevant literature on the topic being studied.
- ❖ It provides an overview of information relating to a particular topic that helps the researcher to comprehend what is already known about the topic and what needs to be investigated further.
- ❖ Literature can be sourced through books, journals, research reports, newspapers, magazines, indexes, abstracts and computer-assisted searches.
- ❖ Review of literature guides the researcher to plan study methods (selection of tools, data collection methods, and analysis) and prepare conceptual framework.
- ❖ The researcher should collect most important and up-to-date information on the topic.

4. **Develop a theoretical or conceptual framework**
- ❖ Theoretical framework is a broad, general explanation of the relationships between the concepts of the research study based on an existing theory.
- ❖ Developing theoretical and conceptual framework helps the researcher in selection of variables, their operationalization; formulation of hypothesis and interpretation of findings.
- ❖ It helps to provide a scientific base for all the study variables and add to the scientific knowledge.
- ❖ A purely descriptive research may not require a theoretical framework.
- ❖ A research without theoretical base simply provides a set of isolated facts.

5. **Identify the study assumptions and acknowledge the limitations of the study**
- ❖ Assumptions are overt and/or innate beliefs held by the researcher about phenomenon that is accepted as truth without proof or empirical evidence.
- ❖ Each research study is based on certain assumptions that influence the questions asked, data collected, methods used to gather it and its interpretation.
- ❖ Assumptions should be stated clearly.
- ❖ *Limitations* are uncontrolled variables or shortcomings in a study, usually beyond the researcher's control that may adversely affect the credibility and generalizability of the findings.
- ❖ The researcher should identify the study limitations and explicitly acknowledge them.

6. **Formulate the hypothesis and define variables**
- ❖ Hypothesis predicts the relationship between two or more variables in a study.
- ❖ Whilst the problem statement raises a question, the hypothesis predicts its answer.
- ❖ It provides direction for research methodology, selecting sampling method, identifying data collection method, conducting analysis and interpretation of findings.
- ❖ It should be stated clearly and testable.
- ❖ A variable is a characteristic, event or response that represents the elements of the research question.

❖ These variables need to be operationally defined so as to enable accurate measurement of the concept and allow replication of the study.

Design and Planning Phase

7. Select the research design
❖ A research design is a specific outline that details the methods and procedures used to conduct the study.
❖ It outlines various aspects of data collection such as "which data is to be collected," "when it is to be collected," and "how it is to be collected," the setting of the study, sample size and sample techniques used.
❖ The quantitative research designs are broadly classified into experimental and nonexperimental designs.
❖ Nonexperimental designs are used to describe, differentiate and examine associations between variables. These include descriptive, correlational and comparative studies.
❖ Experimental designs are used to predict and control the phenomena. These are further classified into true and quasi-experimental designs.

8. Identify the population
❖ The main aim of quantitative research is to conduct study on smaller samples and generalize the research results to a larger population.
❖ Population is the entire group of people about whom the researcher wishes to generalize the study findings.
❖ The research should specify the target population (broad population to which the study results are generalized) as well as accessible population (actual population on which the researches study is being conducted).
❖ By specifying the population, the researcher is clear about the groups on which the study will be conducted and on which the study results can be applied.
❖ For the results to be applied to the target population, the characteristics of the accessible population should be similar to target population.

9. Develop sampling plan and select the sample
❖ In research studies it is not always possible to study an entire population, as studying it in its entirety is very time consuming, costly and requires more resources. Therefore, a subset of subjects which is representative of the given population, termed as sample is selected for the study purpose.
❖ The selected sample characteristics must be similar to population characteristics so as to be able to generalize the results to the population.
❖ The researcher should prepare a sample plan which includes inclusion and exclusion criteria, sample selection method and sample size.
❖ By using inclusion and exclusion criteria the researcher will be able to select prospective subjects for the study.
❖ Sampling techniques or methods outline the strategies used to obtain samples for studies. Commonly the sampling techniques are classified into two types viz. probability (random) or nonprobability (nonrandom) sampling techniques or methods.
❖ Selection of sampling method depends on availability of the resources and nature of the study.
❖ Sample size denotes minimum number of sample needed to detect significant relationships or differences existing among the variables. In quantitative research studies sample size is determined by using power analysis.

10. **Specify methods to measure the research variable**
    - In quantitative research the collected data should be quantifiable, objective, accurate and reliable.
    - In quantitative research variables are measured very accurately and measurements should be accurate, valid and reliable.
    - The selection of data collection method is based on research design and availability of resources.
    - The commonly used quantitative data collection approaches are biophysiologic measurements, self-reports, observation methods.

11. **Ascertain ethical clearance to safe guarding human rights**
    - Majority of research studies in nursing involve human beings as subjects and their rights must be considered before conducting the study.
    - It is essential that all research studies involving human subjects be reviewed by ethical review board to protect the welfare of the study participants.
    - While conducting research involving human subjects it should be ensured that their participation is voluntary, prior consent is obtained, privacy and fair treatment is ensured and are protected from potential harm.

12. **Conduct a pilot study**
    - Pilot study is a trial, small scale study carried out before final research.
    - It is conducted to test, refine or modify research methodology and help in preparing a larger and more comprehensive investigation.
    - Through this pilot study the researcher evaluates the feasibility and acceptability of data collection procedures.
    - Subjects are selected for the pilot study that is similar in characteristics to the sample that will be used for the actual study.
    - Once the pilot study is over the researcher should make necessary revisions before commencing the final study.

Empirical Phase

13. **Collect the data**
    - Variables in a study are measured through data collection procedure. Data collection should be a systematic process and considerable attention is required during this phase to diminish the introduction of bias.
    - Researcher needs to develop data collection plan to specify how, who, where, when and what type of data will be collected.
    - In experimental research studies the researcher needs to develop intervention protocol that describes intervention details like intervention components, timing, frequency, dosage and who will provide the intervention and training of the interventionist. This will allow the standard approach for the conduct of research and enhance internal validity.

14. **Organize the data for analysis**
    - After data collection the collected data needs to be organized for analysis.
    - During this phase questionnaires are checked for completeness, decisions regarding missing data are made and errors in data entry determined.
    - Later the data is entered into a statistical software program for analysis.
    - During this phase the statistician can help to determine which statistical procedures will be appropriate to analyze the data.

Analytic Phase

15. **Analyze the data**
    - In the analytic phase relationships among the data are identified and research

questions answered through the synthesis of numerical data.
- If questions were posed, findings should answer those questions.
- If hypotheses were stated, findings should support or not support them.
- Tables, graphs and line diagrams are helpful to summarize data from which relationships between data items can be observed.
- Analysis techniques conducted in quantitative research include descriptive and inferential statistics.

16. **Interpret the findings**
- Interpretation of research involves describing strengths and weaknesses of the study, implications for nursing and recommendations for future research.
- After data analysis the results need to be interpreted based on the study hypothesis or research question to ascertain the meaning and importance of findings.
- During this phase the researcher should discuss all problems raised during data collection process and limitations of the study.
- The researcher compares the results of the present study with similar previous studies to discuss the findings and add the present knowledge to the existing body of knowledge.

Dissemination Phase

17. **Communicate the findings**

In this phase the researcher prepares research reports with an intention to communicate findings to the appropriate audience. Research findings can be communicated through publication in research journals and presentation in national, regional, state and local conferences.

18. **Utilize the findings**

The final step of a good research study is to plan for its utilization in practice settings. In this phase the researcher lists recommendations about how the present research findings can be integrated into clinical practice. An example of quantitative research process is presented in Flowchart 2.2.

ADVANTAGES AND DISADVANTAGES OF QUANTITATIVE RESEARCH

The main aim of quantitative research is to conduct study on a sample and generalize the results to a larger population. The advantages and disadvantages of quantitative research are presented in Table 2.1.

QUALITATIVE RESEARCH PROCESS

Qualitative research is selected when little is known about the phenomena and the researcher wants to get a more holistic sense of its experience. It is a naturalistic approach to research where the focus is on understanding the meaning of an experience of the individual's perspective or gain insight into people's attitudes, behaviors, value systems, concerns, motivations, aspirations, culture or lifestyles.

"A qualitative study is defined as an inquiry process of understanding a social or human problem, based on building a complex, holistic picture, formed with words, reporting detailed views of informants, and conducted in a natural setting." —**Creswell, 1998**

Characteristics

- Study is conducted in a natural setting.
- It uses multiple approaches to understand the concepts.
- Research design emerges during the research process and is not prespecified.
- Researcher views the social phenomena comprehensively.
- Researcher uses complex reasoning that is comprehensive, repetitive, continuous and simultaneous.
- Researcher becomes intensively involved.

Flowchart 2.2: Phases of quantitative research process

I. Conceptual Phase
1. Problem statement: "Efficacy of Body Mind Spirit (BMS) intervention on well-being, of depressive patients"
2. Determine the purpose and objectives of the study:
   - Assess the level of depression and well-being among depressive patients
   - Evaluate the efficacy of BMS intervention by comparing well-being between experimental and control group subjects
3. Review the literature
4. Develop a conceptual framework:
   - This study is based on integrative BMS model
5. Identify the study assumption:
   - Combined therapies are more effective than monotherapies for depressive patients
   - Nurses can learn complementary therapies very easily and practice them on depressive patients
6. Formulation of hypothesis:
   - There will be a statistically significant decrease in depressive scores among experimental group subjects compared to control group subjects at 6 months follow-up
   - There will be a statistically significant increase in well-being scores among experimental group subjects compared to control group subjects at 6 months follow-up

↓

II. Design and Planning Phase
7. Research approach and design—quantitative approach, true experimental design—pretest-posttest control group design
8. Identify the population:
   - Patients diagnosed with depression
9. Select the sample:
   - Depressive patients who are attending psychiatric OPD at District Hospital, Kolar
   - 120 depressive patients randomly assigned to experimental and control group
10. Specify the methods to measure the research variables:
    - Self-report questionnaires—Beck Depressive Inventory, Body-Mind Spirit, Well-being Inventory
11. Obtained institutional ethical clearance
12. Conducted pilot study

↓

III. Empirical Phase
13. Collect the data:
    - Administered questionnaires and implemented BMS intervention to experimental group participants for one month and assessments done on a monthly basis up to six months for both the group subjects
14. Organize the data for analysis: Data were organized under the following headings:
    - Description of demographic characteristics
    - Pre intervention comparison
    - Post intervention comparison
    - Correlation between dependent variables

↓

IV. Analytic Phase
15. Analyze the data:
    - Descriptive and inferential statistics were used
16. Results were interpreted based on objectives

↓

V. Dissemination Phase
17. Communicate the findings:
    - Prepared research report, published research articles in indexed journals and presented in conferences
18. Utilize the findings:
    - BMS techniques implemented in routine care for depressive patients

Table 2.1: Advantages and disadvantages of quantitative research

Advantages	Disadvantages
• Allows greater objectivity and accuracy of results as it employs structured procedures, randomization and use of reliable and valid tools. • Controls confounding variables significantly and identifies cause and effect relationship. • Enhances generalization of results as it involves greater number of subjects. • Personal bias can be avoided by using randomization techniques while selecting subjects. • Findings are replicable as standard means are used. • Systematic comparisons across categories and time periods can be achieved by analyzing vast sources of information. • Contributes to testing nursing theory.	• Research is conducted in a controlled setting (not a natural setting) resulting in opposed to real world results. • Even though controlled environment is used, confounding variables may continue to be present. • Collects a much narrower and at times superficial data set. • The development of standard questions by researchers can lead to "structural" bias and false representation, where the data actually reflects the researcher's view rather than the participant's. • Results provide numerical descriptions rather than detailed narrative, thus limiting elaborate accounts of human perception.

Purposes of Qualitative Research

The main purpose of qualitative research is to explore, describe and explain the phenomena to gain new insights into the topic being studied. Qualitative research question focuses on describing what is this? Or what is occurring or taking place in the situation? And are more interested with the process rather than the outcome of the study (Ploeg J, 1999). The main purposes are:

❖ Collect and explore an in depth information that cannot be expressed quantitatively.
❖ Describe complex phenomena with rich descriptions.
❖ Facilitate better understanding of the phenomena and gain a new perspective on the topic.
❖ Explore issues that are culturally sensitive and related to difficult to access groups.
❖ Track unique or unexpected events.
❖ Illuminate experience.
❖ Give voice to those rarely heard.
❖ Guide nursing practice by enabling systematic structuring of ideas that emerge from persons who are experts through life experience.
❖ Contribute to instrument development by using the voice of research participants to enable evaluation of existing instruments or creation of new ones.
❖ Build nursing theory by using personal stories to enlighten and enrich understanding of everyday health experience.

STEPS IN QUALITATIVE RESEARCH PROCESS

The process of qualitative research is less formally planned wherein the planning and implementation of research moves hand in hand (Flowchart 2.3). An example of qualitative research process is presented in Flowchart 2.4.

1. **Identify the problem**
   ❖ The researcher identifies the problem that is poorly understood and about which little is known.
   ❖ Researcher begins with a broad research question that is narrowed down and defined once the study gets underway.
   ❖ Research questions focus on open ended questions such as "what is this?" "What is occurring here and why it occurred?" Attention is more on the process rather than the outcome.

2. **Review of literature**
   ❖ Qualitative research describes the phenomena based on participant's view point rather than on any prior information.

Flowchart 2.3: Phases of qualitative research process

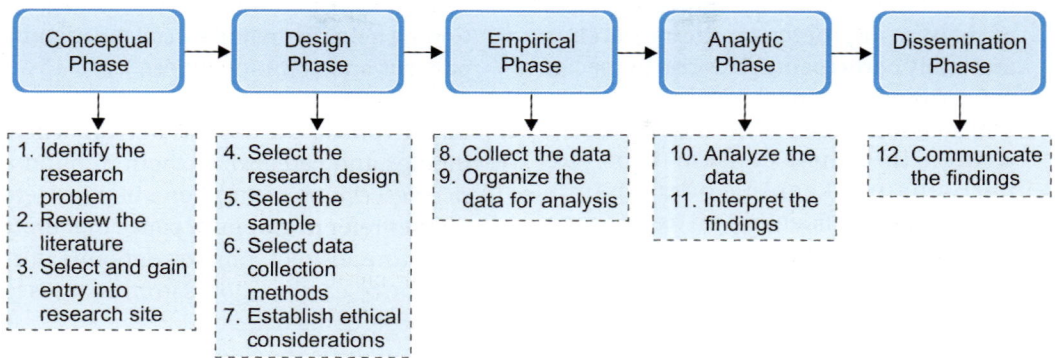

- Some researchers believe that literature review in qualitative studies may become a source of bias.
- While some researchers conduct a literature review during the conclusion stage, others conduct a preliminary literature review upfront to obtain some guidance.

3. **Select and gain entry into research site**
- In qualitative research as the researchers have little understanding of the phenomena and population the entry in research setting is an ongoing process.
- Gaining entry into research setting requires prior permission from concerned authorities and establishing relationship and rapport with key informants (people with important source of information) and study participants.

4. **Select the research design**
- In qualitative studies research design evolves during the process of data collection and is called emergent design.
- Research design is selected based on the nature of phenomenon under study.
- The commonly used designs in qualitative research are phenomenological design, ethnographical design, grounded theory approach and case study.

5. **Select the sample**
- Nonrandom sampling techniques are used to select the sample. Participants are recruited purposefully based on their personal knowledge of experience with the phenomena.
- The sample size is small compared to quantitative research. In-depth inquiries are conducted. The depth and quality of data is more important than quantity of data.
- Sample size is decided based on data saturation, resources; time and study objectives.
- Data saturation occurs when themes and categories in the data become repetitive and redundant resulting in no new information being gathered by further data collection.
- Commonly used sampling methods are quota sampling, purposive sampling and snowball sampling.

6. **Select data collection methods**
- The data in qualitative research studies are participant's thoughts, views, ideas and perceptions.
- The commonly used data collection methods are unobtrusive and obtrusive.
- Unobtrusive methods are simple observation, document analysis, audio and video recording.
- The obtrusive methods include semi-structured and unstructured in-depth interviews, focus group discussions and participant observation.

7. **Establish ethical considerations**
   - In qualitative studies the intimate nature of relationship between the researcher and study participants gives rise to special concerns relating to ethical issues.
   - Ethical issues are dealt with by obtaining written informed consent from the participants, keeping participant's information confidential and maintaining anonymity of the subjects.
8. **Collect data**
   - In qualitative studies the selection of samples, data collection, analysis of data and data interpretation take place simultaneously.
   - The researcher collects data from the participants by talking directly or observing their behavior or examining documents in their natural setting where the participants are experiencing a problem.
   - Multiple data collection methods such as interviews, observations and documents are used to collect data from participants.
   - The researcher uses unstructured data collection methods like interviews and observations which are loosely structured using open-ended questions. These allow the participants to express full range of beliefs, feelings and behavior.
   - Most researchers record or document their data through the use of field notes, tape records.
   - Field notes document the researcher's observations and interviews.
   - Data from interviews or focus groups can be recorded as hand written, field notes or tape-recorded.
   - The research findings are described based on the participants view point rather than researcher's perception which demonstrates the trustworthiness of the data.
9. **Organize the data for analysis**
   - Researcher organizes the data into categories on the basis of themes, patterns or concepts. In order to achieve this, the researcher uses coding process.
   - While coding the researcher assigns a word, phrase or number to each category.
   - Coding helps to organize data and identify patterns and commonalities.
10. **Analyze the data**
    - In this phase the researcher identifies themes and categorizes them to build a rich description of the phenomenon. Here themes refer to groups of codes that unify into more abstract common denominators and the researcher moves from analysis to synthesis of the data.
    - Data analysis involves putting together related themes of narrative information into a logical sequential order.
    - The researcher may work with the participants in developing themes that emerge from the data collection process.
    - As the identification of the themes begins, the researcher writes down the ideas on paper and rewrites it in an attempt to group the data effectively.
    - The researcher uses logical processes and complex reasoning skills throughout the research process that are either inductive or deductive in nature.
    - Through deductive (general to specific) thinking process the researcher builds the themes that are continuously checked against the data.
    - Through inductive (specific to general) process the researcher organizes the data into increasingly more abstract units of information. During this process the researcher works back and forth between the themes and the database until a comprehensive set of themes is established.
    - Data are more easily managed with the use of software programs like Computer Assisted Qualitative Analysis Software (CAQAS). This software is helpful in coding data quickly and schematically depicting on of how codes might form themes.

Flowchart 2.4: Phases of qualitative research process

I. Conceptual Phase:
1. Identify the research problem: Cancer diagnosis affects the various aspects of human life and causes an enormous spiritual crisis. During this stage the person seeks spiritual support
2. Review the literature: Researcher conducted review of literature while concluding the study to understand the spiritual needs of cancer patients
3. Select and gain entry into research site: Researcher obtained permission from the hospital authorities to conduct the study

II. Design Phase:
4. Select the research design: Qualitative approach with phenomenological research design was selected
5. Select the sample Selected 18 cancer patients from the Cancer Institute in Tehran using purposive sampling method. Sampling continued until data saturation is achieved in all categories
6. Select data collection methods: Semi-structured interview schedule was prepared
7. Establish ethical considerations. Obtained informed consent from participants. Participants were also guaranteed that their names (identity) shall not be revealed

III. Empirical Phase:
8. Collect the data: Semi-structured interviews were used for data collection. Interview process was recorded with patient's permission
9. Organize the data for analysis: Recorder information was converted verbatim soon after completion of the interview and analyzed simultaneously. This procedure was followed for all the 18 interviews

IV. Analytic Phase:
10. Analyze the data: Conventional content analysis approach was used for data analysis
11. Interpret the findings: From 1850 initial codes, 4 themes viz. connection, peace, meaning and purpose, and transcendence were identified. These themes contained categories of social support, normal behavior, inner peace, seeking forgiveness, hope, acceptance of reality, seeking meaning, ending well, change of life meaning, strengthening spiritual belief, communication with god, and prayer

V. Communicate the Findings:
12. Published research article: Hatamipour K, Rassouli M, Yaghmaie F, et al. Spiritual Needs of Cancer Patients: A Qualitative Study Indian J Palliat. Care. 2015;21(1):61-7

Ensuring Validity of Qualitative Information

- Throughout data collection and analysis the researchers typically record personal reflections, observations, questions, ideas, hunches and feelings.
- These vital steps help to judge and interpret data and ultimately to construct meanings.
- During data analysis process the researcher goes back to the participants to determine whether the participants recognize the experience as their own. This mechanism is called member checking and a standard called credibility which helps to preserve the integrity of participants' statements.

11. Interpret the findings

- Qualitative researchers try to develop the complex picture of the problem and identify the complex interactions between the factors.
- This involves reporting the phenomena from multiple perspectives and identifying the many factors involved in the situation.

12. Communicate the findings

- Qualitative reports are usually filled with rich verbatim passages directly from participants.
- Qualitative research findings serve as a basis for formulation of hypothesis and development of tools. These are tested using quantitative research.

ADVANTAGES AND DISADVANTAGES OF QUALITATIVE RESEARCH

Qualitative research provides a rich and detailed picture of the phenomenon. The advantages and disadvantages of qualitative research are presented in Table 2.2.

DIFFERENCES BETWEEN QUALITATIVE AND QUANTITATIVE RESEARCH

Qualitative research is slightly different from quantitative research (Table 2.3).

SELECTING QUANTITATIVE VS QUALITATIVE RESEARCH

- If it is found that little is known about a phenomenon and the researcher wants to get a more holistic sense of its experience he needs to select a qualitative study.
- If the purpose is to gain an in-depth understanding of the overall phenomena use a qualitative design as follows:
  - If you are interested in learning cultural patterns—use ethnographic method

Table 2.2: Advantages and disadvantages of qualitative research

Advantages	Disadvantages
• Research study is conducted in a natural setting and focuses on human experiences resulting in real world results. • Encourages participants to detail on their responses thus creating an openness to explore sensitive topics and issues pertaining to difficult to access groups or subcultures. • Explains phenomena comprehensively and gains new perspectives to phenomena. • Data reflects the participant's actual perception. • Results provide a deep and detailed narrative description of complex phenomena. • Contributes to instrument development and builds nursing theory.	• Smaller sample is studied as collection of data is more time consuming and can last for months or even years. • Study results cannot be generalized as small sample is involved. • Measurements are neither objective nor accurate; biased information may be collected. • Qualitative research has very little control; therefore, "confound" variables are a problem. • The researcher interprets the research according to his or her own biased view which distorts the data gathered. • Difficult to make systematic comparisons as the collected data is highly subjective. • Replication of results is much more difficult and in some cases even impossible.

Table 2.3: Differences between qualitative and quantitative research

Qualitative	Attribute	Quantitative
• Multiple realities that can be subjective, occurring within the context of the situation • Soft science	Philosophical perspective	• One reality that can be objectively viewed and measured by the researcher • Hard science
• Naturalist • Constructionism • Focuses on interactive processes	Philosophy	• Positivist • Objectivism • Focuses on variables
• Inductive	Types of reasoning	• Deductive
• Describes and promotes understanding of human experiences related to health • Generate hypotheses • Develops theory	Purpose	• Describes variables. • Tests relationships between variables • Examines cause and effect relationship among variables. • Tests theory
• Personally involved, participative and ongoing	Role of researcher	• Detached, objective, controlled and structured

• Use semi-structured methods
  – In-depth interviews
  – Focus groups
  – Participant observation
	Tools	• Use highly structured methods
		  – Questionnaires
		  – Surveys
		  – Structured observation

• Emergent design and flexible
  – Phenomenology
  – Ethnography
  – Grounded theory
  – Historical
	Design	• Rigid design, controlled and experimental
		  – Descriptive
		  – Correlational
		  – Quasi-experimental
		  – Experimental

• Small sample. • Nonrandom sampling methods • Purposive, convenient, snowball	Sampling	• Large sample • Random and nonrandom sampling
• Nonstatistical (words/narratives)	Analysis of data	• Statistical (Numbers)
• Analyze the words of the participant, finds meaning in the words and provides a description of the experience and helps deeper understanding of the experience	Results	• Estimates the outcomes of intervention • Predicts outcome variable
• Transfer knowledge from case analysis to similar cases	Generalization	• Use inference to generalize from a sample to a defined population
• Interpretive reports that reflect the researcher's construction of the meaning of the data	Report	• Objective, impersonal reports

- If you are interested in understanding human experience—use phenomenological method.
- If you are interested in uncovering social processes—use grounded theory method
- If you are interested in capturing unique stories—use case study method

❖ If substantial knowledge already exists choose a quantitative design as follows:
  - If the purpose of the study is to describe the relationship between specific variables, use a descriptive design.
  - To test an intervention (manipulating the independent variable)—use an experimental design.
  - If some elements of control are missing—use quasi-experimental design.

The selection between qualitative and quantitative forms of research rests on the questions a researcher wants to answer and the practicality of gathering the data that will answer those questions. However, in some situations a combination of both quantitative and qualitative methods are more useful to understand, describe, control and predict the phenomenon.

BIBLIOGRAPHY

1. Burns, N., & Grove, S.K. (2004). *The practice of nursing research*. Philadelphia: W.B. Saunders Company.
2. Hatamipour, K., Rassouli, M., Yaghmaie, F., Zendedel, K., & Majd, H.A. (2015). Spiritual Needs of Cancer Patients: A Qualitative Study. Indian Journal of Palliative Care, 21(1), 61–67. http://doi.org/10.4103/0973-1075.150190
3. Knobf, M.T. (2002). Carrying on: The experience of premature menopause in women with early stage breast cancer. *Nursing research*, 51, 9-17.
4. LoBiondo-Wood, G., & Haber, J. (1997). *Nursing Research: Methods, critical appraisal and utilization* (3rd ed.). Boston: Mosbey.
5. Lusk, B. (2000). Pretty and Powerless: Nurses in advertisements, 1930-1950. *Research in Nursing & Health*, 23, 229-236.
6. Nieswiadomy, M.R. (2008). *Foundations of nursing research*. Boston: Pearson Prentice Hall.
7. Ploeg, J. (1999). Identifying the best research design to fit the question. *Part 2:* qualitative designs. *Evidenced Based Nursing*, 2, 36-37
8. Polit, D.F., & Beck, C.T. (2004). *Nursing research: Appraising evidence for nursing practice*. Philadelphia: Wolters Klower/Lippincott Williams & Wilkins.
9. Polit, D.F., & Beck, C.T. (2009). *Nursing research:* Generating and assessing evidence for nursing practice. Philadelphia: Lippincott Williams & Wilkins.
10. Polit, D.F., Beck, C.T., & Hungler, B.P. (2001). *Essentials of Nursing Research: Methods, Appraisal, and Utilization* (5th ed.). Philadelphia: Lippincott Williams & Wilkins.
11. Polit, D.F., Beck, C.T., & Hungler, B.P. (2006). *Essentials of nursing research: Methods, appraisal and utilization* (6th ed.). Philadelphia: Lippincott Williams & Wilkins.
12. Rungre, Angkulkij, S., & Chesla, C. (2001). Smooth a heart with water: Thai mothers care for a child with schizophrenia. *Archives of Psychiatric Nursing*, 15, 120-127.
13. Schotfetdt, R.M. (1977). Nursing Research: Reflection of values. *Nursing Research*, 26(1), 4-8.
14. Sharif, F., & Masoumi, S. (2005). A qualitative study of nursing student experiences of clinical practice. *Biomed Central Nursing Journal*, 4, 6.
15. Treece, E.W., & Treece, J.H. (1989). *Elements of Research in Nursing*. St. Louis: The C.V. Mosby Company.
16. Wilson, H. (1987). *Introducing research in nursing*. Menlo Park, CA: Addison-Wesley.
17. Wittig, D.R. (2001). Organ donation beliefs of African American women residing in small Southern community. *Journal of Transcultural Nursing*, 12, 203–10.

REVIEW QUESTIONS

I. Long Essays
1. Define nursing research and describe in detail the steps involved in quantitative research process.
2. Describe the steps involved in qualitative research process.

II. Short Essays
1. What are the differences between quantitative and qualitative research?
2. Describe the characteristics of quantitative nursing research.
3. Explain advantages and disadvantages of quantitative research.
4. Enumerate purposes of qualitative research.

III. Short Answers
1. Phases of quantitative research design.
2. Characteristics of quantitative research.
3. Characteristics of qualitative research.

IV. Multiple Choice Questions
1. The first step in research process is the
   a. Development of a research plan
   b. Conducting survey to determine existing problems
   c. Collection of the available sources for needed information
   d. Identifying the research problem and determining the objectives
2. After identifying the important variables and establishing the logical reasoning in theoretical framework, the next step in the research process is
   a. To conduct surveys
   b. To generate the hypothesis
   c. To focus on group discussions
   d. To determine sample size
3. Which of the following is a characteristic of qualitative research?
   a. Deductive process
   b. Control over the context
   c. Fixed research design
   d. Inductive process
4. Qualitative research design involves
   a. Emergent design
   b. Correlative design
   c. Experimental design
   d. Cohort design
5. The following are the characteristics of quantitative research, *except*
   a. Gathers empirical evidence
   b. Has ability to generalize the findings
   c. Concerned with objectivity
   d. Unique case orientation
6. Which of the following steps is involved in conceptual phase
   a. Determine the purpose of the study
   b. Selecting the sample
   c. Collecting the data
   d. Utilizing the findings
7. Dissemination phase includes all of the following, *except*
   a. Presenting the research paper
   b. Preparing research report
   c. Utilize the findings
   d. Organize the data for analysis
8. Which of the following sampling method is commonly used in qualitative research?
   a. Stratified sampling
   b. Simple random sampling
   c. Systematic sampling
   d. Purposive sampling
9. In which of the following phase pilot study is conducted
   a. Conceptual phase
   b. Analytic phase
   c. Dissemination phase
   d. Designing phase
10. The following are the activities involved in analytic phase, *except*
    a. Collecting data for analysis
    b. Analyze the data

c. Interpret the findings
d. Analysis of numerical data

11. Find out which of the following statements distinguishes quantitative research from qualitative research.
    a. Hypotheses are more likely to be tested in quantitative research than in qualitative research
    b. In nursing fewer quantitative research studies have been conducted in the past than qualitative research studies
    c. Quantitative research focuses on subjective data whereas qualitative research focuses on objective data
    d. All of the above

12. Which of the following statement is true when comparing qualitative research with quantitative research?
    a. Qualitative research most frequently uses a deductive approach whereas quantitative research uses an inductive approach
    b. Qualitative research most frequently uses an inductive approach, whereas quantitative research uses a deductive approach
    c. Qualitative research is more difficult to conduct than quantitative research
    d. Quantitative research is more difficult to conduct than qualitative research

ANSWER KEY

| 1. d | 2. b | 3. d | 4. a | 5. d | 6. a |
| 7. d | 8. d | 9. d | 10. a | 11. a | 12. b |

UNIT 3

Research Problem and Hypothesis

The identification and formulation of a research problem is the primary and most important step that every researcher has to carry out. Selection of the research problem begins with identification of potential problem and ends with research question or hypothesis.

MEANING

- Research problem is the topic researcher would like to address, investigate, or study descriptively or experimentally.
- Research problem is a question that indicates gaps in the scope of knowledge needed for professional practice.
- Research problem is the difference between what the researcher knows and what he should know.

SOURCES OF RESEARCH PROBLEM

Identifying a significant research problem that is appropriate for investigation is a difficult step in the research process and consumes a large part of the total time allocated to the research project. Research problems are generated from a variety of sources (Fig. 3.1).

- *Nursing practice:* It offers clinically relevant research problems. Nurses can develop observational or analytical skills that maximize each opportunity for discovering important problems. For example, a nurse finds that structuring ward activities reduces patient anxiety and hallucinatory behavior among mentally ill patients; administration of antipsychotics early in the night before 7 pm helps the patient to get up early in the morning. Such clinical experiences are rich sources for research problems.
- *Literature review*: Reviewing previous literature such as published articles in journals, books, opinion articles, research reports, unpublished dissertations, and thesis can generate ideas for possible areas of research. These sources provide the opportunity to expand on the work of others, stimulate the imagination of the investigator, and also help to find gaps in nursing literature that require research. For example, a researcher studies an article on the spiritual needs of depressive patients. While reading this article, the researcher learns that not many studies have been conducted on spiritual needs of mentally ill patients. This review may provide the basis for formulating a research problem.
- *Theories*: Theory development relies on research and research relies on theory. Reading theories developed in nursing and other disciplines can provide research problems through a deductive process. This aids in the development of hypotheses for empirical testing. These sources provide meaningful contributions to nursing knowledge. Usually, a component or some components of the

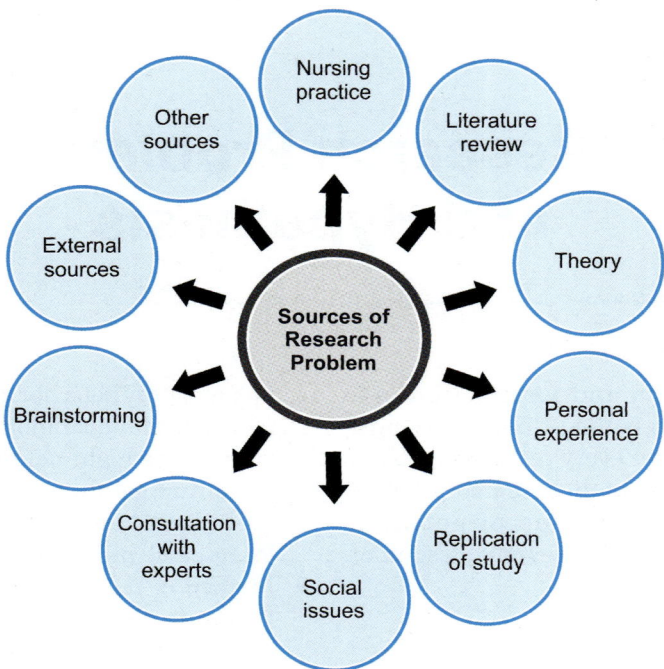

Fig. 3.1: Sources of research problem

theory are subjected to testing in the clinical situation. For example, using Dorothea Orem theory (1985), Anderson 2001 explored the relationship between self-care and self-care agency and well-being among a sample of homeless adults. Using Martha Rogers frame work (1986), Bays (2001) explored the phenomenon of hope and associated factors among stroke patients.

- *Personal experience*: A researcher's personal experience may serve as a rich source of ideas to formulate a research problem. For example, a researcher observed examination anxiety faced by 10th class students. Based on this experience, the research may propose several studies related to examination anxiety among students.
- *Replication of study on new population*: Replication means repetition of research procedures in another study to find out if the same results can be generated. Through replication the researcher can validate some aspects of an established theory and discover results that are in disagreement with previous research results.
- *Social issues*: Social issues can provide topics relevant to healthcare research, which may include domestic violence, sexual harassment, gender discrimination, etc.
- *Consultation with experts*: As experts have sound knowledge in their respective fields, they may help in selection and formulation of a research problem.
- *Brainstorming*: It is a technique where subject experts hold group discussions to generate ideas for formulating an ideal research problem.
- *External sources*: Funding organizations, statutory bodies, and health organizations are also a good source as they suggest

| Box 3.1 | Some of the priority areas of research recommended by the Indian Nursing Council, 2017 |

- Outcome-oriented clinical interventional studies
- Studies involving development of practice standards or guidelines or protocols
- Human resource planning and development studies
- Development of new models for care or educational delivery
- Development and testing of quality assurance models in nursing service and education

Note: Educational interventions are strictly discouraged.

| Box 3.2 | Some of the priority areas of research recommended by Indian Council for Medical Research under maternal health |

- Nutritional disorders among women
- Reproductive health issues
- Healthcare seeking behavior among antenatal women
- Estimating maternal morbidity and mortality rates
- Measuring tools for reducing maternal mortality rate (MMR)

research topics based on their priorities (Boxes 3.1 and 3.2).

❖ *Other sources*: Technological changes, intuition, folklores, and expanded roles of nurses also suggest current problems in the profession.

CRITERIA FOR SELECTING A RESEARCH PROBLEM

Once a problem is isolated, the researcher must be able to determine whether or not his problem is significant for investigation. Selecting a suitable research problem among identified problems involves evaluation of alternatives against certain criteria—internal and external. The criteria for selecting a research problem are presented in Flowchart 3.1.

❖ **Internal criteria**: The researcher should not only have adequate subject expertise in the area of research but also the interest and resources to conduct it.
  ○ *Researcher's interest*: Interest, motivation, and curiosity over the problem develop sustained perseverance. Researcher's qualification and experience play a vital role in developing an interest in the problem.
  ○ *Researcher's competency*: The researcher must be capable of planning and carrying out the research study for which he should have adequate knowledge on subject matter, research methodology, and statistical procedures. The researcher needs to possess personality attributes of creativity, flexibility, and foresight to be able to select a research problem that does not involve objectionable duplication.
  ○ *Researcher's own resources*: As any research work is time consuming and expensive, the researcher should adequately plan his time and financial resources to complete it.

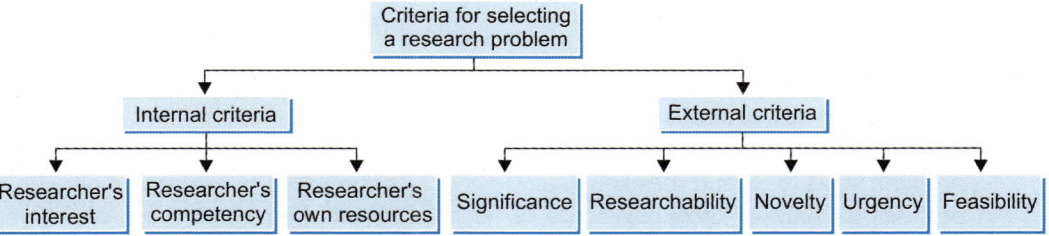

Flowchart 3.1: Criteria for selecting a research problem

- ❖ **External criteria**: The prerequisite of a research problem is that it must be significant, novel, important, and urgent to the profession. Feasibility of the problem is also a significant factor.
  - *Significance of the research problem*: Significance refers to the worthiness of a problem being studied. Research problem is significant when patients, nurses, and healthcare community benefit from this study and:
    - It has the ability to produce or refine relevant knowledge and influence the nursing profession
    - It contributes to the body of organized knowledge in nursing field
    - It builds on previous research
    - It supports theory testing or development
    - It addresses current priorities in nursing
  - *Researchability of the problem*: Research problems are focused on facts rather than on opinion; deal with current and significant issues relevant to the profession, action oriented, and solvable through scientific method. The selected problem should be one that will lead to new problems, is replicable and amenable to further research. Ethical and moral issues though challenging are not amenable for research. For example, a researcher wants to investigate the power of God. Problems of this nature are not amenable to research.
  - *Novelty of the problem*: The problem selected should be novel, so as to avoid wasting time and energy on a problem already researched. Hence, the researcher should select innovative problem so as to extend the growth of professional body of knowledge.
  - *Urgency*: Urgent problems must be given priority because an immediate solution can benefit people.
  - *Feasibility*: Feasibility refers to whether or not a study can be carried out. A problem though significant and researchable may still not be appropriate, if it is not feasible. The feasibility of a study can be assessed by verifying the availability of the subjects, resources (facilities and equipment), time frame, cost, cooperation of others, and ethical considerations.
    - *Availability of the subjects*: The researcher needs to consider whether a sample with specific attributes will be available and agreeable to participate. Sometimes, adequate number of potential subjects may not be available and even if available may not be willing to participate. Carrying out research under such situations will be difficult. Therefore availability of the subjects must be ensured well in advance.
    - *Resources:* Research requires well-resourced library, skilled guidance, facilities for carrying out data analysis, equipment and supplies, etc. Thus accessibility of resources relevant to the problem should be considered in the early phase of the research itself.
    - *Time frame:* Research studies conducted for getting an academic degree or funded by the organization have a time frame for their completion. The feasibility in such studies is linked to the ability to investigate and complete the study in the stipulated time frame.
    - *Cost:* The problems studied are influenced by monetary considerations. Some of the costs associated

with research are printing, purchase of equipment and stationary (paper, envelopes, postage, etc.), transportation, laboratory fee, payment to data collectors, incentive to subjects, statistical analysis charges, literature search charges, and purchase of books and journals. The researcher must appraise the financial resources (funding organizations) available for conducting the study. Receiving funding for a study indicates that it was reviewed by peers who chose to support the project financially.

- *Cooperation of others:* Research project requires support from prospective subjects, institutional authorities, and administrative approval.
- *Ethical consideration:* The research problem must confirm to the ethics, i.e. the subject's rights are protected, reviewed by ethical committee and have followed ethical guidelines.

Hulley and colleagues have suggested the use of the feasible, interesting, novel, ethical, and relevant (FINER) criteria in the development of a good research question (Box 3.3).

Box 3.3	FINER criteria for a good research question

F—Feasible
- Adequate number of subjects
- Adequate expertise
- Affordable in time and money
- Manageable in scope

I—Interesting
- Arouse the curiosity in investigator

N—Novel
- Confirms, refutes, or extends previous findings

E—Ethical
- Amenable to a study that institutional review committee will approve

R—Relevant
- Relevant to scientific knowledge, clinical practice and future research

FORMULATION OF RESEARCH PROBLEM

Formulation means translating the selected research problem into a scientifically researchable question. To formulate the research problem, the researcher should know the subject matter thoroughly, study the relevant literature on the subject and discuss with subject experts. The process of moving from problem selection to problem formulation is a creative process, which involves both, a sharpening of terms of concepts involved and narrowing of scope. The process of formulation involves the following steps (Fig. 3.2):

❖ **Selection of area of interest**: The first step in selecting a problem is to identify a general problem area related to area of expertise. Start with some broad general ideas and choose a topic, which is feasible and significant. Perform brainstorming about topics, issues, or concerns of interested topics and write down all ideas. The next task is to choose an area of interest and begin to refine the topic. Examples of broad areas are:
  ○ Stigma among mentally ill patients
  ○ Body image concerns of obese adolescents
  ○ Experiences of people with depression

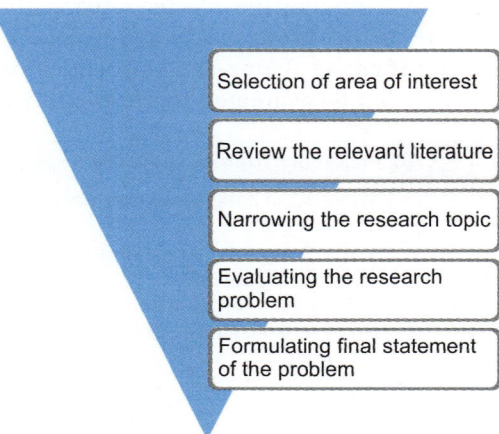

Fig. 3.2: Steps in formulation of research problem

- ❖ **Reviewing the literature**: After selection of a broad area of topic, the researcher should review the literature in order to identify what is already known on the topic. Brief review of literature at this point helps the researcher to identify whether the topic has been well researched and gather what little is known.
- ❖ **Narrowing the topic**: Once the general area of interest is selected, it has to be narrowed down into a researchable. The best way to begin this task is to identify specific aspects of the topic, list out interesting aspects, and find the working definition of the terms. For example, if the interested area relates to stigma among mentally ill patients, begin by asking yourself the meaning of stigma. Are you interested in mentally ill patients? Now consider the selected topic and begin to narrow it down by brainstorming possible questions in a phase wise manner (Box 3.4). During this process some questions will lend themselves to research while others may not. Rule out those questions that are not amenable to research. Discuss with colleagues and prioritize the questions and narrow down the problem.
- ❖ **Evaluating the research problem**: Start by rank ordering the selected researchable questions in terms of relevance or significance. Later, the problem must be carefully evaluated for availability of resources such as time, cost, and subjects; ethical considerations, administrative and peer support, and researcher's competence and interest.
  - ○ Is the researcher having necessary knowledge and skills to conduct research? Is the researcher qualified to undertake the research?
  - ○ Is the researcher motivated to undertake this study?
  - ○ Are adequate funds available for research?
  - ○ Is the problem of current interest? Will the research results have value to clinical practice or nursing education or administration? Is the problem new?
  - ○ Will it be possible to apply the results in practice? Is the problem significant to the profession?
  - ○ Does the research contribute to science of nursing? Is the solution to this problem helpful for the development of further knowledge?
  - ○ Will the research opt for new problems and lead to further research?
  - ○ Is there enough scope left within the area of research?
  - ○ Will it be possible for another researcher to repeat the research?
  - ○ Will it be practically possible to undertake the research?
  - ○ Do you have access to the administrative, statistic, and computer facilities the research necessitates?
  - ○ Is the research free of ethical problems and limitations?
- ❖ **Formulating the final statement of research problem**: Research problem statement is a pronouncement of disparity between what is known and what needs to be known about a topic. After the problem has been selected and its significance determined, the researcher proceeds with the task of formulating or stating the problem in such a specific manner

Box 3.4	Phases of narrowing the research topic
• Phase 1: Why stigma is higher among mentally ill patients?	
• Phase 2: What factors influence stigma among mentally ill patients?	
• Phase 3: What impact the stigma has got on the process of recovery among mentally ill patients?	
• Phase 4: To what extent these factors can be controlled? How effective are nursing interventions in reducing stigma among mentally ill patients?	

Table 3.1: Example of problem statement in declarative and interrogative forms

Declarative form	Interrogative form
Identify the factors that influence stigma among chronic mentally ill patients	What are the factors that influence stigma among chronic mentally ill patients?
Association between stigma and process of recovery among chronic mentally ill patients	What are the effects of stigma on process of recovery among mentally ill patients? or How does stigma affect the recovery process among mentally ill patients?
Efficacy of nursing intervention on decrease of stigma among mentally ill patients	Is nursing intervention effective in decreasing stigma among mentally ill patients?

that it can be subjected to empirical investigation. The statement should be broad enough to cover the concern prompting the study, yet narrow enough to provide direction for designing the study. It can be conceptualized as a declarative sentence (statement) or a question form (interrogative) (Table 3.1).

- The problem statement identifies the specific gap in the knowledge and provides rationale for the study by citing background of the problem and its contributions to practice by using significant literature sources. It also states the goals of the study.
- The research problem should always be stated in grammatically complete sentences, in a readable and understandable way. It should be as brief as possible. The main characteristics of research problem are:
  - It visibly identifies the study variables
  - The variables are expressed in measurable terms
  - Specifies the population under study and research setting
  - It implies the possibility of empirical testing
  - It can be stated clearly and concisely
  - It has a base in the research literature
  - The problem is new and is not already answered sufficiently
  - It has potential significance or importance.

COMPONENTS OF PROBLEM STATEMENT

- In a quantitative study, a well written problem statement comprises of two components: the population of concern and the variable(s) to be studied.
- Consider the PICOT format (participants, intervention, comparator, outcome, and timeframe) for developing a problem statement, which includes population of the study as well as the intervention or comparison interest, the outcome desired and the time limit. For example, a study to investigate the efficacy of empowerment-based nursing intervention to reduce the stigma among chronic mentally ill patients. Application of PICOT format for the above example is presented in Table 3.2.

Critiquing the Problem Statement

- Is the problem clearly stated?
- Is the problem statement written in a single declarative or interrogatory sentence?
- Are the study variables and the population included in the problem statement?
- Is the feasibility of the study apparent when reading the problem statement?
- Is the research problem significant to the nursing profession?
- Is the research problem fit with research priorities?
- Is the research problem fit with previous research?

Table 3.2: PICOT format for developing problem statement

	Criteria	Description	Example
P	Population	• Which specific population interested in? • What are the characteristics of the patient or population? • What is the condition or disease of interest?	Mentally ill population with stigma, their age, duration of illness, area of residence, etc.
I	Intervention	What is the intervention? (for interventional studies only)	Empowered based nursing intervention to reduce stigma
C	Comparison group	What is the alternative to the intervention?	Empowerment based nursing intervention and routine nursing intervention
O	Outcome of interest	What are the outcome measures?	Reducing stigma
T	Time	What is the suitable follow-up time to assess outcome?	Follow-up time to assess outcome

PURPOSES OF RESEARCH STUDY

❖ All research studies have an explicit or implicit purpose statement. It includes variables, population, and setting of the study.
❖ The research purpose states "why" the study is being conducted or what the "goal" of the study is. The goal of a study might be to identify or describe a concept or explain or predict a situation or solution to a situation that indicates the type of study to be conducted (Beckingham, 1974).
❖ The research purpose should be stated objectively without reflecting researcher bias.
❖ The purpose of the study is more commonly seen in journal articles and specifies the type of study to be carried out.
❖ The purpose directs the progress of the study and is generated from the research problem.
❖ While the problem statement indicates what will be examined by the researcher (For example, "decubitus ulcers occur in hospitalized patients despite preventive measures and methods"), the purpose of the study deals with why the study is being conducted (For example, "the purpose of this study was to evaluate the effects of topical application of insulin to promote healing of decubitus ulcers in hospitalized patients").
❖ A few examples of purpose statement verbs with corresponding research methods are:
  ○ Correlation—determine, examine, identify, and understand
  ○ Descriptive—compare, contrast, describe, and identify
  ○ Experimental—determine, examine, investigate, and measure

RESEARCH QUESTION

❖ A research question is nothing but a refined, focused, structured, and well-defined statement of the research topic.
❖ The research question is more precise than the problem statement. These are used interchangeably.
❖ Research question is a simple, brief, and interrogative statement expressed in present tense.
❖ Research question includes study variables and population. It specifies the relationship between the variables to be examined.

- The main purpose of the research question is to define the scope of research and avoid deflection or distraction.
- The main focus of research question in quantitative studies is description of variables, finding the relationship between the variables, finding the differences between two or more groups on selected variables, and to predict the dependent variable.
- Research questions generate from the problem statement and direct the methodology for the study.
- Nonexperimental research designs are generally limited to stating the research question while experimental and quasi-experimental research designs also include hypothesis along with the research question.

RESEARCH OBJECTIVES

Research objective is an active statement, which describes what is to be achieved by the study and how the study is going to answer the specific research question.

Purposes
- Direct the preparation of protocol
- Facilitate development of methodology
- Help the researcher focus on relevant variables in the study
- Guide what information is to be collected
- Help in evaluating whether the research goals have been achieved

Characteristics
A well-worded objective will be specific, measurable, achievable or attainable, realistic, time bound (SMART) (Fig. 3.3)

Other Characteristics
- *Clear:* Clarity should be the main focus of the research objectives. The wording should be clear and defined using simple sentences.
- *Complete:* Each phrase in the research objectives should have a sense of completeness. A complete research objective should have information about the population to be studied.
- *Identify main variables*: In the research objectives, variables should be clearly defined with measurable terms.
- *Based on study purpose*: The objectives should be consistent with identified goals and study purpose.
- *Provide direction*: Objectives should provide direction to the research methodology and interpretation of research results.

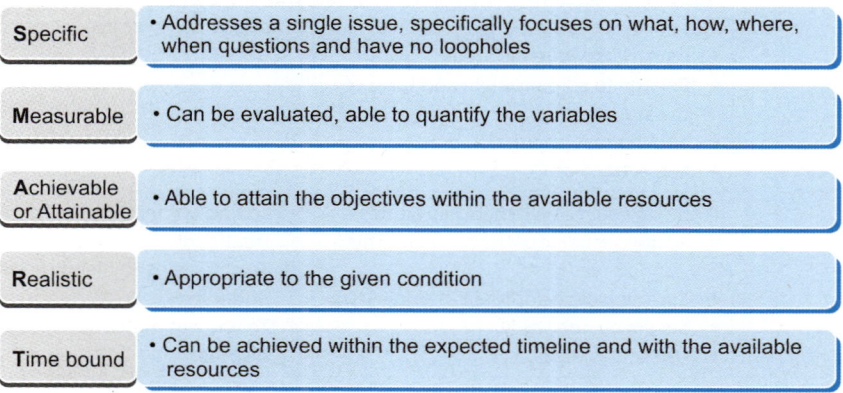

Fig. 3.3: Characteristics of research objectives

❖ *Stated in logical sequence*: The research objectives should be listed in logical sequence.

Types of Research Objectives

There are two types of objectives in a study: broad or main objectives and the specific or secondary objectives. The main objectives lead the research and provide clear, complete, and specific goals to the research study. The specific or secondary objectives are relevant to the research problem and help in attaining main objectives (Table 3.3).

Formulation of Research Objectives

❖ Objectives should be listed in the introduction of the research protocol or report.
❖ Proper action verbs like determine, find out, identify, etc. ought to be used while formulating objectives.
❖ Objectives can be formulated in quantitative as well as qualitative studies.
❖ In quantitative studies, objectives are clear, concise, and declarative statements that provide a direction to investigate the variables. It focuses mainly on measuring the variables, identifying the relationship among themselves, and determine the differences between two or more groups with reference to the selected variables.
❖ In qualitative studies, objectives are more complex and abstract in nature. They focus on obtaining a holistic and comprehensive understanding of the area of the study. The examples for research problem, research question, hypothesis, and objectives are given in Table 3.4.

Example of a problem statement—"Efficacy of holistic group health promotion program on stress and well-being among adolescents".

Examples of research objectives:
❖ To assess the academic stress and well-being among adolescent girls.
❖ To implement innovative holistic group health promotion program for 4 weeks.
❖ To evaluate the effectiveness of intervention by comparing post-test stress and well-being scores of experimental and control group subjects.

Tips for framing research questions and objectives for a research study are presented in Box 3.5.

Table 3.3: Types of research objectives

Types of objectives	Description	Example
Broad or main objectives	These state what is to be achieved by the study in general terms. The key aspects of these objectives are: • Usually only one per study • Related to core problem and topic of the study • Show target population • Use action verb	To determine the factors associated with increased number of diarrhea cases among under-fives in a selected village
Specific or secondary objectives	These objectives systematically address the various aspects of the problem. The key aspects are: • Each objective addresses a single issue • Several in one study • Use action verbs	• To find out methods used for water treatment • To determine the feeding habits of the under fives • To find out methods used for excreta disposal

Table 3.4: Example of research problem, purpose, research question, objectives, and hypothesis

Component	Description	Example
Topic	Broad subject matter being addressed in a study	Relapse prevention among individuals with alcohol use disorder
Research problem	An issue or a problem in the study	Substance abuse and its related problems have become a serious public health issue and conventional therapies have not always been effective. Relapse is highly prevalent among substance abusers following treatment. They need after care interventions.
Purpose	Major intent of the study	To test a holistic-based intervention to reduce relapse rates among individuals with alcohol use disorders
Research question	Questions the researcher would like to answer or address in the study	What is the relative effectiveness of holistic-based intervention on reducing relapse rates among individuals with alcohol use disorders?
Objectives	What is to be achieved by the study	• To develop and implement a holistic-based relapse intervention program • To find out the relative effectiveness of holistic-based intervention program on quantity and frequency of alcohol intake • To determine relapse rates among individuals with alcohol use disorder
Hypothesis	Tentative explanation of the research problem or possible outcome of the research	• Subjects who received holistic-based intervention will exhibit a reduction in quantity and frequency of alcohol intake compared to those subjects who received treatment as usual • Subjects who received holistic-based intervention will have less relapse rates compared to subjects who received treatment as usual

Box 3.5 Tips for framing research questions and objectives for research study

- Carry out a systematic literature review to improve knowledge and familiarity with the topic
- Gather inputs from experts, mentors, and colleagues to refine research question
- Use FINER criteria for developing the research question
- Ensure that the research question follows PICOT format
- Make certain that research question and its objectives are relevant, feasible and answerable
- List primary and secondary objectives
- Develop research hypothesis from the research question.

(FINER: Feasible, Interesting, Novel, Ethical, and Relevant; PICOT: Participants, Intervention, Comparator, Outcome, and Timeframe)

VARIABLES

- A variable is a characteristic, event, or response that represents the elements of the research question in a detectable way (Waltz, Strickland, and Ling, 2004).
- Variable is a factor that can be controlled or changed in an experiment (Wong, 2014).
- In quantitative studies, concepts are usually referred to as variables.
- A variable is something that varies. It refers to measurable characteristics of people, things, and situations that can change or vary, e.g. pulse rate, anxiety level, and degree of pain. These are characteristics of people that can vary from one person to another and also have different values along a continuum.
- Some variables are concrete and clear such as gender, type of blood group, type of residence, etc. while others are abstract and vague such as anxiety, depression, attitudes, etc.
- Some variables are inherent characteristics of people such as age, blood type, or weight, but sometimes the researcher creates a variable for conducting the study, e.g. nursing intervention to reduce pain, various relaxation techniques to reduce anxiety, etc.
- Number of variables that can be measured is unlimited. The complexity of the study increases with the increase in number of variables and longer is the time required for data collection and statistical analysis.
- Depending upon the number of variables, the study can be univariate (one variable), bivariate (two variables), or multivariate (multiple variables).

TYPES OF VARIABLES

Variables can be classified into many types (Fig. 3.4).

1. Independent and Dependent Variables

- The *independent (manipulative) variable* is the stimulus or activity that is applied

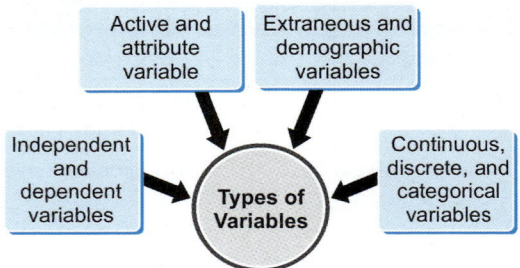

Fig. 3.4: Types of variables

to the experimental situation by the researcher to measure its effects on the dependent variable.
- It is the antecedent and the presumed effect on the dependent variable.
- In experimental research, the independent variable is believed to be the cause or influence, and is manipulated by the researcher to assess its effect on the dependent variable, e.g. in a study to evaluate the efficacy of relaxation on anxiety among adolescent girls, relaxation is the independent variable because the researcher manipulates this variable by providing it to experimental group subjects and withholds it for control group subjects so as to assess the effect of this variable on reducing anxiety (dependent variable).
- In nonexperimental research, the independent variable is not manipulated and is assumed to have occurred naturally before or during the study, e.g. in a study to assess the relationship between gender and somatic symptoms, the gender cannot be manipulated and is observed and measured as it naturally happens.
- *Dependent (criterion) variable* is one that is affected by the independent variable. It is the presumed effect or outcome that varies with a change in the independent variable.
- The researcher would be interested to understand, explain, or predict that changes in the dependent variable are

presumed to be caused by the independent variable.
- The dependent variable is hypothesized to depend on or to be caused by another variable.
- The independent and dependent variables are interrelated and mainly observed in correlational and experimental research studies.
- An independent variable may not be the sole cause for a dependent variable. The dependent variables may have multiple causes or antecedents, e.g. in a study to assess the factors that influence medication adherence among schizophrenia patients, the researcher might consider their attitude, medication side effects, and motivation as independent variables.
- In a study, the researcher may be interested to find out the effect of independent variable on two or more dependent variables, e.g. a researcher may compare the effects of alcoholism on cirrhosis of liver and gastric ulcer. In another study, the researcher would investigate the effectiveness of relaxation therapy on level of depression and wellbeing.
- Variables are not inherently dependent or independent. A dependent variable in one study could be an independent variable in another. Let us consider two studies, *viz.* (1) "effect of exercise on osteoporosis" and (2) "effect of osteoporosis on bone fracture". In the former study, osteoporosis is the dependent variable while in the latter it is the independent variable. Whether the variable is dependent or independent relies on the role it plays in that particular study (Table 3.5 and Fig. 3.5).

2. Active and Attribute Variables
- *Active variables* are created by the researcher. They can also be independent variables, e.g. in a study concerning effectiveness of relaxation in reducing anxiety among children, relaxation

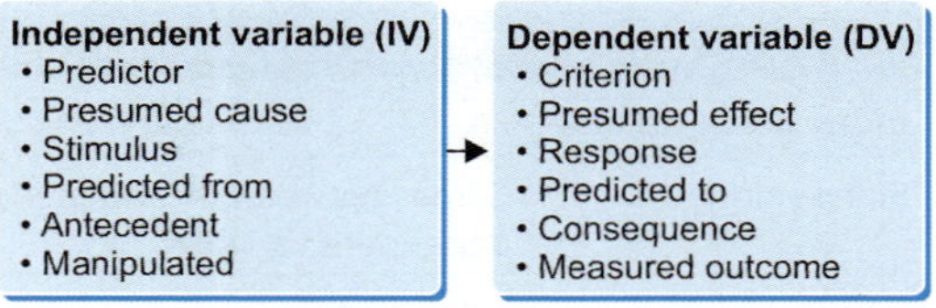

Independent variable (IV)	Dependent variable (DV)
• Predictor • Presumed cause • Stimulus • Predicted from • Antecedent • Manipulated	• Criterion • Presumed effect • Response • Predicted to • Consequence • Measured outcome

Fig. 3.5: Independent versus dependent variable

method is the active independent variable as it is created by the researcher. It can be tailored based on the anxiety level.
- *Attribute variables* are characteristics of the study subjects, which cannot be manipulated, e.g. gender, age, color of eyes, skin color, etc. These variables can also be independent variables with limitation. In a study to examine the presence of the mother in decreasing the anxiety level of a hospitalized child during a painful procedure, age cannot be changed, but we can study anxiety at different age levels. "An active variable in one study could be an attribute variable in another study". Another example is that of the relationship between gender and somatic symptoms where the gender cannot be changed or manipulated, but somatic symptoms between male and female depressive patients can be studied.

3. Extraneous and Demographic Variables
- Variables that may affect research outcomes but have no relevance to the study are termed as extraneous variables.
- Extraneous variables confuse or confound the relationship between dependent and independent variables (Table 3.5 and Fig. 3.6).
- Extraneous variables exist in all studies and can affect the measurement of study variables and the relationship among these variables.
- In interventional studies, the researcher should recognize and control as many extraneous variables as possible.

Table 3.5: Difference between independent, extraneous, and dependent variables

Independent variable	Extraneous variable	Dependent variable
Stands alone	Comes between the independent and dependent variable	Is affected by the independent variables
Cause	May interfere	Effect
Comes first	Can mask the effect of the independent variable	Comes later or last

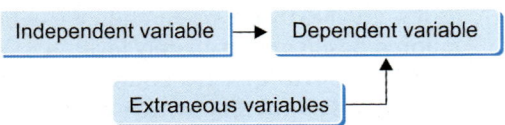

Fig. 3.6: Relationship between independent, dependent, and extraneous variables

- ❖ In the above study, the age and type of procedure will affect the child's anxiety level regardless of whether the parent is present in the room or not. Hence, age and type of procedure are considered as extraneous variables. The researcher can control these variables by limiting the study population to a particular age group and also specifying the painful procedure.
- ❖ Extraneous variables can be classified into recognized or unrecognized, controlled or uncontrolled.
  - ○ When variables are *recognized* before proceeding with the study, they can be measured and controlled by study design or through statistical analysis.
  - ○ When variables are *not recognized* until the study is in process or are recognized before the study is initiated but cannot be controlled are referred to as either *confounding variables* or *biasing variables* or *covariables*.
  - ○ If the extraneous variables are not controlled or measured, they lead to design weakness and hinder the interpretation of the findings.
  - ○ As the control diminishes in correlational, quasi-experimental, and experimental studies, the potential influence of confounding variables increases.
  - ○ Quasi-experimental and experimental designs have been developed to control the influence of extraneous variables.
- ❖ Demographic variables are characteristics of the subjects in the study. Also called as sample characteristics these determine the sample representativeness of the population of interest.
- ❖ These demographic variables cannot be manipulated and are used to describe the study group. These variables also explain their relationship with the dependent variables. Age, gender, educational level, marital status, and religion are some examples of demographic variables.
- ❖ The type of demographic variables collected depends on the purpose of the study.

4. Continuous, Discrete, and Categorical Variables

A *continuous* variable is one which can assume an infinite number of values between two points and not limited to whole number values, e.g. age (1 year, 1½ years, 2 years, and 2½ years), salary (₹ 5,000/-, ₹ 5,600/-, and ₹ 5,700/-), blood pressure (120/80, 122/82, and 124/84), weight (1.1 kg, 1.25 kg, and 1.30 kg, etc.), and height (3′, 3′2″, and 3′3″) are continuous variables.

A *discrete* variable is one that has a finite number of values between any two points, i.e. it can take only whole number equivalents. For example, pulse rate can take only whole number values such as 72 beats/minute, 80 beats/minute, 95 beats/minute, and not fractional values.

Categorical variables are those which assume only a few discrete nonquantitative values. The categorical variables are referred to as dichotomous, trichotomous, or multiple depending upon the number of values they assume (Table 3.6 and Flowchart 3.2).

Measuring Variables

To carry out an analysis, the variables have to be quantified by providing values and a suitable scale. There are four levels of measurements on a continuum of discrete and continuous scale.

1. When variables are classified into two or more categories and there is no difference in size of these categories, they can be measured by a nominal scale, e.g. in gender all are classified as either male or female. There is no difference in maleness compared with femaleness. The only relationship between these categories is that they are different from one another.

2. When variables are classified into categories as well as ranked on a scale from "none" to "a lot" they can be measured by an ordinal scale. For example, levels of anxiety are classified as mild, moderate, and severe. The degree of severity alters with the level of anxiety, severe being more than moderate and moderate being more than mild. It cannot specify how much more the severe anxiety is than the moderate anxiety. In an ordinal scale, categories must be mutually exclusive, i.e. an individual cannot be rated with both mild and moderate anxieties. The difference between the categories must be clearly established so that every person in the sample falls into only one category.

3. When variables are measured on a scale precisely then interval and ratio scales can be used. In these scales, the variables can be categorized and ranked, have equal intervals and represent a range of values. Ratio scales have an absolute zero while interval scales do not.

4. Measurement of scale of variables affects the possibilities for data analysis. Identifying the research variables is the most difficult and time consuming task in planning of a research study. The study can proceed only after identifying the key variables. Examples of research problems and variables are given in Table 3.7.

Table 3.6: Types of categorical variables

No. of values	Type of categorical variable	Variables	Categories
2	Dichotomous	HIV status	• HIV positive • HIV negative
		Gender	• Male • Female
3	Trichotomous	Residence	• Rural • Semiurban • Urban
		Religion	• Hindu • Muslim • Christian
Above 3	Multiple or polytomous	Blood group	• A • B • AB • O

(HIV: Human Immunodeficiency Virus)

Flowchart 3.2: Continuous, discrete, and categorical variables

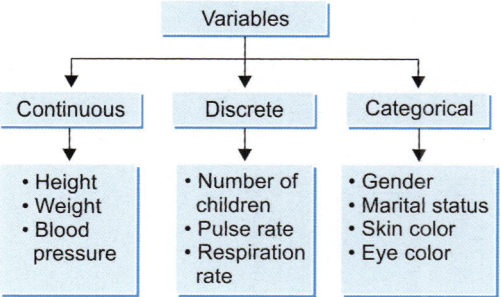

Table 3.7: Examples of research problem statement, objectives, variables, and hypotheses

Type of study	Examples of research problem statement	Objectives	Variables	Hypotheses
Descriptive	A descriptive study on prevalence of lung cancer among adult smokers in a selected industry, Karnataka	◆ Assess the prevalence of lung cancer among adult smokers ◆ Assess the duration of smoking among adult smokers	Research variable: Prevalence of lung cancer	Descriptive studies do not have hypothesis
Exploratory	Smoking-related knowledge, attitudes, behaviors, smoking cessation idea and education level among young adult male smokers in Chongqing, China	◆ Assess the knowledge of smoking-related hazards ◆ Assess the smoking-related attitudes and beliefs ◆ Assess the smoking-related practices ◆ Correlation analyses of knowledge, attitude and behaviors ◆ Find out factors associated with quitting smoking ideas	Research variables: ◆ Knowledge of smoking-related hazards ◆ Attitudes and behaviors related to smoking ◆ Smoking-related practices	◆ Male adults with higher education will have better understanding of smoking being harmful to health ◆ Male adults with higher education will have positive attitude towards smoking related hazards
Correlational	Correlation between human smoking habits and death rates	◆ Assess smoking habits (frequency and duration) among smokers ◆ Assess death rates among smokers ◆ Correlate smoking habit with death rate among smokers	◆ Independent variable: – Smoking habit ◆ Dependent variable: – Death rate	◆ There will be significant positive correlation between smoking habit and death rate among smokers
Comparative	A comparative study of spirometric values among smokers and nonsmokers in a selected hospital	◆ Find out the spirometric values among smokers ◆ Find out the spirometric values among nonsmokers ◆ Compare spirometric values between smokers and nonsmokers	Research variables: ◆ Spirometric values ◆ Smoking habit	There will be significant decrease in spirometric values among smokers compared to nonsmokers

Contd...

Contd...

Type of study	Examples of research problem statement	Objectives	Variables	Hypotheses

Quasi-experimental	A quasi experimental study to assess the effectiveness of selected nursing interventions on health related quality of life and activities of daily living among lung cancer patients in a selected oncology hospital	• Assess the health-related quality of life
		• Assess the activities of daily living
		• Evaluate the effectiveness of intervention by comparing posttest scores on quality of life and activities of daily living of experimental and control group subjects
			• Independent variable:
			  – Selected nursing intervention
			• Dependent variable:
			  – Health-related quality of life
			  – Activities of daily living
				• There will be no significant improvement in quality of life among experimental group cancer patients compared to control group cancer patients

Experimental	An experimental study on efficacy of oral morphine in management of lung cancer pain among advanced stage lung cancer patients admitted in a selected hospice	• Assess pain among advanced stage lung cancer patients both in experimental and control groups
		• Administration of oral morphine to experimental lung cancer patients
		• Implement routine treatment to control group lung cancer patients
		• Compare pain between experimental and control group lung cancer patients
			• Independent variable:
			  – Oral morphine
			• Dependent variable:
			  – Lung cancer pain
				There will be no significant decrease in pain among experimental group lung cancer patients compared to control group lung cancer patients

Conceptual and Operational Definitions of Variables

- A conceptual definition of a variable describes the theoretical meaning and specifies its fundamental characteristics while the operational definition gives precise indication as to what the fundamental characteristics are and how to observe or even measure its characteristics under the study.
- The operational definition of the variable simplifies the concepts into easily understandable terms that can be measured empirically.
- The important feature of operational definition is its ability to indicate what to measure and how to measure, stated in measurable and observable terms, using nonambiguous language precisely and clearly (Table 3.8).

ASSUMPTIONS

- Assumptions are overt and/or innate beliefs held by the researcher about phenomenon that is accepted as truth without proof or empirical evidence.
- An assumption is a realistic expectation, i.e. something that we believe to be true but no adequate evidence exists to support this belief. In a research study, assumptions are out of researcher's control; however, if they disappear the study would become irrelevant.
- Assumptions often are embedded (unrecognized) in thinking and behavior and uncovering these assumptions require introspection and a strong knowledge basis in research.
- In science, hypothesis and assumptions are concepts that are similar in nature. Hypothesis is an argument put forward to explain a phenomenon. Anything taken for granted is an assumption, and a hypothesis is at best a working assumption (Table 3.9). Differences between assumptions and hypothesis are presented in Table 3.10.

Uses of Assumptions

- Assumptions influence the logic of the study, development, and implementation of the research process

| Table 3.8: Examples of conceptual and operational definition of depressive patients ||
Conceptual definition	Operational definition
Depressive patients: Patients who are suffering with depression. Depression refers to both negative affect (low mood) and/or absence of positive affect (loss of interest and pleasure in most activities) and is usually accompanied by an assortment of emotional, cognitive, physical, and behavioral symptoms	In the present study, depressive patients refer to those who meet the criteria for mild or moderate or severe episode according to International Classification of Diseases, Tenth Revision (ICD10) code—F32.0–32.2, F33.0–33.2 and 34
Adolescent: Adolescence is a transitional stage of physical and mental development generally occurring between puberty and legal adulthood	In the present study, subjects chosen are girls studying in selected preuniversity colleges between the age group of 16 and 19 years

| Table 3.9: Relationship between research problem, assumptions, and hypothesis |||
Research problem	Assumptions	Hypothesis
Does higher the IQ of a student, result in better the achievement in learning a foreign language?	There is a correlation between students IQ and their achievement in learning a foreign language.	Higher the IQ the students have, better they achieve in learning a foreign language.

(IQ: Intelligence Quotient)

Table 3.10: Differences between assumptions and hypothesis

Assumptions	Hypothesis
Assumptions are beliefs about the variables	Hypothesis is a prediction about the relationship between two or more variables
Based on these beliefs the researcher attempts to discover the relationship among variables	Predictions between variables are statistically tested
These often have little or no evidence and are statistically not tested	Can be statistically tested, may be accepted or rejected

- Assumptions provide a basis to develop theories and research instruments
- It helps in the objective examination of the phenomenon under study
- It allows for a more vigorous study

Sources of Assumptions
- Universally accepted truths
- Theories
- Nursing practice
- Previous research studies

Types of Assumptions
The four different types of assumptions are:
1. *Universal assumptions:* These are universal truths accepted by majority of the population. These assumptions help us to explain the world around us, e.g. man is a biopsychosocial being.
2. *Empirical based assumptions*: These assumptions are derived from previous research studies. These may be developed to conduct a study, e.g. prevalence of communicable diseases is more common among rural people when compared to urban people.
3. *Theoretical based assumptions*: These assumptions are associated with a specific theory. For example, major assumptions of Orem's theory of nursing are:
    - Self-care is a requirement for every person
    - Universal self-care involves meeting basic human needs
    - Health-deviation self-care is related to disease or injury
4. *Research assumptions*: These are beliefs about the research itself. These are embedded in methodology and statistical analysis.
    - Methodology assumptions: The researcher during survey assumes that the subjects will answer truthfully. While choosing a sample, the researcher assumes that the sample is representative of the population of which inference is to be made. Researchers usually assume that subjects will answer the survey questions sincerely and to the best of their knowledge. It is also assumed that data collection instruments are valid and reliable based upon their previous use.
    - Statistical analysis assumptions: Statistical models in quantitative research designs are accompanied with assumptions. These assumptions generally refer to the characteristics of the data (qualitative and quantitative), distribution of data (normal distribution or not), correlational trends, and variable type (nominal, ordinal, interval, or ratio level variable).

HYPOTHESIS
Once the objectives have been written, the variables defined and the study population determined, it is necessary to refine the written objectives into a set of written testable hypothesis.
- A hypothesis is a declarative statement, which explains the relationship between

two or more variables that predicts a solution to the research problem.
- The hypothesis translates the research problem into a clear explanation or prediction of the expected results.
- It is the basis for scientific investigation and plays an important role in the research process.
- Hypothesis and theories are reciprocal to each other. A verified hypothesis becomes the basis for theory and theory in turn serves as a source for hypothesis generation.

Definitions

"A hypothesis is a conjectural statement of the relation between two or more variables."
—**Kerlinger, 1973**

"Hypothesis is a formal statement that presents the expected relationship between an independent and dependent variable."
—**Creswell, 1994**

"A hypothesis can be defined as a tentative explanation of the research problem, a possible outcome of the research, or an educated guess about the research outcome."
—**Sarantakos, 1993**

"A hypothesis is a statement or explanation that is suggested by knowledge or observation but has not yet been proved or disproved."
—**Macleod Clark J and Hockey L, 1979**

"A hypothesis is a logical supposition, a reasonable guess, and an educated conjecture. It provides a tentative explanation for a phenomenon under investigation."
—**Leedy and Ormrod, 2001**

Characteristics of a Good Hypothesis

A good hypothesis should be simple, clear, relevant, testable, and verifiable (Flowchart 3.3).

Flowchart 3.3: Characteristics of good hypothesis

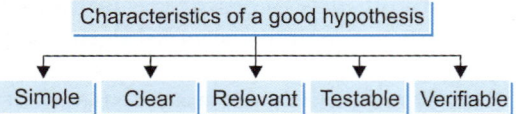

Simple
- The hypothesis should be written in the form of a declarative statement by using present tense in simple and understandable terms.
- It should be limited to a single relationship between two variables so as to add clarity in terms of understanding the intended relationship and the conclusions that follow data analysis.
- It is neither too specific nor too general.

Clear
- A clearly stated hypothesis includes the variables, population, and proposed outcomes for the study.
- A good hypothesis should have a clearly defined independent variable to ensure accurate and consistent implementation of the intervention. The dependent variable must be clearly defined to ensure accurate measurement.

Relevant
- It should be relevant to the research problem and objectives.
- It should be consistent with an existing body of knowledge, previous research findings, or other hypothesis.

Testable
Variables included in the hypothesis should lend themselves to observation, empirically tested by direct or indirect measures.

Verifiable
- It should be verified in practical terms.
- It is considered valuable even if proven false.

Purposes

- Provides a bridge between theory and practice by allowing theoretical propositions to be examined in the real world. Hypothesis sometimes follows directly from a theoretical framework and tests these hypotheses in the real

world. The validity of the theory is never examined directly. The worth of the theory can only be evaluated through hypothesis testing.
- ❖ Provides the reader with a perceptive of the researchers expectations of study before the actual data collection process begins.
- ❖ By stating the anticipated results, it stimulates the researcher's thinking process in the right direction.
- ❖ Provides direction for research methodology, sampling method, data collection, analysis process, and interpretation of findings.
- ❖ Provides an understanding of the predictable study results to the researcher.
- ❖ Links the dependent and independent variables.

Support or Reject Hypothesis
- ❖ Hypothesis cannot be proved or disproved, but can only be supported or not supported.
- ❖ Even if a hypothesis is not supported by the data, it can lead to further investigations. Negative and positive findings are equally important and act as a guiding factor for future research in that field.
- ❖ If a hypothesis is continually supported, it may eventually evolve into a theory.
- ❖ A theory that is continually validated over time by a growing body of data, becomes a law.

Sources of Hypothesis
Hypotheses can be derived from various sources. The major ones include examining the theory, personal experience, imagination and thinking, observation of phenomenon, reviewing research literature or previous research findings, customs, and beliefs (Fig. 3.7).
- ❖ *Theory*: Theory explains all the facts related to a problem. It is one of the main sources of hypothesis generation. Logical deduction from theory or conceptual framework leads to new hypothesis.

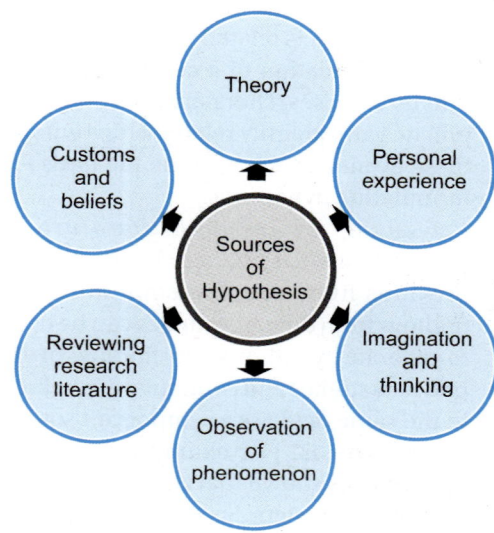

Fig. 3.7: Sources of hypothesis

Through a deductive approach, these hypotheses are drawn from theory for testing. The following hypothesis has been deduced from operant conditioning theory.
  - ○ Chronic mentally ill patients who are appreciated by the nursing personnel for self-care activities require less assistance in activities than patients who are not appreciated.
  - ○ Children who were ignored by nursing personnel for their temper tantrums exhibit less temper tantrums in the future than children who were not ignored for such behavior.
- ❖ *Personal experience*: On the basis of personal experience, the researcher uses his intellect to generate a good hypothesis. Nurses can derive many hypotheses from clinical experience. Greater the researcher's experience higher is the degree of formation.
- ❖ *Imagination and thinking*: Personal ideas and thinking capabilities of the researcher would lead to greater number of hypothesis formulation as well as control over the problem.

❖ *Observation:* The collection of previous and current facts related to a problem lead to the formulation of a good hypothesis. The nurse researchers observe events in practice and identify relationships among these events, which become the basis for formulating hypothesis.

❖ *Reviewing the research literature or previous research findings:* Reviewing the previous literature and combining the findings from different studies can be used to generate hypothesis. The findings of the previous studies and continuity of research in the same field are an important source of hypothesis. For example, previous research has shown that stress can impact the immune system. So, a researcher might state a specific hypothesis as: "People with high stress levels are more likely to catch a common cold after being exposed to the virus than people who have low stress levels".

❖ *Customs and beliefs*: Researchers might look at commonly held beliefs or folk wisdom. "Birds of the same feather flock together" is one example of folk wisdom. Based on this folk wisdom, the researcher might pose a specific hypothesis that "people tend to select partners who are similar to them in interests and educational level".

Types of Hypotheses

The type of hypothesis being developed is based on the research problem and purpose of the study. The common types of hypotheses are listed in Figure 3.8.

Simple vs Complex Hypothesis

A simple hypothesis predicts the relationship between two variables. It contains one independent variable and one dependent variable.

Example: Consider the hypothesis—2-hourly position changing of a fully bedridden patient will prevent bedsore. In the above

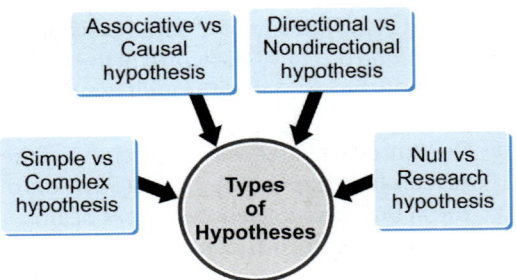

Fig. 3.8: Types of hypotheses

hypothesis, 2-hourly position changing is the independent variable and bedsore prevention the dependent variable. The statement shows that there exists a relationship between 2-hourly positioning and bedsore prevention.

A complex hypothesis predicts the relationship among three or more variables.

Example: Consider the hypothesis—for a fully bed ridden patient 2-hourly position changing, 2-hourly back care, and a high protein diet will build up body resistance, promote blood circulation, and prevent bedsore. In the above hypothesis, the three independent variables are 2-hourly position changing, 2-hourly back care, and high protein diet. The three dependent variables are—(1) promotion of blood circulation, (2) building up of body resistance, and (3) prevention of bedsores.

Associative vs Causal Hypothesis

The relationship in hypotheses is identified as associative or causal. Associative hypothesis predicts an associative relationship between the dependent variable and the independent variable without manipulation. When there is a change in any one of the variables, corresponding changes also occur in the other variable. The association may be positive or negative. Researchers state associative hypothesis when the focus of their study is to examine the relationship and not determine cause and effect. This hypothesis is used in correlational research studies.

Example: Positive relationships exist among affective disturbances, attention impairment, and alogia in schizophrenia patients.

Causal hypothesis examines a cause and effect interaction between two or more variables, referred to as independent and dependent variables. It predicts the effect of an independent variable on a dependent variable specifying the direction of the relationship.

The independent variable is manipulated by the researcher to show an effect on the dependent variable. The dependent variable is measured to examine the effect produced by the independent variable.

Example: Schizophrenia patients who receive social skill training exhibit greater improvement in social relations when compared to those who receive usual care.

Directional ($H_0: \mu_1 > \mu_2$) vs Nondirectional Hypothesis ($H_0: \mu_1 \neq \mu_2$)

Directional hypothesis predicts the direction of the relationship between the independent and dependent variables. These hypotheses are developed from theoretical statements, findings of previous studies, and clinical experience. As the available knowledge increases, the researcher is able to predict the direction of a relationship between study variables. Terms such as less, more, increase, decrease, positive, negative, greater, and smaller indicate the direction of relationships in hypotheses. Generally, the directional hypothesis is preferred as it forces the researcher to think critically. Directional hypothesis can be associative or causal and simple or complex.

Example: There is a positive relationship between knowledge level and drug compliance among schizophrenia patients. Older patients are at a greater risk for falls than younger patients.

Nondirectional hypothesis predicts the relationship between the dependent variable and the independent variable but does not specify the direction of the relationship. When researcher has no clear indication of the nature of the relationship he states a nondirectional hypothesis.

Example: There is a relationship between the age of a patient and the risk of falling.

Null ($H_0: \mu_1 = \mu_2$) vs Research Hypothesis

The null hypothesis (H_0) also referred to as a statistical hypothesis is used for statistical testing and interpretation of results. It states that no relationship exists between dependent and independent variables. A null hypothesis can be simple or complex and associative or causal. An associative null hypothesis states that there is no relationship between variables being studied. For example, "patient's age is unrelated to their risk of falling" or "older patients are just as likely as younger patients to fall". The causal null hypothesis states that the experimental group which received the independent variable is no different from the control group for the dependent variable. For example, "there is no difference in social relations among patients who receive social skills training and those who receive usual care".

A research hypothesis (H_1) is the alternative to the null hypothesis. The research hypothesis states that there is a relationship between two or more variables and it can be simple or complex, nondirectional or directional, and associative or causal. An example of simple, nondirectional, and associative hypothesis is—"there is a relationship between age and risk of falling among patients". An example of simple, non-directional, and causal hypothesis is, "there is a difference in social relations between those who receive social skills training and those who receive usual care". An example of simple, directional and associative hypothesis is, "there is a positive relationship between smoking and incidence of lung cancer".

A hypothesis is not required, if only one variable is being examined. Failure to reject

Research question	Null hypotheses ($H_0: \mu_1 = \mu_2$)	Alternative non-directional hypotheses ($H_0: \mu_1 \neq \mu_2$)	Alternative directional hypotheses ($H_0: \mu_1 > \mu_2$)
Does the change of position have an influence on the development of decubitus ulcers among incontinent patients?	Incontinent patients who receive two-hourly change in position are just as likely to develop decubitus ulcers as those receiving 4-hourly position changes	Frequency of change in position of incontinent patients is related to the development of decubitus ulcers	Incontinent patients who receive two-hourly change in position are less likely to develop decubitus ulcers compared to those receiving daily position changes

Table 3.11: Example of hypotheses

the null hypothesis implies that there is insufficient evidence to support the idea of a real difference in the dependent variable. Examples of null, alternative, directional, and nondirectional research hypotheses are presented in Table 3.11.

Formulation of Hypothesis

The hypothesis is formulated before the study is actually conducted. It flows from the research question, literature review and theoretical framework. Hypotheses are usually formulated in quantitative research studies. The quasi-experimental and experimental studies should be directed by hypothesis. Some correlational studies focus on predicting relationships and may include hypothesis. Researchers employ inductive and deductive reasoning on available theory and knowledge to formulate a hypothesis. It is better that one hypothesis contains only a single prediction about relationships of study variables. The following are the criteria for writing a hypothesis:

- *Written in declarative sentence*: Hypothesis presents an answer or tentative solution to the problem and is written in the form of a sentence.
- *Written in present tense:* Hypothesis is tested in the present and so should be written in the present tense, e.g. there is a positive relationship between the level of depression and suicidal attempts among depressive patients.
- *Contain the population*: The population needs to be specifically identified in the hypothesis, just as it is in the problem statement.
- *Contain the variables*: The variables may be made clearer in the hypothesis.
- *Based on research problem*: It should be relevant to the research problem and purpose of the study.
- *Empirically testable*: A well-stated hypothesis has to be testable. Variables included in the hypothesis lend themselves to observation, measurement, and analysis.

Type I Error

The rejection of a null hypothesis that is actually true, i.e. saying an intervention is effective when it is actually not.

Type II Error

The acceptance of a null hypothesis that is actually false, i.e. saying an intervention is ineffective when it actually is.

Level of Significance (*p*)

The level of significance for rejecting the statistical null hypothesis should always be stated prior to data collection. The level of significance is usually set by the researcher in view of the serious consequences that might arise on account of making a mistake in accepting a "false" research hypothesis. It is set at .05 or .01; this means that the researcher is willing to risk being wrong to the extent of 5% or 1% (five chances in 100 of making a mistake in accepting research hypothesis when it is actually false or one chance in 100 of making a mistake in accepting the research hypothesis). Generally, the aim of the researcher is to reject the null hypothesis because it provides support for the research hypothesis.

Guidelines for Critiquing Hypothesis

- Is the hypothesis written using a declarative sentence?
- Is hypothesis written in present tense?
- Is hypothesis clearly and precisely worded?
- Does the hypothesis contain the population being studied?
- Is each hypothesis directly related to the study problem?
- Is each hypothesis empirically testable?
- Is it apparent that each hypothesis contains only one prediction?

DELIMITATIONS

Delimitations are choices made by the researcher, which should be mentioned. They describe the boundaries set for the study and explain the things not being done, literature not being reviewed, the population not being studied, and the methodological procedures not being used.

- Delimitations are factors that affect the study over which the researcher generally does have some degree of control.
- Delimitations describe the scope of the study or choices made by the researcher. They depict the boundaries of the study and state what the study will include or exclude.
- Delimitations state the extent to which the study may be generalized in the field of practice, and also how these delimitations affect issues of external validity.
- Delimitations frequently include limits on the sample selection and technique, extent of the geographic area from which data are collected, use of tools in data collection, and time frame for the study. Examples of delimitations are presented in Table 3.12.

Delimitations of the study are generally described in the introductory chapter of the thesis or dissertation and at times in the discussion chapter also. Delimitations need to

Table 3.12: Examples of delimitations

Delimitations	Examples
Limits on sample selection and technique	• Due to nonavailability of sampling frame, study used nonrandom sampling technique • To maintain homogeneity in the sample selection, the study included only treatment seeking sample of out-patient department and those meeting specific criteria
Limit on extent of geographic area from which data are collected	• Due to the large number of potential participants in the population, the current study focused only on members located within a selected district
Limits on use of tools for the study	• In order to deal with collected data, the study utilized a survey tool with multiple choice questions and did not include open-ended questions
Limited time frame for the study	• Due to time constraint in the present study, subjects were followed up to 1 month only • Due to time constraint in the present study the data was collected over telephone
Literature not being reviewed	• Due to time constraints the present study included literature pertaining to last 5 years only

be described in detail and reasons explained for not considering certain parameters in the study. The researcher should mention impact of delimitation in relation to overall findings and conclusions of the study.

Uses of Delimitations
- Setting of delimitations and validating them facilitate the researcher in maintaining objectivity in the study.
- Delimitations aid the researcher in reconstructing a study and advance future research on the same topic.
- Delimitations offer the scope for a researcher to conclude the findings and determining a study's reliability or external validity.

LIMITATIONS
- Limitations are restrictions or shortcomings in a study, usually beyond the researcher's control that may decrease the credibility and generalizability of the findings. These affect the results of the study or how the results are interpreted. Examples of limitations are presented in Table 3.13.
- Limitations are weaknesses related to decisions made in a study regarding sampling technique, data collection strategy, instrument used, population chosen (in terms of accessibility), time, and resources.
- All the studies have some inherent limitations and such limitations that might influence the results should invariably be mentioned in the research report.
- Limitations are generally described in the discussion section so that the interpretation of results is done with the knowledge of potential impact on the limiting factors.
- Limitations should be better covered and their discussion typically encouraged when the conclusions of a study are formulated and recommendations made for future research. Otherwise it could lead to an important loss of context for the scientific literature.
- Various points to be considered while stating limitations include—statistical analysis, nature of data collection, instruments utilized, sample, time constraints, etc.
- There are two types of limitations: theoretical and methodological.
    - Theoretical limitations restrict the abstract generalization of the findings, which are reflected in the conceptual and operational definitions of the variables and the study framework. Theoretical limitations might include, research question, objectives, variables or hypothesis that lack a clear link to a relationship (or proposition) expressed in the study framework.

Table 3.13: Examples of limitations

Limitations	Examples
Improper representation of the target population	• The sample size was small, thereby limiting the generalizability of the findings to the larger population • Due to the length of the study, a significant number of respondents available in the pretesting were unavailable or unwilling to participate in the posttest. This restricted the generalizability of the findings
Limited outcomes	• The outcome measures included in the study relied on self-report with subjects. Results cannot always represent the actual occurrence in a generalized form • Outcome measures were assessed during the limited time period due to unavailability of the subjects

Table 3.14: Differences between delimitations and limitations

Delimitations	Limitations
To determine the parameters or scope of the study	To determine the weaknesses associated with decisions made in the study
Delimitations point to the limits beyond which the researcher does not wish to probe. It includes those boundaries that the researcher placed in the study prior to gathering the data	Limitations indicate the weakness of the entire study as the researcher perceives them
Delimitations are set during the planning phase	Limitations are experienced during the implementation phase
There is a level of control over where to draw the boundaries	Difficult to control, these uncontrollable elements are reported in research report

- Methodological limitations can limit the generalizability of the findings. These might include weak design, single setting, unrepresentative sample, limited control over treatment implementation, measuring instruments with limited reliability and validity, limited control over data collection, and improper use of statistical analyses.

Importance of Stating Limitations

- Limitations help the reader to get an accurate sense of what the study results indicate and how widely results can be generalized.
- May be useful for readers as they acknowledge the possible shortcomings while interpreting the study results.
- Evidence generated by the research study is strengthened by identifying limitations.
- Delimitations are different from limitations (Table 3.14).

While it is imperative that limitations are duly recognized for putting the research findings in context, interpreting the validity of the research work and attributing a credibility level to the conclusions of published research, delimitations make the study more feasible and practical by defining the boundaries, and providing the reader an idea of generalizability of the research findings.

BIBLIOGRAPHY

1. Amin, S.S., Daxini, A.B., Patel, D.S., & Modh, D.A. (2015). A Comparative Study of Spiro Metric Values Among Smokers and Non-Smokers. *International Journal of Research Medicine,* 4(4), 16-21.
2. Beckingham, A.C. (1974). Identifying problems for nursing research. International Nursing Reviews, 21(2), 49-52.
3. Burns, N., & Grove, S.K. (2004). *The practice of nursing research.* Philadelphia: W.B. Saunders Company.
4. Claribel, P.L., Simmons, Nicholas MacLeod., & Barry, J.A.L. (2012). Clinical Management of Pain in Advanced Lung Cancer. *Clinical Medicine Insights Oncology,* 6, 331-346.
5. Creswell, J.W. (1994). *Research design: Qualitative and quantitative approaches.* Thousand Oaks, CA: SAGE Publications.
6. Hammond, E.C., & Horn, D. (1954). The relationship between human smoking habits and death rates: a follow-up study of 187,766 men. *Journal of American Medical Association,* 155(15), 1316-28.
7. Hulley, S., Cummings, S., & Browner, W. et al. (2007). *Designing clinical research.* (3rd ed.). Philadelphia (PA): Lippincott Williams and Wilkins.
8. Kerlinger, F.N., & Pedhazur, E. (1973). *Multiple regressions in behavioral research.* New York, NY: Holt, Rinehart and Winston.
9. Kerlinger, F.N. (1973). *Foundations of Behavioral Research* (2nd ed.). Holt, NY: Rinehart and Winston.

10. Kerlinger, F.N. (1977). The influence of research on educational practice. *Educational Researcher*, 16, 5-12.
11. Kerlinger, F.N. (1979). *Foundations of Behavioral research: A conceptual approach*. Holt, New York: Rinehart and Winston.
12. Leedy, P., & Ormrod, J. (2001). *Practical research: Planning and design*. Upper Saddle River, NJ: Merrill Prentice-Hall.
13. LoBiondo-Wood, G., & Haber, J. (1997). *Nursing Research: Methods, critical appraisal and utilization* (3rd ed.). Boston: Mosbey.
14. Macleod-Clark, J. (1983). Nurse-Patient communications: an analysis of conversations from surgical wards. *Nursing Research: Ten studies in patient care,* Chichester: John Wiley & Sons.
15. Macleod-Clark, J., & Hockey, L. (1979). *Research for Nursing, A guide for the Enquiring Nurse.* London: HM Publishers Holdings Ltd.
16. Nieswiadomy, M.R. (2008). *Foundations of nursing research*. Boston: Pearson Prentice Hall.
17. Polit, D.F., Beck, C.T., & Hungler, B.P. (2001). *Essentials of Nursing Research: Methods, Appraisal, and Utilization* (5th ed.). Philadelphia: Lippincott Williams & Wilkins.
18. Polit, D.F., Beck, C.T., & Hungler, B.P. (2006). *Essentials of nursing research: Methods, appraisal and utilization* (6th ed.). Philadelphia: Lippincott Williams & Wilkins.
19. Sarantakos, S. (1993). *Social Research*. South Melbourne: MacMillan Education Australia pty. Ltd.
20. Treece, E.W., & Treece, J.H. (1989). *Elements of Research in Nursing*. St. Louis: The C.V. Mosby Company.
21. Waltz, D., Strickland, O., & Ling, E. (2004). *Measurement in nursing and health research.* Spring Hill, MA: Springer Publishing Company.
22. Wong, G. (2014). Research Questions. In V. Wright-St Clair, D. Reid, S. Shaw and J. Ramsbotham (Eds.), *Evidence-based Health Practice.* South Melbourne: Oxford University Press.
23. Xianglong, Xu., Lingli, Liu., Sharma, M., & Zhao, Y. (2015). Smoking-Related Knowledge, Attitudes, Behaviors, Smoking Cessation Idea and Education Level among Young Adult Male Smokers in Chongqing, China. *International Journal of Environment Research Public Health,* 12, 2135-2149.

REVIEW QUESTIONS

I. Long Essays

1. What is a research problem? How do you select a problem for research? Explain the characteristics of a research problem and list the criteria for evaluating the research problem.
2. What is research hypothesis? Describe types of hypothesis with an example.
3. List the sources of a research problem and explain the steps in its formulation.

II. Short Essays

1. Explain steps in formulation of a research problem.
2. What is hypothesis? List characteristics of a good hypothesis.
3. Explain about limitations and delimitations in research.
4. Describe research objectives and criteria for writing objectives.
5. Explain types of variables with suitable examples.
6. What are assumptions and explain their use in research?

III. Short Answers

1. Assumptions
2. Limitations
3. Delimitations
4. Variables

IV. Multiple Choice Questions

1. Variables are
   a. The main focus of research in science
   b. Something that we can measure

c. Something that can vary in terms of precision
d. All of the above
2. A dependent variable refers to
   a. The variable being manipulated
   b. The variable varied in some way by the researcher
   c. The variable which shows us the effect of manipulation
   d. A variable with a single value that remains constant in a particular context
3. The following are the synonyms for an independent variable, *except*
   a. Stimulus
   b. Manipulated
   c. Consequence
   d. Presumed cause
4. A variable that is presumed to cause a change in another variable is called
   a. Categorical variable
   b. Dependent variable
   c. Independent variable
   d. Intervening variable
5. Which of the following includes examples of quantitative variables?
   a. Age, temperature, income, and height
   b. Grade point average, anxiety level, and depression level
   c. Gender, religion, and ethnic group
   d. Both a and b
6. Which of the following constitutes discrete variables?
   a. Pulse rate
   b. Age
   c. Gender
   d. Height
7. Which of the following is a continuous variable?
   a. Height
   b. Heart rate
   c. Gender
   d. Type of family
8. Which of the following constitutes a dichotomous variable?
   a. Blood pressure
   b. Age at death
   c. Gender
   d. Weight
9. The following are the synonyms for a dependent variable, *except*
   a. Response
   b. Measured outcome
   c. Antecedent
   d. Presumed effect
10. A variable that is not influenced by or not dependent on other variables in experiments is called
    a. Independent variable
    b. Dependent variable
    c. Experimental variable
    d. Response
11. A variable that may affect research outcomes but have no relevance to the study is called
    a. Research variable
    b. Active variable
    c. Dependent variable
    d. Extraneous variable
12. What is the difference between a research question and research objective?
    a. The question is worded by the researcher, the objective is not
    b. No difference, they are the same
    c. The wording of one is likely to be more specific than the other
    d. One of these is proposed by a supervisor
13. Which word fills all the blanks in this extract: we talk about generating ____, testing _____, and rejecting _____.
    a. Questions
    b. Aims
    c. Hypothesis
    d. Objectives
14. A research hypothesis:
    a. Predicts accepted results or outcomes of the study

b. Defines theoretical framework for the study
c. Identifies the sources of the problem under study
d. Clarifies the concepts used in the study

15. What type of hypothesis is the following? "Normal saline flush with heparin is more effective than normal saline flush alone in maintaining patency of on intermittent intravenous site".
    a. Simple hypothesis
    b. Causal hypothesis
    c. Associative hypothesis
    d. Complex hypothesis

16. What type of hypothesis is the following? "Cancer patients who receive music therapy complain less frequently of pain and require less pain medication than those who are not receiving music therapy."
    a. Complex directional hypothesis
    b. Simple associative hypothesis
    c. Simple non-directional
    d. Complex null hypothesis

17. The hypothesis that there is no relationship between the independent and dependent variable is
    a. Directional hypothesis
    b. Null hypothesis
    c. Simple hypothesis
    d. Associative hypothesis

18. Factors which place restrictions on methodology and affect the results of the study are termed as
    a. Objectives
    b. Delimitations
    c. Limitations
    d. Methods

19. The boundaries of the study for the researcher are
    a. Hypothesis
    b. Assumptions
    c. Limitations
    d. Delimitations

20. Which of the following would identify the specific goal of the study based on identified problem?
    a. Research purpose
    b. Literature review
    c. Methodology
    d. Assumptions

21. An operational definition specifies
    a. The data collection techniques used in the study
    b. Levels of measurement to be used in the study
    c. How the variables are defined and measured in the study?
    d. How the outcome of the research objectives for the study will be measured?

22. Basic principles that are accepted on faith or assumed to be true without proof or verification is referred as
    a. Hypothesis
    b. Assumptions
    c. Aim
    d. Objectives

23. The following are the criteria for selecting a research problem, *except*
    a. Researcher interest
    b. Researcher competency
    c. Researcher's own resources
    d. Researcher assumptions

24. Which of the following is not a component of hypothesis?
    a. Dependent variable
    b. Independent variable
    c. Extraneous variable
    d. Study population

25. Sources of researchable problems can include
    a. Researchers' own experience
    b. Practical issues that require solutions
    c. Theory and past research
    d. All of the above

26. The statement of the belief and ideas which are considered to be true without evidence?
    a. Hypothesis
    b. Assumptions

c. Conceptual definition
d. Operational definition
27. Which of the following is an example of an operational definition?
   a. A numeric rating scale is used to measure pain intensity
   b. Family is defined as the blood relatives having legalized relation of a person and carryout roles
   c. Analysis of concept of hope reveals that it has eight separate components
   d. Physiological needs are defined as being the most basic needs of human
28. Which of the following are measured in research?
   a. Variables
   b. Definitions
   c. Samples
   d. Data
29. Term used to describe the specific goal or aim of the study
   a. Research topic
   b. Research problem
   c. Study purpose
   d. Design
30. The statement "people want to control their own health problems" is an example of which of the following?
   a. Assumptions
   b. Framework
   c. Methodological limitation
   d. Theoretical limitation

ANSWER KEY

1. d	2. c	3. c	4. c	5. d	6. a
7. a	8. c	9. c	10. a	11. d	12. c
13. c	14. a	15. b	16. a	17. b	18. c
19. d	20. a	21. c	22. b	23. d	24. c
25. d	26. b	27. a	28. a	29. c	30. a

UNIT 4

Review of Literature

Undertaking literature review is one of the primary functions of a researcher. Nursing research is a continuous process wherein knowledge obtained from previous studies is an integral part of research in general. Before starting a quantitative study, it is essential to determine what previous knowledge exists on the study topic. American Psychological Association 6th edition says, "Literature reviews are tutorials in that the authors define and clarify the problem, summarize previous investigations to inform the reader of the state of the research, identify relations, contradictions, gaps and inconsistencies in the literature and suggest the next step in solving the problem."

A literature review examines and critically evaluates scholarly articles, books and other relevant sources to describe and summarize information related to particular issue/topic or research area. It provides an overview of information relating to a particular topic and explains to the reader how the present study fits within a larger field of study.

DEFINITIONS

A literature review is a synopsis of other research. Moreover, it is a critical appraisal of other research on a given topic that helps to put that topic in context.
—**Machi and McEvoy, 2009**

"A literature review is an objective, thorough summary and critical analysis of the relevant available research and nonresearch literature on the topic being studied".
—**Hart 1998 cited in Cronin, Ryan and Coughlan 2008**

IMPORTANCE OF LITERATURE REVIEW

The important aspects relating to literature review in research are:
- Presents information in a sequential order.
- Evaluates the sources and directs the reader to most recent and relevant information.
- Identifies gaps in the existing literature and concludes how a problem has been researched to date.
- Gives a new explanation to old material or combine new explanations with the old ones.

PURPOSES OF LITERATURE REVIEW

Review of literature provides an in-depth analysis of recently published research findings in a specified area of interest. It provides healthcare professionals latest and accurate information for proper management of patients. The literature review is undertaken for research and non-research reasons:

Research Reasons
- To update the reader on a topic with current literature and form the basis for research.

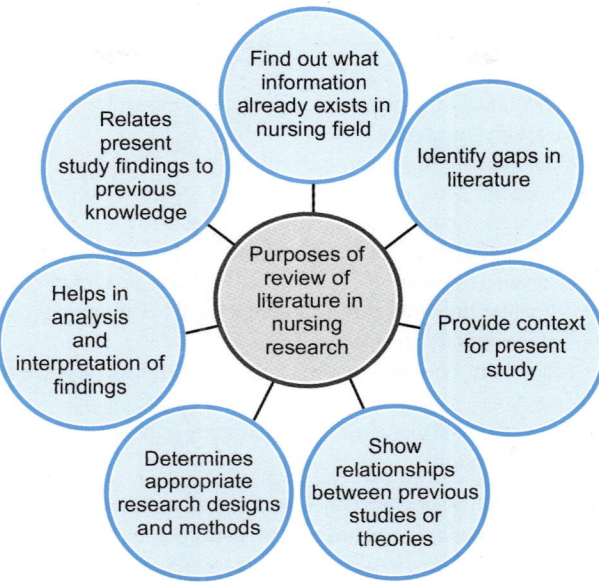

Fig. 4.1: Purposes of review of literature in nursing research

* To critically evaluate the relevant findings that have emerged from previous studies to provide rationalization for proposed research.

Non-research Reasons
* To extract information for developing policies
* To evaluate existing practices
* To develop and revise practice guidelines
* To gain evidence-based knowledge on a subject or topic
* To update present knowledge and practice on a subject matter or area
* As a part of academic assignment
* To develop and revise nursing curricula
* To develop a theory or conceptual framework.

The main purposes of literature review are presented in Figure 4.1.

Purposes of Review of Literature in Quantitative Research

Quantitative research studies are undertaken based on the previous knowledge with a definite research question in mind. The review of literature is useful in all phases of quantitative research (Table 4.1).

Purposes of Review of Literature in Qualitative Research

According to qualitative research method, the phenomena should be explained based on participant's viewpoints rather than on any prior information. While some researchers conduct literature review at the end of the study to avoid bias, a few others conduct preliminary review upfront to obtain a little guidance. The purposes of literature review in various qualitative studies are presented in Table 4.2.

ELEMENTS OF A LITERATURE REVIEW

Review of literature should not just be a simple narrative of previously published summaries. It should—
* include critical discussion reflecting insight and an understanding of conflicting opinions, theories, and approaches.

Table 4.1: Purpose of review literature in quantitative research

Phases	Purpose of review literature
Conceptual	• Encourages and generates new ideas by highlighting inconsistencies/gaps in existing knowledge • Defines, refines and limits the research problem or hypothesis being worked on • Finds out what information already exists in the nursing field • Identifies new ways to interpret prior research • Locates present research within the context of existing literature • Prevents duplication of effort by identifying areas of prior research • Provides the researcher a comprehensive background for understanding contemporary knowledge • Highlights how best the new knowledge can add value to the existing base of evidence • Describes the relationship of each study to other research studies under consideration
Designing	• Helpful in identifying conceptual or theoretical frameworks for a research problem • Determines appropriate research designs and methods (selection of instruments, data collection methods, sampling techniques) for answering the current research question
Empirical	• Directs the data collection process
Analytic	• Gives ideas to researcher about how to classify and present the data. • Helps in analysis and interpretation of findings
Dissemination	• Identify new ways to interpret the study findings and throw light on any gaps in previous research • Helps in relating present research findings to previous knowledge and recommends further research • Assist in developing implications and recommendations • Put one's original work in the context of existing literature • Helps in writing research report • Justify how present research helps to answer some of the questions

Table 4.2: Purposes of literature review in qualitative studies

Type of qualitative study	Purpose of review literature
Ethnography	Provides background for conducting the study as in quantitative research
Phenomenological	Determines current knowledge of phenomenon
Grounded theory	Helps to explain, support and extend the theory generated in the study
Historical research	Develops a research question and is a source for data in the study
Case study	Determines current knowledge relating to the phenomenon

- include synthesis and analysis of the relevant published work linked to the researcher's own purpose.
- be organized around and directly related to the topic/area.
- identify areas of disagreement in the literature and areas which need further clarification.

According to Caulley (1992) of La Trobe University, the elements of literature review are as follows:
- Group authors who draw similar conclusions
- Note areas in which authors are in disagreement
- Compare and contrast different authors' views on an issue
- Criticize aspects of methodology
- Highlight exemplary studies
- Highlight gaps in research
- Describe how the present study relates to previous studies and to the literature in general
- Conclude by summarizing what the literature says.

TYPES OF LITERATURE REVIEWS

There are two types of literature that support the research: the "narrative" review and the "systematic" review (Table 4.3).

Narrative reviews: These are publications that illustrate and discuss a specific topic from a theoretical viewpoint. These reviews are conducted by subject experts; however, they may be subject to bias due to their preconceived ideas.

Table 4.3: Main differences between narrative and systematic reviews

Characteristics	Narrative reviews	Systematic reviews
Question	Broad; hypothesis not stated	Specific; hypothesis is stated
Authors	One or more authors who may be topic experts	Two or more authors who may be topic experts
Characteristics	Describes and evaluates previous work	Extracts and synthesizes previous study findings
Search strategy	Search is conducted using keywords, no detailed search strategy	Comprehensive search is conducted by developing strategy
Purpose	• To provide a broad overview of the literature in a selected topic • To identify gaps in existing research • To develop conceptual framework • Refine research question (Cronin et al. 2008, 38)	• To produce a comprehensive list of the entire literature on a topic • To separate the topic based on predefined criteria • Identifies, appraises and synthesizes all available research that is relevant to a particular review question (Cronin et al. 2008, 38)
Advantages	Provides rationale for new research	• Resolves disagreement between contradictory findings • Provides a reliable base for decision making
Source of literature	Published and unpublished articles are included.	Websites, databases, practice guidelines, published and unpublished sources
Source and selection	Usually not specified, potentially biased	Explicit search approach, criteria-based selection
Evaluation	Methods not specified	Explicit methods used

Contd...

Contd...

Characteristics	Narrative reviews	Systematic reviews
Synthesis	Qualitative	Quantitative (includes meta-analysis)
Inferences	Sometimes evidence based	Usually evidence based
Update	Not updated periodically	Periodically updated
Reproducibility	As conclusions are subjected to bias, results cannot be reproduced independently	With accurate documentation method, results can be reproduced
Limitations	Bias in selection of literature	Narrowly framed review questions provide only limited answers
Example	Kitson A et al. 2013 conducted a narrative review to identify the common core elements of patient-centered care (PCC) in medical and nursing literature. The data was gathered from patient organizations, policy documents, medical and nursing studies related to PCC in the acute care setting. The search sources were Medline, CINAHL (Cumulative Index to Nursing and Allied Health Literature), SCOPUS, texts and primary policy documents. Sixty papers were included in the review wherein three core themes were identified: patient participation and involvement, the relationship between the patient and the healthcare professional, and the context where care is delivered. The study concluded that different professional groups tend to emphasize different elements within the themes. This may affect the success of implementing PCC in practice.	Rathert C et al. 2013 conducted a systematic review on PCC literature to examine the evidence for PCC and outcomes. Three databases were searched for all years through September 2012. 40 articles were analyzed. Results found mixed relationships between PCC and clinical outcomes, i.e. some studies found significant relationships between specific elements of PCC and outcomes but others found no relationship. There was stronger evidence for positive influence of PCC on satisfaction and self-management.

Systematic reviews: These are publications that summarize the evidence on a particular research topic. These reviews are conducted using rigorous methodological approaches like critically appraising and synthesizing results of primary research studies.

- ❖ These provide a comprehensive list of all published and unpublished studies concerning a specific area.
- ❖ There is evidence that systematic reviews improve the reliability and accuracy of the conclusions.
- ❖ These reviews provide systematic and accurate evidence thus facilitating clinicians and policy makers to assess relevant information easily so as to improve patient outcomes.
- ❖ These are published in websites of professional organizations to encourage dissemination of information. Cochrane collaboration (www.cochrane.org) is a professional organization that encourages dissemination of systematic reviews related to healthcare interventions.
  - ○ Meta-analysis is a kind of systematic review. It is typically a statistical technique used in quantitative research designs.
  - ○ It is the analysis of analyses. It involves taking the findings from several studies

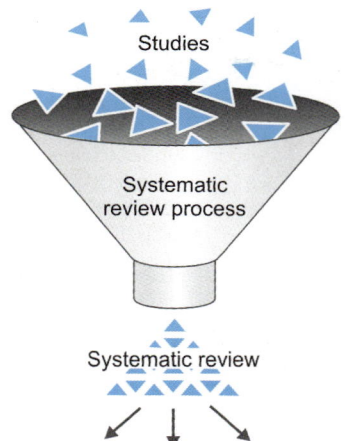

Fig. 4.2: The concept of a systematic review

on peer-reviewed journals. Primarily two types of information are cited in the literature review for research. These are theoretical and empirical.

Theoretical literature: It includes models, theories, conceptual frameworks related to selected research problem and purpose. This literature helps in understanding concepts of research problem and facilitates developing study framework.

Empirical literature: It includes research studies in journals, books, thesis and dissertations related to selected research problem.

The published literature includes primary and secondary sources. The examples of these sources are presented in Table 4.4.

Primary sources in research literature refer to a description of research study written by the original researcher. Usually found in journal articles, these include original, peer reviewed and published research journal articles reported by the researcher. These are direct sources where from first-hand information can be obtained. For example, the journal of advanced nursing publishes research study results written by the original researcher. Predominantly, primary sources need to be employed in developing research proposals and reports.

on the same subject and analyzing them by using standardized statistical procedures. This helps to draw conclusions and detect relationships between findings (Polit and Beck, 2006).
- It offers a possibility to classify and measure the conditions and results of studies in a more precise and rigorous way when compared to verbal descriptions of research (Fig. 4.2).

❖ *Meta-synthesis* is the nonstatistical technique, to evaluate and interpret the findings of multiple qualitative research studies. This involves analyzing and synthesizing key elements in each study with the aim of transforming individual findings into new conceptualizations and interpretations (Polit and Beck, 2006).

SOURCES OF REVIEW OF LITERATURE

The term source refers to material, either print, electronic or visual, essential for research. A comprehensive literature is compulsory for any type of dissertations regardless of the research area and educational institution. The literature should be based on a wide range of trustworthy sources with particular focus

Secondary sources in research literature refer to description of a research study written by someone other than the original researcher. These include the comments and summaries of multiple research studies on one topic, for example, systematic reviews, meta-analysis and meta-syntheses. This content is quoted from the primary source. An inherent problem with secondary sources is that the author has interpreted the work of someone else and this interpretation is purely based on author's perception, giving rise to a likelihood of bias. It is necessary to review primary sources whenever possible to ensure accuracy. Secondary sources are generally utilized in the event of unavailability of primary sources.

Table 4.4: Examples of primary and secondary sources			
Source	Definition	Examples	Potential search tools and sources
Primary	Sources that publish the findings of original research and other types of studies in their first and original form	• Journals • Books • Monographs • Dissertations/theses • Description of theories by the individual • Autobiographies, letters, diaries, speeches, photographs, artifacts • Case reports, anecdotes, clinical description	• CINAHL (Cumulative Index to Nursing and Allied Health Literature) • MEDLINE • PsycINFO • Cochrane Library
Secondary	Sources that synthesize, summarize or comment on original research	• Systematic reviews • Meta-analysis • Integrative reviews • Reviews of individual's articles • Clinical practice guidelines • Reports from Government agencies and professional organizations • Conference proceedings	• CINAHL • MEDLINE • PsychINFO • Cochrane Library • Government guidelines • Professional association databases of practice guidelines

Literature reviews combine primary and secondary sources to document and analyze both published and unpublished material on any given topic over a period of time. Selected sources of literature review are presented in Figure 4.3.

- *Journals*: Peer-reviewed journals can be used to review original research articles. These journals are rich in scholarly articles and can be an effective source to keep up to date with the recent trends and developments in the research area.
- *Dissertations and thesis*: These are research reports that contain details of research done on a particular topic. It is a good source of detailed information and further reference.
- *Conceptual or theoretical papers:* These are associated with an explanatory account of theories or concepts related to the topic.
- *Anecdotes*: These refer to opinions and beliefs about the subject not related to research, review or theory.
- *Autobiographies:* These refer to the telling and documenting of one's own life. They include life narratives, oral stories, diaries, videos, photos, and documents—both official and personal.
- *Description of clinical situations*: These are case studies and clinical reports from the clinical setting.
- *Literature review, bibliographies and journal abstracts*: These are review articles or summary of a particular topic described by somebody other than the original researcher.
- *Textbooks, monographs, and encyclopedias*: Textbooks remain as the most important source to find models and theories related

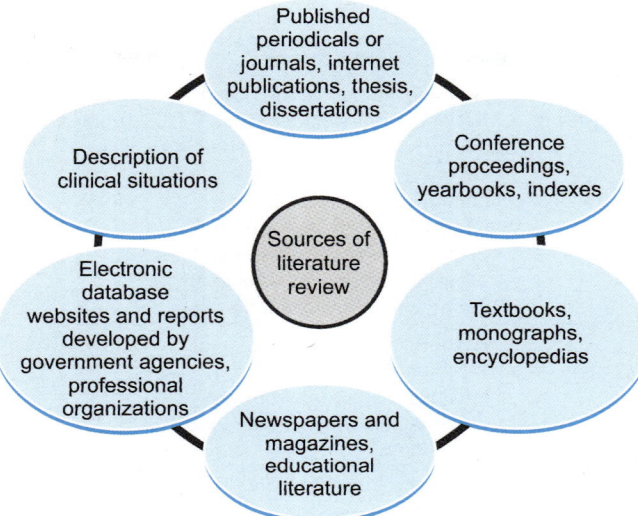

Fig. 4.3: Selected sources of review of literature

to the research area. The material in books are presented in a more ordered and accessible manner than in journals.
- *Newspapers, magazines, and educational literature*: These can be referred to as the main source of up-to-date news.
- *Conference proceedings, yearbooks, and indexes*: Specific theme synopses are published in these reports.
- *Reports*: From Government agencies and professional organizations.
- *Electronic literature searches:* Electronic databases are bibliographic files that can be accessed through online search and retrieved more easily and quickly compared to a manual search. Various electronic databases relevant to nursing profession are presented in Table 4.5.

Table 4.5: Electronic databases relevant to nursing profession		
Database	Main content	Source for access
British Nursing Index	Leading UK nursing database providing bibliographic references to journal articles from all the major British nursing and midwifery journals.	www.rcn.org.uk/elibrary (Royal College of Nursing Library e-library)
CINAHL (Cumulative Index to Nursing and Allied Health Literature)	It covers nursing and allied health journals as well as books, nursing dissertations, conference proceedings in nursing and allied health fields. It covers material dating from 1982 till date.	http://www.cinahl.com
Cochrane Library	Systematic reviews of literature related to medicine, nursing and allied health professions.	http://www.cochrane.org

Contd....

Contd....

Database	Main content	Source for access
PubMed or MEDLINE (Medical Literature Analysis and Retrieval System Online)	It was developed by the US National Library of Medicine (NLM). It includes bibliographic coverage of the biomedical literature. It incorporates information from index medicus, international nursing index and other sources. It covers material dating from 1966 till date.	http://www.ncbi.nlm.nih.gov/PubMed
PsycINFO	It belongs to American Psychological Association and covers literature from psychological and related disciplines.	http://www.psycinfo.com
Registry of nursing research	It was developed by Sigma Theta Tau International Honor Society of Nursing, available through Virginia Henderson International Nursing Library.	http://www.nursinglibrary.org

CRITERIA FOR SELECTION OF SOURCES

Certain norms to be followed while selecting the sources are:

- *Use of most recent sources*: Use of sources to be as current as possible is particularly true for medical and scientific disciplines where research conducted becomes outdated as and when new discoveries are made.
- *Use evidence*: The sources must be based on evidence. It demonstrates validity.
- *Be selective*: Only the most important review sources must be selected. The type of information chosen should relate directly to the research problem. The selection of sources should be based on scope and purpose of the study.
- *Use relevant sources*: Sources should include relevant primary sources or data or studies. If necessary, appropriate secondary sources may also be used.
- *Exercise care while rephrasing*: While rephrasing a source that is not own, the author's information or opinion should be represented accurately and suitable citation of that work provided.
- *Describe search procedure*: The researcher should explain the search procedure used to identify the review literature.
- *Balanced coverage of available sources:* Based on a wide range of trustworthy sources, keeping the scope and purpose of the study in mind, choose only the key points from each source. Literature should include enough material to show the development and limitations in the particular area.
- *Referencing accurately:* The researcher should provide accurate references for all sources of literature.

STEPS IN LITERATURE REVIEW PROCESS

A literature review is a systematic and orderly process which is organized in nature. It is done to elicit information for developing policies and evidence-based practices. Preparation of literature review includes the following steps (Fig. 4.4).

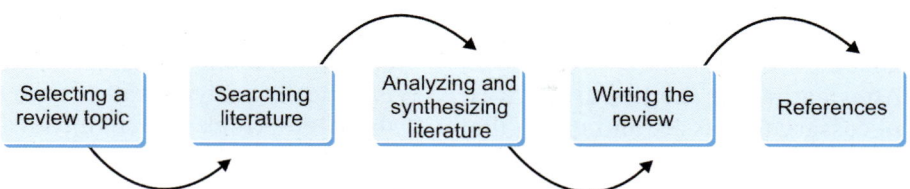

Fig. 4.4: Steps in literature review process

1. **Selecting a review topic**: The selection of a review topic is directed by a research objective or research problem. This step involves understanding the concept of research problem and identifying the key search terms and developing a structure for the review.
2. **Searching literature**: Once the topic is selected, the researcher searches for appropriate literature in a structured way.
    - Literature search should involve both primary and secondary sources, and also theoretical or anecdotal papers related to the topic.
    - Existing literature and systematic reviews are also significant sources of data as they provide an overview of the research undertaken and offer the bibliographic references for the topic (Ely and Scott, 2007).
    - During this step, comprehensiveness and relevance need to be considered and more specific the literature is to the research question, the more focused the result will be. In order to avoid generation of overwhelming information, the review topic needs to be narrowed down.
    - Presently, literature searches are carried out usually using electronic databases and computers. Manual search of journals specifically related to the topic can also be done.
    - Usually, a search should include 5–10 years of age work.
    - The researcher needs to identify relevant databases related to the topic.
    - Keyword searches are the universal and most widespread methods of identifying literature. The keywords need to be cautiously selected so as to generate the data being sought. Alternate keywords with similar meaning may be considered for eliciting further information. For example, while undertaking a review on body-mind-spirit intervention, one would need to include terms such as holistic intervention, alternative and complimentary therapies, etc.
    - An alternate approach is to combine the keywords. To facilitate such combinations, most databases use "Boolean operators". The most common Boolean operators are "AND" (Look for articles that include all the identified keywords), "OR" (Look for articles that include any of the identified keywords) and "NOT" (Exclude articles that contain this specific keyword) (Ely and Scott, 2007).
    - It is essential to keep a record of the keywords and methods used while conducting literature search so as to describe the search procedure (Timmins and McCabe, 2005).

    A thorough literature search enables the researcher to broaden the knowledge on a selected topic and also position the research question in the context of current knowledge.
3. **Analyzing and synthesizing the literature**:
    - At the beginning, the researcher should carry out a first read of the collected

articles to understand what it is all about.
- After gathering the literature, it is necessary to classify and group the articles based on their type of source.
- This needs to be followed up with a further systematic and critical review of the content.
- Cohen, 1990; proposed a simple method for systematic review identified as PQRS system—preview, question, read and summarize. This method facilitates easy identification and retrieval of material.
  * In the *preview stage*, the researcher identifies relevant reviews based on the purpose. Reading the abstract appearing at the beginning of the paper helps the researcher to decide whether further reading or inclusion is necessitated.
  * In the *question stage*, questions are posed of each publication. It is desirable to have an indexing and summary system including the title of the article, author, purpose and methodology utilized, findings and outcomes of the research study. It is also useful to list out the comments or key thoughts on the researcher's response to the article after it has been reviewed. The source and full reference may also be included.
  * *Reading* is an ongoing process during which above specified questions are answered for each article.
  * In *summary stage*, evidence needs to be summed up and logically presented, comparing and contrasting findings, and presenting new insights where possible. It comprises of key observations, remarks, strengths and weaknesses of the article. This forms a basis for writing the review.

While writing the final review, it is essential that the necessary information is critically analyzed rather than merely detailed. Heck and Langton (2000) focused on the criteria of quality, credibility and accuracy for evaluating the literature. While quality and credibility issues are linked to the journal, the peer review process, reputation of the author and the statements made; content is assessed for its accuracy and coherence with existing knowledge on the subject.

4. **Writing the review**: Once the literature is analyzed and synthesized, focus must be on structuring and writing the review. Writing the review of literature involves selection of relevant resources, organization of these sources and writing the review.

Selection of reviews: Reviews or sources are selected for inclusion in literature review based on their quality and relatedness to purpose of the study.

Organization of reviews:
- The reviews that provide background, significance and justification for the study are included in the introduction chapter.
- Studies with similar methodology and supported studies are presented in review of literature chapter.
- Studies with similar findings need to be included in discussion chapter.

Writing the reviews:
- Reviews need to be presented in a clear, logical and consistent manner. The method of writing a literature review differs based on the type of review undertaken. The systematic reviews have a specific format to write.
- While writing reviews, long and confusing words may be avoided, use of terminology minimized, short sentences with clear messages used, spelling and grammar are correct.

- Before starting to write, a framework may be developed.
- The length of the literature review (word limit) should be in accordance with the guidelines prescribed by the university or institute.
- A well-organized literature review consists of
   - Introduction
   - Main body
   - Conclusion

Introduction: It introduces the central topic by including the brief overview of the problem. It outlines the organization of literature, key search items used and the boundaries. It provides a concise evaluation of the literature on the topic by outlining what has been studied till date, how adequate and dependable those studies are, what gaps are there in existing body of research, and what contribution the new study will make.

Main body: Findings from the literature are discussed in the main body of the literature review. The various approaches or methods for structuring the main body (Carnwell and Daly, 2001) are presented in Table 4.6.

- Dividing the literature into themes or categories
- Describing the literature in a chronological order based on time period
- Discussion on theoretical literature followed by discussion on potential empirical research
- Describing theoretical and empirical literature in two different subsections.

Key points to be considered while writing the review:

- The empirical and theoretical sources must be presented in a *concise and accurate manner.*
- The researcher should *discuss in depth* those studies that are more relevant in guiding the present investigation.
- The findings from the study should be *logically built* on each other so that the reader can rationalize how the body of knowledge in the research area evolved.
- *Ethical issues* must be considered while presenting the sources. The content from the sources must be presented honestly and not by distorting the facts to support the selected problem.

Table 4.6: Various methods of framing review

Method/approach	Advantages and disadvantages
Dividing the literature into themes or categories—here literature is discussed based on the theme	• Most common method • Permits integration of theoretical and empirical literature • Helps to know how closely the themes are related to the literature
Describing the literature in a chronological order based on time period	Useful when investigating how a topic emerged over a period of time
Discussion on theoretical literature, followed by discussion on potential empirical research	• Useful when available literature is mostly theoretical in nature and not empirical • Can be used to identify the need for investigation
Describing theoretical and empirical literature in two different subsections	Might likely end up being a description of review rather than a critique

- The review should not be a succession of quotes or abstracts and must be written in *researcher's own words*.
- While describing the study findings, use language that describes *tentativeness* of the results rather than making a definite statement (Polit and Beck, 2006).
- It is desirable to incorporate a *critical review of the methodologies* while detailing empirical literature.
- When few studies in the area of interest are available, the review should incorporate the *analyses of methodologies* utilized in all the studies.
- When using thematic approach, the description should flow logically from one theme to another to maintain uniformity and continuity (Beyea and Nicoll, 1998).
- The researcher should *summarize and evaluate evidence* about a topic, *outlining the similarities and differences,* explanations on *inconsistencies and uncovered topics* (Polit and Beck, 2006).
- The review should be presented like a critical evaluation of the available information highlighting and *comparing the results* from other sources.
- The review should also address *inconsistencies, contradictions, strengths and weaknesses* present in the literature (Colling, 2003).
- The review should *identify major trends, patterns and relationships* among studies.

Conclusion: It is a brief summary of the findings that depicts current knowledge and offers a justification for carrying out future research. It should be written in own words including relevant information and significant findings related to the topic. It should specify gaps in the knowledge and inconsistencies in the methodology.

5. *References:* The literature review should include all the references that have been referred—books, journals, articles, reports and other sources. All the citations in the text must be mentioned in the reference section. Every effort should be made to ensure its accuracy.

GENERAL GUIDELINES FOR REVIEWING THE LITERATURE

- Reviewed literature should be related to the research problem or question.
- The purpose and objectives of the study should guide the selection of literature.
- The researcher should safeguard against replication of the read information.
- Researcher should also use sources like newspapers, magazines and other reports.
- The use of most recent references is important.
- It is imperative to record the bibliographical data on any material that is read so as to ensure proper citation in the reference section.
- Literature review without appropriate references amounts to plagiarism.
- Long lists of nonspecific references may be avoided.
- A wide variation or inconsistency in previous study results may be cited separately.
- In the review section of the thesis, dissertation or the journal article, all the relevant references should be cited.
- The depth and breadth of the literature review (number and quality of the sources) depends on the background of the researcher, the complexity of the research project, amount of literature available on the selected problem and the nature of document being prepared.

Critiquing the Literature Review in a Published Study

- Have the most recent and relevant studies been included?
- Is the current knowledge about the research problem described?
- Does the literature review identify the gap in the knowledge?
- Does the literature review provide the basis for study conducted?
- Is the literature review clearly organized, logically developed and concisely written?
- Are the references cited accurately?

BIBLIOGRAPHY

1. Burns, N., & Grove, S.K. (2004). *The practice of nursing research*. Philadelphia: W.B. Saunders Company.
2. Campbell, M., Young, P.I., Bateman, D.N., Smith, J.M. & Thomas, S.H. (1999). The use of atypical antipsychotics in the management of schizophrenia. *British Journal of Clinical Pharmacology*, 41, 13-22.
3. Carnwell, R., & Daly, W. (2001). Strategies for the construction of a critical review of the literature. *Nurse Education in Practice*, 1, 57-63.
4. Cronin, P., Ryan, F., & Coughlan, M. (2008). *Undertaking a literature review*: a step-by-step approach, *British Journal of Nursing*, 17(1), 38-43.
5. Ely, C., & Scott, I. (2007) *Essential Study Skills for Nursing*. Elsevier, Edinburgh.
6. Fink, A. (2014). Conducting Research Literature Reviews: From the Internet to Paper (4th ed.). Thousand Oaks, CA: Sage *publications, Inc.*
7. Fink, A. *(2005).* Conducting Research Literature Reviews: From the Internet to Paper (2nd ed.*).* Thousand Oaks, CA: Sage publications, Inc.
8. Fletcher, R.H., & Fletcher, S.W. (1997). Evidence-Based Approach to the Medical Literature. *Journal of General Internal Medicine*, 12, 5-14. doi:10.1037/0278-6133.24.2.225.
9. Galvan, J. (2006). *Writing literature reviews: a guide for students of the behavioral sciences* (3rd ed.*).* Glendale, CA: Pyrczak Publishing.
10. Galvan, J.L. (2013). *Writing literature reviews: A guide for students of the social and behavioral sciences*. Glendale, CA: Pyrczak Publishing.
11. Gillet, A. (2012). Using English for academic purposes: a guide for students in higher education, Reporting—paraphrase, summary and synthesis [online], available: http://uefap.com/writing/writfram.htm [accessed 4 September 2012].
12. Hart, C. (1998). Doing a Literature Review: Releasing the Social Science Research Imagination. Thousand Oaks, CA: Sage Publications.
13. Hek, G., & Langton, H. (2000). Systematically searching and reviewing literature. *Nurse Researcher,* 7(3), 40–57
14. Jesson, J. (2011). Doing Your Literature Review: Traditional and Systematic Techniques. *Thousand Oaks,* CA: Sage publications, Inc.
15. Khan, K.S., Terriet, G., Glanville, j., Sowden, A.J., & Kleijnen, J. (2001). Undertaking systematic reviews of research on effectiveness: CRD's guidance for carrying out or commissioning reviews (2nd ed.). New York: NHS Centre for reviews and dissemination. University of York, 2000. [CRD Report No. 4]. Available from: http://www.york.ac.uk/inst/cdr/report4.htm.
16. Kitson, A., Marshall, A., Bassett, K., & Zeitz, K. (2013). What are the core elements of patient-centered care? A narrative review and synthesis of the literature from health policy, medicine and nursing. *Journal of Advanced Nursing,* 69(1), 4–15.
17. Leucht, S., Pitschel-Walz, G., Abraham, D., & Kissling, W. (1999). Efficacy and extra pyramidal side-effects of the new antipsychotics olanzapine, quetiapine, risperidone, and sertindole compared to conventional antipsychotics and placebo. A meta-analysis of randomized controlled trials. *Schizophrenia Research,* 35, 51-68.
18. Marder, S.R. (1999). Antipsychotic drugs and relapse prevention. *Schizophrenia Research,* 35, 87-92.
19. Murray, R. (2006). *How to Write a Thesis.* UK: Open University Press.
20. Persaud, N. (2010). *Primary data source: Encyclopedia of research design* (2nd ed.). Thousand Oaks, CA: SAGE Publications, Inc.

21. Polit, D.F., Beck, C.T., & Hungler, B.P. (2006). *Essentials of nursing research: Methods, appraisal and utilization* (6th ed.). Philadelphia: Lippincott Williams & Wilkins.
22. Rathert, C., Wyrwich, M.D., & Boren S.A. (2013). Patient-centered care and outcomes: a systematic review of the literature. *Medicine Care Research Rev*, 70(4):351-79. doi: 10.1177/1077558712465774.
23. Ridley, D. (2012). The Literature Review: A Step-by-Step Guide for Students (2nd ed.). Los Angeles, CA: SAGE.
24. Rother, E.T. (2015). Systematic literature review X narrative review. Acta paul.enferm. [Internet].2007 June [cited 2015 Dec 25]; 20(2): v-vi. Available from: http://www.scielo. br/scielo.php?script=sci_arttext&pid=S0103 21002007000200001&lng=en. http://dx.doi.org/10.1590/S0103-21002007000200001.
25. Timmins, F., McCabe, C. (2005). How to conduct an effective literature review. *Nurs Stand,* 20(11): 41-7
26. Treece, E.W., & Treece, J.H. (1989). *Elements of Research in Nursing* (2nd ed.). St. Louis, CV: Mosby Co.
27. Paul, W., & Vogt, A. (2005). *Dictionary of Statistics & Methodology: Secondary Source.* (3rd ed.). Thousand Oaks, CA: SAGE Publications.
28. Weidenborner, S., & Caruso, D. (1997). *Writing research papers: A guide to the process*. New York: St. Martin's Press.

REVIEW QUESTIONS

I. Long Essays
1. Define review of literature; narrate purposes of literature review in quantitative research.
2. What are the sources of literature review? Explain with examples.
3. Narrate steps in writing review of literature.

II. Short Essays
1. Explain importance of review of literature.
2. Explain the purpose of literature in qualitative research.
3. Explain types of review of literature.
4. Explain the differences between narrative and systematic reviews.

III. Short Answers
1. Define review of literature.
2. List out the sources of literature.
3. Expand CINAHL, MEDLINE and BNI.
4. Difference between primary and secondary sources.
5. What are electronic databases?

IV. Multiple Choice Questions
1. Literature review is a
   a. Brief critical discussion about the merits and weaknesses of a literary work
   b. Study-by-study or article-by-article description of studies previously done
   c. Summary of current knowledge about particular practice or problem and includes what is known and unknown about the problem
   d. A compilation of all positive results on research
2. When conducting a review of literature on a particular subject, the researcher should
   a. Read all available material on the subject
   b. Read the whole journal article and then decide whether or not it is useful
   c. Read strategically and critically
   d. Read fully only those contents that appear to agree with his/her point of view
3. The purpose of literature review is
   a. To clarify importance of a research problem
   b. To identify the gaps
   c. To identify strengths and weaknesses of previous studies
   d. All of these
4. The literature review section of a research report might include a summary of which of the following?

a. Empirical literature
b. Funding sources
c. Proposed methods and design
d. Description of study sample

5. What are the sources of review of literature?
   a. Books
   b. Abstracts
   c. Journals
   d. All of the above

6. Which of the following represents a primary source?
   a. The results of a computer search related to the primary topic of interest
   b. A report of a study written by the researcher who conducted the study
   c. A published summary of the relevant research in a primary care area
   d. The keywords to use in a computer search

7. At what point is the literature review conducted in a qualitative investigation?
   a. Prior to study implementation
   b. During study implementation
   c. After study completion
   d. Depends on the type of study

8. How many years is it necessary to go back in the literature for an evidence-based project?
   a. 3 years is sufficient
   b. 5 years is preferred
   c. 7 years is expected
   d. All literature is to be included

9. Of the following, which is the most efficient tool to use for scholarly literature searches
   a. Web browsers
   b. Online journals
   c. Search engines
   d. Government websites

10. Why do you need to review the existing literature?
    a. To enjoy reading the academic research on a specified topic
    b. Because without it, researcher could never reach the required word count
    c. To find out what is already known about specific area of interest.
    d. To have a long list of references.

11. A systematic literature review
    a. Summarizes best available evidence
    b. A replicable, scientific, and transparent process
    c. Provides exhaustive list of all published and unpublished studies
    d. All of the above

12. A narrative review is
    a. Subjective summary of research findings
    b. Describe and evaluate previous work
    c. Overview of the literature in a selected area
    d. All of the above

13. The first step in doing a literature review is
    a. Selection of a review topic
    b. Searching for literature
    c. Analyzing and synthesizing the literature
    d. Writing the review

14. When might a researcher not carry out a full review of literature at the start of a study?
    a. In qualitative research designs, when the researcher believes that review of literature may create a source of biasness
    b. In quantitative research designs, when the researcher believes that review of literature may waste his time and resources
    c. If the literature is old and will not provide a firm basis for the study
    d. In mixed method design, when the researcher believes that review of literature may not be required

15. Which of the following is a primary source of published literature?
    a. Books
    b. Manuals
    c. Original research articles
    d. Encyclopedias

16. Which of the following is a secondary source of published literature?
    a. Dissertations
    b. Original research articles
    c. Anecdotes
    d. Conference proceedings

17. In published research literature, a primary source refers to
    a. The first author in a multi-authored study
    b. An article written by the people who conducted the study
    c. A report given by subjects who provided the data
    d. A clinical report on the effectiveness of primary care

18. Which of the following indexes is the most helpful in locating sources for a nursing research proposal?
    a. CINAHL (Cumulative Index to Nursing and Allied Health Literature)
    b. Hospital literature index
    c. International nursing index
    d. Nursing studies index

ANSWER KEY

1. c	2. a	3. d	4. a	5. d	6. b
7. d	8. b	9. b	10. c	11. d	12. d
13. a	14. a	15. c	16. d	17. b	18. a

UNIT 5

Theory and Conceptual Framework in Nursing Research

One of the reasons for conducting research in nursing is to develop a body of knowledge unique to nursing through generating or testing of theory. To develop such a body of knowledge, the research should be based on theoretical or conceptual framework that guides the research in a systematic and orderly fashion.

If the research study undertaken is based on a theory, it directs the nurse researcher to select and define basic concepts of the study, identify variables and determine relationships between variables. However, if the study is not based on theory, it limits both the use of research results in practice and the capacity to construct future research studies from the results. This justifies the argument that nursing research and practice should be theory based.

OVERVIEW OF THEORIES

The word "theory" is derived from the Greek word *theoria,* which denotes vision or speculation. Theories are always tentative and by no means regarded factual or valid. These theories describe and explain phenomena which can further be subjected to expansion or modification. If the theory is not supported by empirical evidence, it may even be discarded.

Definitions of Theory

A theory is a set of interrelated constructs, definitions and propositions that present a systematic view of phenomena by specifying relations among variables, with the purpose of explaining and predicting the phenomena.
—**Kerlinger, 1986**

Theory is an integrated set of defined concepts and propositions that present a view of a phenomenon. Theories can be used to describe, explain, predict or control the phenomenon. —**Burns and Grove, 2005**

Theory can also be defined as an organized set of interrelated statements or concepts that explain the relationship between variables leading to a better understanding of the phenomena.

Definitions of Nursing Theory

Nursing theory is a set of concepts, depositions and propositions that project a systematic view of phenomena by designating specific interrelationship among concepts for the purpose of describing, explaining, predicting and/or controlling phenomena.
—**Chinn and Jacobs, 1983**

Nursing theory is an articulated and communicated conceptualization of invented or discovered reality in or pertaining to nursing for the purpose of describing, explaining, predicting or prescribing nursing care.
—**Meleis, 1991**

Basic Elements of Nursing Theories

Nursing has identified its domain in a paradigm that includes four linkages. The four major concepts that describe any nursing theory are (Fig. 5.1):

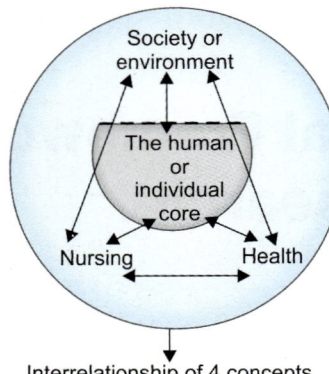

Fig. 5.1: Elements of nursing theories

1. The human or individual
2. Society or environment
3. Health
4. Nursing actions

Characteristics of Nursing Theories

George (1990) proposed various characteristics of nursing theories. George suggested that the nursing theories should:
- be logical in nature.
- include interrelated concepts in such a way that they facilitate a different perspective of the phenomena.
- provide a basis for hypotheses development and testing.
- be simple, yet generalizable.
- be consistent with other validated theories, laws and principles.
- increase general body of knowledge.

Purposes of Theories

Theories serve several purposes in the development of science and clinical practice:
- Theories provide a direction for actual research.
- They provide a meaning to isolated facts, observations and empirical findings.
- Theories pull together the results of observations allowing researchers to make general statements about variables and the relationships among variables
- Having a theoretical base for research study provides credibility and develops nursing knowledge.
- Theories provide the nurse with a sound basis to describe, explain and predict factors influencing nursing care.
- They provide professional autonomy and authority.
- Theories guide education, research and practice and distinguish nursing practice from other disciplines
- As a profession, it is only the development of theoretical knowledge based on research findings that can establish and nurture nursing practice.

Components of Theory

The theories are composed of concepts, constructs, propositions and models.

Concepts are not only the basic components but also the building blocks of theory. A concept is considered to be an abstract idea that is used to describe or identify phenomena.

It is a complex mental formulation of an object, property or event that is derived from individual perception and experience (Chinn and Jacobs, 1983, p. 200).

Concepts assist us in formulation of a mental image about the object or situation, help us to name things and occurrences in the world and assist us in communicating with each other about the world. Theories are formulated by linking concepts together. Concepts are said to be "empirical, inferential or abstract depending on their ability to be observed in the real world" (George, 1990) (Flowchart 5.1).

At a broad or high level of abstraction, a concept is known as a construct while at a narrow or more concrete level the concept is known as a variable.

Construct is a highly abstract, complex phenomenon that cannot be directly observed but must be understood by less abstract indicators of the phenomenon, e.g. wellness, self-esteem, assertiveness, etc.

Flowchart 5.1: Types of concepts

- **Empirical**
  - These are observed directly in the real world
  - For example: Size and color of the wound, edema, height of the patient bed
- **Inferential**
  - These are indirectly observed
  - For example: Pain, temperature
- **Abstract**
  - These are difficult to observe directly or indirectly and may have more than one meaning
  - For example: Stress, state of health

Once the concepts are thoroughly defined these then connected with statements about the expected relationship among themselves will be termed as propositions.

A proposition is a statement or assertion that may indicate a relationship between concepts. It is a structural element of theory. Based on the theorist's view, propositions are stated and concepts arranged together to indicate how one affects the other. Propositional statements can be described as the positive or negative relationship, direct or indirect effects or linear or nonlinear associations among concepts. For example, there is a positive relationship between stress and anxiety level; there is negative relationship between pain and quality of sleep; microorganisms cause diseases in human being.

In the above proposition, the concept of sleep is related to concept of pain which can be stated as "severe pain predisposes to sleeplessness".

Propositions are symbolically represented by *models*. These models help in explaining theory concepts using symbols and facilitate the understanding of concepts and their relationship. Theory focuses on propositional statements of the phenomena, while model emphasizes on components and structure of the phenomena.

"Models are the representation of the interaction among and between the concepts showing patterns" (George, 1990, p. 5).

Example: In agent-host-environment model, the concepts are agent, host and environment and a triad drawn among these concepts illustrates the model of agent-host-environment representing a relationship between these concepts.

Classification of Theories

Based on the complexity and level of abstraction in addressing the person, environment, health and nursing, the nursing theories are classified into grand theory, middle range theory and practice theory (Table 5.1).

Nursing theories can also be classified based on purpose as descriptive, explanatory and predictive theories (Table 5.2).

Development of Theories

Commonly two approaches are used in developing theories (Flowchart 5.2). The researcher may move from specific observations to theory (inductive reasoning) or from a theory to observations (deductive reasoning).

Inductive reasoning involves collecting observations that lead to development of hypothesis and later to theory. This approach begins with specific observations and moves to general statement that can be tested through research. In qualitative research approaches, inductive reasoning process is used.

Deductive reasoning generates the theory beginning with validation of an existing

Table 5.1: Classification of theories based on level of complexity/abstraction

Type of theory	Description	Level of complexity/abstraction	Examples
Grand theories	They attempt to explain broad areas and are applicable to all areas of the profession. They include numerous concepts that are not well defined and have ambiguous and unclear relationships. For empirical testing and theoretical verification, these grand theories need further simplification	It is the most complex and broadest in scope, not amenable to testing, provide foundation for a mid-range theory	• Dorothea E Orem's self-care deficit nursing theory • Sister Callista Roy's adaptation model • Martha Rogers' science of unitary and irreducible human beings
Middle range theories	These focus more narrowly on specific aspects of the profession and provide basis for generating testable hypotheses and have a strong relationship with practice and research	These theories are moderately abstract; contain clearly defined limited number of concrete variables. Variables are operationally defined in which the nature and direction of relationships are specified and organized within a limited scope	• Patricia Benner's model of skill acquisition in nursing • Merle H Mishel and Margaret F Clayton—theory of uncertainty in illness • Elizabeth R Lenz and Linda C Pugh—theory of unpleasant symptoms
Practice theories	These are also termed as prescriptive theories, situation-specific theories or micro theories. These theories describe, explain and provide an understanding of the patient experiences of the specific phenomenon. Practice theories can include a particular element of a specialty such as operating room nursing, obstetric nursing, mental health nursing, pediatric nursing, etc. These theories typically describe elements of nursing care and their impact	Compared to middle range theories, these are less complex, more specific and narrow in scope. They contain few easily understandable and measurable concepts limited to specific populations and explain a small aspect of reality	Riegel B and Dickson VV—a situation-specific theory of heart failure self-care

Table 5.2: Classification of theories based on purpose

Type of theory	Purpose	Type of research	Examples
Descriptive theories: They describe and classify specific characteristics of individuals, groups, situations or events. Example: Peplau's theory of interpersonal relations	These type of theories are put to use when very little is known about the phenomenon in question	To test descriptive theories, the researchers conduct descriptive research studies	Bond et al. (2011) conducted a study on "A univariate descriptive analysis of 5 years' research articles". This study used King's dynamic interacting system and goal attainment theory as an organizing framework because it includes three systems and their interactions. In the above study three systems included are individual nursing theory, integration of theory into scientific research and interaction of many theories to help build nursing's scientific knowledge
Explanatory theories: These specify associations among the dimensions or characteristics of individuals, groups, situations or events. Example: Watson's theory of human caring	These explain how the parts of phenomenon are related to one another and also to what extent do two or more characteristics tend to occur together	These theories are tested using correlational research	Munro (1983) conducted a study to find out the correlates of job satisfaction among recent graduates of nursing program. This study used Herzberg's theory of job satisfaction and dissatisfaction
Predictive theories: These propose to predict the precise relationships between the dimensions or characteristics of a phenomenon or differences between groups. *Example:* Orlando's theory of deliberative nursing process	These types of theories address cause and effect relationship and find out why changes occurred in the phenomenon	These theories are tested using experimental or quasi-experimental research designs	Ziemer (1983) conducted an experimental study to find out the effects of procedural, sensory and coping strategies information on postoperative coping behaviors. This study used theory of cognitive imagery

Flowchart 5 2: Development of theories

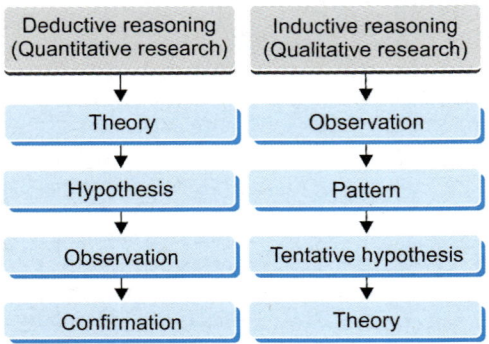

theory and moves to specific observations. It is an approach used to test predictions and validate existing relationships or theories. Specific hypothesis can be deduced from a theory that serves as a more general statement of interrelated phenomenon. These hypotheses are tested by research study. Deductive reasoning helps to reveal existing relationships.

The validity of nursing knowledge generated or theory developed through inductive and deductive reasoning depends on the accuracy of information. Conclusions are valid if statements on which they are based are valid.

Theory Testing in Nursing Research

Theory is a collection of concepts which are connected to each other by way of statements called propositions. Research hypotheses are derived from these propositions and tested by conducting research study to validate propositions in the underlying theory. This information contributes to the evidence in support of the theory and develops the science related to the concepts being studied.

THEORETICAL FRAMEWORK/ CONCEPTUAL FRAMEWORK

To develop a sound base of scientific knowledge to nursing, the research studies should be based on theory or conceptual framework. This enables the findings of the study to be positioned within the existing professional knowledge that provide a base to the nursing profession. The best approach to obtain a body of knowledge specific to nursing profession is by conducting research studies based on theory and develop on the work of other researchers who used the same theoretical base. Even a small research study turns out to be reasonably significant when the study findings can be added to those of others who have used the same theoretical frame. The terms "conceptual model" and "theoretical framework" are often used interchangeably, but a theoretical framework generally incorporates at least a part of the specific theory as the basis for the study.

The *theoretical framework* is a collection of interrelated concepts that depicts pieces of theory to be examined as a base for research studies. It describes relationships between the concepts based on an existing theory.

A theoretical framework often includes propositional statements describing the relationships among variables and has received more testing than the more tentative conceptual model (Polit and Beck, 2004).

Some theoretical frameworks used in nursing:
- Interpersonal theory: Peplau (1988)
- Health promotion model: Pender (1987)
- Goal attainment theory: King (1981)
- Self-care deficit theory: Orem (1991
- Theory of unitary human beings: Rogers (1970)
- Adaptation theory: Roy (1984)
- Systems model: Neuman (1972)
- Conservation model: Levine (1973)

CONCEPTUAL MODELS

A conceptual model is an identical conceptual framework made up of concepts and propositions that state the relationship between the concepts. These concepts are abstract in nature and are not readily observable in the real world. Person, environment, health and nursing are general concepts identified in nursing models. At the beginning of the research project, the researcher should thoroughly review the literature and identify the theoretical or conceptual framework for the study.

A *conceptual model* is defined as a set of abstract and general concepts that are assembled to address a phenomenon of central interest.

A conceptual model or theoretical framework provides a coherent, unified and orderly way of predicting related events or processes relevant to a discipline (Fawcett, 2005).

Compared to theories the conceptual models are loosely structured, but provide a framework for communicating a particular perception of the world and put specific ideas or notions into a meaningful framework for viewing the world.

Importance of Using a Conceptual/Theoretical Framework to Guide a Research Study

The Indian Nursing Council and Nursing Departments of various Universities have made the use of conceptual and theoretical frameworks mandatory to guide nursing research and incorporate them in research reports for the award of certificates and degrees.

Utilization of conceptual or theoretical framework might involve the use of already existing theories or conceptual models as basis or guide for the study to generate predictions that could be tested empirically (Akpabio and Ebong, 2010).

The use of theoretical or conceptual framework as basis for the research study has following advantages:

1. Guides the research process from the formulation of research question, design selection, to interpretation of findings.
2. Provides skeleton for the research study which serves as a source for principles, assumptions and ideas to frame the study design and methods (Hanson, 2011).
3. Guides in testing hypotheses based on the assumptions of the theory.
4. Places the research findings within the realm of existing professional knowledge which provides a base for the nursing profession.
5. Interprets the research findings based on conceptual framework (Radwin and Fawcett, 2002; Polit and Beck, 2004).
6. Makes practical application of study findings easier.
7. Enables the researcher to merge the facts together such that the interpreted relationship would direct practice.
8. Allows the researcher to build upon one another's work thereby building a body of knowledge (George, 2009).
9. The research findings have broad significance and utility as well as relevant assumptions to direct the study (Kaiser, 2009).
10. The relationship between theory and research is reciprocal and a mutually beneficial one. Theory guides the research study by helping the researcher in understanding the study concepts, their relationships with each other and provides framework to conduct study. Research helps in developing and testing theory.
11. Kaiser (2009) highlighted the use of theories in research as follows:
    - To help in identification of meaningful and relevant areas for study
    - To develop or refine the study
    - To define the concepts and propose relationships between them
    - To provide general framework for data analysis
    - To interpret research findings
    - To generate nursing diagnosis and guide implementation of findings
    - If the research is conducted in isolation of the relevant theory, it results in

disconnected information which does not add to the accumulated knowledge of the discipline

Identification, Selection and Development of Conceptual Framework in Nursing Research

- While conducting a research study, selecting an appropriate conceptual model or theoretical framework is an important step as it provides guidance to the researcher.
- The nurse researchers can use either nursing or non-nursing theories or conceptual frameworks to provide a conceptual context for the study.
- Akpabio and Ebong (2010) state that before selecting theoretical or conceptual frameworks, there is a need to evaluate the different theories or frameworks available within the selected area of interest.
- The selected conceptual model should provide adequate description of its constructs and provide guidance and base for the research study.
- The concepts contained in the framework or theory should be clearly identified, defined and the relationships between variables clearly stated to bring about their meanings.
- The relationships among the variables in the conceptual framework or theory should then be used as a guide to identify and relate variables in the study.
- The assumptions and beliefs reflected in the framework or theory should be identified and clearly stated and also used to guide the development of assumptions in the study.
- In addition, the researcher should identify and clearly state how the concepts and assumptions in the theory or framework are applicable to the research study through justification on the relationships among variables in the theory as well as those in the research.
- For a descriptive or exploratory research study, the theory or model should be descriptive in nature; for a correlation study, the explanatory theory or model can be adopted; while for experimental or quasi-experimental studies, predictive theories or models should be chosen (Polit and Hungler, 2014) (Table 5.2).
- To develop conceptual framework, the researcher should have knowledge of theories, related field experience and be aware of findings from previous studies on similar topics. He or she should have the skill to identify and establish the relationship among two or more study concepts, conceptualization of abstract ideas and ability of linking these abstract ideas with logical scheme to generalize the facts.
- Researcher should also have the inductive and deductive reasoning abilities to develop conceptual framework.
- The conceptual model or framework fits in both quantitative and qualitative research studies. In quantitative research, the conceptual framework is developed or identified at the beginning of the study which then leads to the formulation of hypotheses which are later tested (Flowchart 5.3). In qualitative research study, the conceptual framework or theory may evolve as data are gathered in the field (Flowchart 5.3). Conceptual framework emerges after the research is complete.
- Kaiser (2009) outlined measures to be considered while applying conceptual framework in research study (Box 5.1).

Steps in the Application of Conceptual Framework/Theory in Research

Stember (2015) provided systematic and comprehensible steps for application of conceptual framework in research. Initially the researcher should search the literature for suitable theories and examine for appropriateness and select the theory that

Flowchart 5 3: Conceptual framework in quantitative and qualitative research

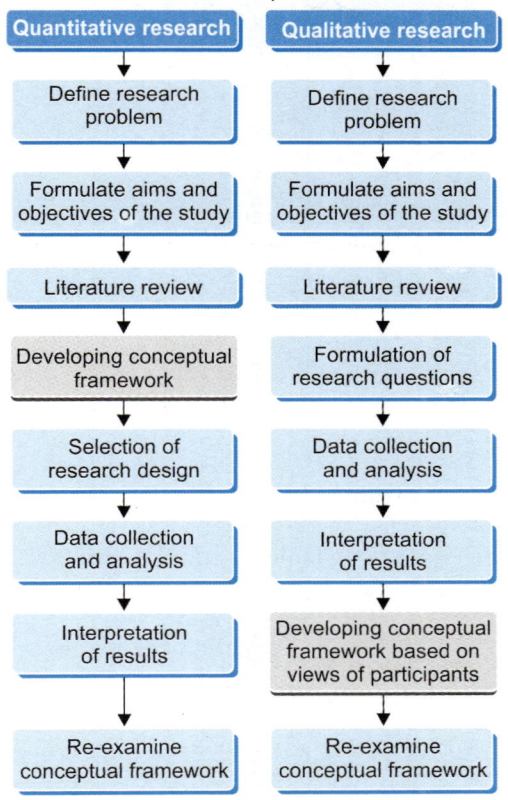

| Box 5.1 | Measures to consider while applying conceptual framework in research study |

- The selected research problem should fit into the chosen framework to lead and enhance the study results
- The strengths and weaknesses or limitations of the framework must be identified and addressed where possible
- The conceptual definitions should be construed from the framework
- The data collection tools should be matching with the framework
- The findings of the research study should be interpreted based on the framework
- Implications derived from the study should be based on the framework

will guide and direct the research process. The description of various steps is presented in Table 5.3.

Research study example 1: Mock et al. (2007) conducted a study on effect of exercise on fatigue and physical functioning in cancer patients which used theoretical framework based on Levine conservation model. This model was used to guide investigation of exercise intervention to lessen cancer-related fatigue among cancer patients. Levine conservation model was adopted for the above study because it included principles that help explain cancer-related fatigue and support exercise as a potential intervention for fatigue (Fig. 5.2). Levine conservation model proposes general mechanism underlying biobehavioral symptoms, such as fatigue that necessitates a response or adaptation from the individual to maintain unity and integrity (Levine, 1996). According to Levine, the goal of an individual is conservation or preserving an integrated and balanced whole person (Levine, 1973). The concepts included are energy, social integrity, personal integrity and structural integrity.

Research study example 2: Rentala S (2013) conducted a study to evaluate the efficacy of body-mind-spirit (BMS) intervention on process of recovery and well-being among depressive patients. The theoretical framework for this study was based on integrative body-mind-spirit (IBMS) model which was developed as a holistic approach that ties Eastern philosophy and its practical techniques to Western forms of therapy. It focuses on the mind-body-spirit relationship, recognizes spirituality as a fundamental domain of human existence. The goal is for healing and capacity building. This model was used to guide evaluation of holistic intervention to improve process of recovery among depressive patients. The concepts included in IBMS model are engaging, nurturing, shifting, integrating and transforming. Applications of IBMS model concepts in research study are presented in Table 5.4 and Figures 5.3 and 5.4.

Table 5.3: Steps in development of conceptual framework—Levine conservation model

Steps	Description	Examples
Identification of concepts	Initially the researcher identifies the general concepts of the study. These concepts may be based on previous research findings, real life observations or experiences, existing theories or models.	In the above study, variables are fatigue, sleep disturbance, physical functioning, emotional distress, quality of life and social functioning.
Establishing relationship between concepts	Researcher gathers relevant information from the existing theories and previous research findings to establish relationship between concepts. Gathering relevant information about concepts enables the researcher to judge the amount of empirical support the theory has received.	• There is a significant relationship between changes in levels of physical functioning and fatigue, difficulty in sleeping, emotional distress, quality of life and social functioning. • Regular exercise decreases fatigue, sleep disturbance and emotional distress as well as increases physical and social functioning and quality of life.
Formulate hypotheses	Based on the relationship among variables (propositions), the researcher formulates hypothesis.	• Cancer patients receiving radiation therapy or adjuvant chemotherapy who participate in a regular exercise program demonstrate significantly higher levels of quality of life, physical and social functioning compared to similar patients who do not participate in regular exercise. • The amount of change in physical functioning from baseline to post exercise program was correlated with the amount of change in level of fatigue, difficulty in sleeping, emotional distress, quality of life and social functioning.
Select instruments	Based on the framework, researcher selects instruments that are used to measure variables or concepts.	• Conservation of energy was represented by variables fatigue and sleep. While fatigue was measured by modified Piper Fatigue Scale (Piper et al., 1998), quality and quantity of sleep were measured by the Pittsburgh Sleep Quality Index (Buysse et al., 1989). • Conservation of structural integrity was represented by physical functioning and this variable was measured by pedometer and accelerometer (measures steps taken and speed movement); self-perceived physical functional ability was measured by physical functioning subscale (Ware and Sherbourne, 1992).

Contd...

Contd...

Steps	Description	Examples
		• Conservation of personal integrity was represented by the study variables—emotional distress and quality of life. While emotional distress was measured by the Profile of Mood States Scale (POMS), quality of life was measured by Medical Outcome Study (MOS) 36-item Short-form Health Survey (SF-36). • Conservation of social integrity was represented by social functioning and was measured by MOS SF-36 social functioning subscale. • The exercise intervention tested in this study included the conservation of energy component within the Levine model in which the focus is on balancing the individual's energy resources with energy expenditure.
Describe the findings	Study findings are explained based on the theory.	• During the cancer treatment, patients with regular exercise exhibited lower fatigue level compared to patients without regular exercise. These lower fatigue levels were a result of energy conservation. • Patients with regular exercise improved in functional capacity compared to nonexercisers. This improvement in functional capacity was attributed to conservation of structural integrity. • Regular exercises presented lower mood distress scores and higher quality of life scores. This improvement was attributed to conservation of personal integrity. • Regular exercisers presented improved social functioning scores compared to nonexercisers. This improvement was attributed to conservation of social integrity.
Take decision	Based on the results, a decision is taken about whether the theory is supported by the results of the study or not. Based on the theory identify implications of the study results. Make recommendations for future research to include use of theory.	Levine conservation model proved to be a useful organizing framework for the study of a nurse-directed exercise intervention to manage fatigue in cancer patients.

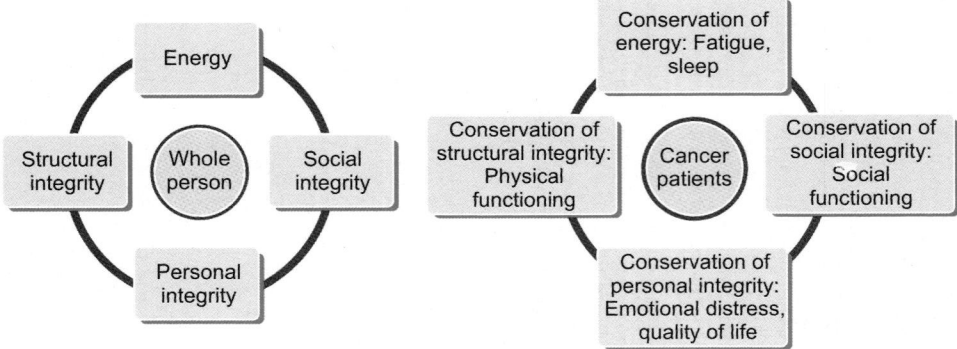

Fig. 5.2: Application of Levine conservation model—conceptual framework concepts and study variables

Table 5.4: Application of integrative body-mind-spirit (IBMS) model to research study		
IBMS concepts	Description	Application to research study
Nurturing	IBMS model is about facilitating unconditional self-acceptance and self-appreciation, as well as an education on techniques in nourishing the body, mind and spirit.	In the present study, nurturing activities include self-love techniques, ten techniques of longevity, hand massage techniques, mindful meditation. All these activities nurture the body-mind-spirit.
Shifting	It is believed that problems arise because of disconnection or stagnation in one or more of the physical, mental, or spiritual domain, or the disconnection or imbalance between the domains. Therefore, facilitating reconnection is the first subcomponent of BMS intervention.	In the present study, shifting represents change from negative affect to positive affect, reconnecting physical, mental and spiritual health with various nurturing activities. The activities include connecting the participants to immediate somatic experiences recognizing the emotional strength and internal resources.
Integrating	It involves anchoring of learning and integrating changes in the physical, mental, spiritual domains into the total being of the self.	In the context of present study, integration represents integrating all these nurturing activities in the day-to-day life to improve physical, mental and spiritual health. The integration activities included in the present study are developing action plan, practicing self-affirmative techniques, homework exercises, practice sessions, daily spiritual practices (meditation, mindfulness, etc.), group discussion, etc.
Transforming	Transforming intervention helps participants to search for their idiosyncratic meaning and purpose in life, to enhance their ability to embrace pain and live in the moment, and to deepen connection with the authentic self and the transcendence. The individuals expand into higher levels of consciousness and decide to transform the role and identity from victim to survivor, or even advocate for the betterment of the other people.	In the present study, transforming intervention includes encouraging the subjects to verbalize experiences and growth, appreciation of their self-capacity to accommodate suffering, accepting pain rather than eliminating pain. During this phase, participants develop purpose in life and accept reality.

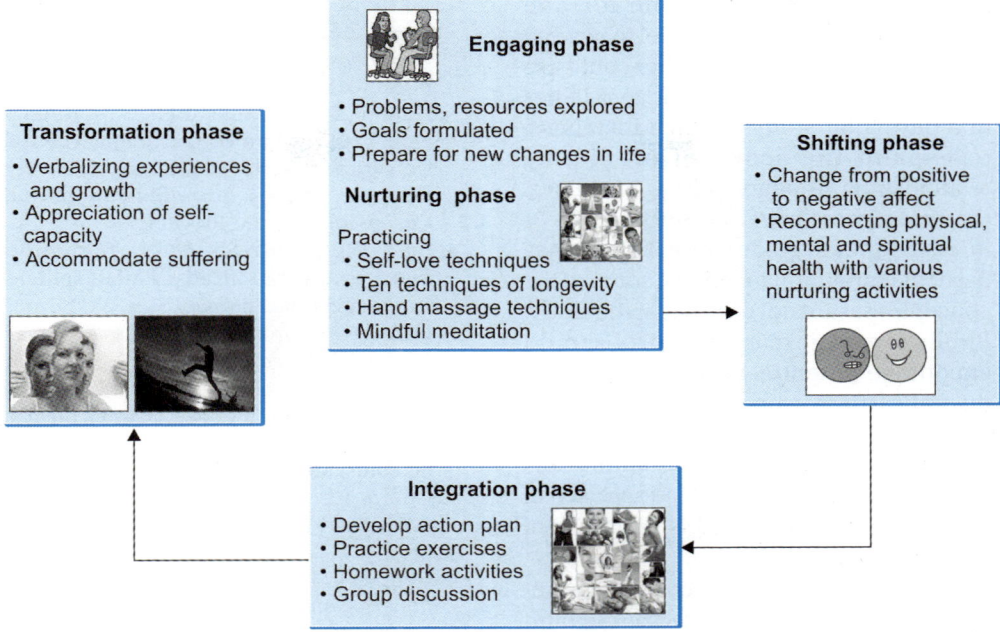

Fig. 5.3: Application of IBMS model

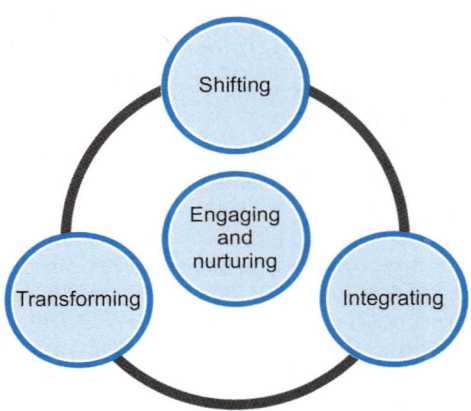

Fig. 5.4: Components of integrative body-mind-spirit (IBMS) model

Challenges associated with Utilization of Conceptual Framework/Theory in Nursing Research

In 2010, Akpabio and Ebong listed challenges associated with use of conceptual or theoretical framework. These are as follows:

❖ Many researchers lack adequate knowledge regarding theories and how to apply them in nursing research.
❖ Limited knowledge in understanding concepts of theories, lack of skills in explaining relationship among variables based on theoretical framework.
❖ Inability to identify and understand assumptions within the model and relate them to the research variables.
❖ Inadequate skills in evaluating the conceptual framework for strengths and weaknesses.
❖ Lack of interest in applying a model to guide a research study.

Overcoming the Challenges

❖ There is a need for the researcher to strengthen interest towards the application of conceptual or theoretical framework. Interest could motivate the desire and improve skills necessary in applying theories to guide studies.

❖ Sometimes, it is impossible for one theoretical framework or model to have all the concepts that the researcher could use to predict relationships among variables in a particular study. In such instances, to expand the scope of predicting relationships among variables in studies, the researchers usually combine two or more theories to guide a research and pay particular attention to remove some of the concepts that are not relevant in the study.

❖ Publishers of research reports should encourage potential authors to include theoretical frameworks in research reports submitted for publications. This helps readers to understand interrelationships among variables and assumptions used in the study, thus making implementation of research findings easier.

Once a theoretical or conceptual framework is selected, it should be used throughout the study. This means that it should guide the entire research process.

Critiquing the Theoretical Framework

❖ Is the theoretical framework clearly defined?
❖ Is the theoretical framework consistent with purpose of the study?
❖ Are the concepts clearly and operationally defined?
❖ Do they reflect the area of investigation?
❖ Is the theoretical basis for hypothesis formulation clearly articulated?
❖ Are the relationships among propositions clearly defined?
❖ Is the instrument used to measure the variables consistent with the theoretical framework?
❖ Are the study findings related to the theoretical rationale?

BIBLIOGRAPHY

1. Akpabio, I.I., & Ebong, F.S. (2010). *Research Methodology and Statistics in health and behavioral sciences.* Calabar: University Printing Press.
2. Barbara, R. (2008). A situational specific theory of heart failure self-care. *Journal of Cardiovascular*, 23(3), 190-196.
3. Bond, A.E., Eshah, N.F., Bani-Khaled, M., Hamad, A.O., Habashneh, S., Kataua, H., et al. (2011). Who Uses Nursing Theory? A Univariate Descriptive Analysis of Five Years' Research Articles. *Scandinavian Journal of Caring Sciences*, 25, 404-409.
4. Burns, N., & Grove, S.K. (2001). *The practice of nursing research* (4th ed.). Philadelphia: WB Saunders Publications.
5. Burns, N., & Grove, S.K. (2005). *The Practice of Nursing Research: Conduct, Critique and Utilization* (5th ed.). St. Louis, MO: Elsevier.
6. Chinn, P.L., & Kramer, M.K. (2011). *Integrated knowledge development in nursing.* (8th ed.). St. Louis: Mosby.
7. Chinn, P.L., & Jacobs, M.K. (1983). *Theory &Nursing: A systematic approach.* St. Louis: Mosby.
8. George, J. (1990). *Nursing Theories: The Base for Professional Nursing Practice.* Norwalk, Connecticut: Appleton & Lange.
9. George, J.B. (2010). Nursing Theories-The base for professional Nursing Practice (5th ed.). Upper Saddle River, N.J.: Prentice Hall.
10. Kaiser, P. (2009). *Nursing Research and Theories.* Retrieved on 12 November, 2014 from http://www.currentnursing.com/nursingtheory/r.
11. Kerlinger, F. (1986). *Foundations of behavioral research* (3rd ed.). New York: Holt, Rinehart & Winston.
12. Ketefian, S. (2001). *Issues in the application of research to practice.* St. Louis: Elsevier-Mosby.
13. Levine, M.E. (1973). *Introduction to Clinical Nursing* (2nd ed.). Philadelphia, PA: FA Davis.
14. Levine, M.E. (1996). The conservation principles in nursing: a retrospective. *Nursing Science Quarterly*, 9, 38–41.
15. Meleis, A.I. (1991). *Theoretical nursing: development and progress* (2nd ed.). Slough: Lippincott.
16. Mock, V., Ours, C., Hall, S., Bositis, A., Tillers, M. et al. (2007). Using a Conceptual model in nursing research: Mitigating fatigue in cancer patients. *Journal of Advanced Nursing*, 58(5), 503-512.
17. Munro, B.H. (1983). Job satisfaction among recent graduates of school of nursing. *Nursing research*, 32(6), 350-355.

18. Polit, D.E., & Hungler, B.P. (2014). *Doing your research project: A guide for the first time researchers.* Retrieved on 12 February 2015 from http://books.google.com.ng/books?isbn=0335264476.
19. Polit, D.F. and Beck, C.T. (2004) Nursing Research: Principles and Methods. 7th Edition, Lippincott Williams & Wilkins, Philadelphia.
20. Radwin, L., & Fawcett, J. (2002). A conceptual model based program of nursing research: retrospective and prospective applications. *Journal of Advanced Nursing,* 40(3), 355-60.
21. Riegel, B., & Dickson,V.V. (2008). A situation-specific theory of heart failure self-care. *Journal of cardiovascular nursing,* 23(3), 190-196.
22. Rentala, S. (2013). *A study to evaluate the efficacy of Body-Mind-Spirit (BMS) intervention on process of recovery and wellbeing among depressive patients* (Doctoral dissertation, Rajiv Gandhi University of Health Sciences, Bengaluru, Karnataka).
23. Stember, M. (2015). *Theoretical framework. A little bit about frameworks.* Retrieved on 13 February 2014 from http://users.Ipfw.edu/Stember/339/framework.html
24. Younas, A., & Sommer, J. (2015). Integrating nursing theory & process into practice. *International journal of caring sciences,* 8(2), 443-490.
25. Ziemer, M. M. (1983) Effects of information on post-surgical coping. *Nursing Research,* 32(5), 282-287.

REVIEW QUESTIONS

I. Long Essay
1. What is conceptual framework? Explain advantages of using conceptual framework in a research study. Describe steps in development of conceptual framework with suitable research study.

II. Short Essays
1. Conceptual framework
2. Characteristics of theory
3. Role of theory in nursing research

III. Short Answers
1. Theory
2. Model
3. Concepts
4. Constructs
5. Propositions

IV. Multiple Choice Questions
1. Nursing has used theories from
   a. Sociology
   b. Psychology
   c. Anthropology
   d. All of the above
2. Grand theory means
   a. Most complex and broadest in scope
   b. Moderately abstract
   c. Prescriptive theories
   d. None of the above
3. Which of the following is a building block of theory?
   a. Concept
   b. Construct
   c. Theoretical propositions
   d. All of the above
4. The word theory is derived from which of the following words?
   a. Theoria
   b. Theorium
   c. Theoretia
   d. Theoryia
5. It is a set of abstract and general concepts that are assembled to address a phenomenon of central interest termed as
   a. Conceptual model
   b. Theoretical propositions
   c. Grand theory
   d. Meta theory

ANSWER KEY

| 1. d | 2. a | 3. d | 4. a | 5. a |

UNIT 6

Research Approaches and Designs

A research approach or method is a general framework guiding the research study that includes broad assumptions, methods of data collection analysis, and interpretation. It depends upon the nature of the research problem being investigated. There are three basic methodologies or approaches used in any research, viz. qualitative, quantitative, or mixed methods.

Research design is a specific outline detailing how chosen method or approach will be applied to answer a particular research question. It is a framework used for the planning, implementation and analysis of the research study intended to connect the conceptual research problem to the achievable empirical research. It has two levels. The first level is concerned with the decisions on what evidence is needed to answer the research problem. The second level concerns with methods of collecting evidence (what type of data, what method of data collection, what sampling strategy, and so on) (Flowchart 6.1).

MEANING AND DEFINITION

Research design is a blueprint or master plan specifying the methods and procedures for conducting a research study involving the description of research setting of the study, sample size, sampling technique, tools and methods of data collection, and analysis to answer specific research questions or test the research hypothesis.

On the whole, a research design is a plan to investigate a research problem covering description of all methods and materials that have a bearing on the quality of evidence the study yield.

Flowchart 6.1: Levels of research design

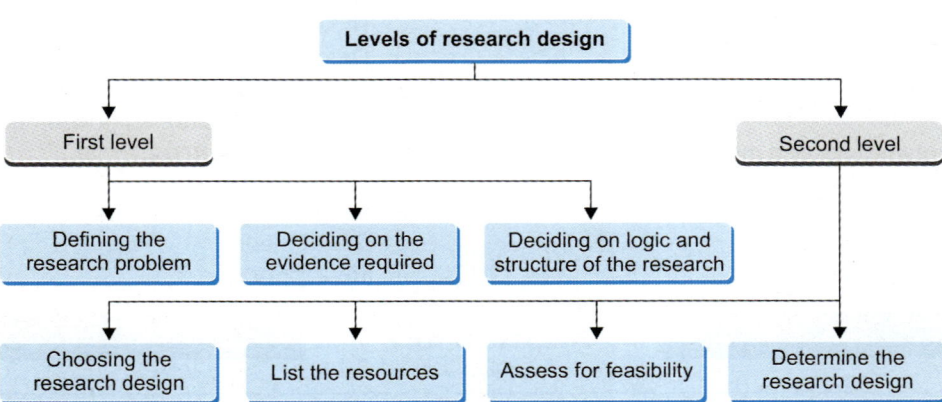

A research design includes strategies and methods for data collection and analysis to meet the research purpose.

Research design is "a plan that describes how, when, and where data are to be collected and analyzed" (Parahoo, 1997).

PURPOSE OF A RESEARCH DESIGN

The main purpose of a research design is that it:
- Allows smooth implementation of various research processes, making research efficient with minimal outlay of resources.
- Guides the researcher in planning and implementing the study in a way to answering the research question.
- Helps the researcher to arrange the ideas in a systematic way so as to get a glimpse of flaws and inadequacies.
- Specifies the controlling mechanisms that will be used in the research study. The control provided by the design increases the probability that the study results are accurate reflection of reality.
- Provides a set of instructions to the researcher regarding study setting, sample size and techniques, time period, selection of variables, tools and methods of data collection, data analysis, and style of research report preparation.
- Research design has a great bearing on the reliability of the results arrived and constitutes a firm foundation for the entire structure of the research work. Preparation of research design should be done with great care as any error in it may upset the entire research process.

CHARACTERISTICS OF A QUANTITATIVE RESEARCH DESIGN

A quantitative research design must always build on previous findings. The main characteristics of a research design are presented in Figure 6.1.

- **Appropriateness to the research problem:** A research design should be appropriate to the research question and usually involve the consideration of the following factors: the methods of obtaining information, skills of the researcher and availability of time and money for research work.
- **Controls extraneous variables:** The best design should control extraneous variables, i.e. isolate the variables that are under the study from all other variables and measure them accurately, so that the collected data are reliable and valid.
- **Lack of bias:** It is an influence that produces a distortion in the study results. Bias can occur either during designing the research or selection of subjects or data collection or the analysis phase.

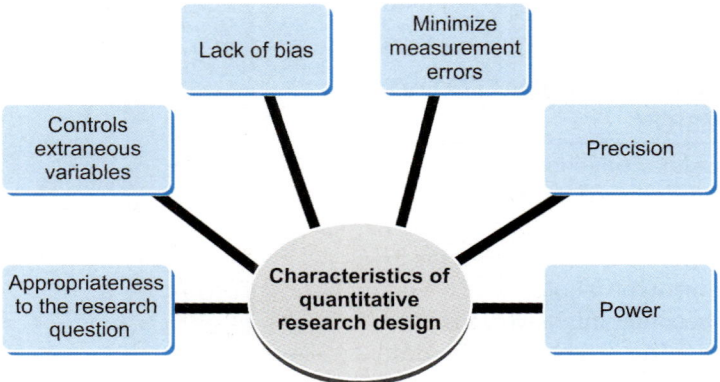

Fig. 6.1: Characteristics of quantitative research design

Selection bias in quantitative research can be reduced by randomization and double-blind procedures while in qualitative research observer's bias can be reduced by triangulation method.

- ❖ **Minimize measurement errors**: The best design should minimize the measurement errors.
  - ○ If the purpose of the study is to explore or discover the ideas and the insights, the design should be flexible enough to include the different aspects of the phenomenon.
  - ○ If the purpose of the study is to describe the phenomena, the design should minimize bias and maximize the reliability of the evidence collected.
  - ○ If the research study involves the testing of hypothesis of a causal relationship between variables, the design should permit inferences about causality in addition to the minimization of bias and maximization of reliability.
- ❖ **Precision**: In research design, precision refers to an ability to obtain the most accurate effect of treatment variable on an outcome variable. It can be achieved through the use of precise measuring tools and a design that controls over extraneous variables.
- ❖ **Power**: It is the ability of the research design to detect the relationship among variables. Power increases when a large sample is used.

CHARACTERISTICS OF A QUALITATIVE RESEARCH DESIGN

- ❖ Uses various data collection strategies
- ❖ Is flexible, rather than tightly predicted
- ❖ Takes place in natural setting
- ❖ Tends to be holistic, determined for an understanding of the whole
- ❖ Researcher becomes intensively involved
- ❖ Requires ongoing analysis of the data to formulate subsequent strategies and determine when data collection needs to be completed.

KEY ELEMENTS OF RESEARCH DESIGN

Research design describes methods and materials used to investigate the research study keeping in view the objectives of the research and availability of resources. The key elements of research design are presented in Figure 6.2.

- ❖ **Research problem**: The first step in the research process is the selection of research problem. It is also the most important step as the further steps depend on this selection of the problem. Hence, the research design should include a clear statement of the research problem.
- ❖ **Approaches and methods**: It should include research approaches (qualitative, quantitative, or both), description of population, subjects, sample, sampling techniques, variables, time duration, setting of the study, intervention, comparisons, controls for extraneous variables, communication with the subjects.
- ❖ **Data collection methods**: One of the elements of research design includes measures and methods used for gathering

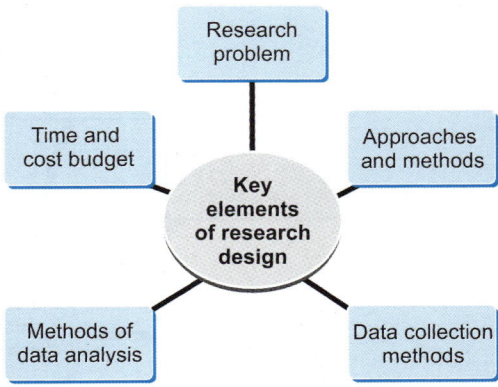

Fig. 6.2: Key elements of research design

data. It comprises of tools and methods of data collection (questionnaire, observation, interview, etc.), time and location of data collection and study setting.
- **Methods of data analysis**: It must include a plan for data analysis and methods (quantitative or qualitative data analysis techniques) used in processing and analyzing the data.
- **Time and cost budgets**: The time and cost budgets are important components of research design as these are two of the constraints under which most research is done.

SELECTION OF RESEARCH DESIGN

A number of considerations influence the selection of research design. The researcher should select the most appropriate design to meet the objectives of the study. Selection of research design is influenced by several factors. Some of them are listed in Figure 6.3.

Current Knowledge of the Research Problem

- The choice of a research approach depends to a great extent on the nature of the research problem that has been identified. Quantitative approaches are appropriate when the purpose of the study is to find out the effect of an intervention (evaluating the effect of spiritual intervention on depression among cancer patients), test the relationship between the variables (correlation between well-being and spirituality among cancer patients), or describe a phenomenon with precision (determining the incidence of depression among fourth stage cancer patients).
- Qualitative approaches are appropriate when the purpose of the study is to understand the meaning of a phenomenon about which little is known (understanding the spiritual needs of end-stage cancer patients).
- A mixed method is appropriate when a combination of meaning and control is needed. Frequently, this method is used when a qualitative approach is used to design an instrument (development of spiritual needs assessment tool using qualitative interviews) or an intervention that is subsequently tested for effectiveness by using quantitative methods (assessment tool is used to measure the spiritual needs of cancer patients).

Knowledge and Experience of the Researcher

- Researchers' knowledge and experience play a key role in the selection of research approach. A researcher with scientific

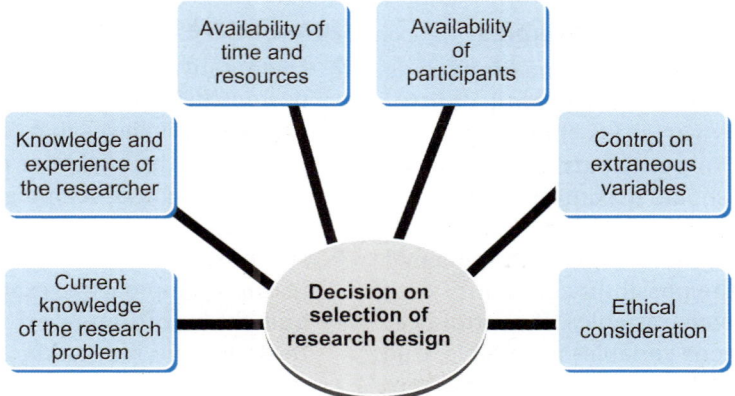

Fig. 6.3: Factors influencing the selection of research design

knowledge, skillful in scientific writing, familiar with statistical packages, and quantitative journals would most likely select a quantitative design.
- On the other hand, a researcher efficient in conducting interviews, making close observations, and writing narrative descriptions prefers the qualitative approach.
- If the researcher is efficient in both qualitative and quantitative methods, he would prefer the mixed methods research.

Availability of Time and Resources

- Resources like equipment, facilities, and support from colleagues are important for conducting research. Availability of resources for a research study affects the selection of research design.
- Time is also an important factor in selection of a research design. For example, longitudinal studies require more time than cross-sectional studies do.

Availability of Participants

The selection of research design may be influenced by number and availability of study subjects. If only few subjects are available with specific characteristics, a qualitative research approach may be selected. On the other hand, if a large sample is available, the researcher can select quantitative research.

Control on Extraneous Variables

- An efficient design can maximize true results, decrease error, and control extraneous variables that may affect outcome. To get accurate results, the researcher should maximize control.
- The selection of research design is either true experimental or quasi-experimental based on the possibility of control over the extraneous variables. If control over the extraneous variables is possible, true experimental designs can be chosen. However, if the researcher is unable to control the selected extraneous variables, quasi-experimental designs can be selected.

Ethical Considerations

- These include respect for participants, informed consent, and protection from harm.
- The consideration of ethics may affect the selection between an experimental design and a nonexperimental design.

DECISION ON SELECTION OF RESEARCH DESIGN

- Make a written list of the pros and cons of each design
- Balance the factors involving time, cost, ethical issues, and integrity of the study
- Anticipate alternative research findings and consider whether design adjustments might affect the results
- Seek the advice of research experts
- Write out a rationale for design decisions

TYPES OF RESEARCH DESIGNS

Different types of research designs cater to different types of questions or hypothesis. They are often classified as quantitative or qualitative or mixed designs. Various types of research designs are presented in Flowchart 6.2.

Quantitative Research Designs

- Quantitative research designs rely on the postpositivist paradigm philosophy. This philosophy believes that causes probably determine the effects or outcomes and emphasizes on developing and testing of theories.
- Postpositivists normally use deductive reasoning approach to examine the cause and their influence on the outcome. In deductive reasoning approach, the researcher selects the theory or framework where concepts have already been

Flowchart 6.2: Types of research designs

Types of research designs

- **Quantitative research design**
  - Nonexperimental design
    - Based on purpose:
      - Descriptive
      - Correlational
    - Based on time of data collection:
      - Cross-sectional
      - Longitudinal
    - Based on time of event being studied:
      - Retrospective
      - Prospective
  - Experimental design
    - True experimental
      - Post-test only control group design
      - Pre-post-test control group design
      - Solomon four group design
      - Crossover design
      - Factorial design
      - Randomized block design
    - Quasi-experimental
      - Nonequivalent control group pre-postdesign
      - After only nonequaivalent control group design
      - One group pre-postdesign
      - Time series design
- **Qualitative research design**
  - Ethnography
  - Phenomenological design
  - Grounded theory approach
  - Historical research
  - Case study design
- **Mixed method design**

reduced to variables. These variables are then tested to support the theory.
❖ Quantitative research is designed to collect numerical data, which can be transformed to usable statistics for answering research question or hypothesis.
❖ Quantitative research designs are well structured and specify the research methodology in detail which includes sample characteristics and selection, setting, nature of intervention, tools to measure the variables, methods used to control extraneous variables, time and type of data collection, methods used for data collection, and information to be shared with the participants.

Flowchart 6.3: Schematic diagram depicting the selection process in research design

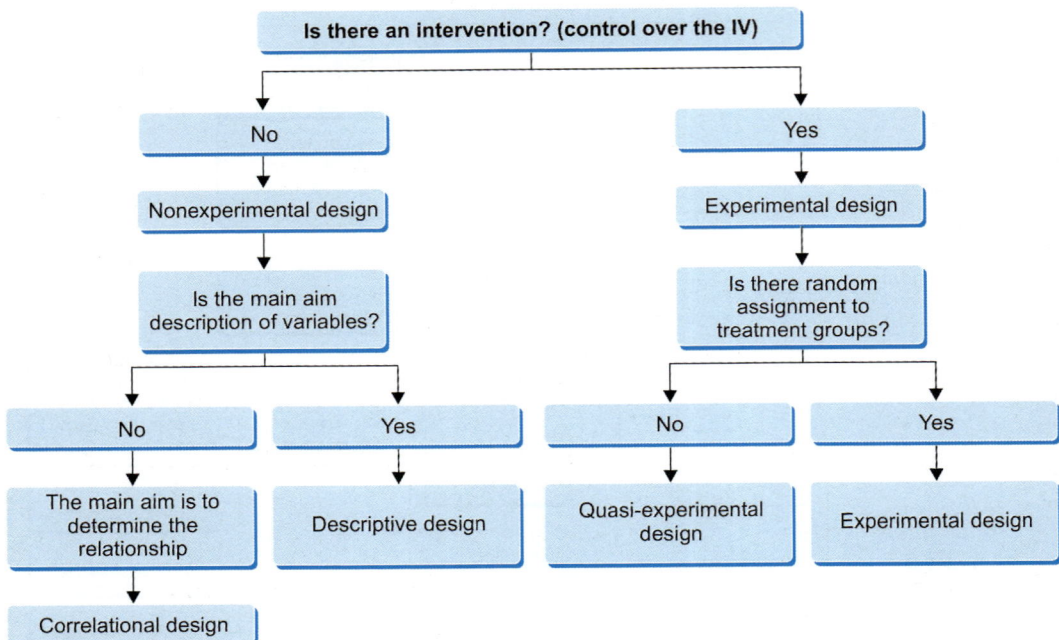

Types of Quantitative Research Designs

A variety of research designs are used in nursing research, which are categorized differently by different authors. According to Dickoff and James (1968), the four most commonly used types are: (1) descriptive, (2) correlational, (3) quasi-experimental, and (4) experimental research designs. While descriptive and correlational designs are referred to as nonexperimental designs, quasi-experimental, and true experimental research designs are referred to as experimental designs. Flowchart 6.3 helps in the selection process of research design.

NONEXPERIMENTAL DESIGNS

- ❖ Nonexperimental designs focus on examining variables, as they naturally occur in the environment and not on the implementation of a treatment by the researcher.
- ❖ Nonexperimental designs describe, differentiate, or examine associations among the variables.
- ❖ These designs do not use control groups, manipulation of independent variable, or random assignment of sample to the groups, as it only employs observation.
- ❖ This type of research is also a rich source of data that helps the researcher to formulate questions for use in experimental or quasi-experimental designs.

Reasons for undertaking nonexperimental designs

- ❖ In many instances, some variables are not amenable to experimental manipulation or randomization (height or gender).
- ❖ In some instances, no control over the independent variables is possible as they have already occurred.

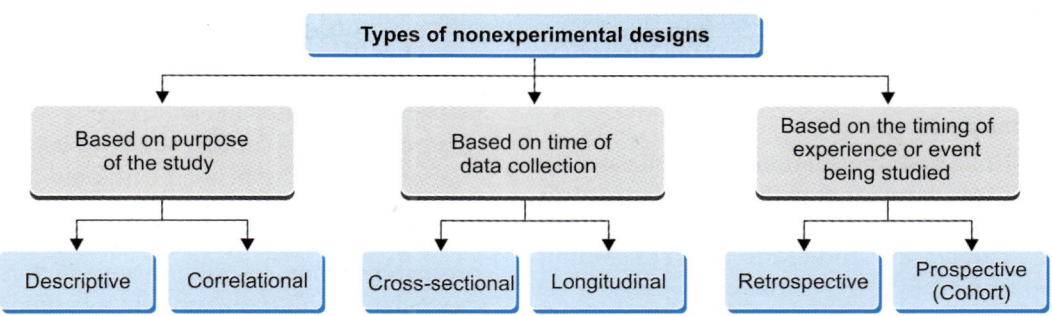

Flowchart 6.4: Types of nonexperimental designs

- At times, there are practical constrains or ethical considerations to manipulate variables.
- To get a realistic understanding of the phenomena as it exists in the natural setting, the researcher deliberately chooses not to manipulate the variables.

Types of nonexperimental designs: The three basic categories of nonexperimental designs are presented in Flowchart 6.4.

Classification based on purpose of the study: Based on the purpose of the study, non-experimental designs can be classified into either descriptive or correlational.

1. DESCRIPTIVE OR EXPLORATIVE DESIGNS

The main aim of descriptive research is the accurate depiction of individual characteristics, events, or groups and the frequency of occurrence of phenomena using statistics to describe and summarize the data (Polit and Hungler, 2013).

The purpose of descriptive research is the exploration and description of phenomenon in real life situations. It describes what actually exists, determines the frequency of occurrence, and categorizes the information. Instruments used to obtain data in descriptive studies include questionnaires, interviews (closed questions), and observations (checklists, etc.). Sample subjects are chosen who represent the population at large. No attempt is made to explain or predict what the situation might be in future or how it might change. In a descriptive design, bias can be controlled through:

- Conceptual and operational definitions of variables
- Sample selection and size
- Use of valid and reliable instruments
- Following appropriate procedure in data collection

Purposes

- These designs are used to develop theories, identify problems and trends in illness
- Explore new areas of research
- Describe situations as they exist in the world
- Provide knowledge base for other types of quantitative research methods

Thus, descriptive studies can provide valuable evidence regarding disease prevalence, nature, and intensity. In nursing, the only way to understand the beliefs and values of different individuals and groups is by describing them. This descriptive knowledge helps in developing nursing interventions that benefit individuals, families, or groups so as to obtain desirable and predictable outcomes.

Advantages

- More flexible and broad in scope
- Can focus on range of topics and also applicable to any population

- Great deal of information can be obtained from a larger population
- Its methodology can be explicitly stated making it easier to evaluate and replicate

Disadvantages
- Collected information is superficial. The breadth rather than depth of information is emphasized.
- Large-scale studies are time consuming and costly.

Types of Descriptive Designs

Descriptive designs can be classified into typical descriptive, exploratory, and comparative descriptive designs (Flowchart 6.5).

Flowchart 6.5: Types of descriptive design

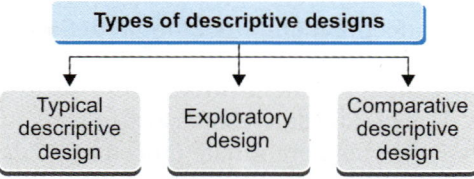

- *Typical descriptive design*: This design is used to examine variables in a single sample, which includes identifying the variables, measuring the variables, and describing them. Schematic presentation of typical descriptive design is presented in Figure 6.4.
  Example: A study to assess the pain experiences among patients with rheumatoid arthritis. In this study, the researcher describes the intensity and frequency of pain among patients.
- *Exploratory design*: This design is used to explore related factors of the existing phenomenon in order to enhance the understanding of the less understood phenomena. This includes identifying the variables and related factors, measuring frequency of occurrence and describing them with an in-depth explanation. Schematic presentation of exploratory design is presented in Figure 6.5.
  Example: An explorative study to assess various factors associated with pain and coping measures among patients with rheumatoid arthritis. In this study, the researcher may describe various factors associated with pain and related coping mechanisms, measure those factors and provide an in-depth explanation.
- *Comparative descriptive design*: In this design, two or more groups are compared on the basis of selected variables. This includes measuring the differences in variables occurring naturally between the two or more groups and comparing them on selected variables. Schematic presentation of comparative descriptive design is presented in Figure 6.6.
  Example: A comparative study on pain symptoms among male and female patients suffering with rheumatoid arthritis.

2. CORRELATIONAL DESIGNS

It involves the analysis of two variables to describe the strength and direction of the relationship between them. These studies are used to answer questions about relationships or associations. Correlational research assesses the inter-relationships among study variables without any active intervention by the researcher (Polit and Hungler, 2013).
- These designs are used to examine relationships between or among, two or more variables in a single group without any intervention.

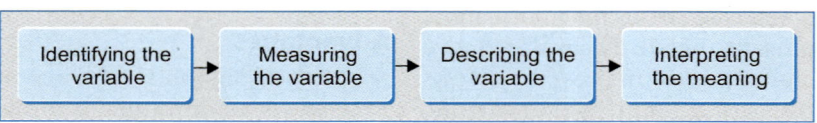

Fig. 6.4: Schematic presentation of typical descriptive designs

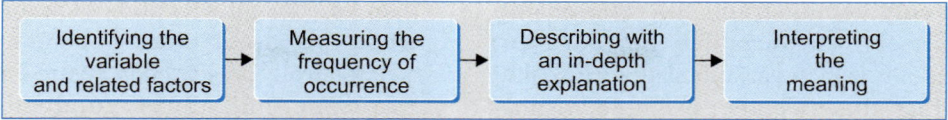

Fig. 6.5: Schematic presentation of exploratory design

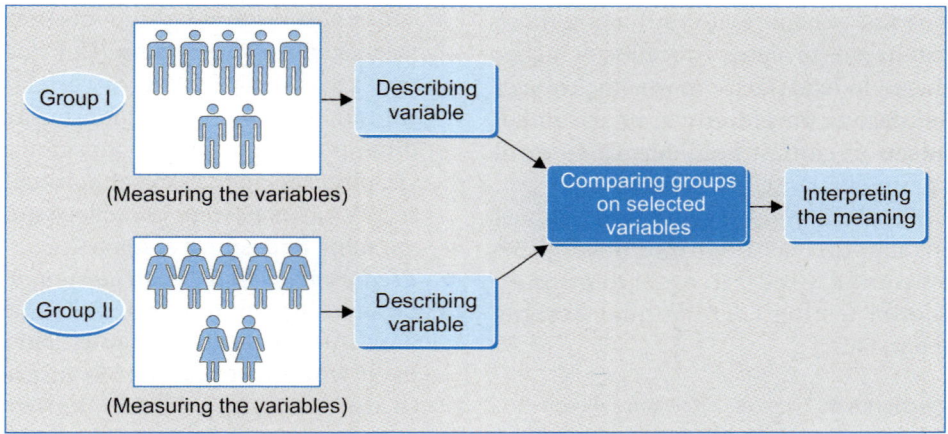

Fig. 6.6: Schematic presentation of comparative descriptive design

- Correlational designs are usually cross-sectional.

Purposes

- These designs study whether changes in one or more variables are related to changes in another variable (covariance).
- Correlations assess direction and degree (magnitude and strength) of the relationships, or associations among variables.
- Hypotheses are generated from correlational study results, which are tested by quasi-experimental and true experimental studies.

Advantages

- Efficient means of collecting a large amount of data about a problem and discover a large number of inter-relationships in a relatively short period of time.
- Correlational research usually takes place in a natural setting and thus better suited to solve practical problems in everyday life.
- Relatively uncomplicated to plan and implement.
- The researcher has the flexibility in exploring the relationships among variables.
- Demonstrates strength and direction of a relationship between the variables, which helps the researcher to narrow down on the findings and determine cause-and-effect relationship by conducting experimental studies.

Disadvantages

- These studies lack randomization and control between the variables. Thus they are susceptible to faulty interpretation of relationships.
- As correlation research only uncovers a relationship and cannot manipulate variables of interest, causality cannot be established, i.e. it cannot provide a conclusive reason for why there is a relationship.

- It only demonstrates the relationship between the variables, but does not explain, which variable is the cause and which the effect. For example, a study demonstrated that education and wealth are highly correlated. However, the study does not explain whether having more wealth leads to higher education or higher education leads to more wealth. Though the reasons for either can be assumed, causation cannot be determined until experimental research is done.

Types of correlational designs: Correlational designs can be classified into descriptive correlational, predictive correlational, and model testing correlational designs (Flowchart 6.6).

Flowchart 6.6: Types of correlational designs

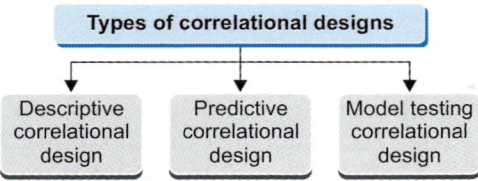

- *Descriptive correlational design*: These designs describe variables and examine the relationship among themselves. This facilitates identification of many inter-relationships in a situation. Researchers do not make any attempt to control or manipulate the situation. In these studies, variables must be clearly identified and defined conceptually and operationally. Descriptive correlational design is schematically presented in Figure 6.7.
  Example: Ahuja (2014) conducted "a correlational analysis of physical, mental, emotional, spiritual, social, and self-consciousness among students pursuing teacher education program". This study is a nonexperimental descriptive correlational study that looks at the relationship among different dimensions of consciousness, viz. physical, mental, social, spiritual, and self. Participants were 135 college students pursuing BEd course at Agra.

- *Predictive correlational design*: These designs attempt to explore what factors may influence an outcome. They are used when a researcher is interested in determining whether knowing a previously documented variable can lead to the prediction of a later variable. These are sometimes called regression studies based on the statistical test used for analysis. The variable to be predicted is termed as the dependent variable while the other is termed as independent or predictor variable. It attempts to predict the level of the dependent variable from the measured value of the independent variable.
  Example: In the following study, self-care behavior (dependent or outcome variable) could be predicted by depressive symptoms of agitation and loss of energy

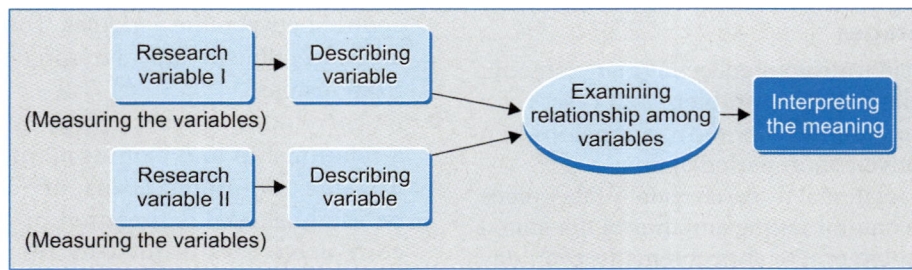

Fig. 6.7: Schematic presentation of descriptive correlational design

(independent variable or predictors) (Fig. 6.8).

Coyle (2012) conducted a predictive correlational study to determine if depressive symptoms were predictive of self-care behaviors in adults who had suffered a myocardial infarction. The results found that depressive symptoms of agitation and loss of energy were significantly predictive of self-care performance in myocardial infarction patients.

Independent variables that are most effective in prediction are highly correlated with the dependent variable but not with other independent variables in the study.

In predictive correlational study, variables are proposed by a theory-based mathematical hypothesis, which is expected to predict the dependent variable effectively. Regression analysis is then used to test the hypothesis.

These studies are tremendously useful in nursing practice because their results can be used to identify early indicators of complications, disease, or other negative outcomes facilitating preventive action.

* *Model testing correlational design:* These studies examine proposed relationships for a model or theory, i.e. hypothesize on how various elements in the patient care environment interact, how these variables can be measured, and direct and indirect effects of variables on outcomes. A large heterogeneous sample is required to measure all the variables relevant to the model. The researcher identifies all the ways to express relationships between

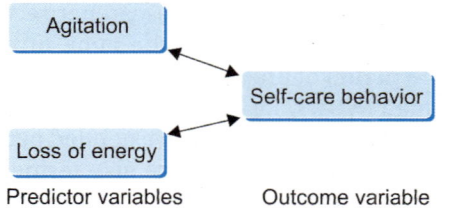

Fig. 6.8: Example of predictive correlational design

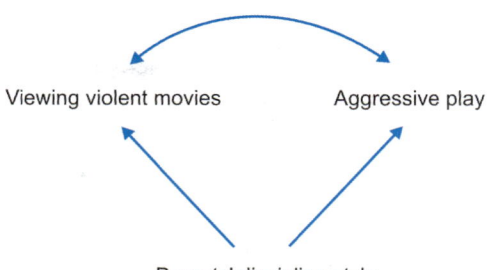

Fig. 6.9: Variables in model testing correlational design

concepts and develops a conceptual map. The analysis determines whether the data are consistent with the model.

Example: In the below presented model (Fig. 6.9), the relationship between aggressive play, viewing violent movies, and parents' discipline style is depicted. To test this model, the researcher assesses parents' discipline style, viewing violent movies behavior, and aggressive play (variables), and performs statistical analysis to determine whether the data are consistent with the model.

Classification Based on Time of Data Collection

Nonexperimental designs can be classified as either cross-sectional or longitudinal based on time of data collection.

1. CROSS-SECTIONAL DESIGN (DATA COLLECTED AT ONE POINT IN TIME)

Cross-sectional studies involve observing a single phenomenon across multiple populations at a single point in time without any follow-up for determining the relationship between variables (Fig. 6.10). This design is an observational one, meaning the researcher records information about the subjects without manipulating the study environment. This design is appropriate for describing the characteristics or status of a disease in a population and also relationships among risk factors and conditions at a time point.

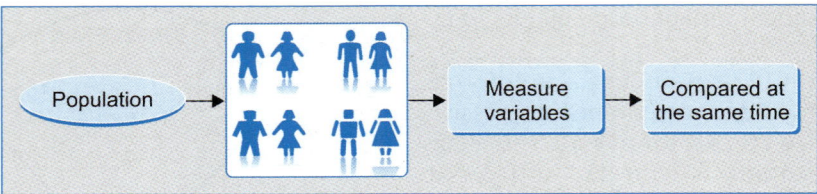

Fig. 6.10: Schematic presentation of cross-sectional design

Retrospective studies are typically cross-sectional, wherein exposure and outcome are measured at same time point, i.e. data on dependent and independent variables are collected simultaneously. In nursing, cross-sectional designs are used to understand the association between variables pertaining to individuals and their health status.

Example: In a study to assess the cholesterol level among daily walkers and nondaily walkers, the cholesterol level is assessed among two age groups and genders at one time between daily walkers and nondaily walkers. The study compared the cholesterol levels of daily and nondaily walkers among two age groups, i.e. over 40 and under 40, both in male and female categories at a given time point.

This cross-sectional study allows the researcher to compare the educational level, income and diet patterns in relation to walking and cholesterol level without any additional cost. However, it may not offer specific information about cause-and-effect relationships as such studies offer information at one single time point and do not consider what happened before or after the said time point. Therefore, the researcher is not sure, if the daily walkers had low cholesterol before the walking routine or daily walking helped them to reduce the previously high cholesterol level. The outcome in a cross-sectional study needs to be replicated using a longitudinal design to validate these differences and assure they are truly activity related.

Advantages

- Suitable for describing the phenomenon at a fixed time point
- Only one testing period is needed
- Less time consuming, inexpensive, and easy to conduct
- Large amounts of data can be collected at a single time point; the results are readily available
- Allows researchers to compare many different variables at the same time
- Confounding variables like maturation resulting from the elapsed time is not present
- Ethical, as it involves minimum risk to subjects
- These studies enable the exploration of health conditions affected by human development
- There is no loss of subjects due to study attrition

Disadvantages

- Cause-and-effect relationship cannot be established
- As different individuals are involved, the personal characteristics may differ
- Cannot study the dynamics of the phenomenon over time

2. LONGITUDINAL DESIGNS (DATA COLLECTED AT MULTIPLES TIME POINTS)

In a longitudinal design, researcher records numerous observations of the same subjects over a period of time, which at times may last for many years, i.e. the data is collected at multiple time points over an extended period. Therefore, these studies are also termed as repeated measures or cohort studies. These designs study the changes in the phenomenon over time and describe the chronology of phenomenon for establishing causality. Collection of data at multiple time points strengthens causal inferences. In longitudinal studies, the nature of the study and available resources decide the number of data collection points and the time intervals between them. When the changes in the phenomenon are rapid, frequent data collection points with relatively short intervals may be required to understand the trend. These studies usually focus on nonclinical population.

Example: A study to assess the effect of daily walking on cholesterol level among men and women included 40-year-old daily walkers and nondaily walkers. The study assessed the initial cholesterol level and followed up for 20 years to find out the daily walking effect on cholesterol level.

These designs are also used for follow-up studies of a clinical population to assess the subsequent status of people with a specified condition or who received a specific intervention (Fig. 6.11).

- *Example 1*: A longitudinal study to assess the cognitive development among Down syndrome infants. In this study, infants with Down syndrome were assessed for cognitive development and later followed up for 18 years to assess the subsequent cognitive development.
- *Example 2*: A longitudinal study to assess the incidence of cardiovascular diseases among individuals. In this study, diabetics and nondiabetics were followed up for 5 years and the results compared to know the incidence of cardiovascular disorders.
- *Example 3*: A longitudinal study to assess the effect of holistic relapse prevention intervention among individuals with alcohol dependence. In this study, the subjects received holistic relapse prevention and were followed up for 1 year to know the relapse status.

Advantages

- As same subjects are followed throughout the study, the personal factors are same
- Can study dynamics of phenomenon over time
- Can document a causal factor and preceded outcome, hence strengthening hypothesis about causality.

Disadvantages

- As research takes years to complete, the probability of subject drop out (attrition) is high
- The effect of testing may influence the result
- Expensive

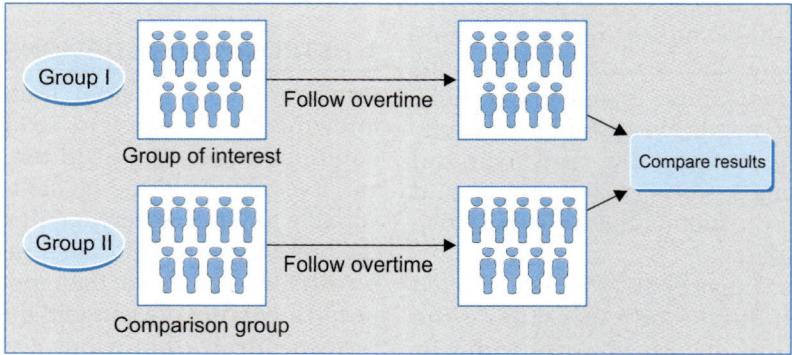

Fig. 6.11: Schematic presentation of longitudinal study

Types of longitudinal studies: Longitudinal studies can be classified into three types: (1) trend (2) panel and (3) follow-up studies (Flowchart 6.7).

Flowchart 6.7: Types of longitudinal studies

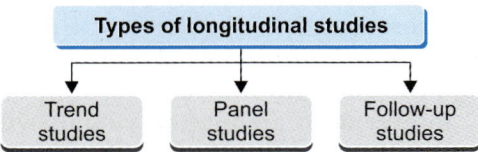

- *Trend studies*: In such studies, different samples are selected at repeated intervals from the same population and studied overtime with respect to the phenomenon. These studies allow the investigators to study the patterns and rates of changes overtime and predict future developments based on previous patterns.
  Example: Analyze the number of students entering nursing program to forecast future supplies of nurses.
  Hasson D et al. (2010) conducted a 4-year longitudinal study on trends in self-rated health among nurses to find out the transition from nursing education to working life. The aim of the study was to monitor the self-rated health (SRH) among nurses, beginning from the final semester at the university till they entered working life.
- *Panel studies*: The term panel refers to sample of subjects who are the source of data. In these studies, the same sample supplies the data at various time points. As the same sample is studied over time, the researchers are in a position to identify the subjects "who did" and "who did not change" over a period of time and examine the factors that sets these two groups apart.
  Example: Tanya et al. (2006) conducted a longitudinal study to examine the influence of changes in work conditions on stress outcomes as well as influence of changes in stress outcomes on work conditions. This study used panel design with a time interval of 3 years. The sample consisted of 381 hospital nurses with different functions, working at different wards. Same set of nurses were assessed for stress outcomes at different intervals for 3 years and working conditions compared with stress levels.
- *Follow-up studies*: These are undertaken to find out the subsequent development of individuals who have a specific problem or who have received a special intervention.
  - *Example:* Kremer (2014) conducted a study to assess longitudinal spiritual coping with trauma in people with HIV. This 10-year study examined how people with HIV use spirituality to cope with life's trauma on top of HIV-related stress.
  - *Example:* Brown et al. (2014) conducted a longitudinal study to evaluate the effectiveness of group-based self-management treatment for HIV patients. This study assessed the longitudinal changes in spirituality and optimism after participation in group-based HIV intervention.

Classification based on timing of event being studied: Nonexperimental designs can be classified as either retrospective or prospective based on timing of the experience or the event being studied.

1. RETROSPECTIVE DESIGNS

Retrospective (Ex post facto—is from after the fact) means the study has been conducted subsequent to the dependent variable being affected by the independent variable and the researcher attempts to link the present events with the past events. The researcher collects the data on an outcome occurring in the present and then linking it retrospectively to previous circumstances (Fig. 6.12). Retrospective studies are typically

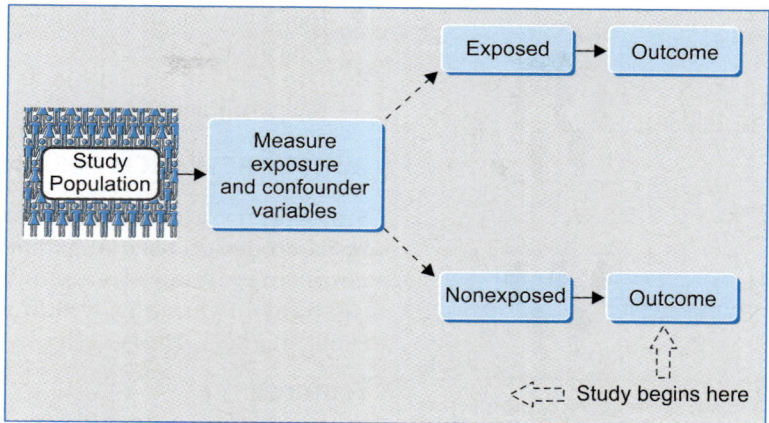

Fig. 6.12: Schematic presentation of a retrospective study

cross-sectional, i.e. data about both present outcomes and past events and occurrences are collected at a single time point.

Example: A retrospective correlational study was conducted among alcoholic liver cirrhosis patients to find out alcohol consumption pattern. In this study, dependent variable cirrhosis of liver had already occurred. Here, the researcher collects the alcohol consumption pattern and links it to the present diagnosis.

Features

- ❖ The study proceeds backwards from effect to cause
- ❖ Both exposure and outcome have occurred before the start of the study
- ❖ It uses the control or comparison group to approve or disapprove the inference

Advantages

- ❖ Less time consuming, inexpensive, and easy to conduct
- ❖ No risk for subjects
- ❖ Several etiological factors can be studied at the same time
- ❖ Ethical, as it involves minimum risk to subjects
- ❖ Can cover extended past periods without losing subjects in less time
- ❖ Can investigate rare conditions
- ❖ Risk factors can be identified
- ❖ Prevention and control programs can be established

Disadvantages

- ❖ Study depends on the respondents memory and knowledge
- ❖ Validation of collected information is difficult
- ❖ Selection of control group is difficult
- ❖ Cause-and-effect relationship cannot be established
- ❖ Not suitable for evaluation of intervention

2. PROSPECTIVE DESIGNS

This study begins with identification of presumed cause (alcohol consumption) and goes further in time to observe the presumed effects (cirrhosis of liver). Prospective studies are those in which data are collected about events as they occur moving forward in time. The researcher initially collects the data about presumed cause (independent variable) and subsequently the effect on outcome is measured (occurrence of dependent variable) (Fig. 6.13). These studies though similar to longitudinal studies, not all prospective studies are longitudinal and vice-versa. For example, intervention studies are prospective in nature, i.e. the researcher introduces the

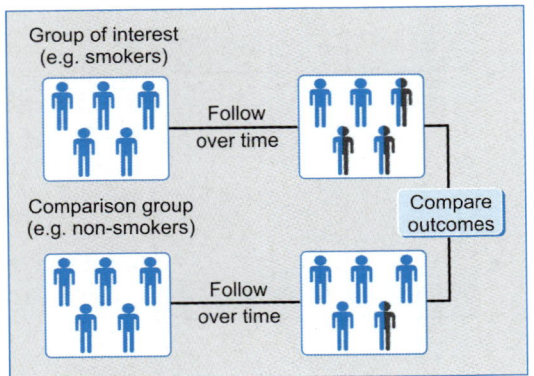

Fig. 6.13: Schematic presentation of prospective design

intervention and then determines its effect. The data collected 1 day after the intervention would be prospective but not longitudinal. Prospective designs yield better quality evidence than retrospective designs.

A good example for nonexperimental prospective study would be—a researcher wanting to assess the incidence of rubella during pregnancy and related malformations in the offspring. In this study, the researcher would begin with a sample of pregnant woman who have been infected with rubella disease during their pregnancy while others have not. Then, the subjects are subsequently followed up for the occurrence of congenital anomalies in their newborns.

Another example would be a researcher wanting to test the hypothesis that the incidence of smoking is related to lung cancer. In this study, the researcher would begin with subjects who have been smoking while others have not. Then, the smokers and nonsmokers are subsequently followed-up for the occurrence of lung cancer.

Advantage
- Collects specific exposure data.

Disadvantages
- Time consuming and expensive
- Repeated testing and changing environment threaten the study results
- Inefficient for investigating diseases with long latency periods
- Drop out of the subjects due to long follow-up period

SURVEY RESEARCH DESIGNS

Surveys are a form of nonexperimental research design used to gather information about prevalence, frequency, and interrelations of variables within a population (Polit and Beck, 2014).

Features
- Surveys tend to collect information pertaining to activities, beliefs, preferences and attitudes, actions, opinions, behaviors, awareness, and practices by usually asking the sample of people a few direct questions.
- Samples are selected from a defined population and data is collected at a particular time point.
- Collects data from various subjects within a defined population having similar characteristics.
- Mostly sample is selected by random sampling technique to ensure representativeness of the whole population to which the results will be generalized.
- Where the survey involves a sample—it is called sample survey and where the entire population is involved—it is called population survey such as census.
- Surveys may be conducted by phone, mail, or through personal contact with the subjects.
- Questionnaires and personal interviews are most commonly used data collection methods in survey research.
- In surveys, subjects may be studied using a cross-sectional or a longitudinal approach. In cross-sectional surveys, both exposure and outcome of events are studied simultaneously at one point in time. In longitudinal surveys, subjects are followed over an extended period of time.

❖ The tools used may be questionnaires or interview schedules. It is essential that these tools are reliable and valid.

Types of Surveys

Surveys can be classified based on both the basis of nature of phenomenon under study and methods of data collection (Flowchart 6.8).

Based on nature of phenomenon under study surveys can be classified as descriptive, exploratory, comparative, or correlational.

- ❖ *Descriptive survey*: It is carried out to describe the frequency of occurrence of a phenomenon.
  Example
  - A study to assess the perception and practice of selected contraceptive methods among target population in selected areas of Mumbai.
  - The survey of nurse's knowledge and attitude towards cancer pain management: Application of Health Belief Model.
- ❖ *Exploratory survey*: It is undertaken to describe the phenomena and find out the related factors about which much is not known.
  Example: An exploratory survey to assess the knowledge, practice, and prevalence of polycystic ovarian syndrome among women attending gynecology outpatient department (OPD) of selected hospital in Delhi.
- ❖ *Comparative survey:* It is undertaken to compare and contrast the existence of a certain phenomenon in two or more groups.
  Example: To compare the body-mass index of adolescent boys and girls.
- ❖ *Correlational survey*: It is undertaken to find out the relationship between two or more variables in a natural setting without manipulation or control.
  Example: Factors related to academic stress among adolescent girls: a descriptive correlational research study.

Based on methods of data collection, surveys can be classified as written, oral, and electronic.

- ❖ *Written survey*: Data is collected in a written form using structured questionnaires, opinionnaires, etc.
- ❖ *Oral survey*: Data from respondents is collected using face-to-face interviews or telephonic conversation.
- ❖ *Electronic survey*: Data is gathered using electronic means such as electronic mail messages (e-mails), web forms, and mobile short message services (SMSs), etc.

Advantages of Survey Design

- ❖ Survey design can be applied to different populations and topics

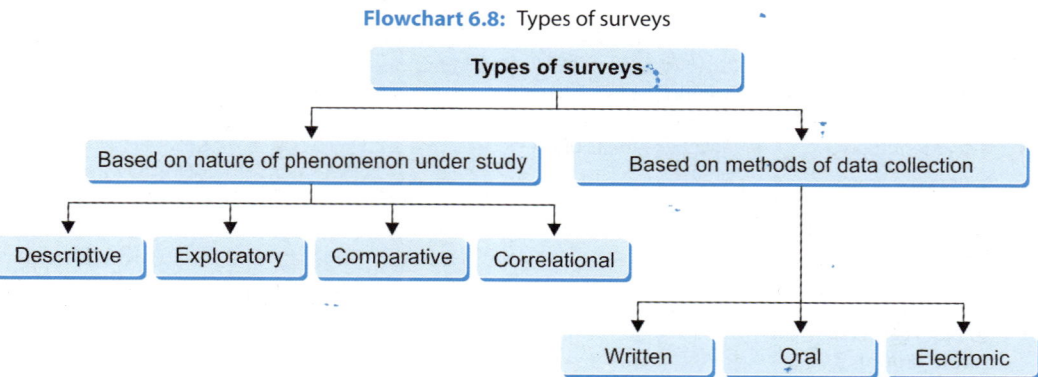

Flowchart 6.8: Types of surveys

- Broad in scope
- Economical way of gathering data
- Takes less time to conduct the study because they do not require follow-up

Disadvantages of Survey Design
- Tends to gather superficial data rather than probe in-depth.
- Cause-and-effect relationship cannot be established as information on both exposure and outcome is collected simultaneously, i.e. whether outcome followed the exposure or exposure resulted from the outcome.
- Self-reported responses may be unreliable as people may provide socially acceptable responses.

EXPERIMENTAL RESEARCH

Experimental research is an objective, systematic, and controlled investigation carried out to predict and control phenomena, wherein the researcher manipulates and controls one or more variables while observing the effect of manipulation on other variables.

VALIDITY OF EXPERIMENTAL DESIGNS

Study validity measures the truth or accuracy of the findings obtained from a study. The validity of the study's design is central to obtaining quality results and findings from a study. Strengths and threats to a study's validity provide a major basis for making decisions about which findings are accurate and might be ready for use in practice (Brown, 2014).

Shadish et al. (2002) described four types of validity:
1. Internal validity
2. External validity
3. Construct validity
4. Statistical conclusion validity.

Understanding these types of validity and their possible threats are important in critically apprising quasi-experimental and experimental studies. The different types of threats to validity are listed in Table 6.1.

Table 6.1: Types of threats to validity

Threats to internal validity	Threats to external validity	Threats to construct validity	Threats to statistical conclusion validity
• Selection bias • Attrition • History • Maturation • Testing • Instrumentation changes • Contamination • Compensatory rivalry • Compensatory equalization of treatment • Demoralization of control group	• Hawthorne effect (expectancy effects) • Novelty • Setting • Experimenter effect • Reactive effects of the pretest	• Inadequate definition of construct • Mono-operation bias	• Low-statistical power • Violated assumptions of statistical tests • Low reliability of the measures • Low reliability of intervention implementation

1. Internal Validity

Degree to which one can infer that the independent variable is truly causing or influencing the dependent variable and that the relationship between these two variables is not the effect of an extraneous variable (Campbell and Stanley, 1963). It is the extent to which changes in the dependent variable (effect) can be attributed to the independent variable (cause). To maximize the effectiveness of the results internal validity demands a strict control over the study. Any study can contain threats to internal validity. Threats to internal validity compromise researcher confidence in saying that a relationship exists between the independent and dependent variables. Some of the common threats to internal validity are selection bias, attrition (mortality), history, maturation, testing, instrumentation, contamination, compensatory rivalry, compensatory equalization of treatment, demoralization of the control group.

- *Selection bias*: If random selection of subjects or random assignments to groups is not followed in the study, the researcher will have difficulty in attributing causality to the experimental treatment. For example, subjects assigned to the control group would vary from subjects assigned to the experimental group. This variation in assignment could result in different reactions among groups to the treatment. In this case, the treatment would not have caused the difference in group outcomes. The researcher should take steps to ensure that subjects in all treatment groups are as similar as possible. Random selection and assignment will decrease the potential for selection to be a threat to validity.
- *Attrition (mortality)*: Attrition involves participants who drop out from the study before its completion. Subject attrition becomes a threat when:
  - There is a disparity between type of people dropping out of the experimental group or control group.
  - Subjects from one group have dropped out at a disproportionate rate.

  As the sample attrition rate increases, the remaining sample will be less representative of the target population. For example, in an experimental group, where subjects with severe depressive symptoms dropped out of the study at a greater rate than those in the control group, the average depression scores on the posttest for the experimental group might be unrepresentatively low. In this context, the researcher may erroneously conclude that the intervention is effective. The longer a study lasts, the greater is the chance for subject drop out. To overcome this threat, the researcher should make the participants realize the importance of their continued participation in the particular study.
- *History*: History is an event that is not related to the study but occurs during the span of the study, i.e. between pretest and posttest period. History could influence the responses of the subjects to the treatment and alter the outcome of the study. For example, the researcher is conducting a study on health education program regarding prevention of dengue fever. Around the same time, the subjects watch a television program on prevention of dengue fever. During the posttest, the subject's scores show an improvement. However, the researcher may not be able to determine whether the change in the knowledge scores is a result of the health education program or a result of watching the television program. This historical event could create a threat to the study's internal validity. History can be controlled by having a control or comparison group in the study.
- *Maturation*: In the research context, maturation relates to time and its effect on the study subjects. Long periods of

experimental research may lead to certain biological or psychological changes in subjects as a result of passage of time rather than effect of treatment or certain external events. These include physical growth, emotional maturity, fatigue, bodily changes, etc. For example, in a study where the researcher is evaluating the efficacy of medicated dressing on wound healing in postoperative patients, if the experiment is conducted over a period of time, it is difficult to evaluate whether the effect on wound healing is due to dressing or maturation (natural healing). A comparison group helps control for this threat.

- *Testing (reactive effects of the pretest)*: In a research context, testing refers to the effect of pretest on subject's performance in posttest. Subjects who take a pretest in an experiment may learn from their testing experience, which will improve their posttest performance on the dependent variable. Pretesting might also alter the subject's sensitivity or responsiveness to the dependent variable. If comparison group is not included in the study, it is difficult to study the testing affect, i.e. segregate the effects of pretest on posttest. Solomon four-group design is used to isolate pretest intervention effects on intervention.

  For example, in subjects who take the IQ test the second time, the score results in a 3–5 point increase than in those taking it the first time. This is due to the pre-test cues about the posttest.

- *Instrumentation changes*: Threat to internal validity can be due to alteration in the precision of the instrument or the investigator's ratings rather than a result of the experimental treatment. The investigator may record observations inaccurately due to fatigue. For example, if the researcher used one weighing scale at pretest and a different weighing scale at follow-up or if the same measuring tool yields less accurate measures at posttest compared to pretest, it could bias the results. Instruments like thermometer, weighing scale, blood pressure (BP) measurements, etc. should be checked for accuracy at regular intervals and same instruments or tools should consistently be used throughout the study to minimize instrument-related errors. Training sessions for investigators and check for fatigue factors may also help control instrumentation changes.

- *Contamination*: It occurs when the control group is exposed to some of the treatment given to the experimental group. For example, while testing the efficacy of exercise program on weight loss, if some of the control group subjects are exposed to experimental group treatment during the study period, the effect of the experimental program may be obscured.

- *Compensatory rivalry*: Subjects involved in the study may want to produce the best possible outcome for the investigator. In this scenario, subjects receiving no treatment may try to perform as well as the subjects in the treatment groups. This would obscure the differences between groups.

- *Compensatory equalization of treatment*: Researcher involved in an experimental study may feel the need to compensate for the lack of treatment benefit in the control group. Accordingly, he may provide an alternative type of care to the control group that equalizes the benefit, thus obscuring the effect of the experimental treatment.

- *Demoralization of control group*: The control group subjects who realize that they are not receiving the desired treatment become unhappy about it. They may exaggerate their illness symptoms while the true differences may be much lower.

2. External Validity

It is concerned with the extent to which study findings can be generalized beyond the sample used in the study (to other settings or samples) (Shadish et al., 2002). Single studies have narrow generalizability, whereas multiple replications of a study using different samples from different populations in different settings have broader generalizability.

If the study has external validity, the researcher may argue that the intervention is applicable to other populations and in other settings. Threats to external validity compromise researcher confidence in stating whether the study's results are applicable to other groups. Some of the common threats to external validity are Hawthorne effect (expectancy effects), novelty, and setting.

- *Hawthorne effect*: The Hawthorne effect is the tendency of the study participants to modify their behavior merely because they are aware of being observed. The change in the study outcome is related to its mere monitoring as subjects are aware that researcher is interested in that outcome. For example, in a study conducted by Dr Amici et al. (2000), the investigator informed the preoperative patients that they are being involved in a research study and thus would be closely monitored in the postoperative period for complications and pain levels. These patients were likely to report lower levels of pain and other complaints compared to control group patients (those consented for surgery in routine manner). This effect can be controlled using double-blind experiment. In this, neither the researcher nor the research participants are aware of the group to which they belong.
- *Novelty*: When a treatment is new, the subjects and researcher might change their behavior in various ways. They may either be enthusiastic or watchful towards the new treatment method. Results may reflect reactions to novelty rather than to intervention. Once they are familiar with the treatment, the results might get altered.
- *Experimenter effect (Rosenthal effect)*: It refers to a phenomenon where the interviewer attributes influence the respondent's answers. For example, interviewer's gender, attire, and appearance may influence study participants' responses in nonexperimental studies.
- *Setting*: It is essential for the researcher to consider the setting in which the study is conducted. There may be significant differences between the study setting and other settings where the researcher wants to apply the results. For example, people residing in hilly areas have higher hemoglobin levels (Hb) as requirement of oxygen is more at higher altitudes, due to which there is greater production of red blood cells (RBCs). However, the Hb level of people living on the plains is lower in comparison; so a generalization for people in hilly areas does not apply to people living on plains.

3. Construct Validity

Construct validity examines whether conceptual definitions and operational definitions of variables fit together. Threats to construct validity include inadequate definition of constructs, mono-operation bias.

- *Inadequate definition of construct*: A deficiency in the conceptual or operational definitions leads to low construct validity.
- *Mono-operation bias*: Mono-operation bias occurs when the researcher uses only one method of measurement to assess a construct. This one method of measurement assesses few dimensions of the construct, which may lead to under representation of the constructs of interest. If the researcher uses more measures, the construct validity will improve. For example, if pain were a dependent

variable, it could be measured by more than one measure such as verbal reports of pain, observation of behavior that reflect the pain, and pain rating scale. This leads to validity with pain.

4. Statistical Conclusion Validity

Statistical conclusion validity is concerned with whether the findings about relationship between variables or differences between the groups derived from statistical analysis accurately reflect the real world. False findings cause threats to statistical conclusion validity. These are of low-statistical power, violation of assumptions of statistical tests, low reliability of the measures, and low reliability of intervention implementation.

- *Low-statistical power*: Statistical power refers to the ability of the design to detect differences, if at all they exist in reality. Low-statistical power increases the probability of concluding that there are no significant differences between samples while an actual difference exists (Type II error). This type of error is most likely to occur when sample size is small. Adequate statistical power is achieved by using a large sample size.
- *Violated assumptions of statistical tests*: Many statistical tests, such as "t" test and "ANOVA", rely on the outcome data to be normally distributed that is to fall under a bell-shaped curve. Others such as a chi-square require an appropriate distribution between "condition present" and "condition absent". Empty cells in a 2 × 2 table are difficult to analyze. Forcing statistical tests onto inappropriate data can generate findings that are not true.
- *Low reliability of the measures*: Measuring tool must be reliable to reveal true differences. The measurement is reliable, if the tool provides the same result for the variable each time it is measured. For example, a depression scale is reliable, if it gives similar scores when depression is repeatedly measured over a short time period. Threats occur when the researcher uses measuring tool with low reliability and poor accuracy and consistency.
- *Low reliability of intervention implementation*: If the treatment is not implemented according to the standardized protocols, the variability in treatments will lead to variability in subject's responses. In other words, if the method of administering a research intervention varies from one person to another the chance of detecting a true difference decreases. The inconsistency in implementation of study intervention creates a threat to statistical conclusion validity. This must be controlled by having standardized protocols for administration of treatment to subjects.

Researcher strives to design studies that confirm to all the above four types of study validity. In some situations, meeting the requirements for one type of validity interferes with the possibility of achieving others. For example, homogeneity for controlling extraneous variables and control over consistency of conditions strengthen internal validity but limit external validity. When there is a conflict between internal and external validities, it is desirable to opt for strong internal validity. If the findings are not internally valid, they cannot possibly be externally valid too. When the findings are themselves not valid it makes little sense to generalize them to a larger population.

ELEMENTS OF EXPERIMENTAL RESEARCH

Experimental research designs deal with investigation of the effect of independent variable on the dependent variable where the independent variable is manipulated through intervention or treatment and the effect of these interventions (independent variable) is observed on the dependent variable.

This design is powerful for testing hypothesis of casual relationship among variables, i.e. to find out the exact relationship between cause-and-effect in a most efficient way. To examine the cause, the researcher must eliminate all the factors influencing the dependent variable other than the independent variable being studied (minimizing the effect of extraneous variables). Experimental design provides greatest amount of control with the least error possible. The following are the elements of experimental research:

- Random assignment of subjects to groups
- Precisely defined independent variable
- Manipulation of independent variable
- Having a comparison group
- Clearly identified sampling criteria
- Carefully measured dependent variables
- Controlled environment for conducting study

The experimental designs are classified into true experimental and quasi-experimental designs.

TRUE EXPERIMENTAL DESIGNS

True experimental designs investigate the cause-and-effect relationship between independent (predictor) and dependent (outcome) variables under controlled conditions. In these designs, researchers have control over the extraneous variable, which allows them to confidently predict that the observed effect on the dependent variable is only due to the manipulation of the independent variable. Some of the symbols regularly used in research studies are:

- R—random assignment of the subjects to groups
- O—observation or measurement of dependent variable
- X—experimental treatment or intervention.

Essential characteristics of true experimental design: Characteristics of true experimental design are presented in Figure 6.14.

- *Manipulation:* It means administering the treatment or intervention to some participants and withholding it from others (by administering alternative treatment or no treatment). Here, the researcher intentionally controls the independent variable and observes its effect on the dependent variable.
  - *Example*: A study evaluated the effectiveness of gentle back massage on improving quality of sleep among depressive patients. Receiving gentle back massage is the independent variable in this example. This could be manipulated by giving back massage to some patients and withholding it for others. Later patient's quality of sleep (dependent variable) is compared among the two groups to infer whether differences in receiving the intervention resulted in differences in quality of sleep.
- *Randomization*: Randomization means introduction of chance into the selection or assignment of subjects to treatments. Randomization can occur at two levels:

Characteristics of true experimental design		
1. Manipulation It refers to conscious control of independent variable by the researcher through treatment or intervention to observe its effect on dependent variable	2. Randomization It refers to every subject having an equal chance of being assigned to either the control or experimental group	3. Control It refers to use of control group and controlling the effects of extraneous variables on the dependent variable

Fig. 6.14: Characteristics of true experimental design

(1) random selection and (2) random assignment. Random selection refers to the process of drawing the sample from a population for study by way of chance. It can be simply put as "each subject in the population has an equal chance of selection". In other words, it refers to the random assignment of subjects to different groups or treatment conditions. Here "every subject has an equal chance of being assigned to any of the experimental or control groups". Random assignment is sufficient for a study to be referred to as experimental. Through this random assignment systematic bias is eliminated.

Example: In the above example, if 60 depressive patients are selected among 100 available depressive patients by using lottery method or random number table, it denotes random selection. Now, if the selected 60 depressive patients are randomly assigned to experimental and control groups by using toss of a coin or random number tables or computerized random number generators, it denotes random assignment.

❖ *Control*: Control means use of control group and controlling the effects of extraneous variables on the dependent variable.
  ○ The control group refers to a group of subjects or conditions that match as closely as possible with an experimental group, but is not exposed to any experimental treatment. The subjects in both control and experimental groups are similar in characteristics. While the experimental group receives planned treatment or intervention, the control group receives no experimental treatment or may receive any other intervention. Later, comparison is made between control and experimental groups to observe the effect of this treatment or intervention.

Example: In the above example, experimental group subjects receive gentle back massage while the control group subjects do not. Later, quality of sleep is compared between the groups.
  ○ The effects of extraneous variables on dependent variable can be controlled by manipulation, randomization, use of strict protocols, blinding, and matching.
    ◆ Strict protocol refers to identical management of treatment group subjects with respect to administration of intervention, which can be achieved by a well-designed protocol.
    ◆ Blinding refers to the concealment of group allocation from study participants, i.e. being unaware of which group, control or experimental they are in.
      – In single-blind experiments, it is only the study participants who are kept unaware of their status as members of the control or experimental groups. For example, in a study to investigate the effect of a new drug, the researcher administers new drug to experimental group participants and placebo (sugar pill) to the control group participants. In this study, the subjects are unaware of whether they are receiving the new drug or the placebo.
      – In double-blind experiment, both the investigator (individual implementing the intervention) and the participants are unaware of which participant is allotted to the experimental group, i.e. who is receiving the real treatment. This is done to improve the reliability and validity of the experiment. For example, to investigate the effect of a new drug, both the researcher

and the study participants are unaware of who is receiving the new drug and who is receiving a placebo.
- Matching is a technique wherein the subjects are matched based on a particular variable and then put into groups. The researcher matches every subject in one group with an equivalent in another group, thus creating equivalent groups for the study. It reduces the bias by controlling the confounding variables.
  – *Example*: In a study to evaluate the effectiveness of daily exercise on reducing cardiovascular disorders, the researcher matches the subjects based on their age, gender, and smoking habits.

Types of commonly used true experimental designs: The six types of commonly used true experimental designs are depicted in Flowchart 6.9.

1. POSTTEST ONLY CONTROL GROUP DESIGN (AFTER ONLY DESIGN)

In this design, dependent variable is measured only once after the experimental treatment has been administered.

Steps

i. Subjects are randomly assigned (R) to either of the control or experimental groups.
ii. The subjects are not pretested
iii. Experimental group subjects receive the experimental treatment or intervention (X). The control group receives the routine treatment or no treatment.
iv. Posttest observations (O) are carried out on both the groups to assess the effect of manipulation (Fig. 6.15).

Example: A study to evaluate the effectiveness of antenatal exercises on labor outcome among antenatal mothers.

Advantages

❖ This design is helpful in situations where pretest is not feasible for the subjects. In the above example, the antenatal mothers are assigned to experimental and control groups. Experimental group antenatal mothers are given exercise program and labor outcome is compared between the two groups. In this study, labor outcome is the dependent variable that cannot be assessed at antenatal period.

In another study "To assess the effects of immediate versus delayed pushing by women in the second stage of labor on fetal well-being", the fetal well-being is the dependent and outcome variable of interest, which cannot be assessed before labor.

❖ The posttest comparison with randomized subjects controls for the main effects of history, maturation, and pretesting. It is because without a pretest, the interaction effect of pretesting cannot be observed.

Disadvantage

Though random assignment should ensure equality of groups, in the absence of pretest, the researchers are not definite whether the groups are similar.

Flowchart 6.9: Types of true experimental designs

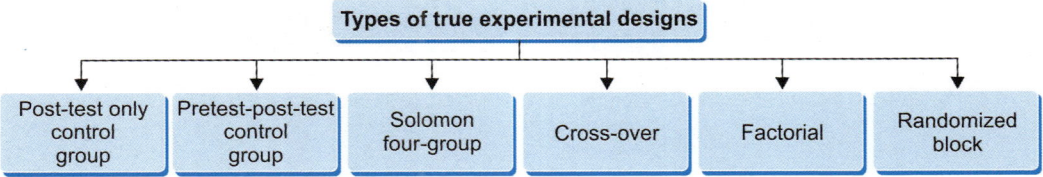

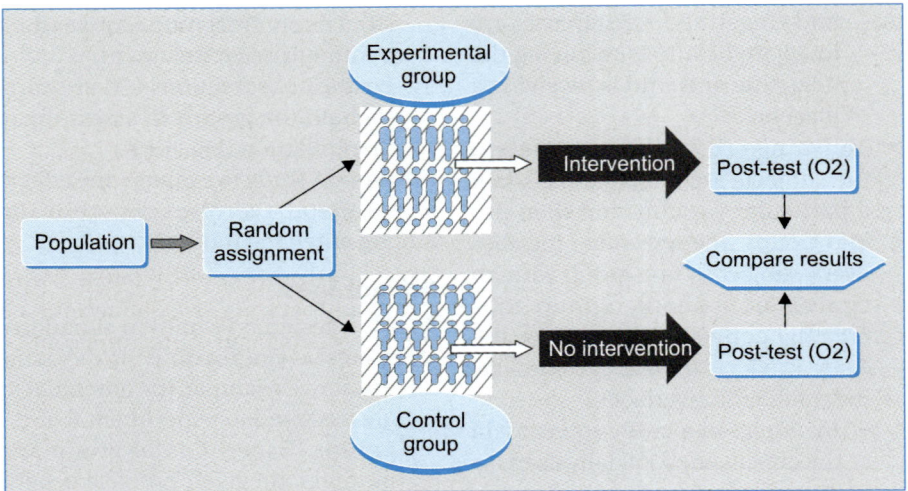

Fig. 6.15: Schematic presentation of posttest only control group design

2. PRETEST-POSTTEST CONTROL GROUP DESIGN

This is a classic experimental design wherein the dependent variable is measured at two points in time, i.e. before and after the experimental intervention.

Steps

i. Subjects are randomly assigned (R) to either a control or an experimental group.
ii. The subjects in both the groups are pretested (O1).
iii. Experimental group subjects receive the experimental treatment or intervention (X). The control group receives the routine treatment or no treatment.
iv. Both the groups are posttested (O2).

Researchers often use this design to assess change from the pretest to the posttest as a result of a treatment or intervention (Fig. 6.16).

Example: The efficacy of body-mind-spirit intervention on well-being and quality of life among depressive patients from the pretest.

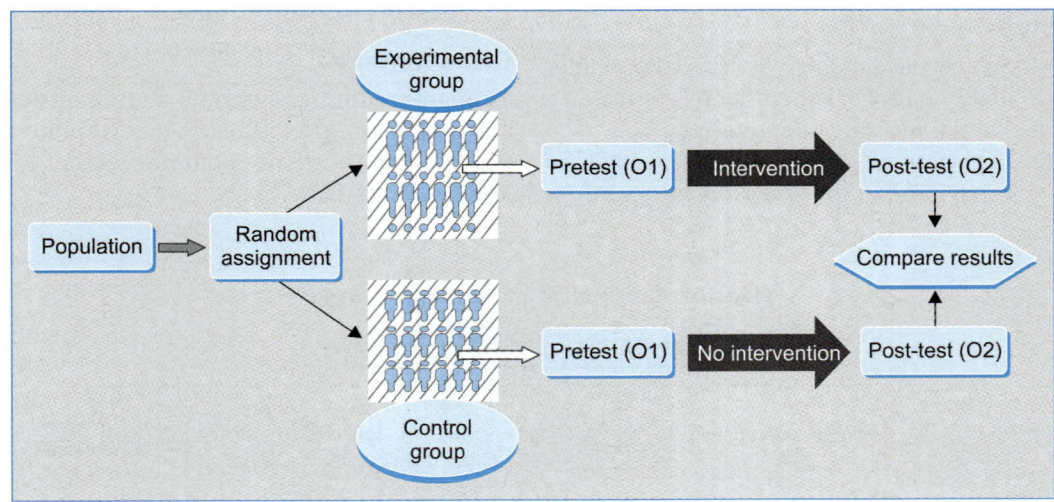

Fig. 6.16: Schematic presentation of pretest-posttest control group design

Advantages

❖ The main advantage is the randomization. Through randomization it can be assured that both the groups are equal in all the characteristics and any change in the posttest could be the result of the treatment or intervention.
❖ This design controls for all threats to internal validity.

Disadvantage

The external validity or generalizability of the study is limited by the possible effect of pretesting.

3. SOLOMON FOUR-GROUP DESIGN

This design has four groups—two experimental and two controls. While one experimental and one control group are administered pretest, the other two groups are not. Posttest is conducted for all the groups.

Steps

i. Subjects are randomly assigned (R) to one of the four different groups.
ii. The subjects in experimental group one and control group one are pretested (O1).
iii. Two experimental group subjects receive experimental treatment or intervention (X). The two control group subjects receive routine treatment or no treatment.
iv. All the groups are posttested (O2) (Fig. 6.17).

In studies where pre and postassessments are done, the pretest measure has the potential to distort the posttest results. The change in posttest measures may not solely be due to treatment but also by the exposure to the pretest. To avoid reactive effects of the pretest, this design has two experimental and control groups. One experimental and control group each is administered pretest while other two groups are not. This allows the effects of the pretest measure and intervention to be segregated.

Example: Nursing students completed a questionnaire measuring their knowledge scores on drug calculation as a pretest. Later, the students might look up for answers to some unknown questions. This might result in scoring better on the posttest compared to scoring without taking the pretest. This example suggests that pretest sensitization had an influence on posttest scores. To avoid this sensitization, Solomon four-group design is used.

Advantages

❖ It minimizes the threat to internal and external validity.
❖ This design is helpful in reducing the effect of pretest measures on posttest (reactive effects of the pretest).
❖ Any differences between the experimental and control group posttest scores

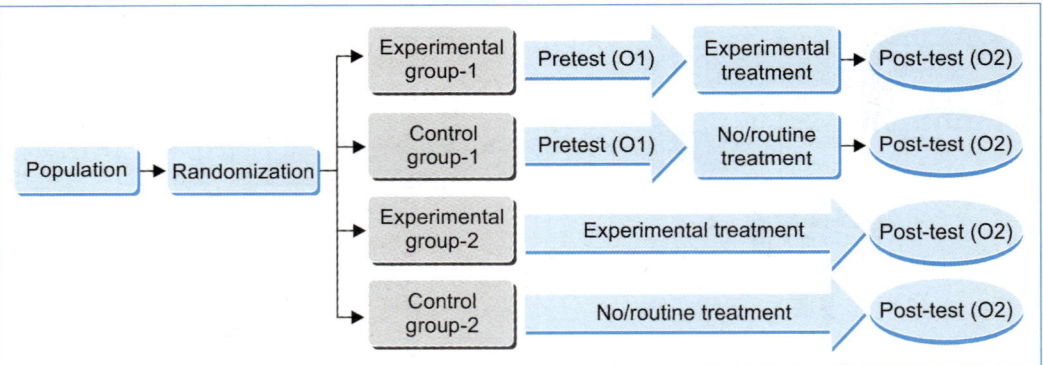

Fig. 6.17: Schematic presentation of Solomon four-group design

can be confidently associated with the experimental treatment.

Disadvantages
- It requires more samples
- Data analysis is complicated

4. CROSS-OVER DESIGN

Cross-over design is also known as repeated measures design. In this design, same subjects are exposed to more than one experimental treatment, i.e. subjects are administered two treatments, one experimental, and the other control or reference. The subjects are randomly assigned to one of the two groups. While one group receives the experimental treatment initially the other group receives the reference treatment first. After a certain time period, the treatments are crossed over thereby allowing the subjects to serve as their own controls. Multiple cross-over designs involve several treatments.

Steps
i. Subjects are randomly assigned (R) to one of the two groups
ii. Subjects in both the groups are pretested (O1)
iii. Experimental group subjects receive first set of treatment (X1)
iv. The control group subjects receive second set of treatment (X2)
v. Both the groups are posttested (O2)
vi. After a period of time, the treatments are swapped among the experimental and control groups [experimental group subjects receive second set of treatment (X2) and control group subjects receive first set of treatment (X1)]
vii. Both the groups are posttested (O3) (Fig. 6.18).

Example: A study to compare the effectiveness of massage and music therapy on the development of premature infants. In this study, some infants are randomly assigned to receive massage therapy first and music therapy later. However, the other infants receive music therapy first and massage therapy later.

Advantage
- It is used to test multiple hypotheses in a single study.

Disadvantage
- Cross-over effects (when subjects are exposed to two different treatments, the

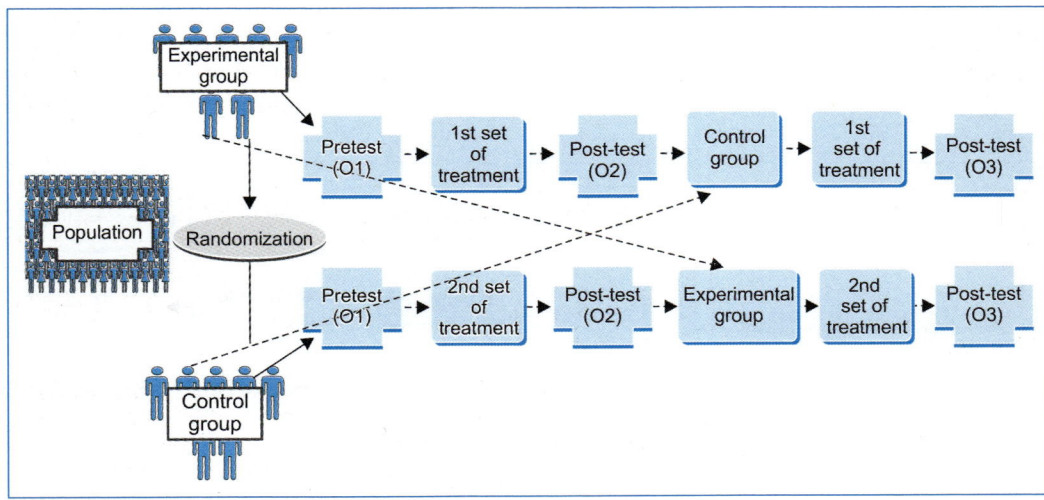

Fig. 6.18: Schematic presentation of cross-over design

likelihood of being influenced during the second treatment due to their experience with the first treatment is high).

5. FACTORIAL DESIGN

Independent variables are sometimes called factors. When the researcher uses multiple independent variables in a study, it is called factorial design. In this design, two or more independent variables are manipulated by the researcher simultaneously to observe their effects on the dependent variable. In such designs, the researcher studies the effect of each independent variable on the dependent variable as well as the effect of interaction between independent variables on the dependent variable. It incorporates 2 × 2 or 2 × 3 factorial, which can be in any combination. This facilitates testing of several hypotheses in a single study.

Steps
i. Subjects are randomly assigned (R) to four groups (A, B, C, and D).
ii. Subjects in all the groups are pretested (O1)
iii. Group A subjects receive intervention 1 and 2 (X1 + X2)
iv. Group B subjects receive intervention 1 only (X1)
v. Group C subjects receive intervention 2 only (X2)
vi. Group D subjects receive no intervention
vii. Subjects in all the groups are posttested (O2) (Table 6.2 and Fig. 6.19).

Example: In a study to evaluate the effectiveness of relaxation and distraction on reduction of pain among cancer patients, a 2 × 2 factorial design with four cells (A, B, C, and D) are used. Each cell contains equal number of subjects. Cell A subjects receive distraction and relaxation intervention, cell B subjects receive only distraction intervention, cell C subjects receive only relaxation intervention, cell D subjects receive no intervention and serve as a control group. Cell A subjects allow the researcher to examine the interaction between two independent variables, relaxation and distraction.

Advantage
❖ Factorial designs allow the examination of theoretically proposed inter-relationships between multiple independent variables.

Table 6.2: Schematic presentation of factorial design

Levels of relaxation	Levels of distraction	
	Distraction (Intervention X1)	No distraction
Relaxation (Intervention X2)	Group A (X1 + X2)	Group C (X2)
No relaxation	Group B (X1)	Group D (No intervention)

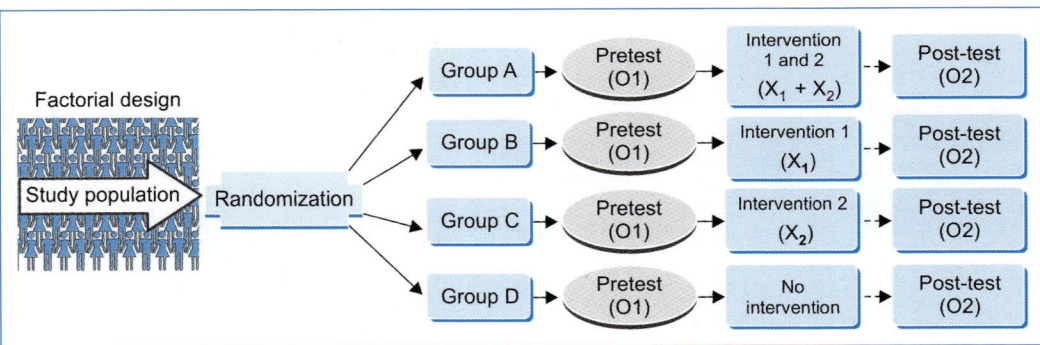

Fig. 6.19: Schematic presentation of factorial design

Disadvantage

❖ These designs require large samples.

6. RANDOMIZED BLOCK DESIGN

In this type of design, the researcher divides the subjects into subgroups or blocks such that the variation within the blocks is less compared to the variation between them. This is followed by random assignment of subjects within each block. Randomized block design is most useful in situations where in the experimental subjects are heterogeneous and it is possible to divide the experimental subjects into homogeneous groups or units called blocks. In these designs, there are two independent variables (factors). While one independent variable can be manipulated, and the other cannot be manipulated experimentally called the blocking variable. When the researcher is comparing the effects of vaccine versus placebo therapy for male and female individuals, the design could be 2 × 2 (four cells) experiment with type of intervention as one factor and gender as the other. Gender cannot be manipulated known as the blocking variable.

Steps

i. Subjects are divided into homogenous subgroups (Block A—males and Block B—females)
ii. Subjects within each block are randomly assigned to experimental and control groups (each block has experimental and control groups)
iii. Subjects in each block are pretested (O1)
iv. Block A and B experimental group subjects receive experimental treatment (X)
v. Block A and B control group subjects do not receive experimental treatment
vi. Subjects in all the groups are posttested (O2) (Table 6.3 and Fig. 6.20).

Example: In a 2 × 2 experiment, 500 male subjects and 500 female subjects are available for the study. The researcher makes two blocks based on gender (male and female). Subjects from each block are randomly assigned to either vaccination or placebo thereby having 250 subjects in each cell. 250 men and women get the placebo and the other set of 250 men and women get the vaccine.

Table 6.3: Schematic presentation of randomized block design

Gender	Treatment	
	Placebo (Control group)	Vaccine (Experimental group)
Male (Block A)	250	250
Female (Block B)	250	250

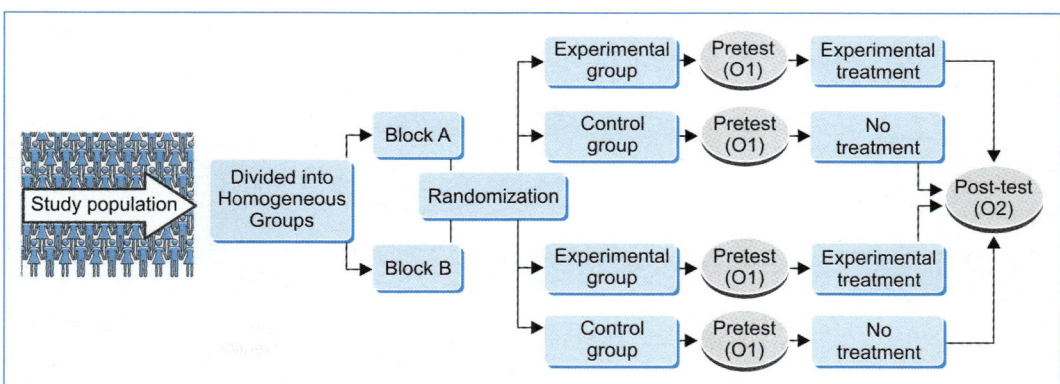

Fig. 6.20: Schematic presentation of randomized block design

Men and women are born physiologically different and react differently to vaccination. In the above example, the design eliminates gender as a potential source of confounding variable since each treatment condition has an equal number of male and female in vaccine and placebo cells. This ensures that differences between treatment conditions cannot be attributed to gender.

Advantage
- Reduces the variation in the treatment by a homogeneous combination of subjects through randomized block design.

Disadvantage
- These designs require large samples.

RANDOMIZED CONTROLLED TRIALS

Well-designed randomized controlled trials (RCTs) are considered the gold standard for measuring the intervention effect. This method is used in various fields such as medicine, psychology, education, and administration. In the field of medicine, these designs are used to evaluate the effectiveness of prevention strategies, screening and diagnostic tests, treatment procedures, and educational modules.

Randomized controlled trials are quantitative, comparative, controlled experiments wherein the investigator evaluates the effect of intervention by administering it to subjects who have been randomly assigned to either of the intervention or control groups.

Steps
i. Subjects are randomly assigned to intervention or control groups.
ii. The intervention to be tested is called the experiment and the group receiving this intervention is called the experimental group. The other intervention is regarded as a standard of comparison or control and the group which receives it is called the control group.
iii. Subjects in one group receive the treatment being tested; the other receives an alternate treatment or placebo or no treatment.
iv. Both the groups are followed up and outcomes measured at specific intervals.
v. These outcome measures are statistically compared to assess the difference in response between the groups so as to study the effect of experimental treatment.

Randomization procedure ensures that all the subjects have an equal chance of being allocated to intervention or control groups, characteristics of the subjects are similar in both the groups and any significant differences between groups in the outcome measures can be attributed to the intervention.

Advantages
- The most powerful way to find out cause-and-effect relationship
- Blinding is possible
- Completely removes effect of extraneous variables
- Strict protocols are followed

Disadvantages
- Recruitment of sample may be difficult
- Costly and time consuming
- Hawthorne effect

CLINICAL RESEARCH

Clinical research is basically the study of health and illness among people. It deals with the scientific investigation of etiology, prevention, diagnosis, or treatment of human disease using human subjects or materials of human origin. Clinical research helps to generate new information and translate basic research into new and effective treatments to enhance patient care.

Clinical trials are a type of clinical research performed on large group of individuals to evaluate the effectiveness and safety of new treatments or drugs by following a predefined plan or protocol. The subjects by consenting to participate in such clinical trials not only play an active role in improving their health condition but also contribute to medical research.

- Any of the government health agencies, researchers affiliated with a hospital or university medical program, independent researchers, or private industry may conduct clinical trials.
- Generally, approval or disapproval of new treatments by the government is based on clinical trial results.
- Through clinical trials the harmful treatment being provided to the public can be prevented.
- To investigate the effectiveness of the treatment, the participants in these trials are assigned to two or more groups. Participants in experimental group receive experimental treatment while the participants in the control group receive placebo therapy to compare the effectiveness of treatment.
- Volunteers are recruited to take part in clinical trials and paid.

Drug clinical trials usually proceed through four phases (I, II, III, and IV), which may run to many years. Each phase of the drug approval process is treated as a separate clinical trial. If the drug successfully passes through the first three phases, it usually gets the approval of the regulatory authority for use among human beings. Postapproval studies are conducted in the fourth phase. Extensive preclinical studies need to be conducted by pharmaceutical companies before they can start clinical trials on a drug.

A clinical trial can have four possible outcomes:
  i. *Positive trial*: It shows that the new treatment is largely beneficial and better than the standard treatment.
  ii. *Noninferior trial*: It shows that the new treatment is same as the standard treatment effect.
  iii. *Inconclusive trial*: It shows that the new treatment is neither clearly superior nor clearly inferior to standard treatment.
  iv. *Negative trial*: It shows that the new treatment is inferior to standard treatment.

Advantages

- Clinical research provides opportunities for patients to receive promising new therapies free of cost, which otherwise are not readily available.
- Participants will be monitored closely in event of adversities.
- Clinical research trials may at times be lifesaving.
- Participants will be contributing to advancements in healthcare and medical research thereby serving fellow patients.
- Though participating in clinical trial is not a source of income, however, it comes with certain benefits in the form of reimbursements relating to travel expenses, medical care, food, and sundry expenses.

Disadvantages

- The new treatment may not be better than the current treatment
- Patients may need to stick to the trial schedule and make frequent visits
- In rare conditions, serious side effects may occur due to new treatment, which may not be covered by medical aid from the employer or be eligible for insurance claim.

Strengths of True Experimental Designs

- It is most scientific in nature
- True experiments because of their rigor, precision, and control properties are considered the most powerful methods for testing hypothesis of cause-and-effect relationship between variables
- Randomized controlled trial is placed at the highest level on the evidence-based practice pyramid

Limitations of True Experimental Designs

❖ Experiments are sometimes criticized for their artificiality
❖ Due to ethical reasons certain manipulations cannot be done in human studies
❖ Pretest can affect the response of posttest

QUASI-EXPERIMENTAL DESIGNS

Quasi-experimental designs facilitate the examination of causality in situations in which complete control is not possible. In these designs, one of the components of true experimental design, i.e. either the random assignment of subjects to groups or control groups for comparison are typically lacking. Due to this, they are not as powerful as true experimental designs in establishing the cause-and-effect relationship between independent and dependent variables. Degree of control that the researcher has over the subjects and the study variables is the major distinction between the true and quasi-experimental designs. Though these designs are conducted in natural settings, they may be exposed to many threats, which may reduce the generalizability of the study findings.

Types of quasi-experimental designs: The four types of commonly used quasi-experimental designs are depicted in Flowchart 6.10.

1. NONEQUIVALENT CONTROL GROUP PRETEST POSTTEST DESIGN

This design is similar to pre–post control group design except that the participants are not randomly (NR) assigned to groups. Both experimental and control group subjects are pretested (O1); the experimental group subjects receive experimental treatment (X) and comparison group subjects receive standard care; both the groups are posttested (O2).

Steps

i. Nonrandom assignment (NR) of subjects to either a control or an experimental group
ii. The subjects in both the groups are pretested (O)
iii. Experimental group subjects receive the experimental treatment or intervention (X). The comparison group receives the routine treatment or no treatment
iv. Both the groups are posttested (O) (Fig. 6.21).

Example: In a study to evaluate the effectiveness of therapeutic environment on conflict and containment rates among schizophrenia patients, the experimental group and comparison group subjects were admitted to different psychiatric wards. As the ward environment is manipulated for the study purpose, the researcher preferred different

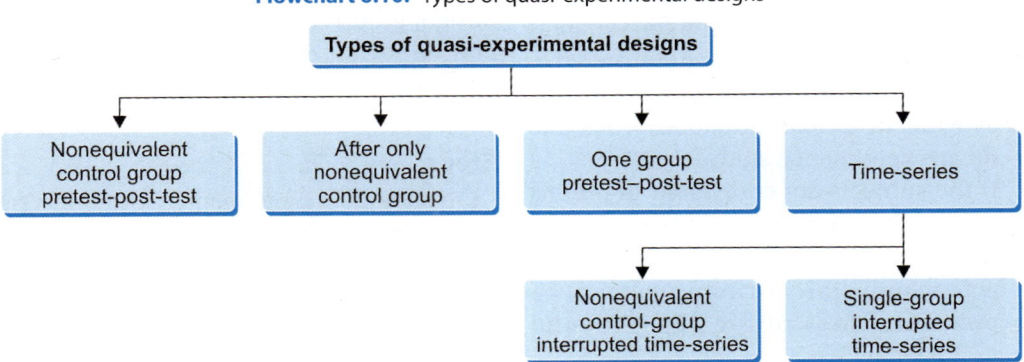

Flowchart 6.10: Types of quasi-experimental designs

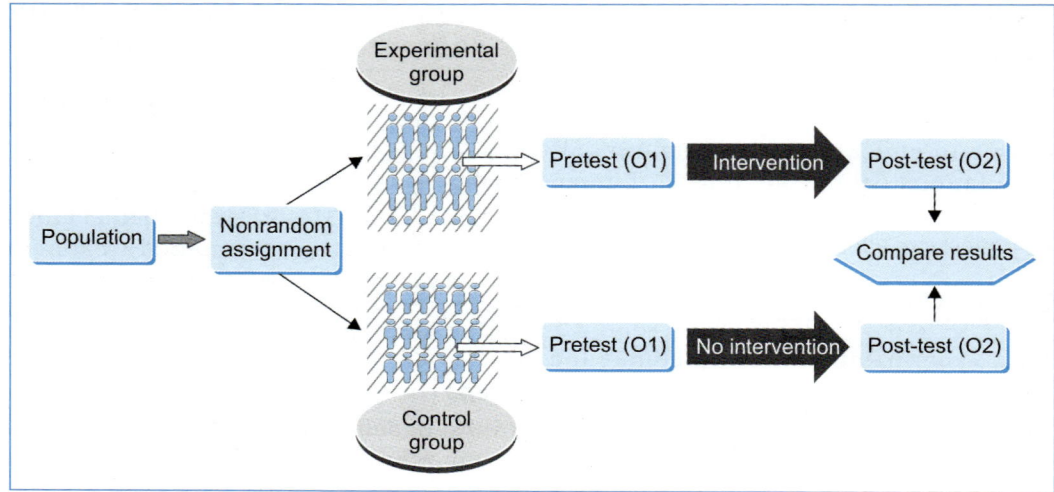

Fig. 6.21: Schematic presentation of nonequivalent control group pretest–posttest design

wards for experimental and control subjects to avoid contamination of treatment conditions. With pretest, the researcher ensured that the two groups were equal in demographic parameters, conflict, and containment rates.

In another study to evaluate the effectiveness of group therapy on well-being of diabetic patients, the researcher chose experimental group and control group subjects from two different hospitals to avoid intervention contamination.

Advantages

❖ This design is relatively strong because the gathering of data at the time of pretest allows the researcher to compare the equivalence of the two groups on variables before the intervention is administered.
❖ It is used in situations where random assignment or control group is not possible for an experimental study.
❖ If the subjects are equivalent in pretest scores, it will allow the researcher to infer that it was the intervention that was responsible for improvement in posttest scores of the experimental group subjects.

Disadvantages

❖ Due to lack of randomization, it can no longer be assumed that the groups are equivalent.
❖ The biggest threat to internal validity in selection bias.
❖ If differences exist in pretest scores, it is difficult to infer the effectiveness of the intervention. It can only be controlled statistically in the analysis.

2. AFTER-ONLY NONEQUIVALENT CONTROL GROUP DESIGN

In this design, the dependent variable is measured only once after the experimental treatment has been introduced. For this design, groups must be similar or one must control for these differences to make valid comparisons and conclusion regarding the effect of intervention.

Steps

i. Nonrandom assignment (NR) of subjects to either a control or an experimental group.
ii. Experimental group subjects receive the experimental treatment or intervention (X). The comparison group receives the routine treatment or no treatment.

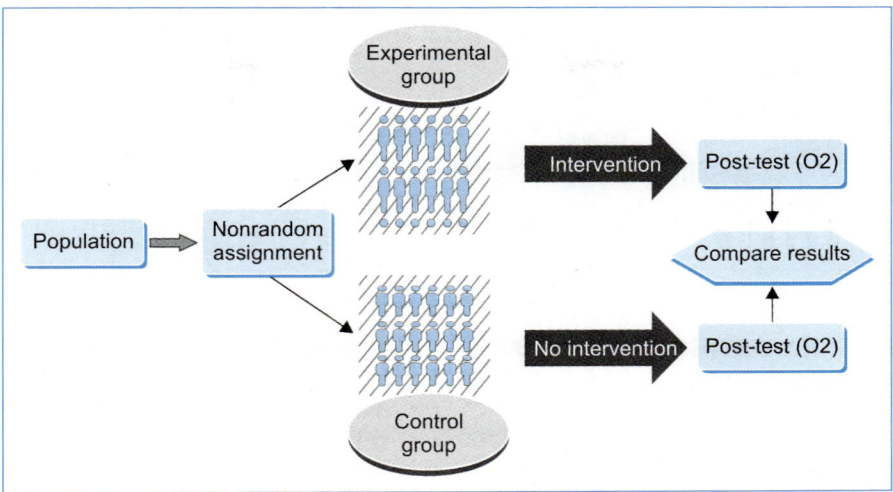

Fig. 6.22: Schematic presentation of after only nonequivalent control group design

iii. Both the groups are posttested (O) (Fig. 6.22).

Example: "A study to evaluate the efficacy of distraction in reducing pain perception among children". In this study, the researcher provides distraction to the experimental group children while no distraction is provided to the control group children during the painful procedure. He then examines the differences in amount of pain during the procedure between the subjects in two groups. In this study, it is not possible to pretest the amount of pain before the procedure.

Advantage
- This design is used in situations in which a pretest is not possible.

Disadvantage
- Selection bias may occur.

3. ONE GROUP PRETEST POSTTEST DESIGN

This design is used when only one group is available for study. Dependent variable is assessed (pretest) before implementation of the intervention to the subjects followed by posttest observation. Pre–post assessments are compared to assess the effect of intervention on subjects. In this design, both randomization and control are absent. It is considered very weak because the researcher has very little control over the experiment. Evidence generated from this type of design is interpreted with careful consideration because of design limitations. In some textbooks, this design is considered as pre-experimental design.

Steps
i. The subjects are pretested (O1)
ii. Receive the experimental treatment or intervention (X)
iii. Subjects are posttested (O2) (Fig. 6.23)
   Example: In a study on sexual behavior in teens, behavior is measured baseline (pretested), a nurse-based educational intervention is administered and subsequent behavior is measured again (posttest).

Advantage
- This design can be used, if no control group is available for an experimental study.

Disadvantages
- Effectiveness of the intervention cannot be proved on account of threats to internal validity
- Results cannot be generalized

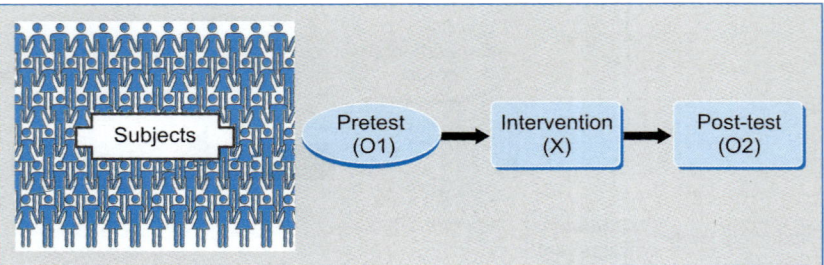

Fig. 6.23: Schematic presentation of one group pretest–posttest design

4. TIME-SERIES DESIGN (REPEATED MEASURES DESIGN)

In this design, the researcher collects data multiple times at pretest level, i.e. before introduction of treatment to establish a baseline point of reference on outcomes. Later, subjects are administered experimental treatment, which is followed by collection of data at multiple time points to determine the change from baseline. Multiple data collection points help to rule out the history effects. These designs may be experimental, quasi-experimental, or nonexperimental.

Advantage
- Several observations of the dependent variable help strengthen the validity of the design.

Disadvantage
- History and testing are the greatest threats to validity.

Commonly used time-series designs are nonequivalent control group interrupted time-series design and single-group interrupted time-series design.

- **Nonequivalent control-group interrupted time-series design**: In this design, subjects are not assigned randomly to groups. Here, the researcher collects data multiple times at pretest level after which subjects are administered experimental treatment followed by collection of data at multiple time points.

Steps
  i. Nonrandom assignment (NR) of subjects to either a control or an experimental group.
  ii. The subjects in both the groups are pretested at multiple times (O1, O2, and O3).
  iii. Experimental group subjects receive experimental treatment or intervention (X), whereas the comparison group receives the routine treatment or no treatment.
  iv. Both the groups are posttested at multiple times (O4, O5, and O6) (Fig. 6.24).

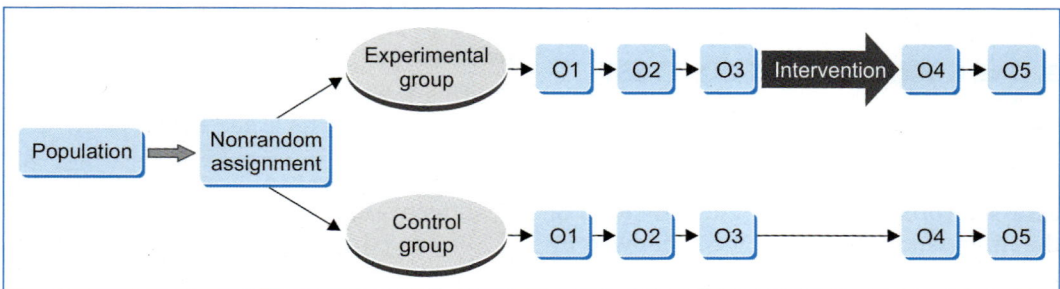

Fig. 6.24: Schematic presentation of nonequivalent control-group interrupted time-series design

Examples: A researcher may evaluate anxiety levels of school students studying in class 10. After assessing for anxiety levels for 3 weeks at weekly intervals (both the groups), the subjects in experimental group are provided cognitive behavioral therapy to reduce anxiety. The anxiety levels are again evaluated for the next 3 weeks.

A researcher evaluated experimental and control group children's school work on a weekly basis. Experimental group children were introduced to new teaching method while the control group children received routine teaching. The school work of children from both groups was evaluated on a weekly basis.

- **Single-group interrupted time-series design**: This design consists of a single group, wherein the researcher collects data multiple times at pretest level. Later, subjects are administered experimental treatment, which is followed by collection of data at multiple time points.
  Steps
  i. The subjects in group are pretested at multiple times (O1, O2, and O3)
  ii. Subjects receive the experimental treatment or intervention (X)
  iii. Subjects are posttested at multiple times (O4, O5, and O6) (Fig. 6.25).

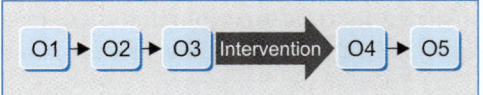

Fig. 6.25: Schematic presentation of single-group interrupted time-series design

Examples: A researcher may evaluate pain levels of arthritis patients. After assessing for pain levels for 3 weeks at weekly intervals, the subjects are provided physiotherapy to reduce pain. The pain levels are again evaluated for the next 2 weeks.

Strengths of quasi-experimental designs
- Feasible, practical, and generalizable
- More adaptable to the real-world practice setting than true experimental designs
- For some hypotheses, these designs may be the only way to evaluate the effect of the independent variable of interest
- Introduce some research control when full experimental rigor is not possible

Limitations of quasi-experimental designs
- There is no control over extraneous variables influencing the dependent variable
- Lack of randomization or absence of control group makes the results of the study less reliable and weak for establishing the cause-and-effect relationship between independent and dependent variables.

Experimental designs are considered level I and quasi-experimental designs are considered level II evidence.

EPIDEMIOLOGICAL RESEARCH DESIGNS

Epidemiologists measure the occurrence of disease or other health-related events in a population. They assess whether an exposure is associated with a particular disease. Epidemiological studies are generally classified as interventional (experimental) or observational (nonexperimental) studies (Flowchart 6.11).

Interventional Studies

In these studies, subjects are assigned to groups randomly. The commonly used epidemiological interventional studies are: (1) clinical trials and (2) field trials.

Clinical trials
Clinical trials are usually carried out in healthcare settings by involving patients to evaluate the efficacy of new treatment or intervention in treating the disease or condition.

Example: The women's nutritional intervention study was conducted among breast cancer women to assess whether a low-fat diet will reduce cancer recurrence and improve survival rate. This study spanned over 5 years, where a total of 2,000 postmenopausal women with breast cancer were recruited and

Flowchart 6.11: Types of epidemiological research designs

```
Epidemiological research designs
├── Interventional studies
│   ├── Clinical trials
│   └── Field trials
└── Observational studies
    ├── Cohort studies
    ├── Case-control studies
    └── Cross-sectional surveys
```

randomized to receive standard treatment plus a low-fat dietary intervention or standard treatment alone. The standard treatment included radiation therapy or chemotherapy (Chlebowski and Grosvenor, 1994; Henderson, 1995).

Field trials

Field trials are conducted in the field or community among healthy individuals to evaluate the efficacy of intervention in reducing the risk among healthy individuals.

Example: A study was conducted involving 48,000 postmenopausal women in USA to determine whether a sustained low-fat diet will reduce the incidence of breast cancer. The subjects with no prior history of cancer (colon or breast) were randomized to the intervention and control groups. The dietary intervention was designed to reduce fat intake to 20% of total kilocalories and increase intake of fruits and vegetables. This study followed the subjects for 11 years (Chlebowski and Grosvenor, 1994; Henderson, 1995).

Observational Studies

In these studies, the researcher merely observes the happenings by making a note of who is exposed or not exposed and who has or has not developed the disease. The commonly used epidemiological observational studies are: (1) cohort studies (2) case–control studies, and (3) cross-sectional surveys.

1. Cohort studies

Cohort studies are conducted to find whether exposure precedes the outcome. These studies begin with identification of normal subjects who are assessed for their exposure and nonexposure to risk factors. The subjects are followed over time and the incidence of disease is measured and compared among exposed and nonexposed group to find the causative factors for a particular disease (Fig. 6.26). In cohort studies, as exposure is

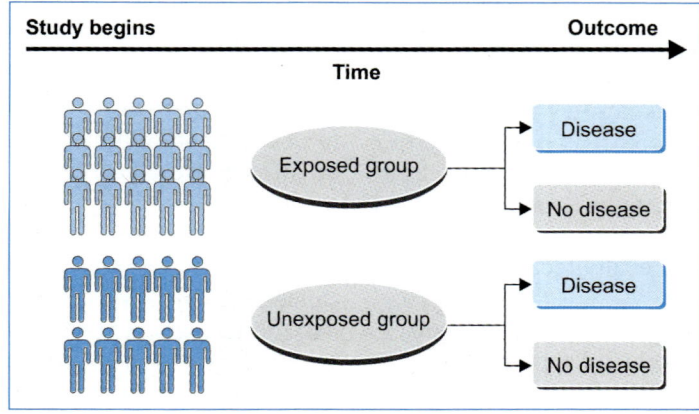

Fig. 6.26: Schematic presentation of a cohort study

identified before the outcome, they provide a sequential relationship between exposure and outcome, thus having the potential to provide strong scientific evidence. These study designs are similar to experimental studies except that allocation of subjects to the exposure is not controlled by the researcher.

Example: In 1987, Willett et al. conducted a study on 89,538 registered nurses aged between 34 and 59 years with no past history of cancer. They initially completed a dietary questionnaire designed to measure individual consumption of total fat, saturated fat, linoleic acid, and cholesterol as well as other nutrients. Depending on fat intake, these nurses were classified into five groups and followed up. The incidence of breast cancer in each of these groups was measured and compared.

- ❖ *Advantages*
  - ○ Facilitates investigation of rare exposures among the population because subjects are selected by their exposure status
  - ○ Allows calculation of absolute risk and relative risk
  - ○ Investigator can examine multiple outcomes simultaneously
- ❖ *Disadvantages*
  - ○ Requires more samples
  - ○ Long follow-up duration
  - ○ More time consuming and expensive
  - ○ Confounding variables are the major problem in analysis
  - ○ Subject selection and drop out are the potential causes for bias

2. Case–control studies

Case–control studies investigate the risk factors for diseases. The study begins with identification of individuals with disease (cases) and without disease (controls). These individuals (cases and controls) are compared for risk factors (Fig. 6.27). Case–control studies require less samples compared to cohort studies.

Example: In 1992, Chuang et al. conducted a case–control study involving 128 histologically or cytologically confirmed cases of hepatocellular carcinoma and 384 controls without the disease. The study was carried out to assess whether hepatitis B infection played a role in the etiology of primary hepatocellular carcinoma. Of the cases, 77% were carriers of the hepatitis B surface antigen (HbsAg) compared with only 28% of the controls.

- ❖ *Advantages*
  - ○ Generates more information from few subjects
  - ○ Only feasible option when there is a long latent period between an exposure and the disease

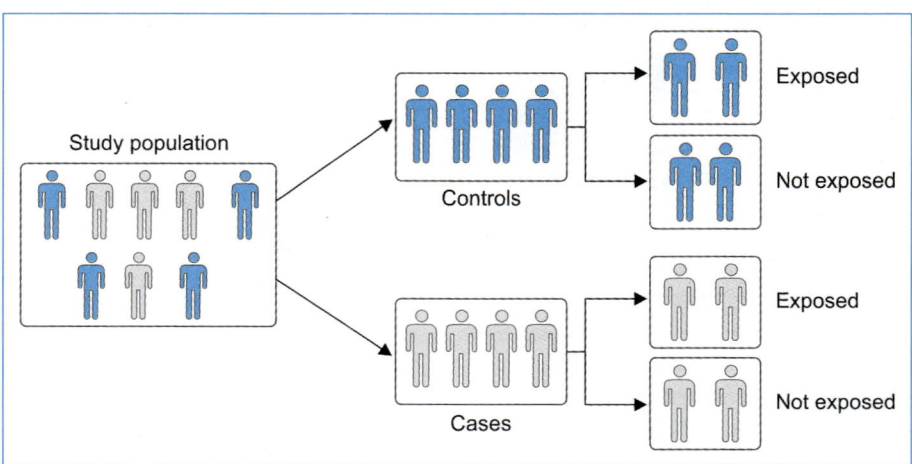

Fig. 6.27: Schematic presentation of a case–control study

- Only few subjects are required
- Useful for generating hypothesis that can be tested using other types of designs

❖ *Disadvantages*
- Confounding variables are the major problem in analysis
- Subject selection is potential cause for bias

3. Cross-sectional surveys

These are used to estimate the prevalence of diseases. In these studies, sample are selected from a defined population and data collected at a particular time point. The researcher obtains information on both the exposure and outcome of the event simultaneously (Fig. 6.28). In this type of study, samples are selected using random sampling techniques to ensure that the selected subjects are representative of the whole population with a view to generalize the study results.

Example: Fukao et al. (1993) conducted a cross-sectional survey to find out the association between *Helicobacter pylori* infection and chronic atrophic gastritis among 1,815 randomly selected healthy blood donors in Japan. Blood samples were taken from all the study subjects and measurements made of serum *H. pylori* IgG antibodies and serum pepsinogen I and II (markers of chronic atrophic gastritis). The prevalence of antibodies against the bacterium among subjects with chronic atrophic gastritis was then compared with the prevalence among individuals without chronic atrophic gastritis.

❖ *Advantage*
- Takes less time to conduct study because they do not require follow-up.

❖ *Disadvantage*
- Since information on both exposure and outcome is collected simultaneously, it is not possible to identify whether the outcome followed the exposure or exposure resulted from the outcome. In the example above, it is not possible to establish whether *H. pylori* infection preceded or followed chronic atrophic gastritis.

Critiquing Quantitative Research Design

❖ Is the research design appropriate for the purpose of the research study?
❖ What means were used to control for threats to internal and external validity in the use of experimental design?
❖ Can the researcher draw cause-and-effect relationship between the variables using the research design?

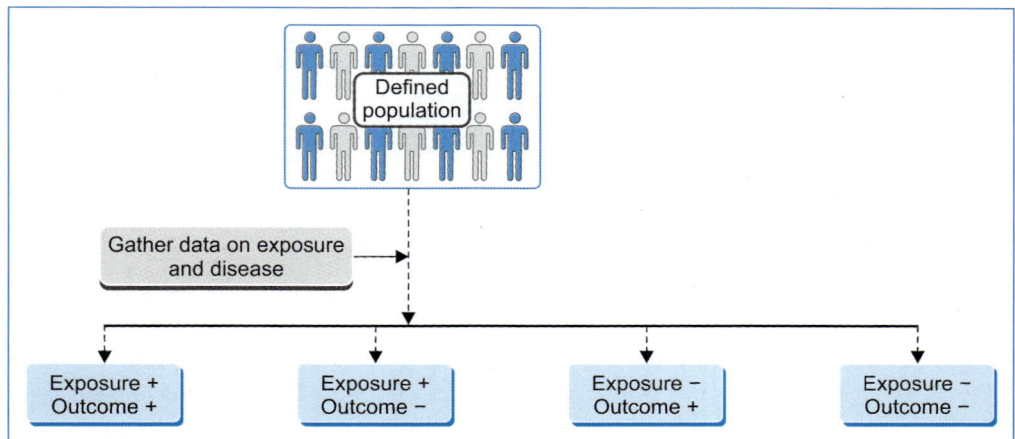

Fig. 6.28: Schematic presentation of cross-sectional survey design

Qualitative Research Designs

A qualitative design is selected when little is known about a particular phenomenon, experience, or concept. These designs are based on the naturalistic paradigm philosophy (reality is subjective, not objective, and that multiple realities exist rather than one). This approach typically uses inductive reasoning, wherein it begins with assumptions and specific observations of a particular instance, which are then combined into a large whole or general statement leading to development of concepts and themes. Once the concepts or themes are identified, these themes are grouped into a theory, which can then be tested using a quantitative design. Qualitative designs primarily involve the analysis of words. Research design in a qualitative study is not concrete. As the data is being gathered, the researcher makes deliberate modifications in line with new findings.

Types of Qualitative Research Designs

The four types of qualitative research designs most often used to conduct nursing research include—(1) ethnography, (2) phenomenological design, (3) grounded theory approach, and (4) case study (Flowchart 6.12).

ETHNOGRAPHY

Ethnography means study and description of a culture of a particular group of people. It involves collection and analysis of data about cultural or social groups.

- *Research problem and question*: The research problem in ethnography research focuses on describing and understanding a specific culture.
- *Conducting research*: The planning and implementing of an ethnographic research study takes place in three stages—(1) pre-fieldwork, (2) fieldwork, and (3) post-fieldwork.
    1. *Activities in pre-fieldwork*
        - Choose the problem and people
        - Search the literature and gather information on the problem and people
        - Formulate a systematic plan of investigation
    2. *Activities in fieldwork*
        - Focuses on making contacts and gaining entry, establishing relationships, and beginning to describe the culture experience.
        - As a participant observer, the researcher enters into the everyday life and activities of the people of the culture being studied.
        - The researcher studies the group's apparent and learned patterns of behavior, sociocultural practices and traditions mainly focusing on culture, and how people interact with each other.
        - Researcher spends over a year in the field setting long enough to see a full cycle of activity on emic (insiders views about their culture) and etic (outsiders view about experiences of that culture) perspectives to gain a better understanding of behavior, values and social relationships. This spending of extended time with respondents in their native culture is termed as prolonged engagement.
        - Data collection methods used in ethnography are census taking (collection of basic demographic data), mapping (identifying the location of people, culture, environmental features), document analysis (vital statistics, records, newspapers, personal diaries), life histories (comprehensive biography of an informant's life), and event analysis (detailed written and photographic documentation of events as wedding, funeral, and festivals). Techniques used are observation, unstructured in-depth interviews, records, physical evidences like diaries, letters, photographs, etc.

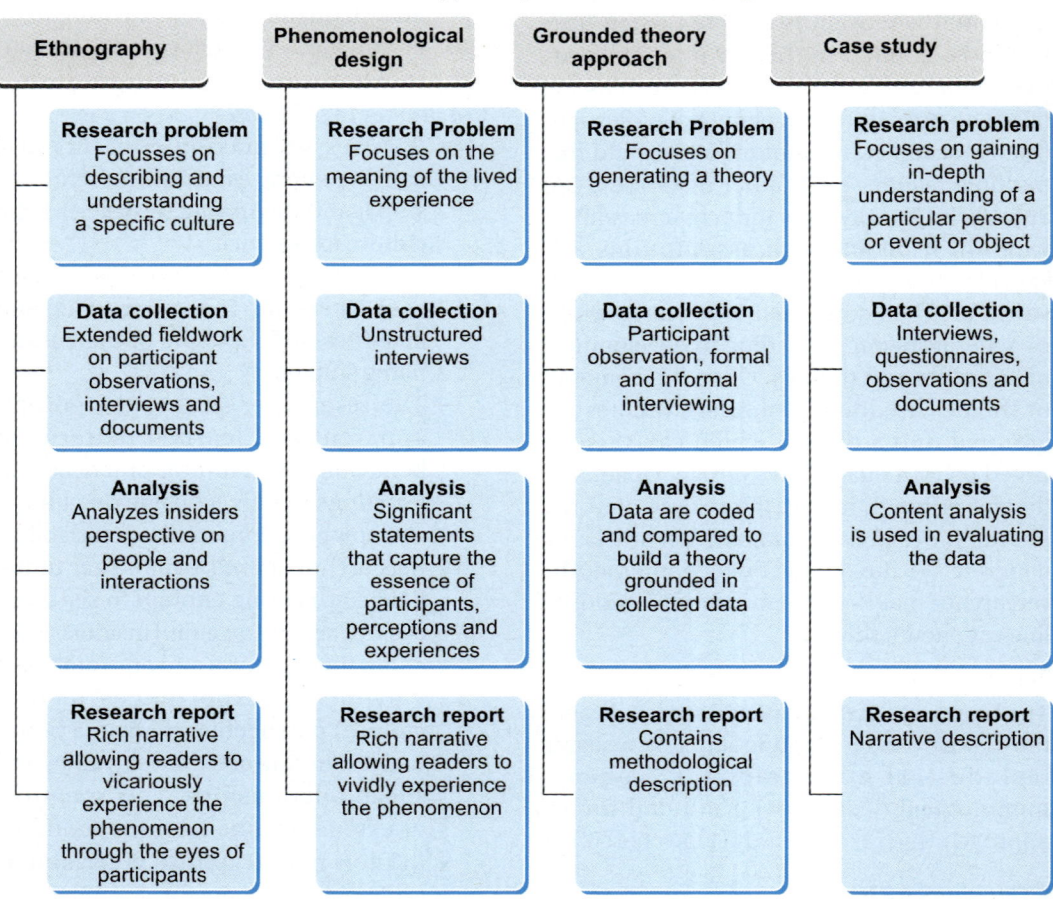

Flowchart 6.12: Types of qualitative research designs

- Identify emerging themes and categories and analyze general features of the culture.
- Refine the theme by double checking and monitoring the field information, evaluating gathered data to broaden understanding of how representative the research findings are of members of the culture.

Ethnographers usually seek three broad types of information:
  i. Culture behavior (what people do)
  ii. Culture artifacts (what members of the culture make use of)
  iii. Culture speech (what people say)

3. *Activities of post-fieldwork*
Ethnographic research report includes a rich and holistic description of the culture under study and provides access to health beliefs, health practices, and cultural problems. It begins with a brief overview of the setting and the people being studied, followed by a review of the specific problem being addressed and a discussion of the fieldwork.

Example: Wittig (2001) conducted an ethnonursing study involving 10 African-American women focusing on organ donation beliefs among their community in the rural area. He conducted in-depth interviews during his numerous visits to the site.

PHENOMENOLOGICAL DESIGN

It is the study of phenomenon, wherein the researcher describes the subjective reality of an event as perceived by the study participants. Phenomenology systematically uncovers and describes the meaning or essences of an experience. In phenomenological terms, these experiences are called the lived experience. Nursing phenomenological studies have contributed greatly to our knowledge about human experiences in health and illness, healing, and dying (for example, loss of an unborn child, recurrence of cancer), and the meaning of these experiences to the patients.

- *Research problem and question*
  - The research question focuses on the meaning of the lived experience.
  - The main goal is to develop rich, full, and insightful description of the lived experience.
- *Sample*
  - Commonly purposive sample is selected from persons who have actually lived the experience under study and are able and willing to describe the experience.
  - Participants are requested until there is redundancy in the data or saturation. Saturation refers to the participants descriptions becoming repetitive with no new or different ideas or interpretations emerging.
- *Data collection*
  - Data is collected using unstructured interviews and written description. Interaction between the researcher and participant is focused on achieving a full description of the lived experience.
  - Researcher often starts by identifying participant perceptions or expectations about the phenomenon to be studied and then attempts to consciously bracket them—hold them separate—so that they will not color either the data collection or the analysis process.
  - Bracketing is a reflective self-assessment methodological device in phenomenological inquiry where the researcher deliberately puts aside one's own belief about the phenomenon under investigation or what one already knows about the subject prior to and throughout the phenomenological investigation (Carpenter, 2007).
  - The researcher must be an empathetic and skilled listener and encourage full description.
  - Interviews are recorded and transcribed verbatim.
- *Data analysis*
  - Read the entire disclosure of the lived experience straight through to obtain a sense of the whole
  - Reread the disclosure to discover the essences of the lived experience under study
  - Formulate a consistent description of the lived experience for all participants

Example: Rungreangkulkij (2001) conducted a phenomenological study involving 12 Thai mothers' having adult schizophrenic children. The study focused on the experiences of the mothers in caring for their schizophrenic children.

GROUNDED THEORY APPROACH

Grounded theory is the discovery of theory from data that have been systematically obtained through research. It combines both inductive and deductive research methods. With the use of inductive processes, theory emerges from the data. Deduction is then used to test the theory empirically. The research process ends with a theoretical formulation or integrated set of conceptual hypotheses. Grounded theorists study social processes in everyday human life and interactions.

For nurse researchers, the grounded theory approach facilitates the development of mid-range theory grounded in the life and language of people living with illness conditions.

- *Research problem and question*: The goal of grounded theory approach is to generate a theory, propose theoretical propositions or models that illustrate the theory.
- *Sample*: Sample is determined by generated data and analysis. Sampling is continued until the categories are saturated.
- *Data collection*
  - Grounded theorists must view the environment as informants do and focus on the interaction under study.
  - Participant observation, informal interviewing, and formal interviewing are the three main sources of data generation.
  - The grounded theorist writes field notes and also uses audio-taped records to capture the participant's interview word for word.
- *Data analysis*
  - The process of data collection and analysis occurring simultaneously is referred to as constant comparison. Here, the previous data are constantly compared to current data as they are being gathered.
  - Significant concepts are identified and codes assigned. These concepts are constantly reviewed as new interpretations of the data are made.
  - Once the concepts have been identified and their relationship specified, the researcher reviews the literature to find out if any similar associations have already been investigated.

Example: Knobf (2002) sought to develop a substantive theory to explain women's responses to chemotherapy-induced premature menopause within the context of breast cancer.

CASE STUDY

Case study is an approach to qualitative research that focuses on gaining an in-depth understanding of a particular person or object or an event at a specific time. This design is used for intensive exploration of a single unit of study such as a person, a very small number of subjects, family, group, community, or institution.

- Case study may be quantitative or qualitative depending on the purpose of the study and the design chosen by the researcher.
- In qualitative case studies, the researcher must be interested in exploring the meaning of experiences from the subjects perspective rather than generalizing the results to other groups of people.
- *Data collection*
  - Data are collected using a variety of means and methods such as interviews, questionnaires, observations, audio and video recordings, and documents.
  - During data collection, the researcher examines all the variables that have an impact on the situation being studied.
  - The researcher explores the subject's history and previous behavioral pattern in detail. Both quantitative and qualitative information are likely to be integrated into the case–study design.
  - The case studies can be classified into single case versus multiple case. In a single case, the focus is on a particular person or an event at a specific time; while in a multiple case (collective case), the focus is on more than one person or an event at a specific time or over different time periods.
- *Data analysis*: It involves examination of communicated messages. Content analysis method is used to analyze the data from case studies.

Example: A study to determine the responses of diabetic patients in use of insulin pump. In this study, one patient or few patients with diabetes are studied for a time to understand their experiences in use of insulin pump.

Mixed Method Designs

Designing quantitative experimental studies with controls may provide strong external validity but at times may have limited internal validity. Qualitative studies may have strong internal validity but weak external validity. Any one approach to measure the concept may be inadequate.

Researchers are more likely to capture the essence of the phenomena by combining qualitative and quantitative methods. In mixed methods, research elements of both qualitative and quantitative approaches are present. In this approach, representativeness and generalizability of quantitative research and in-depth contextual nature of qualitative research are combined in a single research study.

Meaning

Mixed methods research is a research approach that combines philosophical assumptions of both qualitative and quantitative approaches and goes beyond simply collecting and analyzing both kinds of data. It uses both approaches in tandem, so that the overall strength of the study is greater than either qualitative or quantitative research (Creswell and Plano Clark, 2007).

The benefits of combining the qualitative and quantitative methods can increase the confidence in study data, expand understanding of the phenomena and integration of theories. Denzin (1989) believed that combining multiple theories, methods, and data sources can assist researchers in overcoming the bias that comes from single method. He defines triangulation as the combination of two or more theories, data sources, methods, or investigators in the study of a single phenomenon.

Triangulation method evolved to include using multiple data collection and analysis methods, multiple data sources and multiple theories. Triangulation can be done in four basic ways:

1. **Data triangulation:** It refers to use of multiple data sources to validate conclusions. It includes time, space, and person triangulation. In time triangulation, data on the same phenomena is collected at different times. In space triangulation, the researcher collects data on the same phenomenon at different sites. In person triangulation, data is collected from different types of subjects. Collection of data from many sources widens the perspective on the phenomenon of interest.
2. **Methods triangulation:** It refers to use of multiple data collection methods to collect the information.
3. **Researcher triangulation:** In this, more than one researcher may collect the data to ensure the validity of the collected information and minimize the researcher bias.
4. **Theory triangulation:** In this, the researcher uses more than one theory or hypothesis to analyze and interpret the data. This helps the researcher to avoid preconceived ideas to guide data analysis and interpretation.

Example: Daaleman TP et al. (2008) conducted a qualitative study to explore spiritual care needs among end-life patients. The main aim of this study was to explore the views of medical professionals on spiritual care provided to dying patients and their family members. This study collected information from 12 clinicians and other healthcare providers by conducting interviews.

Other Types of Research Designs

Numerous other designs exist that do not fit into the aforementioned classification system.

Usually, these designs originate from specific questions arising from unique purpose.

Historical Research

Historical research is the systematic collection, critical evaluation, and interpretation of historical evidence. It answers questions relating to causes, effects, or trends relating to past events that may throw light on the prevalent behavior or practices. Many nurse researchers have undertaken biographical histories to become aware of the prevailing values and beliefs that may have shaped the successive developments in nursing. Data sources include records, video tapes, photographs and interviews, review of published reports, etc.

Lusk (2000) conducted a historical research to evaluate the relative status of nurses in advertisements by analyzing their images in advertisements from 1930 to 1950. She hypothesized that nurses relative status in advertisements would be higher in 1940 (when women were encouraged to enter nursing as a patriotic duty) than in 1930 or 1950.

Methodological Studies

These are conducted to develop, validate, test, and evaluate the research instruments and methods.

Tejero (2010) conducted a methodological study to develop and validate an instrument to measure nurse–patient bonding.

Secondary Analysis

It uses previously gathered data to test new hypotheses, explore new relationships among variables, or create new insights. Because the process of data collection is time consuming and extensive, use of secondary data is an efficient way to create new insights and new knowledge. The various clinical nursing databases available as management and policy tools serve as important sources of data for secondary analysis.

Harris et al (2016) conducted secondary analysis by using existing data to find out patients' experiences of psychiatric care in emergency departments.

Meta-analysis

In this technique, findings from several studies are utilized to create a data set that may be analyzed as a single piece of datum. It is the analysis of analyses. It involves taking the findings from several studies on the same subject and analyzing them using standardized statistical procedures. This helps to draw conclusions and detect relationships between findings. It offers a possibility to classify and measure the conditions and results of studies on a more precise and rigorous way compared to verbal descriptions of research.

Zangaro and Soeken (2007) conducted a meta-analysis of studies of nurses' job satisfaction. 31 studies were included in meta-analysis. This study examined the strength of the relationship between job satisfaction, autonomy, job stress, and nurse–physician collaboration among registered nurses working in staff position.

Outcomes Research

It is a branch of public health research that deals with the end results (outcomes) of the structure and processes of the healthcare system on the health and well-being of patients and population. This research examines effect of interventions on health status of patients (or communities).

- ❖ It describes, interprets, and predicts the impact of healthcare interventions on patient health outcomes, which is important to healthcare providers, government and private agencies, accrediting organizations, and society at large.
- ❖ These studies focus on outcomes, which include quality of life, care satisfaction, and financial burden among patients and caregivers.
- ❖ It relies on various disciplines such as epidemiology, informatics, anthropology, economics, health services research, health policy, and biostatistics.

- These studies utilize both qualitative and quantitative research methods, which include experimental and non-experimental methods, RCTs, meta-analysis, observational methods, prospective cohort studies, retrospective cohort studies, population-based studies, and economical analysis.
- Outcomes studies generally use large representative, heterogeneous sample rather than random samples.
- Outcome studies provide good opportunity to build a strong scientific foundation for nursing practice.
- Outcomes research mainly focuses on evaluating patient outcomes, structural variables, and process of care.
    - *Evaluating care outcomes* includes long-term symptoms, daily activities of living, quality of life, functioning status, etc. Example: Ausserhofer (2013) conducted a cross-sectional survey to explore the relationship between patient safety climate and patient outcomes in acute care hospitals. The organizational variables included in this study were quality of nurse practice environment, nurse staff levels, and skill mix. The patient outcomes were pressure ulcers, falls among patients, iatrogenic infections, and patient satisfaction.
    - *Evaluating structure of care* includes organization and administration elements, patient characteristics that guide the process of care such as nurse staffing, work environment, hospital characteristics, organization of care delivery, etc. Example: Effken (2013) used dynamic network analysis tool to examine handoffs between day and night shifts on seven units in three hospitals. This study examined the relationship between the handoff communication network metrics and a variety of patient safety quality and satisfaction outcomes.
    - *Evaluating the process of care* includes standards of care, practice styles, and cost of care. Example: Cossette (2012) conducted a randomized trial to evaluate efficacy of individual nursing intervention among acute coronary syndrome patients. The study intervention included a one-to-one nurse patient meeting before patient discharge and two follow-ups after discharge over a 10-day period. The outcomes included in this study were illness perceptions, family support, anxiety level, medication adherence, and knowledge on cardiac risk factors among patients.

Critiquing Qualitative Research Design

- Does the research design fit appropriately according to the variables studied and purpose of the study?
- Does the study focus on the subjective nature of human experience?

DEVELOPING RESEARCH PLAN

Once the research problem is identified and defined, the researcher must organize his ideas and put them in a written form which can be described as a research plan.

Advantages of Developing a Research Plan

- Helps the researcher to arrange the ideas in a systematic way so as to get a glimpse of flaws and inadequacies.
- It provides a list of what must be done and which materials have to be collected as a preliminary study.
- This documentation allows to seek critical review from experts.

Components of Research Plan

- The problem to be studied by the research must be explicitly stated

- Research objectives should be clearly stated
- Each concept or variable to be measured should be defined in operational terms
- The plan should include the method to be used in solving the research problem
- Should state the population and methods to select the sample
- Must include data collection measures
- The plan must also state the details of the techniques to be adopted. For example, interview method or observation technique, etc.
- Pilot study results should be mentioned
- Should include the time and cost budget
- The plan must also include data processing methods

BIBLIOGRAPHY

1. Ahuja, S. (2014). Correlational Analysis of Physical, Mental, Emotional, Spiritual, Social and Self-Consciousness. *Indian journal of applied research*, 4(6), 1-4.
2. Amici, D., Klersy, C., Ramajoli, F., Brustua, L., & Politi, P. (2000). Impact of the Hawthorne Effect in a Longitudinal Clinical Study: Controlled Clinical Trials. *International Emergency Nursing*, 21(2):103–14. doi: 10.1016/j.ienj.2015.09.004.
3. Ausserhofer, D., Schubert, M., Desmedt, M., Blegen, M.A., De Geest, S., Schwendimann, R. (2013). The association of patient safety climate and nurse-related organizational factors with selected patient outcomes: a cross-sectional survey. *International Journal of Nursing studies,* 50(2), 240-50
4. Brown, J., Hanson, J.M., Schmotzer, B., Webel, A.R. (2014). Spirituality and optimism: a holistic approach to component-based, self-management treatment for HIV. *Journal of Religion Health*, 53(5), 1317-28.
5. Brown, S.J. (2014). *Evidenced-based nursing: the research practice connection* (3rd ed.). Sudbury, MA: Jones and Bartlett
6. Browner, W.S., Newman, T.B., Cummings, S.R., & Hulley, S.B. (2001). *Designing Clinical Research: An epidemiologic approach* (2nd ed.). Philadephia: Lippincott Williams and Wilkins.
7. Burns, N., & Grove, S.K. (2004). *The practice of nursing research*. Philadelphia: W.B. Saunders Company.
8. Campbell, D.T., & Stanley, C.J. (1963). *Experimental and Quasi-Experimental Designs for Research.* Boston: Houghtan Mifflin Company.
9. Carpenter, D.R. (2007). Phenomenology as method. In H.J. Streubert & D.R. Carpenter (Eds.), *Qualitative research in nursing: Advancing the humanistic imperative* (pp. 75- 99). Philadelphia, PA: Lippincott.
10. Chlebowski, R.T. & Grosvenor, M. (1994). The scope of nutrition intervention trials with cancer-related endpoints. *Cancer*, 74, 2734–2738.
11. Chinn, P.L., & Kramer, M.K. (1995). *Theory and nursing: A systematic approach* (4th ed.). St. Louis: Mosby Yearbook.
12. Chuang, W.L., Chang, W.Y., Lu, S.N., Su, W.P., Lin, Z.Y., Chen, S.C., Hsieh, M.Y., Wang, L.Y., You, S.L. & Chen, C.J. (1992). The role of hepatitis B and C viruses in hepatocellular carcinoma in a hepatitis B endemic area. A case–control study. *Cancer*, 69, 2052–2054.
13. Claire, & Selltiz., et al. (1962). *Research Methods in Social Sciences*. New York; Holt, Rinehart and Winston, Inc.
14. Cohen, J. (1988). *Statistical power analysis for the behavioral sciences* (2nd ed.). Hillsdale, NJ: Lawrence Erlbaum Associates.
15. Cossette, S., Frasure-Smith, N., Dupuis, J., Juneau, M., Guertin, M.C. (2012). Randomized controlled trial of tailored nursing interventions to improve cardiac rehabilitation enrollment. *Nurse Research*, 61(2), 111-120.
16. Creswell, J.W., & Plano Clark, V.L. (2007). *Designing and conducting mixed methods research*. Thousand Oaks, CA: Sage.
17. Daaleman, P.T., Usher, M.B., Williams, W.S., Rawlings, M., & Hanson, C.L. (2008). An exploratory study of spiritual care at the end of life. *Annals of Family medicine*, 6(5), 406-411.
18. Denzin, N.K. (1989). *The research act: A theoretical introduction to sociological methods* (3rd ed.). New York: McGraw-Hill.
19. Dickoff, J., & James, P. (1968). A theory of theories: A position paper. Nursing Research, 17(3), 197-203.

20. Effken, J.A., Gephart, S.M., Brewer, B.B., & Carley, K.M. (2013). Using ORA a network analysis tool to assess the relationship of handoffs to quality and safety outcomes. *CIN: Computers, Informatics, Nursing*, 31(1), 36-44.
21. Evans, M., Hastings, N., & Peacock, B. (2000). *Statistical Distribution* (3rd ed.). New York: Wiley.
22. Frey., Lawrence. R., & Carl, L. Kreps. (2000). *Investigation Communication: An Introduction to Research Methods* (2nd ed.). Boston: Allyn and Bacon.
23. Fukao, A., Komatsu, S., Tsubono, Y., Hisamichi, S., Ohori, H., Kizawa, T., Ohsato, N., Fujino, N., Endo, N. & Iha, M. (1993). *Helicobacter pylori* infection and chronic atrophic gastritis among Japanese blood donors: a cross-sectional study. *Cancer Causes Control*, 4, 307-312.
24. Harris, B., Beurmann, R., Fagien, S., & Shattell, M.M. (2009). Patient's experiences of psychiatric care in emergency departments: A secondary analysis. *Nightingale Journal of Nursing*, 47(5):608-15. doi: 10.1016/j.ijnurstu.2009.10.007.
25. Hasson, D., Llindfors, P., & Gustavsson, P. (2010). Trends in self-rated health among nurses: a 4-year longitudinal study on the transition from nursing education to working life. *Journal of Professional Nurse*, 26(1):54-60. doi: 10.1016/j.profnurs.2009.09.002.
26. Henderson, M.M. (1995). Nutritional aspects of breast cancer. *Cancer*, 76 (suppl. 10), 2053-2058.
27. Jackson, S.L. (2011). *Research Methods and Statistics: A Critical Approach* (4th ed.). New York, NY: Greenwood.
28. Kerlinger, F.N. (1979). *Foundations of Behavioral research: A conceptual approach*. New York: Holt, Rinehart and Winston.
29. Knobf, M.T. (2002). Carrying on: The experience of premature menopause in women with early stage breast cancer. *Nursing Research*, 51(1), 9-17.
30. Kremer, H., Ironson, G. (2014). Longitudinal spiritual coping with trauma in people with HIV: implications for health care. *AIDS Patient Care STDS*, 28(3), 144-54. doi: 10.1089/apc.2013.0280.
31. Lusk, B. (2000). Pretty and powerless: Nurses in advertisements, 1930-1950. *Research in nursing & health*, 23, 229-36.
32. MacNealy., & Mary, S. (1999). *Strategies for Empirical Research in Writing*. New York: Longman.
33. Nora-Beata., Erichsen., & Arndt, B. (2013). *Evidenced Based Complement Alternative Medicine*, 3, 635-647. doi: 10.1155/2013/913247
34. Parahoo, K. (1997). *Nursing research: principles, process and issues*. Basingstoke: Macmillan.
35. Polit, D.F., Beck, C.T., & Hungler, B.P. (2006). *Essentials of nursing research: Methods, appraisal and utilization* (6th ed.). Philadelphia: Lippincott Williams & Wilkins.
36. Polit, D.F. and Hungler, B.P. (2013). *Essentials of Nursing Research: Methods, Appraisal, and Utilization* (8th ed.). Philadelphia: Wolters Kluwer/Lippincott Williams and Wilkins.
37. Polit, D.F. and Beck, C.T. (2014). *Essentials of Nursing Research Appraising Evidence for Nursing Practice (*8th ed.). Philadelphia: Lippincott Williams & Wilkins.
38. Rungreangkulkij, S., Chesla, C. (2001). Smooth a heart with water: Thai mothers care for a child with schizophrenia. *Archives of psychiatric nursing*, 15, 120-7.
39. Shadish, W.R., Cook, T.D., & Compbell, D.T. (2002). *Experimental and quasi-experimental designs for generalized causal inferences*. Chicago: Rand McNally.
40. Tanya, G., Doef, M., Leiden, S.M., leiden, V.C. (2006). A Longitudinal Study of Job Stress in the Nursing Profession: Causes and Consequences. *Journal of Nursing Management*, 14, 289-299.
41. Tejero, L.M.S. (2011). The mediating role of the nurse–patient dyad bonding in bringing about patient satisfaction. *Journal of Advanced Nursing*, 68(5), 994–1002.
42. Timothy, P. Daaleman., M.P.H., Barbara, M. Usher., Sharon, W. Williams., Jim Rawlings., & Laura, C.H. (2008). *Annals of Family Medicine*, 6(5), 406–411
43. Tuckman, B.W. (1978). *Conducting Educational Research*. New York: Harcourt Brace Jovanovick, Inc.
44. Willett, W.C., Stampfer, M.J., Colditz, G.A., Rosner, B.A., Hennekens, C.H. & Speizer, F.E. (1987). Dietary fat and the risk of breast cancer. *New Engl J Med*, 316, 22-28

45. Wittig, D. (2001). Organ donation beliefs of African American women residing in a small Southern community. *Journal of Transcultural Nursing*, 12(3), 203-210.

46. Zangaro, A.G., & Soeken, L.K. (2007). A meta-analysis of studies of nurses' job satisfaction. *Research in Nursing and health*, 30, 445-458.

REVIEW QUESTIONS

I. Long Essays

1. Define research design. Explain characteristics of research design.
2. Write the classification of research design. Discuss advantages and disadvantages of experimental research.
3. What is qualitative research design? List out the types and explain any one type with an example.
4. Differentiate between qualitative and quantitative research designs.
5. List various nonexperimental research designs. Explain correlational research designs with examples.
6. List various quasi-experimental designs. Describe its advantages and disadvantages.

II. Short Essays

1. Explain characteristics of true experimental research design.
2. What are the factors to be considered while selecting research methods?
3. Explain descriptive research designs.
4. Differentiate between experimental and nonexperimental research design.
5. Explain in detail about retrospective and prospective designs.
6. What are epidemiological research designs and briefly explain the types?
7. Explain the types of true experimental research design.
8. Narrate survey methods.

III. Short Answers

1. Threats to internal validity
2. Threats to external validity
3. Survey studies
4. Hawthorne effect
5. Observational studies
6. Design
7. Cross-sectional designs
8. Attrition
9. Manipulation
10. Randomization
11. Control

IV. Multiple Choice Questions

1. Blueprint of research work is called
    a. Research problem
    b. Research design
    c. Research tools
    d. Research methods
2. Research design involves description of
    a. Research approach
    b. Setting of the study
    c. Sample size
    d. All of these
3. Which research paradigm is least concerned about generalizing its findings?
    a. Quantitative research
    b. Qualitative research
    c. Mixed research
    d. None of the above
4. What is the key defining characteristic of experimental research?
    a. Extraneous variables are never present
    b. A positive correlation usually exists
    c. A negative correlation usually exists
    d. Manipulation of the independent variable
5. Which of the following best describes quantitative research?
    a. The collection of non-numerical data
    b. An attempt to test the researcher's hypotheses

c. Research that is exploratory
d. Research that attempts to generate a new theory

6. "A study to assess the experiences of patients suffering from rheumatoid arthritis." Which of the following designs is suitable to this study?
   a. Descriptive study
   b. Correlation study
   c. Historical study
   d. Experimental study

7. Which of the designs is suitable for the given example? "A comparative study on pain symptoms between male and female rheumatoid arthritis patients."
   a. Descriptive design
   b. Correlational design
   c. Comparative design
   d. Explorative design

8. The most appropriate research design for testing the cause-and-effect relationship between the variables is
   a. Experimental
   b. Correlational
   c. Descriptive
   d. Qualitative

9. Which of the designs is suitable for the given example? "To assess the cholesterol level among daily walkers and non-daily walkers."
   a. Experimental design
   b. Historical design
   c. Cross-sectional design
   d. Case–study design

10. Which of the following designs is suitable for the given example? "To assess the incidence of cardiovascular diseases among individuals followed up for 5 years."
    a. Retrospective design
    b. Longitudinal design
    c. Cross-sectional design
    d. Explorative design

11. Which of the designs is suitable for the given example? "A study to assess the multifactorial dimensions of pain and coping measures of rheumatoid arthritis patients."
    a. Experimental design
    b. Longitudinal design
    c. Retrospective design
    d. Explorative design

12. A longitudinal or prospective study is also referred to as a/an
    a. Ecological study
    b. Cross-sectional study
    c. Cohort study
    d. Observational study

13. Which of the following are essential characteristics of true experimental design, expect
    a. Manipulation
    b. Randomization
    c. Control
    d. Nonrandomization

14. In _____, you make observations prior to and immediately after introducing your independent variable
    a. Descriptive design
    b. Explorative design
    c. Pretest–posttest design
    d. Posttest only design

15. Which type of research provides the strongest evidence about the existence of cause-and-effect relationships?
    a. Nonexperimental research
    b. True experimental research
    c. Descriptive research
    d. Correlational research

16. A positive correlation is present when _____.
    a. Two variables move in opposite direction
    b. Two variables move in same direction
    c. One variable goes up and down
    d. Several variables never change

17. When two groups, control and experimental take a posttest after intervention without taking a pretest the design is called
    a. Cross-over design
    b. After-only design
    c. Solomon four-group design
    d. Pretest–posttest design

18. Which of the following is a true experimental design?

a. Single-group, posttest-only design
b. Single-group, pretest-posttest design
c. Ex post facto design
d. Factorial design

19. Quasi-experimental designs have
    a. An independent variable and dependent variable
    b. Nonrandom allocation of participants to experimental and control groups
    c. Both (a) and (b)
    d. No manipulation

20. The group that does not receive the experimental treatment condition is the _____.
    a. Experimental group
    b. Control group
    c. Treatment group
    d. Independent group

21. John is conducting research on effects of eating bananas on memory. To investigate this, participants are given a memory test followed by either a rest period with a banana to eat or a rest period alone. They then complete a second memory test. The results of the first and second memory test are compared. This an example of a/an _____ design
    a. Cross-sectional
    b. Longitudinal
    c. Survey
    d. Experimental

22. The term internal validity refers to which of the following?
    a. There is no measurement error inherent in the instruments used in the study
    b. All participants in the study have been given exactly the same treatment
    c. The researcher can be confident that the results of the experiment are due to the experimental manipulation and nothing else
    d. The variables in the experiment are all under the direct control of the researcher

23. Which of the following is an advantage of retrospective design?

a. Several etiological factors can be studied at the same time
b. Suitable for descriptive studies
c. Suitable for evaluation of intervention
d. Cause-and-effect relationship can be established

24. "A study to determine the effect of lack of sleep on attention span of students the following day" is an example of which type of research design?
    a. Descriptive
    b. Correlated
    c. Experimental
    d. Non-experimental

25. The quasi-experimental design does not include
    a. Manipulation of independent variable or control
    b. Random sample or control group
    c. Random or manipulation of independent variable
    d. Manipulation of independent or dependent variables

26. When behavior of the study subjects and study outcome are altered as a result of subjects awareness of being under observation, this phenomena is called
    a. Hawthorne effect
    b. Maturation
    c. History
    d. Contamination

27. When experimental research is carried for a long period of time there may be changes in subjects in different ways like physical growth, fatigue, bodily changes, etc. This phenomena is called
    a. Hawthorne effect
    b. Maturation
    c. History
    d. Contamination

28. Experimental studies differ from other research approaches on account of following
    a. Controlled manipulation of at least one treatment variable
    b. Exposure of all the subjects to the treatment

c. Study participants will be easily available
d. Conducting the study will be easy
29. Case studies may concern an in-depth examination of
   a. Individuals
   b. Group of people
   c. Institutions
   d. All of the above
30. Which of the following designs controls for the sensitization of subjects to a pretest?
   a. Pretest–posttest control group design
   b. Solomon four-group design
   c. Case study
   d. Posttest only control group design
31. Which research is a study of past records and other information source?
   a. Fundamental research
   b. Applied research
   c. Historical research
   d. Basic research
32. .... involves the collection and analysis of the culture of a group.
   a. Phenomenological research
   b. Ethnographical research
   c. Grounded theory
   d. Historical research

ANSWER KEY

1. b	2. d	3. b	4. d	5. b	6. a
7. c	8. a	9. c	10. b	11. d	12. c
13. d	14. c	15. b	16. b	17. b	18. d
19. c	20. b	21. d	22. c	23. a	24. b
25. b	26. a	27. b	28. a	29. d	30. b
31. c	32. b				

UNIT 7

Sample and Sampling Techniques

The selection of a representative sample though comes across as an intricate, confusing, and technical subject; it is still an essential part of any research process. In research reports, the description of sampling process is presented in methods section. Frequently, the misinterpretations in terminology are on account of the contrasting meanings and usage. It would thus be ideal to examine the related terminology so as to make the underlying assumptions more clear.

Population is the aggregation of individuals or objects that possesses similar characteristics defined by the researcher. It includes target and accessible population.

Target population is the entire group of people or objects meeting a set of criteria established by the researcher for which he wishes to generalize the study findings. For example, in "a study to assess the biopsychosocial problems of human immunodeficiency virus (HIV) patients in India", the target population would be all the HIV patients in India.

Accessible population also known as the *study population* is the subset of the target population to which the researcher has reasonable access for selection of subjects to the research study. They may be limited to an institution, city, region, state or a country. In the above example, accessible population will be all the HIV patients taking treatment at a selected district hospital.

In research studies, it is not possible to study an entire population as studying it in its entirety is very time consuming, costly, and requires more resources. Therefore, a subset of subjects which is representative of a given population is selected which is termed as *sampling*. It is the process of choosing a set of people, incidents, or behaviors from a population for conducting the study.

A **sample** is a limited part of a population whose properties are studied to gain information about the whole (Webster, 1985).

- Sample is a group of people, objects, or elements that are taken from a larger population for participation in a study. In research studies, individuals are usually mentioned as subjects or participants.
- The selected sample should be representative of the entire population. By studying the sample the researcher generalizes the results to the population from which the sample has been chosen.
- In the above example, sample will refer to the HIV patients taking treatment at the selected district hospital during the data collection period.

An **element** is the most fundamental unit about which information is collected. In the above example, a single HIV patient refers to the element.

In sampling, the population is divided into a number of parts called *sampling units*.

Sampling frame is a list of the eligible participants who meet the characteristics of the population and are accessible to the researcher. It is the source or list of all the subjects, objects, or elements from which the sample is drawn. It defines the researcher's population of interest. For example, a list of all HIV patients taking treatment at selected district hospital during the data collection period.

Problems in Sampling Frame
- Incomplete sampling frame: This sampling frame does not include all the elements in the population. Such incomplete frames cannot yield representative samples. For example, a list of under-5 age group children in a specific geographic area may not contain the names of all under-5 age group children due to nonregistration.
- Blanks or foreign elements in sampling frame: Some sampling frames have blanks or contain elements not relevant to the target population. For example, the list of members in Trained Nurses Association of a specific state may contain a few members from the other state.
- Duplicate listing: Sometimes elements appear more than once in the sampling frame.

In evaluating the sampling frame, the researcher should consider the above problems and take appropriate remedial action like preparing supplementary list of missing items or preparing a new list.

Examples of target population, accessible population, and their sampling frames are presented in Table 7.1 and Figure 7.1.

Randomization is a procedure which guarantees an equal opportunity to each individual in the population to be a part of the sample so as to minimize the differences among groups by equally distributing them based on certain characteristics.

Representativeness means the sample must be as similar to the population in as many ways as possible. As the representative sample reflects the characteristics of the population, it allows the sample findings to be generalized to the population. Randomization is the best way to achieve representativeness which may either be through random selection or random assignment.

Sampling error is the deviation of the selected sample from the true characteristic of the entire population. This error occurs when the researcher selects a sample that is non-representative of the entire population and the results thus generated do not represent the results that would have been obtained from the entire population.

Table 7.1: Examples of target population, accessible population, and their sampling frame

Target population	Accessible (study) population	Sampling frame
• All depressive disorder patients taking antidepressant treatment in District hospitals	• All depressive disorder patients taking antidepressant treatment in district hospital, Kolar	• A list of all depressive disorder patients taking antidepressant treatment in district hospital, Kolar
• All HIV patients taking treatment in ART centers	• All HIV patients taking treatment in ART centers of Bengaluru city	• A list of all HIV patients taking treatment in ART centers of Bengaluru city
• All institutionalized chronic mentally ill patients	• All institutionalized chronic mentally ill patients in Bengaluru city	• A list of all institutionalized chronic mentally ill patients in Bengaluru city
• All children suffering with autistic disorder	• All autistic children taking treatment in Institute of Mental Health, Hyderabad.	• List of all autistic children taking treatment in Institute of Mental Health, Hyderabad.

(ART: Antiretroviral Therapy; HIV: Human Immunodeficiency Virus)

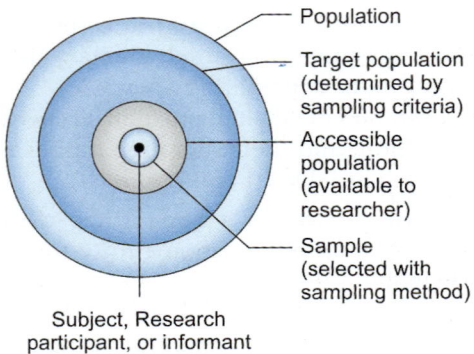

Fig. 7.1: Population and sample

Sampling bias refers to the systematic error in sample selection leading to over-representation or under-representation of a certain section of the population in terms of an attribute related to the research study.

Selection bias occurs when subjects are selected for the study or assigned to groups in a way that is not objective (impartial). This may pose a threat to the validity of the study.

Sampling plan is an explicit plan stating the sampling method, sample size, and the subject recruitment procedure.

Eligibility criteria: It is a criterion defined by the researcher which states who can or cannot participate in the study. It provides a list of characteristics that must be possessed by all the subjects participating in the study. The researcher should narrowly define these criteria to ensure homogeneity in the sample and also control extraneous variables. These criteria have an implication while interpreting the results and generalizing the findings.

Inclusion criteria are predefined characteristics that each subject should possess so as to be included in the sample. These are guidelines for choosing subjects with a predetermined set of characteristics that include major features important to the research question.

Exclusion criteria are characteristics that a population must not possess. These are characteristics that eliminate a potential subject from the study. These characteristics are often considered as extraneous factors that confound the results and present threats to the validity of the study conclusions. The exclusion criteria serve as a control for extraneous and confounding factors and make the sample homogeneous.

In descriptive, correlational, and survey research designs, the eligibility criteria tend to be less restrictive. However, in comparative and true or quasi-experimental designs the eligibility criteria tend to be more restrictive so as to serve as a control for extraneous factors that may confound the results.

"A study to evaluate the efficacy of body-mind-spirit intervention on well-being and process of recovery among depressive patients in a selected district hospital of Karnataka". The eligibility criteria for the above study is presented in Table 7.2.

Advantages of Sampling

- *Economical in nature*: In most cases, measuring the whole population is difficult and impossible because of the large size and part of it being inaccessible. It is economical to collect data from the sample rather than the entire population, when the resources are limited. By using sampling method, the researcher can save time, money, and resources. Sampling provides an economical option for the researcher to generate empirical evidence.
- *More practical*: Sampling is the only practical and convenient method, when the population is infinite. Sampling makes the data collection and interpretation much easier and enables a better understanding of the data.
- *Possible to collect intensive and exhaustive data*: As the number is limited, it is possible to collect an in-depth and comprehensive data. It is also easy to establish better rapport with the subjects.

| Table 7.2: Eligible criteria ||
Inclusion criteria	Exclusion criteria
• Patients who had a current diagnosis of depression confirmed by a psychiatrist that met the criteria of International Classification of Diseases, Tenth Revision (ICD-10) code—F32.0–F32.2 (mild depressive disorder, moderate depressive disorder, and severe depressive episode without psychotic symptoms), F33.0–F33.2 (recurrent depressive disorder—current episode mild, moderate, and severe without psychotic symptoms) and F34.1 (dysthymia) • Aged between 20 and 40 years • Being able to converse, read and write in Kannada or English languages • Recommended antidepressant treatment by the treating psychiatrist • Began antidepressant treatment during the immediately preceding 1-week period	• Depressive patients with psychotic symptoms (ICD-10 F32.3 and F33.3). • Individual with a dual diagnosis or comorbid disorder like cancer, hypertension, diabetes, and other severe life-threatening illnesses • Current drug or alcohol dependence or abuse (within the last 3 months) • Patients who displayed unmanageable behaviors requiring extensive care • Effective ongoing psychotherapy • Pregnancy or breastfeeding • A significant medical condition that could interfere with participation in therapy

* *Greater accuracy and reliability*: Conducting study on an entire population provides the researcher with huge data, making it a burdensome task to maintain the exactness. Thus sampling ensures completeness, precision, and reliability as the magnitude of the process is limited.

Disadvantages of Sampling

* *Chances of bias*: If sample is not selected carefully, it may lead to sampling bias.
* *Difficulty in getting representative sample*: When there are inherent defects in the population, it is difficult to get a truly representative sample.
* *Need for specific knowledge*: The researcher should have specialized knowledge on sampling process and techniques.

Characteristics of a Good Sample Design

For a sample to be more purposeful it should echo the similarities and differences inherent to the population. The main idea behind drawing a sample is to draw inferences about the larger population using the smaller sample. The following are the characteristics of a sample (Fig. 7.2):

* *Representativeness*: It means that the sample, the accessible population, and the target population characteristics are similar in as many ways as possible. The sample characteristics must be reasonably representative of the characteristics of the population. For example, a sample must be representative in terms of demographic characteristics, which may include age, gender, occupation, monthly income, area of residence, type of family, etc. which often

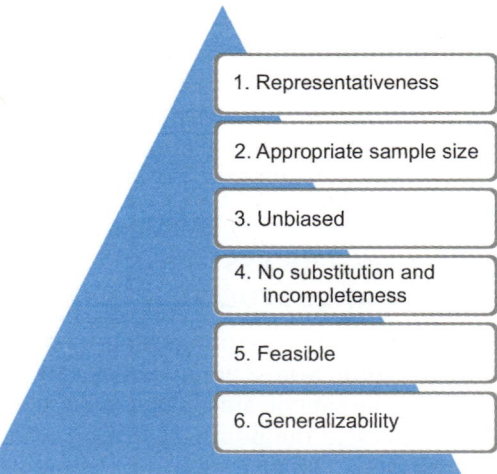

Fig. 7.2: Characteristics of a good sample design

influence the study variables. The sample also needs to be representative relative to the variables being examined in the study. For example, if the study examines attitude towards restraints among nurses, the sample must be representative of the distribution of attitudes towards restraints use among nurses. Representativeness of the sample makes it possible to generalize the findings to the population.

- *Appropriate sample size*: In quantitative studies, the sample size should be adequate to get reliable results. As the sample size increases, the representativeness of the sample also increases. This increase in sample size automatically decreases the sampling errors.
- *Unbiased*: Sample should be free from errors or bias. A sample is unbiased, if every individual in the population has an equal opportunity of being selected. This sample is representative of the population. Bias is introduced into the sample when the sample is selected nonrandomly.
- *No substitution and incompleteness*: Once the sample is selected, it is neither replaced nor is it incomplete in any aspect of research interest.
- *Feasible in the context of funds and time available*: Sample design must be feasible in terms of available resources and time.
- *Generalizability*: Sample should be such that the results obtained from the sample data can in general be applied to the larger population with a reasonable level of confidence.

SAMPLING PROCESS IN QUANTITATIVE STUDIES

Sampling is the process of choosing a subset of the population from a population of interest. Studying the sample aids in generalizing the results back to the population from which it was taken. The two important principles in sampling process are selecting right people and right number to have an accurate representativeness of the population and minimize sampling errors. In quantitative studies, sampling plan is formulated in advance so that the researcher can anticipate the feasibility, precision, and cost in sample selection. The carefully carried out sampling process helps to draw a representative sample from the population. The major steps in sampling process are listed in Figure 7.3 by way of an example. Let us consider the study "evaluate the efficacy of body-mind-spirit intervention on well-being and process of recovery among depressive patients in a selected district hospital of Karnataka".

- *Identifying and defining the target population:* Once the study topic is finalized, the researcher usually has some idea about the target population based on the area of interest.

  A review of the literature reveals the target populations studied in the past and their relation to the present study. The problem statement describes purpose of the study, variables, population, and setting. The researcher has to then define elements, sampling units, extent, and timing (Table 7.3).

  In the above study, the target population can be all depressive disorder patients between the age of 20 and 40 years and on antidepressant medication.
- *Describing the accessible population*: The accessible population is a subset of target population to which the researcher should have reasonable access for selection of subjects. It may be restricted to a region, city, or an institution. For example, all depressive disorder patients taking antidepressant treatment at a selected district hospital in Karnataka. While determining the accessible population, the researcher should consider the available resources like money, time, location, and willingness of the subjects to participate in the study.

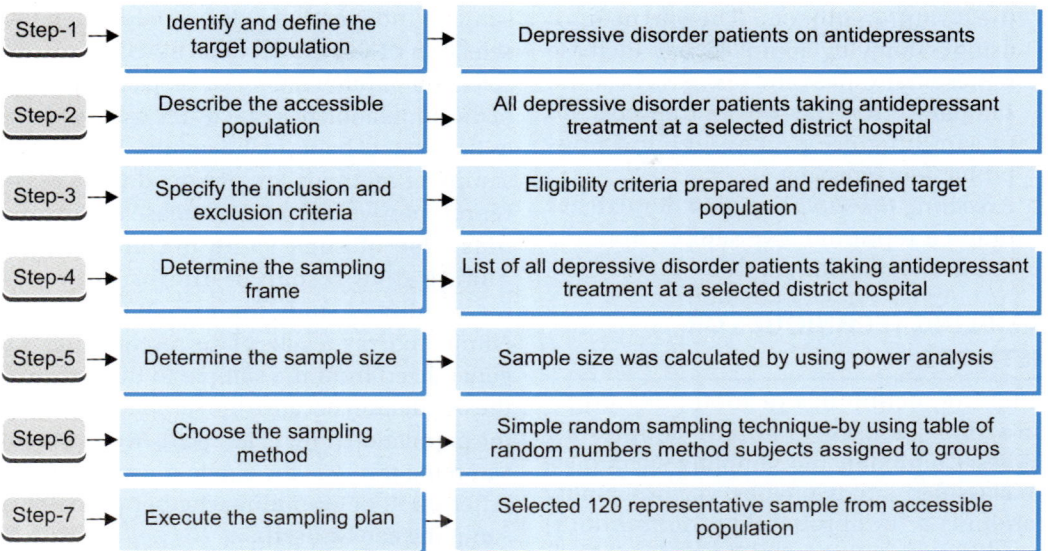

Fig. 7.3: Steps in quantitative sampling process

Table 7.3: Examples of defining elements, sampling units, extent, and timing			
Elements	Sampling units	Extent	Timing
Individuals	Individuals over 20 years	Individuals over 20 years of age having tobacco chewing habit	Individuals over 20 years of age having tobacco chewing habit for the last 5 years
Families	Families with kids	Families with two kids	Families with two kids and residing in a specified area for the last 1 year
Patients	Patients with depressive disorder	Patients who are suffering with depressive disorder for the last minimum 1 year	Depressive disorder patients taking antidepressant treatment in a district hospital during a specified time period

❖ *Specifying the inclusion and exclusion criteria*: In this step, the researcher specifies the characteristics of the population by detailing inclusion and exclusion criteria. The sample should meet all the inclusion criteria. This eligibility criterion helps the researcher to redefine the target population.

❖ *Determining the sampling frame*: In this step, the researcher identifies elements in the accessible population and makes a list of all the participants. A list of sampling unit and setting is also prepared. For example, preparing the list of all depressive disorder patients taking antidepressant treatment at a selected district hospital in Karnataka.

❖ *Determining the sample size*: In this step, the researcher decides how many elements of the accessible population are to be chosen for the study. The selection of sampling method and sample size depend upon the time and funds available for conducting research.

❖ *Choosing the sampling approach or method*: The researcher must decide on the method or technique for selecting the sample subjects. The purpose of using a sampling approach is to increase representativeness and decrease bias and sampling error. The two basic approaches to sampling are probability and non-probability sampling.

❖ *Executing the sampling plan*: Researcher draws a representative sample from the accessible population.

SAMPLING TECHNIQUES OR METHODS

Sampling techniques or methods outline the strategies used to obtain samples for studies. Commonly the sampling techniques are classified into two types, viz. probability (random) or nonprobability (nonrandom) sampling techniques or methods (Fig. 7.4).

Probability Sampling Techniques or Methods

In probability (random) sampling technique, elements are randomly selected from a given population. In this method, every member of the available population has an equal and independent chance of being selected for the sample. Independence is ensured when the selection of one subject has no effect on the selection of other subjects, i.e. each member of the population has exactly the same chance as the other of being in the sample. Probability sampling methods are designed to increase representativeness and decrease systematic bias. Use of such sampling methods in quantitative research studies improves the validity of study findings. When bias is eliminated, the results of the research may be generalized from the sample to the whole of the population because the sample represents the population (Frey et al. 2000). Availability of sampling frame is the single most important criterion in determining whether probability sampling can be used.

Types of Probability Sampling Techniques

The four most commonly used probability sampling methods are (1) simple random, (2) stratified random, (3) systematic, and (4) cluster.

1. *Simple random sampling technique:* It is the simplest of the probability sampling techniques. In this technique, the researcher randomly selects the sample from a sampling frame. Each member of the accessible population has an equal chance of being chosen as a subject. The prerequisites for implementing, this technique must include a homogenous population and availability of the sampling frame (list of the members of accessible population) (Fig. 7.5). The advantages and disadvantages of simple random sampling technique are presented in Table 7.4.
   Selection process
   ○ Identify and define the population
   ○ Decide the desired sample size
   ○ List all members of the population
   ○ Assign consecutive numbers to all members on the list
   ○ Choose any of the following methods to select sample

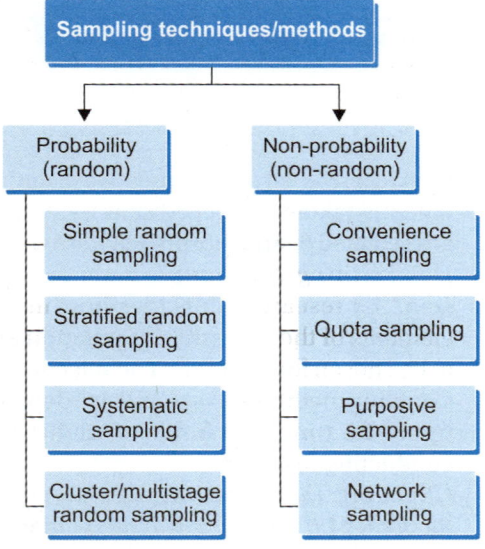

Fig. 7.4: Types of sampling methods or techniques

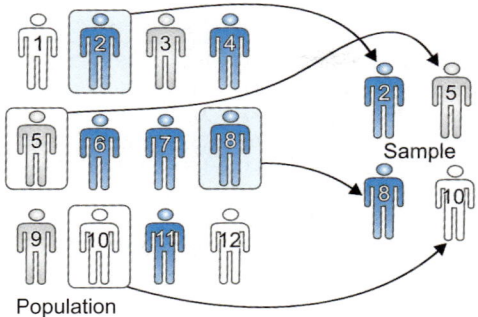

Population

Fig. 7.5: Simple random sampling technique

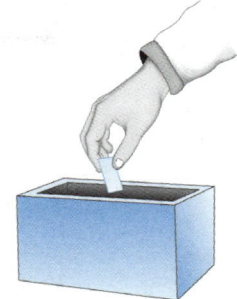

Fig. 7.6: Lottery method of sampling

Table 7.4: Simple random sampling technique—advantages and disadvantages	
Advantages	Disadvantages
• Easy to select sample • Eliminates researcher bias • Provides a means for estimating sampling error • Greater likelihood of getting a representative sample • Meets assumptions of many statistical procedures	• Researcher should have the list of all the members of the population, which is not always possible • Large sample size is compulsory • Time consuming especially if the population is large • Monetary costs are high • Laborious process—developing a sampling frame, numbering all the elements • Easy to get the data wrong just as easy it is to get it right

Methods: In simple random sampling technique, the sample can be selected using the following three methods:

i. *Lottery method:* The researcher can use the lottery method when the sampling frame is small. In this method, the researcher write names on slips of paper, place them in a box, mix them well and draw them one at a time until the desired sample size is arrived. All such selected names become the subject for the study. This lottery method can be carried out in either replacement or nonreplacement manner. In replacement method, the chosen name slips are replaced back in the box, while in the nonreplacement method the chosen name slips are not replaced back in the box (Fig. 7.6).

ii. *Table of random numbers method:* In this method, the researcher selects the subjects by using random number table. This random table includes several numbers in rows and columns. The researcher places a finger on the random table with his eyes closed. That number is the starting place. The numbers are further identified by moving the finger up, down, right, or left till the desired sample size is obtained. If the researcher comes across similar numbers, they are ignored and subsequent number considered. For example, if the researcher wants to select 30 subjects from a population of 250 subjects and the first number 22 is selected as a starting point, the subsequent 29 numbers will be those running in any of the specific directions. For example, in Box 7.1, the first number selected being 22 the subsequent numbers will

Basics in Nursing Research and Biostatistics

Box 7.1   Table of random numbers

43	239	210	67	190	222	**22**	154	58	245	114	138	169	85	109
145	151	69	2	19	61	168	74	237	126	240	205	232	206	93
199	42	135	157	247	112	29	152	196	208	6	200	213	236	123
220	64	132	55	94	141	170	87	88	217	113	76	57	39	26
18	28	184	63	207	227	62	179	131	177	224	31	159	161	158
79	133	107	66	49	91	56	102	189	182	73	229	171	155	215
197	191	172	89	166	111	99	248	250	146	65	27	219	50	96
192	35	47	221	103	37	40	243	14	117	48	3	101	122	82
7	121	204	75	212	30	137	164	241	20	188	68	198	235	36
52	201	116	25	16	148	51	108	90	119	216	163	174	8	13
110	214	181	233	95	167	238	10	54	150	162	149	33	21	117
98	228	32	246	23	9	165	203	24	44	118	127	12	153	176
70	226	160	11	136	115	84	147	178	45	242	97	124	193	183
211	185	105	139	218	34	81	186	225	38	223	15	92	244	142
195	80	140	77	46	128	83	144	100	180	173	187	5	194	234
134	175	129	59	4	249	156	209	78	125	41	230	72	231	202
86	71	106	120	143	53	130	68	154	65					

be 154, 58, 245, 114, 138... (right side); or 168, 29, 170, 62, 56, 99, ... (down).

iii. *Use of computer generated numbers:* Random number generator is a computer software program commonly used when the target population is large. These programs generate random numbers which can be categorized into true random numbers and pseudorandom numbers. While generating true random numbers, no prediction can be made about the generation of subsequent random number. However, while generating pseudorandom numbers, a prediction of the subsequent number can be made using specially designed algorithms. Hence, it is not really a random number.

2. *Stratified random sampling technique:* In this technique, the accessible population is subdivided into homogenous subsets or strata from which an appropriate number of elements are selected randomly. To prepare these subsets or strata, the researcher should be able to identify some significant characteristics of the population necessary to achieve representativeness. The strata are divided based on the selected characteristics of the population such as gender, occupation, diagnosis, geographical region, etc. Stratification ensures that all the identified characteristics are adequately represented in the sample (Fig. 7.7). By using this technique, the researcher can employ a smaller sample size to attain or meet the same degree of representativeness. The advantages and disadvantages of stratified random sampling technique are presented in Table 7.5.

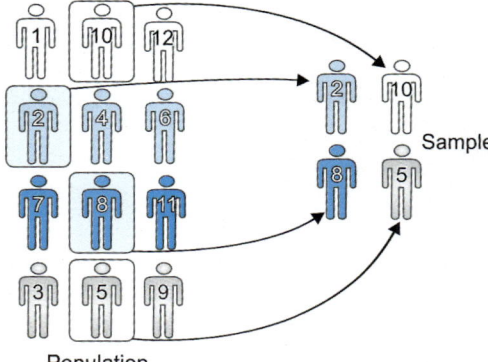

Fig. 7.7: Stratified random sampling technique

Procedure
- Identify and define the population
- Decide the desired sample size

Table 7.5: Stratified random sampling technique—advantages and disadvantages

Advantages	Disadvantages
• Ensures representative sample in heterogeneous population • Ensures accurate results compared to simple random sampling as the group differences within the subgroups are lesser compared to the differences while dealing with the entire population • Utilizes less resources in terms of time-money and effort as it deals with small sample size	• Requires a prior knowledge of the target population • Difficult to identify all members of the population • Difficult to identify all constituents of the subgroups • More laborious

- Recognize the characteristics and subgroups (strata)
- Assign the population to each of the identified subgroup (strata) based on the characteristics
    - Strata include mutually exclusively subgroups of population based on known characteristics such as gender, economic status, etc.
- Take a random sample of participants within each stratum.

Stratified random sampling technique can be classified into proportionate and disproportionate stratified sampling techniques. In *proportionate stratified random sampling,* the population is divided into small groups or strata based on common attributes or characteristics. Random samples are taken from each stratum in proportion to the population from which the strata were created. This is widely used, when the target population is heterogeneous. For example, if the population was diabetic patients in a hospital that had 10% children, 30% females, and 60% males, then a proportionate stratified sample of 100 patients with demographic background as the stratifying variable would consist of 10 children, 30 females, and 60 males from the respective strata. This ensures same sampling proportion in each stratum irrespective of the strata size. In simpler terms, it refers to selecting a sample that is specific to the relative proportions of the subgroups within the population (Table 7.6).

Table 7.6: Example of proportionate stratified random sampling

Stratum	Children	Female adults	Male adults
Population size	100	300	600
Sampling portion	10%	10%	10%
Sample size	10	30	60

In *disproportionate stratified random sampling,* the sample selected from each stratum is not in proportion to the size of the total population in that stratum, i.e. each stratum has different sampling portions. The generation of accurate results is based on the allocation of sampling portion by the researcher. This type of sampling is generally determined by three factors—(1) size of strata, (2) internal variances among strata, and (3) sampling costs. The single difference between proportionate and disproportionate stratified random sampling is their sampling portions (Table 7.7).

Reasons for undertaking stratified random sampling technique:
- When the researcher wants to emphasize on small but important subgroups within the population, this

Table 7.7: Example of disproportionate stratified random sampling

Stratum	Children	Female adults	Male adults
Population size	100	300	600
Sampling portion	10%	30%	60%
Sample size	35	35	35

technique guarantees the presence of the key subgroup within the sample.
- When a researcher attempts to observe existing relationships between two or more subgroups using a simple random sampling technique, the researcher is not confident about equal representation of the subgroups within the sample.
- When researcher wants to represent the most inaccessible subgroups in the population.
- When certain groups are heterogeneous the other are homogenous.
- When it is expected that the difference in response rates among the subgroups of the population will be appreciable.

3. *Systematic sampling technique:* It is a type of probability sampling method used when list of all the elements of the population is available. It is also called ordinal sampling or pseudo-simple random samples. The selection of the sample from the population list is made by randomly selecting a beginning and choosing every kth name (MacNealy, 1999) (Fig. 7.8). The advantages and disadvantages of systematic random sampling technique are presented in Table 7.8.

In this technique, the sample is selected from a larger population by first selecting a random starting point and a fixed periodic or sampling interval. This interval is calculated by dividing the entire population size by the desired sample size. For example, if a researcher wants to select about 100 subjects from a total population of 300, the total number of population (300) is divided by the number of samples required (100). The answer is 3 which is the fixed periodic interval. This effectively means that researcher is going to select every 3rd subject from the population list. First of all, the researcher should prepare the list of 300 members and then determine the random starting point between 1 and 3. For example, if the random starting point is "2", then select

Table 7.8: Systematic sampling technique—advantages and disadvantages

Advantages	Disadvantage
◆ Easy to carry out ◆ Inexpensive	◆ May lead to a biased sample, if a hidden periodic trait exists in the population

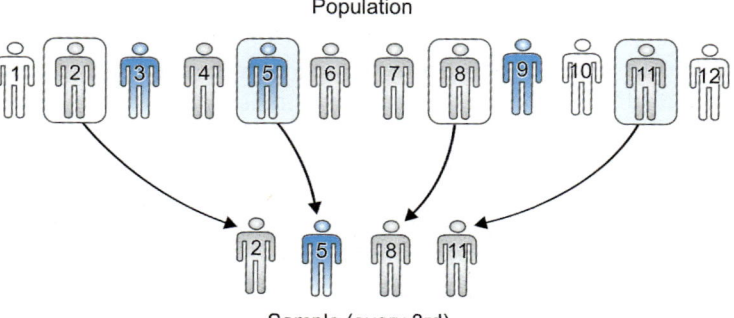

Fig. 7.8: Systematic sampling technique

every 3rd subject (5, 8, 11,.....) until the required 100 subjects have been selected.

Calculation of periodic interval:

$$k = \frac{\text{Number of subjects in the target population}}{\text{Sample size}} = \frac{300}{100} = 3$$

Procedure
- Identify and define the population
- Determine the desired sample size
- Prepare the list of members of the target population (sampling frame)
- Determine periodic interval or kth interval by dividing the size of the population by the desired sample size
- Select the first subject randomly from the list
- Take every kth individual on the list.

4. *Cluster sampling technique (multistage sampling):* Cluster sampling is a technique in which clusters of participants that represent the population are identified and included in the sample (Jackson, 2011). In this technique, randomly selected intact groups sharing similar characteristics form the sampling unit and not the individuals within the defined population, i.e. a group of subjects or elements form the sampling unit instead of a single subject or element. In this technique, instead of selecting all the subjects from the entire population, the researcher takes several steps to gather a sample. First the population is divided into subgroups known as clusters. From the subgroups, sample is selected randomly using simple random sampling technique or stratified random sampling technique. Thus subgroups of the population form the sampling unit (Fig. 7.9). If a sample is selected in single stage, it is called one stage sampling, but if random selection continues through several stages, it is called multistage sampling. For example, if a researcher wants to collect data from intensive care

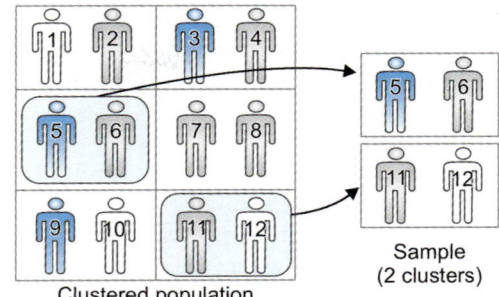

Fig. 7.9: Cluster sampling technique

unit (ICU) nurses, he divides all the hospitals in the city into different clusters. The researcher then selects the clusters through simple or systematic random sampling. From the randomly selected hospitals (clusters) the researcher can either include all ICU nurses as subjects or select a few ICU nurses using simple or systematic random sampling. This type of selection is called one-stage cluster sampling technique.

In multistage cluster sampling technique, the researcher randomly selects a few cities from a list of all cities in the state. Further, a list of all the hospitals in the randomly selected cities is made, of which a few hospitals are selected randomly. From these randomly selected hospitals, the researcher can either include all ICU nurses as subjects or select a few ICU nurses using simple or systematic random sampling.

Reasons for undertaking cluster sampling technique:
- When the population is large and scattered
- When the researcher cannot identify the individual elements or make the sampling frame.

For example, if the researcher wants to survey the academic performance of under graduate nursing students, the researcher divides the entire undergraduate nurses into different clusters (nursing colleges).

From those clusters, the researcher then selects subjects through simple or stratified random sampling technique (Flowchart 7.1)

Procedure
- Identify and define the population (undergraduate nurses)
- Determine the sample size (10,000)
- Decide the cluster (nursing colleges)
- List all clusters (list all nursing colleges)
- Estimate the average number of sample per cluster (for example 100 students in each nursing college constitute one cluster)
- Determine the number of clusters needed. It can be arrived at by dividing the sample size with the estimated size of a cluster (10,000/100 = 100; 100 clusters are required)
- Randomly select the needed number of clusters (randomly select 100 nursing colleges)
- Include all individuals from each of the selected clusters for the study (include all undergraduate nursing students from each selected nursing college)

Types of cluster sampling
- *One-stage sampling*: All the subjects within selected clusters are selected in the sample. For example, the researcher includes all the undergraduate nurses from all the randomly selected clusters as sample.
- *Two-stage sampling*: A subset of subjects within selected clusters is randomly selected for inclusion in the sample. For example, the researcher first lists all the clusters in the population followed by random selection of clusters. From such clusters subjects are then selected randomly using simple random or stratified random sampling technique.
- *Multistage sampling*: Sampling is done at more than two levels. For example, in studying the academic performance of final year undergraduate nurses in a state, the first stage will be to select a few districts in the state. The second stage will be to randomly select a few government and private nursing institutions for the study from the selected districts. In the third stage, the undergraduate nursing students will be selected from the above institutions. The last stage will be that of selecting final year undergraduate nursing students out of those nursing students (Fig. 7.10 and Table 7.9).

Representative sample can be obtained only through probability sampling methods. This method allows the researcher to estimate sampling error. Though it is the most preferred and valued method of obtaining sample elements,

Flowchart 7.1: Schematic presentation of cluster sampling technique

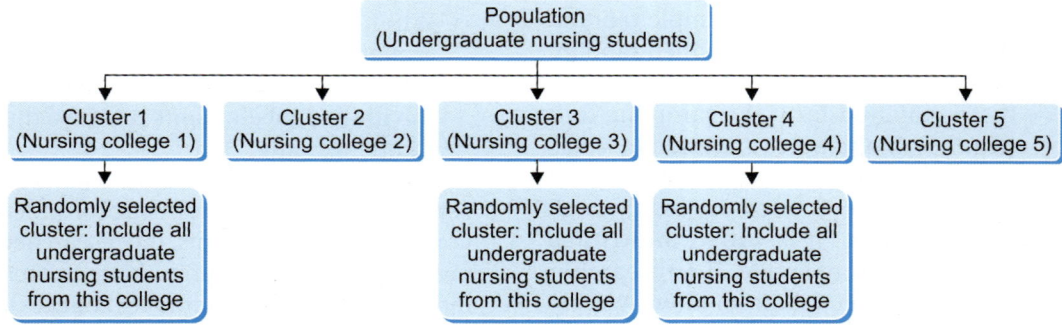

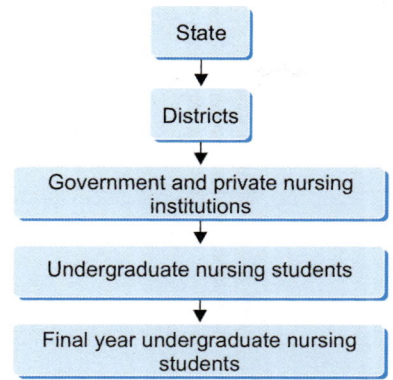

Fig. 7.10: Schematic presentation of multistage sampling

it may at times be impractical. The great drawback of probability sampling is its inconvenience and complexity. Table 7.10 presents the various probability sampling methods and the situations where they can best be employed.

Nonprobability Sampling Techniques or Methods

In nonprobability sampling, every element of a population does not have an opportunity or equal chance to be selected for a study sample. In this method, the elements are chosen by choice, not by chance, which restricts the generalizability of the study findings. Nonprobability sampling methods are useful when the total population is unknown or is not available. For example, where the study defines population as women in menopause it is difficult to find a list of names from any single source.

Generally, it is believed that use of nonprobability sampling methods is more likely to produce a biased sample than probability sampling methods. Nurse researchers must keep in mind that the sample must fit the purpose of the study and best represent the population rather than one that uses the most sophisticated sampling technique.

The four nonprobability sampling methods used most frequently in nursing research are: (1) convenience sampling, (2) quota sampling, (3) purposive sampling, and (4) network sampling.

Convenience Sampling

It is also called accidental sampling wherein the subjects are selected for the study simply because they happen to be in the right place at the right time. It is a nonprobability method of selecting a sample that includes subjects who are available in a convenient way to the researcher. Convenience sampling involves using the most conveniently available people as study participants (Fig. 7.11). To obtain a convenient sample of subjects the researcher simply plans to include those patients who happen to come into the clinic on data collection day. Examples of convenient sampling are patients who attend a clinic on a

Table 7.9: Cluster sampling technique—advantages and disadvantages	
Advantages	Disadvantages
• Very useful when population is large and geographically scattered • The most time-efficient and cost-efficient probability design • Does not need the names of everyone in the population • Larger sample size can be used due to increased level of accessibility of sample group members • A cluster sample would reduce the expense while allowing the results to be generalized	• Requires group-level information to be known • Commonly has higher sampling error than alternate sampling techniques as the clusters in the sample may be composed of similar units leading to large sampling error and reduction in the representativeness of the sample • Sample bias arises when subsets of unequal size are selected • It may not be feasible to apply the findings of this type of sampling to another area

Table 7.10: Summary of probability sampling methods

Method	Selection strategy	Best when	Example	Reliability of conclusions for fixed sample size	Economy	Remarks
Simple random sampling	Each member of the study population has an equal chance of being selected as a sample.	Whole population is available	The target sample included children aged 1–5 years in rural area. A sample of 100 children selected randomly from a list obtained from PHC.	Very good	Expensive	Requires full sampling
Staratified sampling	Each member in the population is assigned to a group or stratum. It is followed by sample selection using simple random sampling technique.	There are specific subgroups to investigate (e.g. demographic groupings)	Children are divided into different strata, e.g. 1 year old children, 2 year old children, 3 year old children, 4 year old children, and 5 year old children. For the study purpose, children are randomly selected from each stratum.	Good	Expensive	Good for non-homogenous population
Systematic sampling	Each member of the study population is listed. A random start is designated followed by selection of members at equal intervals from the population.	A stream of representative people is available (e.g. in the organization).	Prepare a list of children aged 1–5 years in a selected village; calculate sampling interval; first number is randomly selected; then children are selected at equal intervals until the desired number of sample is obtained.	Good	Economical	Sampling frame and size of target population are required
Cluster sampling	Each member of the study population is assigned to a group or cluster followed by random selection of clusters. Thus all members of a selected cluster are included in the sample.	When population groups are separated and access to all is difficult (e.g. population is from various distant cities).	Prepare the clusters, i.e. each village as one cluster which includes children aged 1–5 years; list all the villages; select villages randomly; then include all children aged 1–5 present in that cluster for study purpose.	Poor	Very economical	Very convenient for geographically diverse population

(PHC: Primary Health Center)

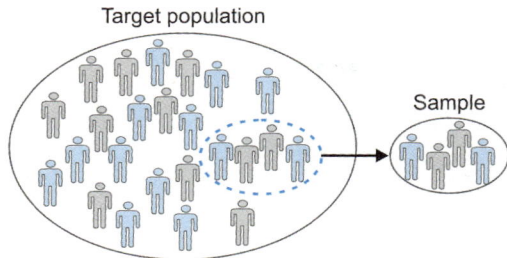

Fig. 7.11: Convenience sampling

specific day, patients who are hospitalized with specific medical diagnosis, students who are present in the classroom on a specific day, etc. The researcher continues to select the subjects until the desired sample size is reached. Though potential bias is difficult to estimate in this sampling method, objectivity can be introduced to reduce deliberate selection of subjects by the researcher. The serious biases are not always present in the convenience samples. This technique is commonly used in healthcare studies because most researchers have limited access to patients who meet study sample criteria. Probability sampling is not possible when the availability of potential patients is limited. By using convenience sampling technique, the researcher includes all the patients who meet the sampling criteria to increase the sample size. The advantages and disadvantages of convenience sampling technique are presented in Table 7.11.

Quota Sampling

The quota sampling technique, divides the population into strata and decides on how many sample are needed from each stratum. This strategy ensures the inclusion of subject types likely to be under represented in the convenience sample such as older adults, uneducated, females, etc. The goal of quota sampling is to replicate the proportions of subgroups present in the target population. This technique is similar to that used in stratified random sampling. Subjects are classified into strata and are selected by nonrandom means. Quota sampling requires that the researcher needs to identify subgroups and their proportions in the target population in order to achieve representativeness for the problem being studied. The quota sample in Figure 7.12 is representative of the gender distribution in the population and not representative of race distribution.

The advantages and disadvantages of quota sampling technique are presented in Table 7.12.

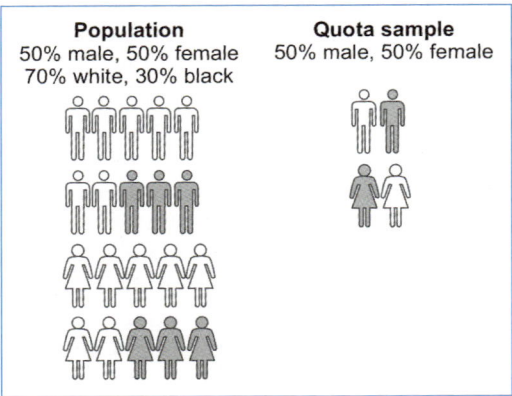

Fig. 7.12: Quota sampling technique

Table 7.11: Convenience sampling technique—advantages and disadvantages

Advantages	Disadvantages
• Easy to implement • Saves time and resources	• Includes atypical participants which results in biased sample • Limits generalizability to the target population

Table 7.12: Quota sampling technique—advantages and disadvantages

Advantages	Disadvantages
• Economically cheap • Ensures that diverse segments of the target population are represented • Overcomes convenience bias	• Results in biased sample • Limits generalizability of results

Procedure
- Divide the accessible population into strata or subgroups
- Subgroups of population may be based on known characteristics such as gender, economic status, etc.
- Determine the proportion of these subgroups in the population
- Choose subjects from subgroups in accordance with their proportion in the population

Purposive Sampling or Judgmental Sampling or Selective Sampling

In this method, the subjects, elements, events, or incidents are chosen with a specific purpose in mind. The selected participants are thought to be typical or atypical participants or similar or varied. Researcher may select participants, who are of different age group, have different diagnoses or illness severity. The main goal of purposeful sampling is selecting information rich cases from which researcher can get needed in-depth information for conducting the study.

For example, researchers describing perceived stress among breast cancer women who are undergoing treatment include women with various stages of breast cancer, with various treatment modalities (only chemotherapy, chemotherapy plus radiation therapy, and only radiation therapy), and with varying ages (<40 years old, 40–50 years old, 50–60 years old, and >60 years).

This method is frequently used by qualitative researchers to gain insights into a new area of study, discover new meaning, or collect an in-depth understanding of a complex experience or situation. This method is also used when the researcher wants to pretest and evaluate the newly developed instruments with a purposive sample constituted by experts from different subjects to collect key information (Fig. 7.13). The advantages and disadvantages of purposive sampling technique are presented in Table 7.13.

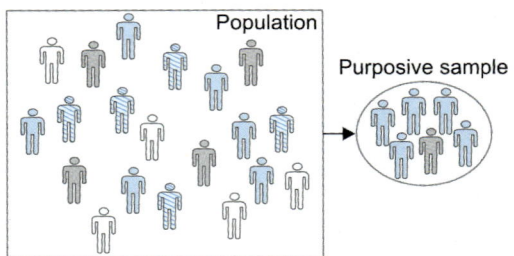

Fig. 7.13: Purposive sampling technique

Table 7.13: Purposive sampling technique—advantages and disadvantages

Advantages	Disadvantages
• Yields selection of typical cases • Useful in explorative studies • Saves resources • Requires less fieldwork	• Highly subjective • Results in biased sample • Limits generalizability

Snowball or Network or Chain or Nominated Sampling

This method is commonly used in social sciences to select potential subjects for the study where subjects are difficult to identify or reach. In this method, investigator asks the subjects to propose another person with a similar trait known to them so that the sample increases in size like a rolling snowball (Fig. 7.14). Snowballing starts with a few eligible study subjects and then proceeds based on referrals from those participants until the desired sample size has been gathered. Snowball sampling is an effective approach for identifying subjects who can provide the greatest insight and essential information about an experience or event that is being studied. This technique is particularly useful while finding subjects in socially devalued population such as individuals with substance abuse and individuals who have committed sexual offenses or criminal acts. The advantages and disadvantages of snowball sampling technique are presented in Table 7.14.

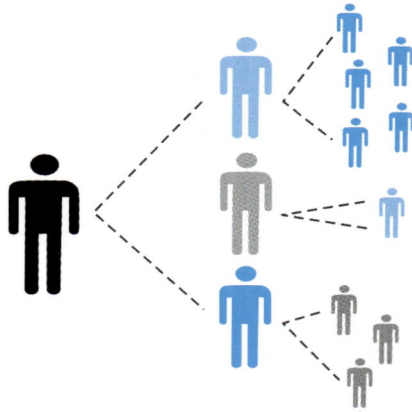

Fig. 7.14: Snowball sampling

Table 7.14: Snowball sampling technique—advantages and disadvantages

Advantages	Disadvantages
• Allows the researcher to reach populations that are difficult to reach • The process is cheap, simple, and cost-efficient	• Representativeness of the sample is not assured • The researcher is not aware of the true distribution of the sample

Example: When carrying out a survey of risk behaviors amongst intravenous drug users, participants may be asked to nominate other users to be interviewed.

Nonprobable sampling methods are commonly used for exploratory or in-depth qualitative research. The samples are rarely representative of the population. Table 7.15 presents the various nonprobability sampling methods and the situations where they can best be employed.

Differences between Probability and Nonprobability Sampling Techniques

Probability sampling is based on the principle of randomization where every member of the available population has an equal chance to be a part of the sample. In nonprobability sampling, the researcher assumes that the characteristics of the sample are evenly distributed within the population. This makes the researcher believe that any sample thus selected would represent the whole population and the results drawn would be accurate. The differences between probability and nonprobability sampling techniques are presented in Table 7.16 and Figure 7.15.

Factors Influencing Sampling

The quality of the research output and the validity of its finding depend upon the appropriateness of the sampling technique selected for the study. The selection of the sampling technique is influenced by the following factors (Fig. 7.16):

Purpose of the Study

- ❖ Probability sampling methods must be selected when the researcher wishes to conduct a study on the sample and generalize the findings to the population.
- ❖ If the researcher is interested in understanding the nature of the phenomena and does not intend to generalize the findings then selection of nonprobability sampling is sufficient.

Type of Research Design

- ❖ Exploratory designs are used to collect an in-depth information from the sample. These designs use nonprobability sampling techniques like convenience sampling or quota sampling in order to find subjects for the study.
- ❖ Comparative designs compare groups to see if they are significantly different on some characteristic or trait. Usually, these studies utilize a stratified random sampling technique.
- ❖ In experimental designs, the investigator must have full control of the variables. As far as the sample is concerned the control is maintained through assignment to groups. The main concern in an experimental design is that the experimental and

Basics in Nursing Research and Biostatistics

Table 7.15: Summary of nonprobability sampling methods

Method	Selection strategy	Best when	Example	Reliability of conclusions for fixed sample size	Economy	Remarks
Convenience sampling	Researcher collects the data from whoever is available and meets the study criteria	Sampling frame is not available and potential participants are limited	Children aged 1–5 years were selected from nearby Anganwadi	Poor	Economical	Used when probability sampling is not possible
Quota sampling	Each member in the population is allocated to a group or stratum. Sample is then selected from each stratum using nonrandom methods	Wide population and subgroups have to be accessed	Children are divided into subgroups or different strata, e.g. 1 year old children, 2 year old children, 3 year old children, 4 year old children, and 5 year old children. For the study purpose, children are selected from each strata by using nonrandom method	Poor	Economical	Good for nonhomogeneous population
Purposive sampling	Researcher hand picks or selects certain cases for the study	A sample which is typical or atypical or similar or varied has to be selected	Selecting children below 5 years of age who have features of Down syndrome	Poor	Economical	Used to gain an insight into the new area of the study
Snowball sampling	Researcher asks the subjects for assistance in identifying people with similar traits after observing the initial subject	Subjects are hard to locate or reach	Researchers seek assistance from mothers of such children in identifying others with features of Down syndrome	Poor	Economical	Used to select subjects from social devalued population

Table 7.16: Differences between probability and nonprobability sampling techniques

Probability Sampling	Non-probability Sampling
• Each person in the population has equal chance of being included in the study	• Each person in the population does not have an equal chance for inclusion in the study
• The results generated are free from bias	• The results generated are more or less biased
• Selection method is objective	• Selection method is subjective
• Used when research is conclusive in nature	• Used when research is exploratory in nature
• These techniques are used in hypothesis testing studies	• These techniques are used in hypothesis generating studies
• Selected sample are representative in nature	• Selected sample are not representative in nature

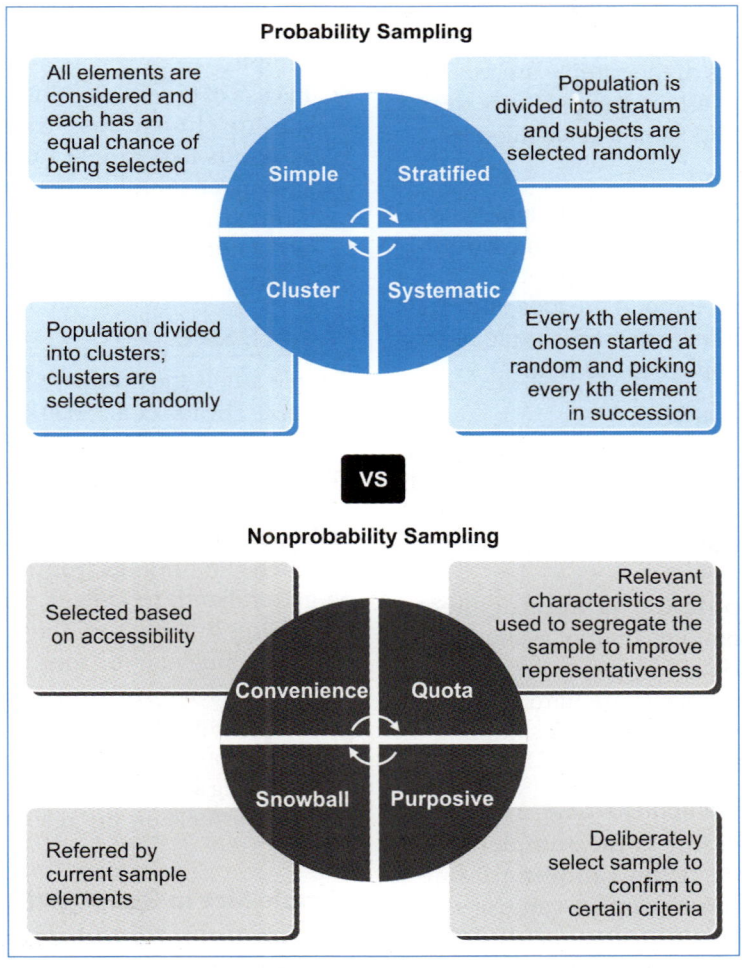

Fig. 7.15: Probability sampling versus nonprobability sampling

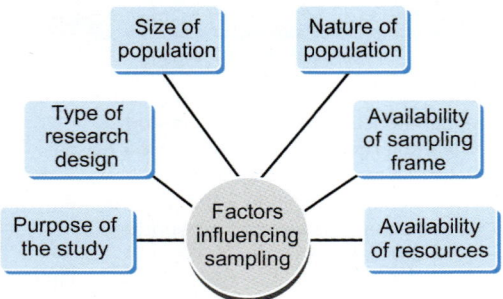

Fig. 7.16: Factors influencing sampling

control groups need to be equivalent at the beginning of the study, so that the effect of the independent variable can be measured. To ensure the equivalence of the groups, the members of the sample are randomly assigned to various groups. These designs use probability sampling techniques.

Size of Population
- When the population is large and scattered multistage cluster sampling would be appropriate.
- On the other hand, if the area and size of the population are small, simple random sampling would be sufficient.

Nature of Population
- If the population is a homogenous sample, it will be representative in most of the variables. Under such condition, simple random sampling will provide accurate results.
- If the population is heterogeneous, stratified sampling or quota sampling will be appropriate.
- Where the subjects are hard to locate or reach, snowball or network sampling will be suitable.

Availability of Sampling Frame
- Sampling frame is the complete list of population. If the sampling frame is available, the researcher can use simple random sampling technique. And if there is no periodic variation or trend present in the above sampling frame then systematic sampling would be preferred.
- Where sampling frame is not available and potential participants are limited the researcher can employ convenience sampling technique.

Availability of Resources (Time and Money)
- If the available finance is limited, the researcher has to choose less costly sampling plan like multistage cluster sampling or quota sampling.
- If the resources are abundant, the researcher can select the most appropriate method of sampling that fits the research objective and the nature of population sample.
- In case of time constraints, the researcher has to choose less time consuming methods like simple random sampling or cluster sampling instead of stratified sampling. Under such conditions, precision is compromised to a certain extent.

SAMPLE SIZE

Sample size is the number of observations in a sample (Evans et al. 2000). It is commonly denoted by n or N. The sample size is an important feature of any empirical study. The subpopulation is studied in order to make an inference to the broader population to which the findings from the study are to be generalized. In census, the sample size is nothing but the population size; but in research, because of time and budgetary constraints a representative sample is generally used. Larger the sample size the more accurate the findings from the study. Determining adequate sample size is the most important decision the researcher needs to take.

Sample Size in Quantitative Research
- Quantitative research deals with accurate measurement of variables, and generalizing

the findings of the sample to the larger population. It can only be ensured by selecting a representative sample.
- Quantitative researchers need to give adequate consideration to the number of subjects needed to test research hypothesis. The larger the sample, the more representative of the population it is likely to be. Smaller samples tend to produce less accurate estimates than larger ones.
- The larger the sample the smaller is the sampling error.

Factors Considered for Determining the Adequacy of Sample Size

By using a small sample size, the researcher will lack precision to provide reliable answers to the research questions. Using a too large sample size will lead to wastage of resources such as time and material. There are several nonstatistical and statistical factors that play a vital role in determining the sample size. The researcher should know all these factors to determine the appropriate sample size.

Nonstatistical factors that are considered to determine the adequacy of the sample size are presented in Box 7.2.
- *Effect size*: The effect size indicates the size of difference between the groups or the strength of the relationship between the two variables.
    1. When the effect size is large, it suggests that a considerable difference between groups or a very strong relationship between variables exists. When a large effect size is present, detecting it is easy and requires only a small sample.
    2. When the effect size is small, it suggests that a small difference between groups or a weak relationship between the two variables exists. Detecting it is difficult and requires larger samples.
- *Nature of the population*: If the population is homogeneous, a small sample adequately represents the population characteristics. As the population homogeneity decreases, the sample characteristics represent the population characteristics less accurately. When the population becomes completely heterogenous, the selected sample characteristics do not represent the population characteristics. In such instances, the chance of occurrence of sampling error is more. By increasing the sample size, the risk of sampling error is reduced.
- *Type of quantitative study*: Descriptive and correlational studies require very large samples as they involve study of multiple variables and the presence of extraneous variables that are likely to affect the subject responses. Researcher comparing the multiple subgroups in a sample such as groups formed by age, gender, area of residence, etc. requires that an adequate sample be available for each subgroup being analyzed.

Experimental studies use small samples compared to descriptive studies. As control in the study increases, the sample size can be decreased. If the study uses matched pairs of subjects, it increases the power to identify group differences and decreases the sample size needed.
- *Sensitivity of the measurements*: When measurement errors are minimal in data collection instruments they are said to be precise.

Box 7.2	Non-statistical factors considered for determining sample size
	• Effect size
	• Nature of population
	• Type of quantitative study
	• Sensitivity of the measurements
	• Number of variables
	• Attrition
	• Data analysis techniques
	• Resources available
	• Sampling procedure
	• Level of significance

- Biophysiological instruments measure phenomena with accuracy and precision. For example, thermometer measures body temperature accurately and precisely. A tool that is reliable and valid measures more precisely than a tool that is less well developed. Tools to measure psychosocial variables tend to be less well developed. For example, a tool to measure anxiety and depression contains a fair amount of error and lack precision.
  - As imprecise measuring tools are susceptible to errors, large samples are required to test the hypotheses adequately.
- *Number of variables*: As the number of variables in a study increases (such as age, gender, education, occupation, etc.), the sample size also needs to be increased in order to detect significant relationships or differences. With the inclusion of multiple dependent variables in the study the sample size needs to be increased. A minimum of 30 subjects is needed for use of the central limit theorem (statistics based on the mean).
- *Attrition*: Attrition refers to a condition where people initially willing to participate fail to continue.
  - Attrition leads to reduction in sample size, which is caused by the failure of participants to complete the study after sample selection. Longitudinal studies and pretest and posttest designs have a higher attrition rate. Attrition can pose a serious threat to the validity of findings when the participants who drop out of the study differ on key variables from those who remain in the study.
  - While planning sample size, attrition needs to be duly considered.
- *Data analysis techniques*: Various techniques are used to analyze the data.
  - Techniques for analyzing variables measured at interval and ratio levels are more powerful in detecting relationships and differences than those used to analyze variables measured at nominal and ordinal levels. Larger samples are needed when variables are measured at nominal and ordinal level as the power of the planned statistical analysis is weak (the ability to detect differences in data is called the power of statistical analysis).
  - The statistical procedures such as t-test and analysis of variance (ANOVA) test (equal group sizes) increase the power as the effect size is maximized.
  - The more unbalanced are the group sizes, the smaller is the effect size. Hence, for unbalanced groups the total sample size should be larger.
  - The chi-square test is the weakest of the statistical tests and requires very large sample sizes to achieve acceptable levels of power.
- *Resources available*: Precision is associated with large samples.
  - Large samples require considerable amount of time and money. For determining the sample size, one needs to consider the available resources also.
  - Sample size is often limited due to practical constraints such as time and subject availability.
- *Sampling procedure*: In cluster sampling and stratified random sampling methods, the sample is divided into several subsamples. For these techniques, a larger sample is needed. When non-probability sampling methods are used even a large sample can include bias. A large sample cannot guarantee accuracy or rectify a faulty sampling design.
- *Levels of significance*: The larger level of significance (alpha between 0.05 and

Box 7.3	Statistical factors considered to determine sample size

- Degree of variability
- Statistical power
- Significance criteria
- One- or two-tailed statistical analysis

0.10 makes it easier to attain statistical significance) requires a greater sample size.

Statistical factors considered to determine the adequacy of sample size are included in Box 7.3:

- ❖ *Degree of variability*: Variability refers to the spread or dispersion of data from the mean. A homogenous population has less variance compared to a heterogeneous population. If the population is homogeneous, smaller is the sample size required to detect the minimum differences between the groups. The more heterogeneous a population is, the larger is the sample size required to obtain a given level of precision.
- ❖ *Statistical power*: It is the ability of the statistical test to reject a false null hypothesis. If the statistical power is high, the probability of making type II error will be less. As the statistical power increases sample size also increases.
- ❖ *Significance criterion*: If a result is statistically significant, it means a true relationship exists between the two variables and it is not an outcome of chance. The statistical significance is denoted by 'p'. The significance criterion is customarily set to .05. As the significance criterion decreases more samples are required to detect the minimum differences between the variables.
- ❖ *One or two-tailed statistical analysis*: If a one-tailed statistical analysis is used, small sample size is required to detect minimum differences between the variables. One-tailed analysis is done when the relationship between variables is in only one direction. Two-tailed analysis requires a larger sample size when compared to the one-tailed statistical analysis.

Strategies for Minimizing the Sample Size

Browner et al. (2001) list the following strategies for minimizing the sample size:

Use Continuous Measurements Instead of Categories

Statistical tests that use continuous values are parametric in nature and are more powerful than those that use categorical values that are nonparametric in nature. Hence, a larger sample is required for a nonparametric test than for a parametric test.

Use more Precise Measurements

When measuring tools are precise and less susceptible to error, small sample is needed to test the hypotheses adequately. If measuring tools are imprecise and susceptible to error, large sample is needed to test the hypotheses adequately.

Use Paired Measurements

Statistical tests like the paired tests are more powerful than unpaired tests. While in paired test each measured value is matched with its own control, in unpaired tests each measured value is compared with other group values. Paired tests require lesser sample size than unpaired tests.

Sample and Statistical Power

- ❖ Sample size is one criterion for determining the statistical power of the study and consequently for reaching correct conclusions or avoiding error of inference from the sample to the target population value.
- ❖ Power is the ability of the statistical test to reject a false null hypothesis, i.e. to detect differences or relationships that actually exist in the population. A large sample size is associated with increased power.
- ❖ The minimum acceptable level of power for a study is 0.8% or 80% (Cohen, 1988).

This power level results in a 20% chance of committing a type II error. The two types of errors that are of concern are:

1. *Type I error*: The sample results fail to reject the null hypothesis at a time when the null hypothesis is true in the population. The researcher draws a conclusion that the intervention had an effect, when in fact it did not. It usually occurs as a result of weakness in design and is considered as a serious flaw and threatens the overall internal validity of the study. It is called alpha (α). The maximum acceptable level of alpha in scientific research is generally 0.05.
2. *Type II error*: The sample results accept the null hypothesis at a time when the null hypothesis is not true in the population. It is the acceptance of a false null hypothesis. The researcher draws a conclusion that there are no differences in the outcomes when in fact there are differences. It is called beta (β).

Methods of Estimating Sample Size

Calculation of sample size is an important step in research process. Different research designs need different methods of sample size calculation. There are several methods to determine the sample size (Subaihi AA, 2003) (Fig. 7.17):

❖ *Using a census for small populations*: One approach to determine the sample size is to include the entire population as the sample. For example, if the population is less than 200, the researcher should measure the variables from every subject in the population to eliminate sample error and to achieve desirable level of precision.
❖ *Thumb rules of estimating sample size*: The sample should be as large as a research project can afford in terms of time and money. Larger the sample size, lesser is

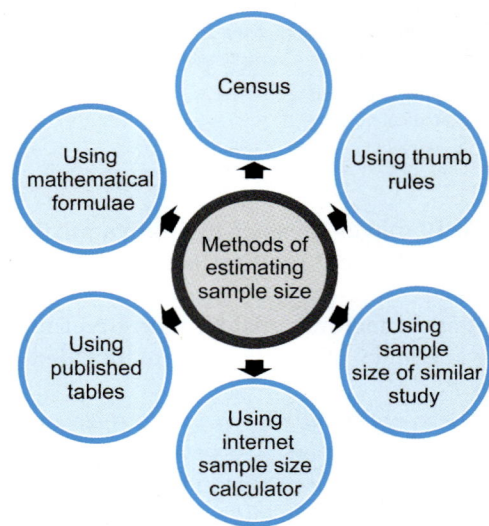

Fig. 7.17: Methods of estimating sample size

the error in generalizing results to the whole population. Based on the power, thumb rules for estimating the sample size is given in Table 7.17.

❖ *Using a sample size of a similar study*: Another approach to determine the size of a sample for a particular study is to use the same sample as those of studies similar to the one under plan, the researcher should know the errors that were made in determining the sample size for a previous study. The literature review can provide

Table 7.17: Sample size rules of thumb

Statistical test	*Reasonable sample size*
◆ t-test or ANOVA—to measure group differences	◆ Cell size of 30 for 80% power, if decreased, no lower than 7 per cell
◆ Correlations and regression— to measure relationships	◆ Approximately 50
◆ Chi-square	◆ At least 20 overall, no cell smaller than 5
◆ Factor analysis	◆ Approximately 300 is "good"

(ANOVA: Analysis of Variance)

guidance on sample sizes that are usually used.

- *Using internet sample size calculator*: Another approach to determine sample is to use one of the internet sample size calculators. The internet websites provide an interactive way to determine the sample size by using precision, confidence level, and variability.
- *Using published tables*: By using published tables, sample size can be estimated. These tables are designed exactly in the same way that the internet calculators are. These tables are fixed and predetermined combinations of precision, confidence level, and variability.
- *Using mathematical formulae*: For descriptive and comparative studies.
  - *Sample size calculation for descriptive study:* Descriptive studies are conducted to describe some specific parameter of population.

  $$\text{Sample size} = \frac{Z^2_{1-\alpha/2} SD^2}{d^2}$$

  $Z_{1-\alpha/2}$—standard normal variate (at 5% type I error (p<0.005) it is 1.96)
  SD—standard deviation of variable (can be taken from previously done study or pilot study)
  d—absolute error or precision

  For example, researcher is interested in knowing the average systolic blood pressure of children in the same city with 95% confidence interval (5% of type I error) and precision of 5 mm of Hg (two tailed). The sample size can be estimated using the above formula as under:
  Based on the previously done studies the SD = 25
  If p< 0.05, the standard normal variate is 1.96
  Absolute error or precision d = 5

  $$\text{Sample size} = \frac{(1.96)^2 (25)^2}{(5)^2} = 96$$

Thus a sample size of 96 is required to estimate the average systolic blood pressure in children.

- *Sample size calculation for experimental studies*: When the variable is continuous data like blood pressure, weight, height, etc. the following formula can be used to compare two mean differences.

  $$\text{Sample size} = \frac{2SD^2 \cdot (Z_{\alpha/2} + Z_\beta)^2}{d^2}$$

  SD—standard deviation = 25 (from previous studies or pilot study)
  $Z_{\alpha/2}$—from Z table
  Z_β—from Z table
  d—effect size–difference between mean values

  For example, a researcher wishes to examine the effect of a new anti-hypertensive drug by comparing it with a placebo. The researcher thinks that if this new drug reduces the blood pressure by 10 mm Hg as compared to placebo then it should be considered as clinically significant. In previous similar studies, standard deviation was found to be 25 mmHg. The researcher selects the level of significance at 5% and the power of the study at 80% and thinks suitable statistical test in this condition will be two-tailed unpaired t-test. The effect size in this condition is 10 mmHg. The sample size can be estimated using the above formula as under:
  Substituting in the formula we get:
  SD—Standard deviation = 25 (from previous studies or pilot study)
  $Z_{\alpha/2}$—$Z0_{.05/2} = Z_{0.025} = 1.96$ (from Z table at type I error of 5%)
  Z_β—$Z_{0.20} = 0.842$ (from Z table) at 80% power
  d = effect size–difference between mean values.

  $$\text{Sample size} = \frac{2SD^2 (1.96+0.84)^2}{10^2} = 98$$

$$= \frac{2(25)^2 (1.96+0.84)^2}{10^2} = 98$$

Thus a sample of 98 subjects is required per group.

SAMPLING BIAS

- It refers to the systematic over-representation or under-representation of certain segments of the population in relation to an attribute relevant to the research study.
- Sampling bias occurs when the chosen sample does not accurately represent the population.
- This error is introduced as the data are collected from a smaller portion rather than the larger whole. There are no sampling errors in a census because the calculations are based on the entire population. For example, in a survey to assess the teenage use of tobacco, high school students were selected as a sample. This sample is biased as it does not include school drop outs.
- A sample is also biased if certain members are under-represented or over-represented relative to others in the population. An example of over-representation can be distribution of a questionnaire to all those visiting a library, which is likely to include more people who are committed to study. An example of under-representation can be using a telephone directory to select the sample as it will not include those without a telephone connection or those not listed in the directory.

Potential Sources of Sampling Bias

- Any deviation from the established sampling rules can introduce bias
- Sampling frame is incomplete or inaccurate
- Some sections of the population are not available or refuse to cooperate
- When nonrandom sampling techniques are used
- Replacing the selected subjects with others
- Low response rate in survey

Measures to Control Sampling Bias

- By using random sampling methods
- By following proper procedure in sample selection
- By ensuring that target population is well defined
- By ensuring that the sampling frame matches the target population as much as possible
- By using large sample size

Systematic Bias

Researcher must remember that there are two causes of incorrect inferences resulting from the data. These are systematic bias and sampling errors.

Systematic bias cannot be eliminated by increasing the sample size as it stems from errors in the sampling procedure. The following factors are responsible for systematic bias (Fig. 7.18):

- *Inappropriate sampling frame*: If a sampling frame is inappropriate, it causes biased representation of the sample. For example, if in conducting a study the researcher interviews only the family, friends, neighbors, colleagues, and none others and later generalizes it to other

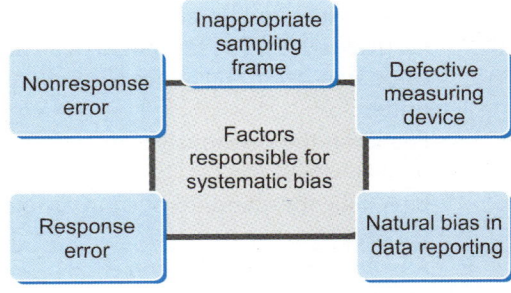

Fig. 7.18: Factors responsible for systematic bias

population, then this sampling frame is inappropriate.
- *Defective measuring device*: If the measuring device is constantly in error, it causes systematic bias. For example, a weighing machine constantly measures the weight of patients 2 kg in excess.
- *Natural bias in the reporting of data*: Generally in surveys people selectively reveal or suppress information rather than giving true information which leads to bias.
- *Response error* is a systematic bias that occurs during data collection, analysis, or interpretation. Different types of response errors are respondent error (e.g. lying, forgetting, etc.), interviewer bias, recording errors, poorly designed questionnaires, and measurement errors.
- *Nonresponse error* is an error that occurs when respondents are different than those who do not respond. This may occur because either the potential respondent was not contacted (unavailable) or they refused to respond (unable or unwilling). For example, the respondent may be on a vacation for the duration of the data collection period or unwilling to take the survey because he simply does not want to take a survey, does not trust the researcher, is uninterested in the subject matter, or fear embarrassment or violations of privacy.

SAMPLING ERRORS

Sampling error is the deviation of the selected sample from the true characteristic of the entire population. It is a statistical value that indicates difference in results found in the sample when compared to the population from which the sample was drawn.

Reasons for Sampling Errors

- When researchers draw different subjects from same population
- When researchers use biased sampling procedure
- When an error occurs by chance (chance error)
- When the sample is nonrepresentative of the entire population

Methods to Control Sampling Errors

- Using appropriate sampling designs
- Selecting large samples
- Multiple contacts to assure representative response

As the sample size increases the sampling error decreases. Increasing the sample size has some disadvantages, viz. collecting data from a large sample is costlier, requires more interviewers, and creates additional burden in selection, training, and control. It also increases systematic bias. If the researcher tries to control sampling errors by using large sample size, it results in systematic bias. The selection of a sampling procedure should guarantee a relatively small sampling error and help to control the systematic bias, effectively.

Problems in Sampling

During the sampling process, the researcher encounters several problems, which include sampling errors, lack of knowledge in sampling process, resources, cooperation from the sample, and representative sample.

- *Sampling error*: This error occurs as a result of collecting the data from a sample rather than collecting it from the whole population. Increasing the sample size reduces this type of error.
- *Lack of knowledge in sampling process:* If the researcher lacks adequate knowledge and experience in research methodology, it may lead to defective sampling frame and selection of inappropriate sampling technique.
- *Lack of resources*: Adequate time, material, and man power are required to implement

sampling process, which otherwise may affect the sampling process.
- *Lack of cooperation from sample:* Researcher requires cooperation from authorities and study subjects. Lack of cooperation causes adverse effect on sampling process.
- *Lack of representative sample*: When the subjects are not selected randomly from the population, the sample may not be representative of the population.

SAMPLING PROCESS IN QUALITATIVE RESEARCH STUDIES

In qualitative research, the researcher collects in-depth information based on subjects' perspective focusing on context. The main intention is to explore and describe the variables rather than generalizing them to other settings. In these designs, decision regarding sampling process and size takes place during the process of data collection. The researchers do not develop any formal sampling plan in advance as in quantitative research. In qualitative studies, the researcher selects a small number of potential participants using purposive sampling technique who are willing to undergo the demands of participation. Common sampling methods used in qualitative research are:

- *Intensity sampling:* Selecting participants who can provide rich or excellent information related to phenomenon of interest.
- *Homogeneous sampling:* Selecting participants who have similar or identical traits such as age or those undergoing similar experience, perspective, or outlook that are useful to a researcher.
- *Criterion sampling:* Selecting participants who meet some predetermined criterion of importance (Patton, 1999).
- *Snowball sampling:* Selecting a few participants who identify future participants from among their acquaintances.

Sample Size in Qualitative Studies
- The main aim of most qualitative studies is to find the meaning, uncover multiple realities, and gain an in-depth understanding of the experiences of the individuals.
- The qualitative researchers deliberately select subjects and determine their number and characteristics in relation to the in-depth understanding needed for their studies.
- Qualitative research focuses on the quality of information obtained from the person, situation, or event rather than on the size of the sample.
- These studies use small and nonrandom samples. Sampling methods used in qualitative research are purposive sampling, snowball sampling, and convenience sampling.
- In a qualitative study, when saturation of study data is achieved it indicates the adequacy of sample size.
- Saturation of study data occurs when additional subjects do not provide any new information but only repetition of previously collected data.
- Verification of study data occurs when researchers are able to confirm their instincts or relationships further.
- In qualitative studies the scope of the study, nature, and quality of information (data) determine the sample size.
  - *Scope of the study*: Study with a broader scope requires larger sample size because researchers will need extensive data to address the study purpose.
  - *Nature of the topic*: If the topic of the study is clear and easily discussed by the subjects then fewer subjects are needed to obtain the essential data. If the topic is difficult to define and awkward for people to discuss then more subjects are required.

- *Quality of the information*: When the quality of the data is high with a rich content, few participants are needed to achieve saturation of data.

GUIDELINES FOR CRITIQUING THE SAMPLING SECTION OF A RESEARCH REPORT

- Is the sample representative of the population?
- Have the target and accessible population been clearly identified?
- Did the researcher select the correct sample to answer the research questions and was the size sufficient to obtain valid results?
- Is the sampling method described?
- Was the method of choosing the sample (probability *vs* nonprobability) appropriate?
- Are potential sampling biases recognized?
- Has subject dropout been explained?
- Are the inclusion or exclusion criteria clearly identified?

BIBLIOGRAPHY

1. Biswas, T., & Charan, J. (2013). How to calculate sample size for different study designs in medical research. *Indian Journal of Psychological Medicine*, 35(2), 121-126.
2. Browner, W.S., Newman, T.B., Cummings, S.R., & Hulley, S.B. (2001). *Designing Clinical Research: An epidemiologic approach* (2nd ed.). Philadephia, PA: Lippincott Williams and Wilkins.
3. Burns, N., & Grove, S.K. (2004). *The practice of nursing research*. Philadelphia: W.B. Saunders Company.
4. Chinn, P.L., & Kramer. M.K. (1995). *Theory and nursing: A systematic approach* (4th ed.). St. Louis: Mosby Yearbook.
5. Cohen, J. (1988). *Statistical power analysis for the behavioral sciences* (2nd ed.). Hillsdale, NJ: Lawrence Erlbaum Associates.
6. Evans, M., Hastings, N., & Peacock, B. (2000). *Statistical Distribution* (3rd ed.). New York: Wiley.
7. Frey, Lawrence R., & Carl L. Kreps. (2000). *Investigation Communication: An Introduction to Research Methods* (2nd ed.). Boston: Allyn and Bacon.
8. Hek, G., and Moule, P. (2006). *Making Sense of Research: An Introduction for Health and Social Care Practitioners* (3rd ed.). London: Sage
9. Jackson, S.L. (2011). *Research Methods and Statistics: A Critical Approach* (4th ed.). New York: Wiley.
10. Kerlinger, F. (1986). *Foundations of behavioral research* (3rd ed.). New York: Holt, Rinehart & Winston.
11. Knobf, M.T. (2002). Carrying on: The experience of premature menopause in women with early stage breast cancer. *Nursing research*, 51, 9-17.
12. LoBiondo-Wood, G., & Haber, J. (1997). *Nursing Research: Methods, critical appraisal and utilization* (3rd ed.). Boston: Mosbey.
13. Lusk, B. Pretty., & Powerless. (2000). Nurses in advertisements: *Research in Nursing & Health*, 23, 229-236.
14. MacNealy., & Mary, S. (1999). *Strategies for Empirical Research in Writing*. New York: Longman.
15. Nieswiadomy., & Rose, M. (2008). *Foundations of nursing research*. Upper Saddle River, NJ: Pearson Prentice Hall.
16. Patton, M.Q. (1999). "Enhancing the quality and credibility of qualitative analysis." HSR: *Health Services Research*, 34(5) Part II. pp. 1189-1208.
17. Ploeg, J. (1999). Identifying the best research design to fit the question: qualitative designs. *Evidenced Based Nursing*, 2, 36-37.
18. Polit, D.F., & Beck, C.T. (2010). *Essentials of Nursing Research: Appraising Evidence for Nursing Practice*. Philadelphia, PA: Lippincott Williams & Wilkins.
19. Subaihi, A.A. (2003). Sample size determination. *Saudi Medical Journal*, 24(4), 323-330.
20. Treece, E.W., & Treece, J.H. (1989). *Elements of Research in Nursing*, The C.V. Mosby Co., St. Louis.

REVIEW QUESTIONS

I. Long Essays

1. Describe in detail the probability sampling methods with an example.
2. Describe in detail the nonprobability sampling methods with an example.
3. Explain the factors influencing sampling.
4. Describe potential sampling bias and measures to control sampling bias.
5. Describe sampling process in quantitative research studies.
6. a. Define the terms—target population, sample, sampling unit, sampling frame, and sampling interval.
   b. Explain the procedure for selecting samples using cluster sampling techniques with simple illustrations.

II. Short Essays

1. Discuss factors to be considered for determining adequate sample size.
2. Discuss the purpose and the use of sampling frames in social work research. Describe how a sampling frame is different from the sample from which it was drawn.
3. Do you believe samples drawn from populations are really representative of the populations from which they were drawn? Why or why not?
4. Discuss the differences between probability and nonprobability sampling. What are their comparative advantages and disadvantages?
5. Discuss how sampling errors vary with the size of the sample.
6. List and discuss the various forms of sampling errors.
7. What suggestions can you provide to minimize nonsampling errors?
8. What is meant by representativeness of a sample? How is it achieved?
9. Describe procedure of lottery method of drawing a sample.
10. Discuss the procedure of generating a random sample.

III. Short Answers

1. Target population
2. Accessible population
3. Sampling frame
4. Sampling bias
5. Eligibility criteria
6. Sampling error
7. Sample
8. Population

IV. Multiple Choice Questions

1. The process of obtaining information about an entire population by examining only a part of it called as study
   a. Sampling
   b. Hypothesis
   c. Pilot study
   d. Ethnography
2. When each individual in a population has an equal opportunity, the phenomenon is termed as
   a. Sampling
   b. Randomization
   c. Sampling frame
   d. Eligibility criteria
3. Which of the following are problems related to sampling frame *except*
   a. Incomplete sampling frame
   b. Duplicate listing
   c. Foreign elements
   d. Complete sampling frame
4. Which of the following sampling methods involve a random start and then proceed with the selection of every kth element from the population?
   a. Simple random sampling
   b. Stratified random sampling
   c. Systematic sampling
   d. Snowball sampling

5. Followings are the advantages of sampling *expect*
   a. More practical
   b. Economy in nature
   c. Greater accuracy
   d. Chance of bias
6. Which of the following is a characteristic of a sample?
   a. Representativeness
   b. Nonbiased
   c. Appropriate sample size
   d. All of the above
7. Sampling error is reduced by
   a. Increasing sample size
   b. Decreasing sample size
   c. Reducing amount of data
   d. None of these
8. Sample is a subset of
   a. Data
   b. Group
   c. Population
   d. Itself
9. Which of the following is a nonprobable sampling method?
   a. Systematic sampling
   b. Stratified sampling
   c. Simple random sampling
   d. Quota sampling
10. The list of all units in a population is called
    a. Random sampling
    b. Sampling Frame
    c. Biased sampling
    d. Parameter
11. Following are the considerations for choosing a sample size *except*
    a. Nature of population
    b. Type of study
    c. Number of variables
    d. Nature of the geographical area
12. Which of the following is true?
    a. The sampling error becomes progressively smaller, with larger the sample size
    b. The sampling error becomes progressively small, with smaller the sample size
    c. The sampling error becomes progressively larger, with larger the sample size
    d. The sampling error is unrelated to sample size
13. When every member of the accessible population has an equal chance of being selected to participate in the study, the researcher is using
    a. Simple random sampling
    b. Snowball sampling
    c. Convenience sampling
    d. Purposive sampling
14. If a researcher selected five schools at random and then interviewed all the teachers in those five schools, the researcher used
    a. Simple random sampling
    b. Stratified random sampling
    c. Cluster random sampling
    d. Two-stage random sampling
15. Which of the following is an example of a random sampling method?
    a. Quota sampling
    b. Convenience sampling
    c. Purposive sampling
    d. Cluster sampling
16. The best sample is one that is
    a. Systematic
    b. Convenient
    c. Representative of the population
    d. Purposefully selected
17. Which of the following is an example of a nonrandom sampling method?
    a. Convenience sampling
    b. Stratified random sampling
    c. Simple random
    d. Cluster random
18. The purpose of stratified random sampling is to make certain that
    a. Every member of the population has an equal chance of being selected for the sample
    b. The sample proportionately represents individuals from different categories of the population

c. The participants chosen for the study are the ones most likely to react to the treatment
d. The sample is more representative of the target population than the accessible population.

19. Population generalizability refers to
    a. Conclusions researchers make about a random sample
    b. Conclusions researchers make about information uncovered in research study
    c. The degree to which a sample represents the population of interest
    d. The degree to which results of a study can be extended to other settings or conditions

20. Hospitals are randomly selected in a region and then nurses in each hospital ICU are asked to participate in the study. Which sampling method is used in this statement?
    a. Systematic sampling
    b. Cluster sampling
    c. Stratified sampling
    d. Simple random

21. When subjects are selected because they happen to be in the right place at the right time the sampling method referred to is
    a. Quota sampling
    b. Purposive sampling
    c. Convenient sampling
    d. Snowball sampling

22. When a researcher in a qualitative study chooses the participants based on what they may be able to contribute to the study the sampling method is called
    a. Quota sampling
    b. Purposive sampling
    c. Convenient sampling
    d. Snowball sampling

23. When every fifth baby born in a hospital is included in a study, the sampling method is called
    a. Systematic sampling
    b. Cluster sampling
    c. Stratified sampling
    d. Simple random sampling

24. A researcher wanted to conduct a study on depression among men working in executive corporate positions; she located 10 subjects by advertising and then invited each of those subjects to refer their acquaintances who meet the study criteria. The sampling technique is called
    a. Quota sampling
    b. Purposive sampling
    c. Convenient sampling
    d. Snowball sampling

25. Which of the following procedures can a quantitative researcher use to estimate sample size requirements?
    a. Weighting
    b. Randomization
    c. Stratification
    d. Power analysis

26. What would be an example of a type one error?
    a. Concluding that there are post-treatment differences between groups when in fact real population differences do not exist
    b. Concluding that there are no post-treatment differences between groups when in fact there are real population differences
    c. Concluding that there are no differences between two groups when in fact there are no real population differences
    d. Concluding that there are differences between groups when in fact there are real population differences

27. Which of the following is true while estimating sample size in a quantitative study?
    a. The sample size can be relatively small if group differences are expected to be large
    b. Smaller sample are needed in experimental than in quasi-experimental research
    c. Large sample size can be compensated for the use of relatively weak sample design
    d. Sample of under 100 subjects are inadequate

28. Which of the following states the major difference between control group and comparison group in experimental research?
   a. Random selection of subjects for the sample and random assignment to groups are hallmarks of true control group
   b. Random assignment to groups is needed to have a true control group
   c. It is less likely that comparison groups will have preexisting differences that may affect results
   d. Most studies in nursing use true control groups

ANSWER KEY

1. a	2. b	3. d	4. c	5. d	6. d
7. a	8. c	9. d	10. b	11. d	12. a
13. a	14. c	15. d	16. c	17. a	18. b
19. d	20. b	21. c	22. b	23. a	24. d
25. d	26. b	27. a	28. b		

UNIT 8

Tools and Methods of Data Collection

After research design and measurement strategies are selected the next step is to identify an appropriate method for data collection. Data collection involves gathering relevant data in order to achieve an answer to the problem stated. It is probably this section in the research process that has been given the most attention than any other.

The word "data" is the plural form of "datum" which means information that is systematically collected in the course of the study. Research data refers to that data which is collected from interviews, observations, surveys, experiments or even from previous literature for the purposes of analysis to produce research results. These results are used to understand a natural phenomenon and predict future events.

Data collection is the process of systematically gathering data and measuring the variables to facilitate answering the research question, hypothesis testing, and evaluating intervention effectiveness.

There are various methods of data collection which can be used by the nurse researchers depending upon the nature of study undertaken. Nurse researchers rely heavily on interviews, focus group discussions, questionnaires, observations, clinical measurements, and use of documents.

PURPOSES OF DATA COLLECTION

- ❖ The collection of data and its analysis assists researchers in discovering answers to their research questions and hypotheses. In some cases it even predicts future outcomes.
- ❖ The results of research are directly dependent on the collected data and its analysis. Accurately collected data ensures that research questions are answered correctly, research is repeatable and validated.
- ❖ A research study can be brilliantly designed, well-controlled and perfectly executed. But if the data collected are not consistent and accurate, the results will be suspicious. The data collection process then is integral to producing reliable evidence for nursing practice. The selection of appropriate data collection tools is therefore a key part of the research process.
- ❖ Data by itself is meaningless as it does not explain or cause change that information does. Through data collection facts are identified, measured, described, and computed for empirical evidences that are objective, reliable, and valid.

CONCEPTS OF DATA COLLECTION

- ❖ To answer the research questions, a researcher requires specific techniques for measuring, observing or recording the data.
- ❖ The data are bits of information or facts that are collected in a research study. It is carried out through data collection procedure.
- ❖ An ideal data collection method should be reliable, valid, sensitive, relevant to the topic and precisely measure the variable.

- Data collection methods are used to gather information in an objective and systematic way. By being objective it means that the data must not be influenced by anyone who collects the information and by being systematic it means that everyone who is involved in the collection procedure must collect the data in the same way.
- First the researcher must be clear about the purpose of the research and information that is needed to answer the research question. Once clarity of purpose and question is achieved the researcher must select the type of data that are required.
- There are many ways to collect data. The choice of a data collection strategy depends on the nature of the research question, the specific information that is being gathered and the resources available to the researcher.
- Irrespective of whether a researcher is conducting a quantitative or qualitative research, it is necessary to identify the best type of data collection method.
- Data collection methods used in quantitative studies are of numeric nature and subject to statistical analysis. These studies use systematic standardized approaches to measure the concept under study. They include measurement, self-report method, and observation.
- The main aim of qualitative studies is to fully explore the concepts under study. Hence, these studies use unstructured methods of data collection. These include focus group discussion and interviews. The collected data are text based in nature and subject to coding.

DATA SOURCES

Data sources are major locations from where the data originates. Data can be numbers, images, words, figures, facts or ideas. Data in itself cannot be understood and to get meaningful information it should be interpreted properly. The design of the research study specifies what type of data are needed and how it can be obtained. These are generally categorized into primary and secondary sources.

Primary sources provide data which are gathered first hand and usually collected by the researcher for a specific research assignment. Here the responsibility of publication, distribution or dissemination remains under the same researcher who originally gathered the data. Data from primary sources are gathered by observation, personal interviews, questionnaires, projective techniques, and biopsychosocial measures. Primary data include original research studies, decennial population census, sample registration system, survey for cause of death and family welfare statistics, letters, diaries, photographs, letters, minutes of meeting.

Secondary sources provide data that have been transcribed or compiled from original sources. Data from secondary sources are gathered by compilation and analysis of original data. Main sources for secondary data are official statistics, patient's medical records, health statistics, web information, historical data, previous research, published and unpublished reports, and records.

DEVELOPING A DATA COLLECTION PLAN

Data collection plans for quantitative studies should be designed to provide meaningful, accurate, unbiased, reliable, and valid data to answer the research question. Various steps involved in data collection plan are listed in Figure 8.1.
- Based on the research question or test of hypothesis the researcher identifies the type of data required.
- Once the type of data is identified the researcher proceeds with selection of data collection method for each variable.
- Researcher should determine if there are instruments available to measure the variable.

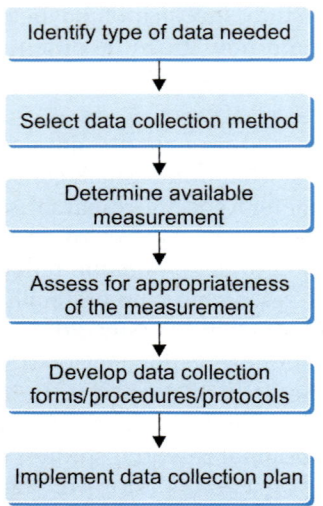

Fig. 8.1: Steps in data collection plan

- Once the suitable instrument is identified, written permission for use in the study may be obtained from the author.
- The potential data collection instruments should be assessed for appropriateness.
- If existing instrument is not suitable the researcher needs to develop a new instrument/tool. Developing a new instrument or tool or measurement should be considered the last resort.
- Researchers who develop a new instrument should refine it by subjecting it to pretesting.
- After the instrument package has been finalized the researcher needs to develop data collection forms, procedures, and data collection protocols.
- Implementing a data collection plan involves selecting data collectors, training them and collecting the data.

DATA COLLECTION PROCESS/PROCEDURE

Data collection is the process of obtaining subjects and collecting the data for a study. The primary goal of a data collection plan is to generate data that are of excellent quality. The data should be clear, unbiased, reliable, and valid. The various steps involved in data collection depend on research design and measuring technique used (Fig. 8.2).

Before commencing the data collection process the researcher decides whether to use existing data or collect it from the participants. Most researchers are usually inclined to collect new data. There are many methods for collecting new data. For example, data can be collected from participants by various methods such as interviews, observing the phenomena, measuring the phenomenon using biopsychosocial measurements. The process of data collection is described in methods section of the research report.

Recruitment of Study Participants

Study participants are usually recruited either in the beginning of the study or throughout the data collection period. The research design determines the method of selecting the participants. In research report the researcher should describe the recruitment process, strategies employed to recruit potential

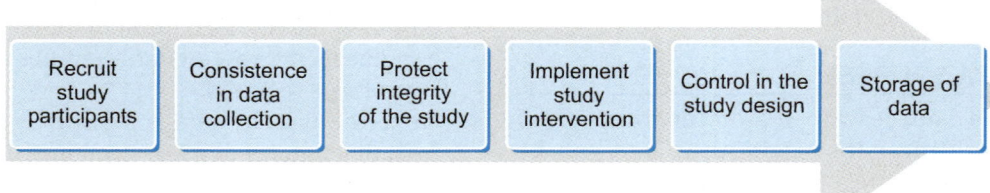

Fig. 8.2: Steps in data collection process

subjects meeting the sampling criteria and specify the number and characteristics of subjects who refused to participate in the study.

Consistence in Data Collection

- In quantitative research studies data is usually collected according to a structured plan. It should indicate what data is required and the way to gather it.
- Consistency is the key to accurate data collection. It involves retaining the same data collection pattern for each collection event as prescribed in the research plan.
- The researcher should specify the source of the data and write a clear, detailed protocol for the data collection process. In addition the researcher should identify the data collectors, train them, and determine ways and means to ensure that relevant data has been collected and missing data or inaccurate responses handled appropriately.
- If the study uses data collectors, researchers need to report the training process and the inter-rater reliability achieved during the training and data collection process.
- Researchers should note even minor deviations and report their effect on the interpretation of study findings in the final study report.
- The researcher needs to describe the approaches used to carry out measurements, time and setting, and a progressive description of how, where and the sequence in which the data should be collected.

During the data collection process the researcher should pose himself the following seven important questions:
- What data to be collected?
- How the data will be collected?
- From whom the data will be collected?
- Who will collect the data?
- Where the data will be collected?
- When the data will be collected?
- How do we ensure that the data are correct?

What Data to be Collected?
Researcher should specify the type of data that will be collected. It depends on the type of study being conducted, hypothesis being tested, and the number of variables involved in the study.

How the Data will be Collected?
Researcher uses instruments or measurements or tools to collect the data. The selection of the measurement is based on the variables that are going to be measured.

From whom the Data will be Collected?
Researcher should identify or select sample subjects for the study, carefully decide on the criteria and make a plan for identifying potential study subjects. He should also consider willingness of the subjects for participation in the study, assuring anonymity and getting permission from the ethical committee.

Who will Collect the Data?
Identify who will actually collect the data. Scientific investigation involves a team of researchers for data collection. Sometimes data collectors are paid for data collection. If only the researcher is going to collect the data it is easy to maintain consistency in data collection. If more persons are involved, training of personnel plays a very important role as they are responsible for collecting the data accurately and completely. The procedure for data collection needs to be pretested. Identify who will be responsible for transferring the data or completing the data entry, describe how anonymity of subjects and confidentiality of the data will be protected.

Where the Data will be Collected?
Depending upon the problem being investigated the researcher needs to select the setting. It is important that optimum conditions

are present for data collection. If self-report questionnaires are being used the researcher might ask the respondents to complete the questionnaire while he remains in same area. This process ensures completeness of the questionnaire. If respondents are tired or the environment is not conducive the answers provided may not be valid.

When the Data will be Collected?

Consider the time of data collection suitable to both the subjects and the researcher. Indicate exactly at what point each piece of data is to be collected and describe if the data will be collected relative to a time or an event. To find out how long the data collection will take place, the researcher should perform a trial run of the procedure. For example, if a questionnaire is being used, it should be pretested with similar potential subjects. If the questionnaire is taking a long time for completion, a decision may be taken to revise the questionnaire.

How do we ensure that the Data are Correct?

Describe accuracy checks and procedures to be followed for dealing with errors and missing data.

Protect Integrity of the Study

Before data collection the researcher reviews the objectives and variables to be considered, conditions to be controlled or eliminated. Usually variables are operationalized in terms of the instruments which are used to measure them. Prior to the data collection process the researcher should get approval from the institutional ethical committee, permission from the setting authorities and also informed consent from the subjects. Before proceeding with the main study a pilot study may be conducted to get a feel of the subjects, setting, methodology, measurements, and implementation of intervention and also identify potential problems. Conducting a pilot study is mandatory in the following situations:

- If the instrument is newly constructed
- Instrument is not used for this population
- Techniques are not familiar to the researcher

Implementing the Study Intervention (in Experimental Studies)

If the study includes an intervention, the relevant details of how it was implemented, nature of treatment, treatment schedule and who implemented the intervention/treatment need to be mentioned in the report.

Control in the Study Design

Control is important in quasi and experimental studies so as to ensure that the intervention is consistently implemented. Researcher builds controls into the study plan to minimize the influence of extraneous variables on the study findings. Researchers need to consider the extraneous variables identified during data collection, data analysis, and interpretation. These variables should be mentioned in the research report so that future researchers are aware of it and attempt suitable control.

In the data collection procedure the researcher should specify the level of significance and how the data is analyzed. Special conditions in the design if any, that will affect the conclusions or generalizations should also find a mention.

Storage of Data

While conducting research on human subjects the investigators have to handle the manner in which the data has to be collected and stored as confidentiality is a major area of concern. It is a sound practice to document the data collection process to preserve the data quality and prepare the research report.

SELECTION OF DATA COLLECTION METHOD

There are many ways to collect data and the selection of a data collection method depends on the following factors (Fig. 8.3):

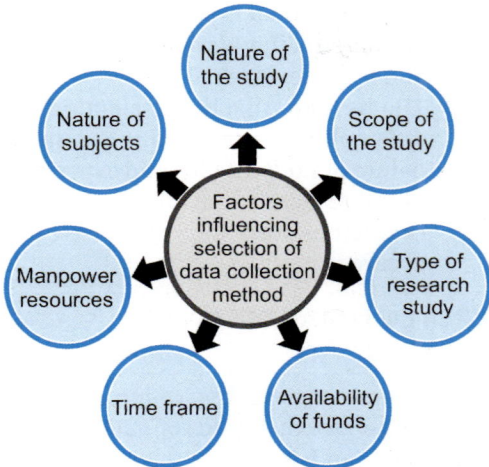

Fig. 8.3: Factors influencing selection of data collection method

1. **Nature of the study**: It is the most important factor affecting the choice of a data collection method. In quantitative studies data collection method is numeric in nature and subject to statistical analysis. In qualitative studies data collection methods are text-based in nature and subject to coding.
2. **Scope of the study**: A research study may either involve a small or a large number of respondents. Face-to-face interview method or observation method are convenient when information is collected from a limited number of respondents. Mail, telephone interview, internet collection methods are convenient when information is collected from large number of respondents.
3. **Type of research study**
   - In descriptive and explorative studies the main aim is to gather more information about the phenomena. The common data collection methods used in these studies are unstructured observation, open-ended interviews and questionnaires.
   - In correlational studies the researcher is looking for relationships among variables and measuring them accurately. The data must be quantifiable so as to arrive at a statistical relationship among the variables. The common methods used in these studies are structured observation, questionnaires, physiological measures, and interviews.
   - In experimental and quasi-experimental studies the main aim is to control the situation and the variables. Therefore the researcher should use precise measures and employ structured methods. The conditions and measurements must be identical for all the subjects. The data must be quantifiable so as to arrive at a cause and effect relationship among the variables. The common methods used in these studies are structured observation, questionnaires, physiological measures, and interviews.
4. **Availability of funds**: Availability of funds should be taken into account while determining the data collection method. When funds available are limited the researcher has to select a relatively cheaper method. For example, observation and interview methods are more expensive compared to questionnaire technique.
5. **Time frame**: Availability of time should also be considered while deciding on the particular data collection method. While methods like face-to-face interviews and observation studies consume more time, methods like self-report and mailing questionnaires take relatively less time.
6. **Availability of manpower resources**: The researcher's knowledge and competence affects the selection of methods of data collection. For example, face-to-face interviews require skilled interviewers; epidemiological studies require researcher with knowledge of statistics; observational and experimental methods require skilled and technically qualified personnel.

7. **Nature of subjects**: If target population is spread in a large geographical area mailed questionnaires are better option, more convenient and cost-effective. If subjects are illiterate, interview method in native language will be more suitable.
    - Each data collection method has its own advantages and none is superior in all situations. For example, a telephone interview method may be considered most suitable in situations where there is shortage of time and funds, and few data items are to be collected without much emphasis on precision.
    - Personal interview method may be relatively better when adequate funds are available and also much information is required.
    - Mailed questionnaire is most preferred in situations where available funds are scarce, constraints on time are few, and information to be gathered is from a geographically dispersed population.
    - In situations that involve huge geographical area, mailed questionnaires along with personal interviews yield optimum results.
    - Secondary data is suitable for investigation only if it is reliable, adequate, and fit for research.
    - The best approach for selection of a data collection method relies on the nature of study, ability, and experience of the researcher, available time and resources and desired degree of accuracy.

TYPES OF DATA COLLECTION METHODS

The various strategies (observation, questioning or measurement) used for gathering the data in a research investigation are known as methods of data collection. Data collection methods are used to gather information in a systematic way.

Once clarity of the research question and purpose are known the researcher must then select the type of data required. These data collection methods are generally classified into primary and secondary data collection methods (Fig. 8.4). Research instrument or a tool is a device used to measure the concept of interest in research study (Table 8.1).

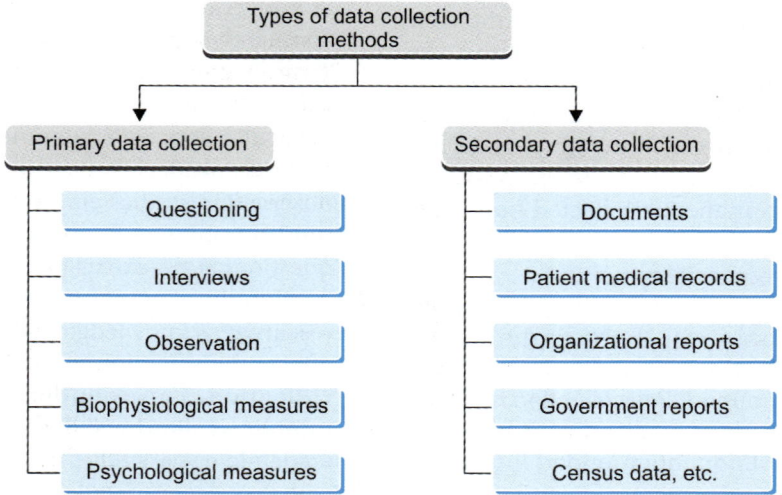

Fig. 8.4: Types of data collection methods

Primary Data Collection

It involves collection of data by the researcher or trained data collector directly from the subjects. The data that are collected are specifically represented for the purpose of the identified research study. The various primary data collection methods include questionnaires, interviews, observations, surveys, projective techniques or biopsychosocial measures.

Advantages
- Data can be collected as per needs
- Completeness of data collection can be ensured
- Accuracy can be verified from the subjects

Disadvantages
- Time consuming
- Introduction of bias on account of inconsistent questions or languages or approaches will create inconsistent data.

Secondary Data Collection

It involves the use of data that were collected for another purpose but used in the current research study. Examples include documents, analysis of newspaper articles, patient's medical records, organizational reports, Government data bases/reports, official statistics, census data, diaries, letters, web information, historical data, previous research, published and unpublished reports and records, etc. The researcher needs to take certain precautions while collecting secondary data such as test the reliability of the data, enquire for suitability of data and check for adequacy of data.

Advantages
- Easier and quicker to collect than primary data
- Electronic data bases are available to retrieve the data

Disadvantages
- Use of secondary data requires a moderate level of skill on the part of the investigator

Table 8.1: Types of data collection methods and tools

Methods	Instrument/tools
Interview	• Interview schedule
Questioning (self-report)	• Questionnaire • Opinionnaire • Attitude scale • Visual analogue scale
Observation	• Rating scales • Observation checklists • Anecdotes • Video tapes/films, electrocardiogram, closed circuit TV
Biophysiological methods/measurements	• In-vivo biophysiological measurements • In-vitro biophysiological measurements • Physical, chemical and microbiological measurements
Psychological measurements	• Projective techniques • Q-sorts • Vignettes • Cognitive and neuropsychological tests
Other methods	• Records, documents and available data

❖ Chance of inaccuracy creeping in during data retrieval process
❖ Data may not be recorded correctly from the primary source.

If the existing data are not available or unsuitable for the research question then the researcher collects new data (primary data).

SURVEY METHOD

Survey method is an approach in which a systematic tool is used to gather information directly from respondents about their experiences, behavior, attitudes or perceptions. When data needs to be gathered from large groups, surveys are the most appropriate form of data collection. Survey tools are often designed by the researcher to capture specific information from a population to answer a particular question (Box 8.1). These surveys are usually conducted in social and behavioral sciences and are an example for field research.

Depending upon the type of questions used a survey method can either be a quantitative or a qualitative method or a mixture of both. In quantitative survey method participant responses are described in numeric terms, while in qualitative survey method the participant responses are described in words. Important characteristics of numeric research surveys are that they use a systematic approach and allow for a quantitative analysis of reliability, validity, and statistical conclusions. Surveys may be conducted on an entire population or on samples. The main methods used in survey data collection are presented in Figure 8.5.

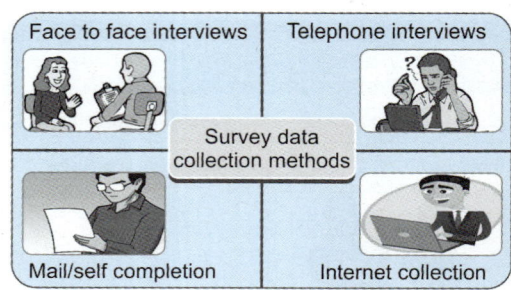

Fig. 8.5: Survey data collection methods

Face-to-Face Interviews

In face-to-face interviews data is collected by a specially trained team of interviewers from the respondents in a face-to-face conversation. Initially the survey organization sends a letter to the respondents informing them that they have been identified for the survey, what the survey is about and why they have been selected. Later the data collector administers the questionnaires at the respondents' homes.

Telephone Interviews

Structured interviews using the telephone are one of the popular methods of data collection. In a telephone interview data is collected by the interviewer by conversing with the respondents over the telephone. In this process the interviewer uses structured questionnaire with less items not lasting more than half an hour. Generally these interviews are used to assess attitude or behavior. This is because people are reluctant to answer personal questions over the telephone when they have not actually met the interviewer.

Mail Survey/Self-completion Data Collection

Mail surveys or postal data collection is an economical method of collecting data from a large sample who are geographically dispersed. In this method the data is collected from the respondents through post. The researcher prepares a structured questionnaire and sends it to the respondents along with a covering

Box 8.1	When to use surveys
	• When information is to be collected from large number of people
	• When answers are needed to a clearly defined set of questions
	• When an in-depth probing of responses is not necessary

letter and a stamped self-addressed envelope. The respondents fill in the questionnaire and send it back to the researcher. Follow up postcards can be sent to boost the response rate. Self report questionnaires can be distributed to participants in specific situations such as when the patient is being discharged from the hospital to get a feedback on the nursing care.

Internet Collection (Web Surveys or E-mail Data Collection)

With greater penetration and popularity of internet among the public it is much simpler to collect data online. It is an economical and speedy way of collecting data without limiting to geographical boundaries, i.e. across states and nations. In this method the data is collected from the respondents through e-mail or online survey. In e-mail data collection method the researcher sends the questionnaire to the respondent through e-mail usually by way of an attachment. The respondent then fills in the questionnaire and mails it back to the researcher.

In web surveys the questionnaires are sent to the respondents by way of a web link in an e-mail or feature as a pop-up window on a website. These web surveys are created using special softwares, which provide a form for the respondents to fill in. On filling up the survey format the respondent submits the data online which then is transmitted to the server with a specific code where it is stored. The data in the server needs to be secured to maintain confidentiality.

The various components, advantages, and disadvantages of survey data collection methods are dealt in Table 8.2.

Epidemiological Survey

- Epidemiological survey conducted in an epidemic focuses to discover the source of an infection, the means by which causative agent was transmitted, and the circumstances that gave rise to the disease.
- The findings are used to devise ways of preventing the disease from spreading. Individuals suffering with the disease and those who have had contact with them are interviewed and undergo laboratory testing.
- Epidemiological surveys use various study designs. At one extreme while a case-control investigation with fewer samples is employed, at the other end large longitudinal studies following up many thousands of people for several decades are employed.
- Data are often obtained by means of records, questionnaires (these may be self administered or administered at interviews), observation, physical examination, and clinical investigations.
- The survey may also include tests on objects from the environment (water, contaminated objects), insects (entomological) and animals (zoonoses).
- In case of intestinal inspections, the restaurants and other places where food is prepared are inspected. The disease characteristics and the number of sick persons determine the type of survey to be conducted.
- The results of the survey are recorded on an epidemiological survey map. The findings determine the actions to be taken with respect to the individuals who have had contact with sick persons (medical observation, isolation, immunization, and chemoprophylaxis).
- They also determine disinfection measures and steps to improve the sanitary conditions and maintenance of water-supply facilities and food service facilities. The findings are also used to study the patterns of distribution of infectious diseases and devise control measures.

QUESTIONNAIRE

Questionnaire is a proforma containing series of questions in a self-report form designed

Table 8.2: Survey data collection methods—components, advantages and disadvantages

Methods of data collection	Sample and sample type	Time taken for data collection	Cost	Response rate	Advantages	Disadvantages
Face to face interviews	Available sampling frames and probability	More	High	High	• High response rate • Better data quality • Capture verbal and nonverbal questions • Collection of in-depth information • Rapport can be established	• Costly process • Interviewers need training and supervision • Interviewer needs to spend long time for data collection • Subjectivity in decision making • Limited sample size
Telephone interviews	Random digit dialing and probability	Less	Medium	Medium	• Cost-effective • Offers convenience for both the interviewer and the subject • Able to reach a large number of geographically spread population • Can be completed in short duration of time • Helps in getting a representative sample due to greater phone connectivity • Quality of data generated can be high if conducted by skilled and experienced interviewers	• Low response rates • Sampling bias may occur • Questions cannot be of long or complex nature • Due to aversion to telemarketers, samples may refuse to participate • Nonverbal communication
Mail survey/self-completion data collection	Available sample frames and probability	Less	Low	Low	• Cost-effective • Ability to reach geographically spread population • Offers convenience for both the interviewer and the applicant	• Low response rate • Poor data quality, where the respondents misinterpret the questions
Web survey and E-mail data collection	Non-probability	Less	Very less	Low	• Low cost • Ability to reach geographically spread population • Facility to use visual aids in web services	• Sampling issues • Poor data quality • Low response rates

to elicit information. Information can be obtained through a written form (paper-pencil approach) or by way of verbal responses of the subjects. It is a structured survey data collection instrument that is self administered by subjects. It is commonly used in nursing research. While a questionnaire is a data collection instrument, questioning is the method or technique to collect the data.

Questionnaires are often employed in descriptive studies to gather a wide range of information from the subjects. These are often developed for a particular study to enable the researcher collect the data from a particular population. Questionnaires can be used with some other tools in a single study, distributed to subjects in a classroom, on the streets, campus, home or at work or through the mail or via the internet. Questionnaire allows access to sample dispersed over large geographic areas. Though the information obtained from a questionnaire is similar to that obtained from an interview, the questions lack depth as there is no much scope to elaborate on the responses or seek clarifications. The researcher cannot exercise probing strategies.

Purposes

- The main purpose of asking questions is to find out what is going on in the minds of subjects: their perception, attitudes, beliefs, techniques, motives, plans, practices, knowledge, opinions, and feelings.
- Through this method the researcher can gather retrospective data about activities and events occurring in the past or gather projections about behavior in which people plan to engage in the future.
- The psychological characteristics of the participants can be captured using self report methods.

Advantages

- Relatively simple, rapid and an efficient way of gathering data and exploring new topics.
- Items can be constructed easily by the beginning researcher.
- It can be given to a large number of people simultaneously; they can also be sent by mail. Therefore, it is possible to cover a widely scattered population.
- Less expensive, particularly in terms of time spent collecting the data.
- Subjects are more likely to express controversial opinions as they feel anonymous.
- Easiest tool to test for validity and reliability.
- Questionnaire can be flexible relating to the type of item, order of items and topics covered by the researcher.
- Subjects will have time to ponder on the response to each of their questions.
- The questions are identical and presented in a consistent manner to each subject thus resulting in more meaningful responses with lesser chance for bias than in an interview.
- Easy to tabulate data from closed items.
- Easy accomplishment of data analysis and interpretation.

Disadvantages

- There is always the possibility that the written question will be interpreted differently by different readers, which is one reason for carefully pretesting questionnaires.
- The validity and accuracy of self-report is a cause for concern as the researcher is not sure if the respondents actually feel and act the way they say or do. The researcher should be prepared to consider these aspects while interpreting the results.
- Inability to probe a topic in-depth unless the questionnaire is lengthy.
- Respondents may skip or disregard a question without providing a suitable explanation. Some items may be misunderstood. The incomplete nature of the data can threaten the validity of the instrument. It is important for the

researcher to describe how the missing data were managed in their study report.
- Some items may force the subjects to choose responses that are not their actual choice (forced-choice items).
- Amount of information gathered is limited by subjects' time and interest span. Usually people do not like to take more than 25 minutes to answer a questionnaire. (Length of questionnaire should not be more than 60 minutes/one hour).
- Printing may be a costly affair if the questionnaire is lengthy and printed on good quality paper.
- Addressing outside envelops and postage are time consuming and expensive respectively.
- Data are limited to information given by the subjects voluntarily. Not all subjects comply with request to participate.
- Subjects' non-verbal cues cannot be observed.
- Response rate of mailed questionnaires is poor when compared to other forms of self report. The representativeness of the sample is doubtful if the response rate is lesser than 50%.

Types of Questionnaires

Questionnaires are developed for a particular study to enable the researcher gather data from a particular population. Questionnaires can be categorized as structured and semi-structured.

1. A *structured questionnaire* contains only predetermined questions and their response options. The subjects are asked to respond to these questions in the same order using the same set of response options so that the order of the questions does not affect the subjects' responses. The questions are standardized to ensure that the subject's answers can be compared. The most structured questionnaires have close ended questions with fixed alternative questions.

2. A *semi-structured questionnaire* contains a mix of open ended and close ended questions. Specific format is followed for obtaining the necessary information. Semi-structured questionnaires are designed to elicit extensive response from the subject.

Types of Questions

Type of questions a researcher chooses depends upon the range of data required and appropriateness to the variable measured. The commonly used questions in a questionnaire are presented in Figure 8.6.

Open-ended Questions

- Open-ended questions are most preferred when the researcher is interested in the subjective aspect of the participant replies and not aware of all the possible responses to the posed questions. Open-ended questions ask for unprompted

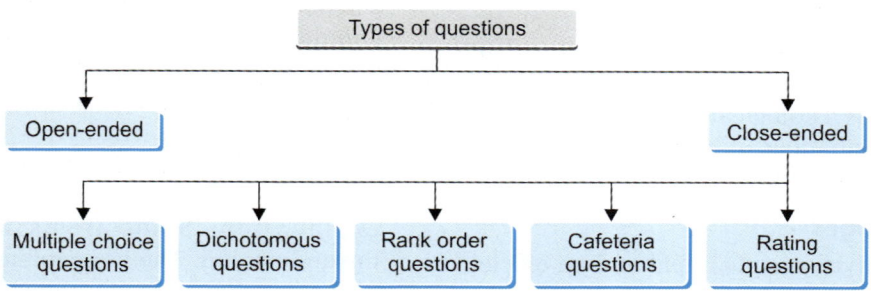

Fig. 8.6: Types of questions

opinions. There are no predetermined answers for the respondents to choose from. Typically, open-ended questions are used in qualitative research by using interviews or focus groups, but may also be used in questionnaires. Responses are analyzed using content analysis to find themes in the words of respondents.

❖ The advantage is that the researcher gets a wide range of responses. Disadvantages of the open-ended questions are that it takes the respondent longer time to complete, misinterpretation of questions by the respondent and longer time required to analyze the data.

Example: What do you like most about nursing profession? Describe the status of a nurse in the society.

Close-ended Questions

❖ Close-ended questions (forced choice questions) are used when the researcher wants the participants to choose from a fixed number of alternative responses. The alternatives may range from a simple yes or no to a complex expression of opinions. As the alternative responses are designed with reference to the requirements of the study, the chances of securing relevant answers are better.

❖ The main advantage is that, closed questions are easier for the respondent to answer, ensure comparability of responses, and facilitate easy analysis. Disadvantages are that they force a statement of response implied in the researcher's terms rather than the respondent's, the limited alternatives may not cover respondent view point, the respondent may be led to choose a response even when he has no knowledge of it. It is also possible that different respondents will interpret the same words and statements differently.

Example: Have you been admitted to the hospital at any time in the past 1 year?
   o Yes
   o No

Commonly used close-ended questions are as follows:

1. *Multiple choice questions*: These questions require the respondents to select a single response from a list of possible answers and are used when the researcher wants respondents to choose the best possible answer among all options presented. Multiple choice questions often have a combination of a right answer along with the wrong answers.
   Example: Which of the following is an important characteristic of a mentally healthy person?
      a. Ability to perform activities independently
      b. Ability to make adjustments
      c. Feeling secure
      d. Changes in behavior
   The list of alternative choices should contain all the possible choices that the respondents would like to have. They should not contain overlapping choices and alternatives should be reasonable. The choices should be conceptually unidimensional. The actual process of designing satisfactory alternative responses to multiple choice questions calls for repeated pretests and revisions.

2. *Dichotomous or two choice questions*: Dichotomous questions are those that can be answered by selecting from one of the only two choices. These typically are used to determine whether a respondent belongs to a particular group or not; whether a trait is present or not. Dichotomous questions yield limited information about the respondent and are difficult to analyze. These questions are most appropriate in situations where other types of questions are not suitable. For example, to which gender do you belong? Male/Female.

3. *Rank order questions:* These questions ask respondents to rank their responses along a continuum ranging from most favorable

to least favorable. Respondents are asked to mark 1, 2, 3 according to their either increasing or decreasing importance.

Example: List the things that you value in your life by placing 1 beside the most valuable alternative, 2 beside the next most important alternative and so on.
- Success
- Family relations
- Health
- Money

4. *Cafeteria questions:* These are special types of multiple choice questions that ask respondents to choose a response that most closely reflects their opinion. For example, the opinion people have about organ donation, electroconvulsive therapy, hormone replacement therapy, etc.

Example: What do you think about electroconvulsive therapy?
   a. It is beneficial and so can be promoted
   b. One should be cautious while taking it
   c. I am uncertain about my views
   d. It is dangerous and so should be avoided.

5. *Rating questions:* These are a set of statements wherein the respondents are asked to express agreement or disagreement on a five-point or seven-point scale or judge something along an ordered dimension. Each response is given a numerical value enabling a total numerical value to be calculated from all the responses.

Example: How satisfied are you with the care provided by the nurses in the hospital?

1	2	3	4	5
Extremely satisfied	Very satisfied	Somewhat satisfied	Dissatisfied	Extremely dissatisfied

Methods of Questionnaire Administration

Questionnaires can be administered through either of the methods—personal administration (individual or group), postal, telephone or electronic.

❖ In personal administration the questionnaire is administered to an individual or a group of respondents through direct contact or over the telephone.
   - Advantage: Here the researcher is available to clarify the doubts/queries that may arise. Response rate is high. Rapport can be established.
   - Disadvantage: Time consuming and costly.

❖ Questionnaires are mailed through postal or electronic means (Q-sort and DELPHI technique). This method is used when the sample is large and widely distributed.
   - Advantages: The cost, manpower, and time involved is less, anonymity of the subjects is maintained.
   - Disadvantages: Low response rate. Some questions may be omitted or misunderstood by the respondents.

The researcher may need to do follow-up for nonresponse by way of sending follow-up letters, making telephone calls and personal visits. The researcher needs to take extra care on aspects such as physical appearance, layout, color, and printing (Fig. 8.7).

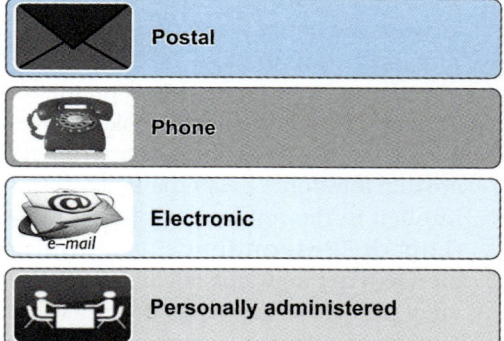

Fig. 8.7: Methods of questionnaire administration

Qualities of a Good Question

Developing questions that suit the maximum number of respondents without losing focus on the information to be collected are the prerequisites for a good questionnaire.

A good questionnaire:
- should be easy to answer
- focus on eliciting necessary information
- use language that is clearly worded and unambiguous and should be interpreted by all subjects in a similar way
- is written at a fifth grade language
- uses words that are familiar
- does not use words that convey more than one meaning
- asks for an answer on only one dimension
- uses correct spelling, grammar and punctuation
- avoids leading and long questions
- should be nonthreatening (should not create a negative reaction)
- does not imply a certain type of answer

Steps in Designing a Questionnaire

The seven steps in designing a questionnaire are presented in Figure 8.8.

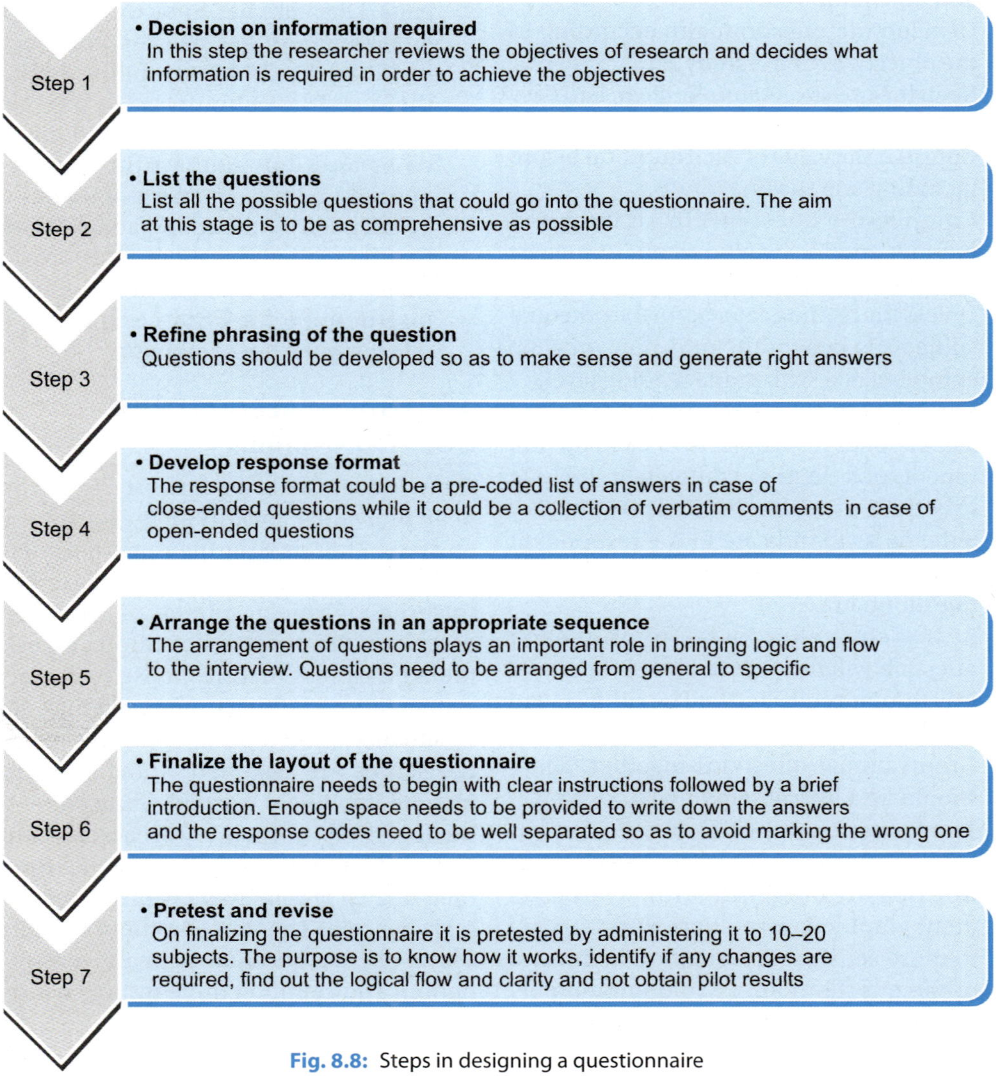

Step 1
- **Decision on information required**
  In this step the researcher reviews the objectives of research and decides what information is required in order to achieve the objectives

Step 2
- **List the questions**
  List all the possible questions that could go into the questionnaire. The aim at this stage is to be as comprehensive as possible

Step 3
- **Refine phrasing of the question**
  Questions should be developed so as to make sense and generate right answers

Step 4
- **Develop response format**
  The response format could be a pre-coded list of answers in case of close-ended questions while it could be a collection of verbatim comments in case of open-ended questions

Step 5
- **Arrange the questions in an appropriate sequence**
  The arrangement of questions plays an important role in bringing logic and flow to the interview. Questions need to be arranged from general to specific

Step 6
- **Finalize the layout of the questionnaire**
  The questionnaire needs to begin with clear instructions followed by a brief introduction. Enough space needs to be provided to write down the answers and the response codes need to be well separated so as to avoid marking the wrong one

Step 7
- **Pretest and revise**
  On finalizing the questionnaire it is pretested by administering it to 10–20 subjects. The purpose is to know how it works, identify if any changes are required, find out the logical flow and clarity and not obtain pilot results

Fig. 8.8: Steps in designing a questionnaire

Simple Suggestions for Designing a Questionnaire

Questionnaires are not easy to construct as they demand a thoughtful, systematic approach. Yet they can be invaluable as a data collection tool for both quantitative and qualitative research.

- Some of the important factors a researcher needs to consider before developing a questionnaire include the type and size of sample, method of administration, cost, and time limit.
- Develop the questionnaire according to the objectives of the study.
- Keep the questions simple, clear, and easy to answer.
- Consider the value of each question before including it in the final draft.
- Compile the questions in an unbiased manner and in a way so as not to suggest the answer.
- Unless the reading capacity of the potential subjects is known the questions may be compiled at a sixth grade reading level.
- Keep the overall questionnaire short and ask the pilot test subjects to estimate the time it took them to complete it. Include this time estimate in the introductory letter so as to indicate to the respondent the time limit available to complete the questionnaire.
- Researcher should know how each question will be analyzed and be sure the way the data collected will be subjected to the specific analytic test.
- Group similar questions together. There should be a logical sequence.
- The questions should be sequenced from general to specific. Start with nonthreatening questions such as demographic information, and work up to more sensitive information at the end of the questionnaire. Avoid emotionally loaded words that may imply a judgment.
- While compiling the rating questionnaire, alternatives that are "neutral" or "undecided" may be avoided as there is often a chance for the respondents to choose this category of alternatives. If a neutral category is required, a separate category may be included that has no numerical value for "not applicable/no answer."
- The printing of the questionnaire should be of a good quality with adequate space for answering. Margin should be provided on both the left and right sides of the page. Due care has to be exercised while finalizing the letter size and font. Section heading should be printed in bold. All the questions should be in one color. Instructions may be printed in different color and font size. At the end of the questionnaire a comment of thanks may be included for the cooperation extended.
- For the mailed questionnaires provide a well-written covering letter with explicit instructions for both completing and returning the questionnaire.

ATTITUDE SCALE/ATTITUDE QUESTIONNAIRE

Attitude represents the inner feeling or belief of an individual towards an object, person or an event. Attitude scale measures the intensity and direction of a subject's feelings or beliefs towards an object, person or situation. It discovers the subject's opinions by asking them to express their response to a series of statements pertaining to an individual, object or situation. Based on the subject's response the scores are assigned. Some statements may be positively worded while some may be negatively worded to reveal the attitude. Respondents indicate their preference through their degree of agreement with statements on a given scale. The items in the scale consist of two parts: a question stem and a response option. The common three response formats are:

- Dichotomous options like yes or no; or agree or disagree following a simple declarative statement.
- Semantic-differential items like bipolar adjectives or pair of descriptive statements that examinees use to select the response option out of a range of values that best matches their agreement.
- Likert formats offer multiple response categories that usually span a 5-point range of responses. For example: 1-strongly agree to 5-strongly disagree.

Response options may be delineated by numbers, percentages or degree of agreement and disagreement. The examples of attitude scales are given in Table 8.3.

OPINIONNAIRE

Opinionnaire, a form of enquiry used to study opinion or belief of an individual on certain important issues. These are usually used in descriptive researches like survey research or public opinion research. It involves various statements or questions pertaining to the research study rated on a three point or five point scale or in the form of yes or no. It uses favorable or unfavorable statements. Though opinionnaires and questionnaires are similar in many ways, the emphasis in opinionnaires is not in seeking facts but in seeking an opinion. Example for an opinionnaire is presented in Table 8.4.

INTERVIEWS

Meaning

- Interview is a method of data collection in which the researcher interacts directly with the participant one-on-one via telephone or in person to get information that is relevant for the research question.
- It is a structured talk between an informant and a researcher. It includes conver-

Table 8.3: Examples of attitude scales

Dichotomous	
Question stem	Response option
Did you regularly attend clinical postings	Yes ( ) No ( )

Semantic differential		
For each pair of statements, choose a number that indicates how well the statement describes	I am reserved 1 2 3 4 5	I am quick to respond

Likert					
Indicate your level of agreement with the following statement: In general, I have a good feeling towards nursing	Strongly agree	Agree	Undecided	Disagree	Strongly disagree

Table 8.4: Participants opinionnaire towards AIDS patients

Please read the following items and indicate your agreement or disagreement.

Sl. No.	Items	Agree	Undecided	Disagree
1.	I am scared of people with AIDS			
2.	I am uncomfortable providing care to AIDS patients			
3.	I am uncomfortable touching people with AIDS			

sations, gestures, facial expressions, and environment of the respondent.

When to Use Interviews

Interviews are used:
- When information is collected from a small geographical area
- To evaluate the program
- When the respondents are illiterate
- To gather an in-depth information in qualitative and descriptive studies
- In situations where complex information or an in-depth information or highly sensitive matter is to be collected. It is also used when high-status respondents are involved

Importance of Interview
- Best suited for assessment of personal qualities
- For diagnosis of emotional problems and therapeutic treatment
- For counseling purpose
- Supplement other methods of data collection
- Probe the views and beliefs of an individual on a particular issue
- Explore the motives of an individual

Advantages
- It is superior to other data collection methods as people are more ready to express their feelings in verbal form than in writing. Development of a good rapport can even elicit confidential information.
- Permits face-to-face contact with a respondent which allows the interviewer to explore the affective as well as cognitive aspects of responses.
- Most appropriate when a detailed and in-depth information is required from a participant.
- The response rate for an interview is higher than for questionnaires which usually allow a more representative sample to be obtained.
- Facilitates collection of data from participants who are unlikely to complete the questionnaire. For example, illiterates, very sick patients.
- It is more flexible, allows the researcher to explore in-depth information, and provides new insight leading to data enrichment. The researcher also has an opportunity to probe further for additional information.
- Explore highly sensitive matters.
- Ambiguity can be clarified and incomplete answers are followed up.
- Interpersonal skills can be used to facilitate cooperation.
- Respondents' own words are recorded.

Disadvantages
- Interviews are time consuming and resource intensive
- Require well-qualified, highly trained interviewers
- Data may be affected by interviewer's biases
- Volume of information is very large; may be difficult to record and reduce data
- Data obtained is affected by age, ethnicity, gender, education, vision, hearing, speech, pain
- Accuracy of the data may be affected by subject's recall error or wish to please the interviewer

Types of Questions Posed in an Interview

The different types of questions that may be posed in an interview are presented in Figure 8.9.

Interviewing Process

Interviews can be conducted by face to face meeting, telephonically or video conferencing. The steps included in interview process are listed in Figure 8.10.

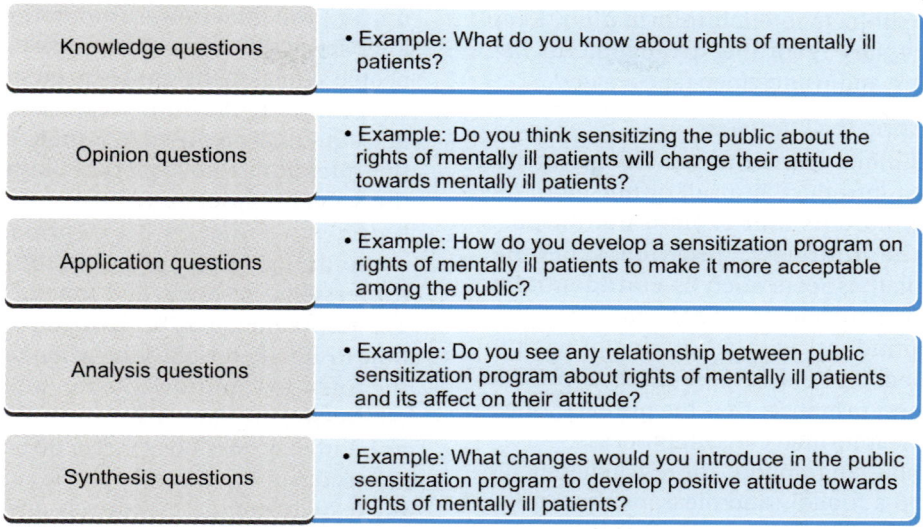

Fig. 8.9: Types of questions posed in an interview

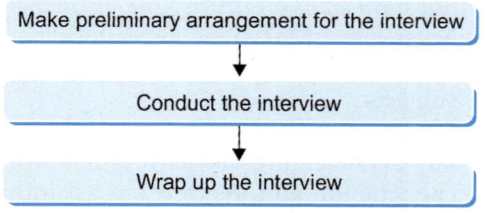

Fig. 8.10: Steps in interview process

Make Preliminary Arrangement for the Interview

- Training the interviewer: The individual conducting the interview needs to be trained on posing the questions in a proper and sequential manner and handle any unanticipated possibilities that might arise during the interview process.
- Preparing for the interview: The researcher has to initially determine as to who is to be interviewed and whether they are willing to participate and provide information. The number of interviewees has also to be determined in order to get reliable information. A plan of the interview along with a schedule or list of questions to be posed has to be determined in advance.
- Pretesting the interview protocol: Researcher needs to establish reliability and validity of the tool and perform pilot testing. Pilot testing helps to identify the design, question sequencing, and recording procedure.
- Familiarity with interview schedule: The interviewer should read the schedule carefully and practice it reading aloud and be familiar with all the questions. Wordings in the questionnaire should be followed exactly as phrased.
- Fix up appointment: The interviewer should fix up the interview as per the convenience of the subjects well in advance. This will save time and allow both the interviewer and the interviewee to be mentally prepared.
- Appearance and dress: The interviewer should look pleasing, relaxed, and friendly. The interviewer should dress in a familiar fashion and with due regard to the sensibilities of the people being interviewed.
- Preparation of environment: Provide privacy and conducive atmosphere to

the subjects to elicit information. Keep necessary recording arrangements like notes, audio and video tapes ready.

Conducting the Interview

- Preliminary introduction: The researcher must introduce himself or herself to the respondents and explain the purpose of the interview, interview schedule, ethical aspects such as confidentiality and anonymity. This provides the respondents with a fair idea of what to expect and encourages them to provide honest responses. It is the primary aspect of the informed consent process.
- Establishing rapport: The researcher should build a friendly and pleasant atmosphere for the subjects and promise them confidentiality. They should be assured about the anonymity of their responses. No pressure shall be laid on the subjects to answer sensitive and embarrassing questions. The conversation may begin with a discussion on general topics.
- Word the questions carefully: Questions shall be worded in a clear, straightforward way. Each question that is asked should relate back to the research question. While questions may be posed using neutral words, those with double meaning may be avoided. Open-ended words such as "how", "why", or "what" may be used. Questions that can be answered with a "yes" or "no" may be avoided.
- Plan the sequence of the questions: An environment may be provided that allows the respondent to answer in a truthful manner. The questions should be as neutral as possible. The interviewer may begin with informational or factual questions that will put the respondent at ease. Questions about the present may be posed before those pertaining to the past or the future. Order the questions from impersonal to personal topics; less sensitive to more sensitive; general to specific. List the questions in the same order to provide consistency and also prevent the interviewer from forgetting. Interviewer should pretest the questions on people similar to the sample to be studied.
- Carrying out the interview: Only one question may be posed at a time. Repeat the question if necessary. Ensure that the subject understands the questions, listen carefully to his replies, and while doing so also observe the facial expressions, gestures, and tone of voice. The respondent may be allowed plenty of time to answer the question while keeping the interview on track. As the interview progresses, the interviewer should remain as neutral as possible. Once a question is asked, the interviewer should be sure that the respondent has completely answered the question before asking a new question. Ask additional questions to follow-up clues or obtain additional information. Do not show signs of surprise, shock or anger. Notes may be taken inconspicuously or a recorder used with due permission of the subjects.
- Communication techniques: The important skills an interviewer requires while carrying out an interview are assuming an open and emotionally neutral body posture, acknowledging with facial expressions like smiling and nodding, appropriate gesturing and looking interested. The appropriate use of silence is effective in getting the respondents to elaborate and reflect over their responses. Other effective techniques like reflecting on remarks, seeking clarification from respondents where necessary can take the interview further.
- Probing: Probing should be used by the interviewer to obtain more information in a specific area of the interview (e.g. When you said you were afraid of going to the psychiatrist what did you actually mean?). Probes should be neutral to avoid the biasing of subject's response.
- Recording the interview: Recording should be done during or immediately after the

interview which can be in the form of handwritten notes, audio or video tape recording. It needs to be done without distracting the interviewee. Tape recording requires permission of the subjects.

Wrap up the Interview

The interview may be wrapped up with a summary of the study followed by a thank you note for the respondents. It is desirable to record the interview and immediately transcribe it verbatim so as to avoid bias and simultaneously produce a permanent testimony of what was said and what was not. Field notes on observations, thoughts, and ideas about the interview during and immediately after each interview support data analysis process. Field notes may be reviewed for additions and revisions.

Types of Interview (Various Approaches to Conduct an Interview)

The format of the interview can be either highly structured or loosely structured depending on the information needed. The types of questions may either be closed, open-ended or probing. Closed questions are similar to those used in questionnaires. The questions may be forced choice or dichotomous. Open-ended questions are also similar to those used in questionnaires. The various approaches to conducting an interview (types of interview method) are presented in Figure 8.11.

Structured Interview (Directive Interview)

In structured interviews the interviewer has a standardized interview schedule, i.e. same set of questions are posed to all the respondents in a similar order. In this method the researcher has the control over the content of the interview and questions are designed before data collection. Interviewers are restricted from changing the specific wording of the questions. The type of questions may be closed. The researcher asks specific questions and enters participant's responses on a paper and pencil

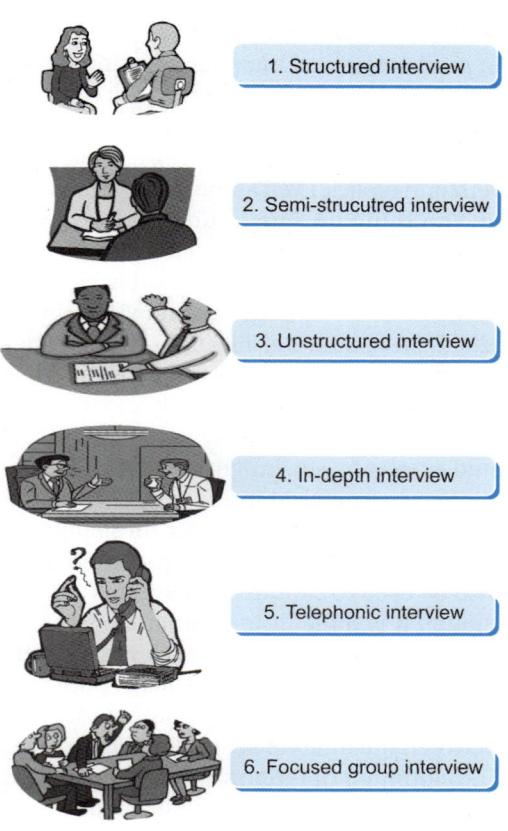

1. Structured interview
2. Semi-strucutred interview
3. Unstructured interview
4. In-depth interview
5. Telephonic interview
6. Focused group interview

Fig. 8.11: Types of interview

instrument or rating scale. Such interviews are appropriate for experimental studies.

Advantages
❖ Quick and easy to administer
❖ Data from one interview can be compared with that of another one
❖ Increases the reliability (degree of consistency) and credibility (truly represents the underlying meaning) of the research data
❖ Attention is focused thus avoiding irrelevant and time consuming conversations
❖ Coding of information and analyzing the data is easy

Disadvantages
❖ Scope for exploration of further information is limited
❖ Limited participant responses

Semi-structured Interview

In semi-structured interviews the interviewer has a flexible interview schedule, i.e. it comprises of predetermined topics and open-ended questions interspersed with gaps for recording verbatim replies. Even as the researcher focuses on the topic on one hand he also has the flexibility to elicit additional information. While the researcher has the capacity to be responsive to the interviewee's agenda and views, he still retains the control and direction of the interview. The interviewer has the liberty to pose questions to each of the participants in a different manner. Such interviews are widely used in qualitative studies so as to gain insight into the topic.

Semi-structured interviews are recorded using tape-recorder and later these tapes are transcribed for analysis. The jotted notes can also be used to capture respondents' answers though it is difficult to simultaneously focus on both conducting an interview and jotting the notes. This approach results in poor notes and also distracts the development of rapport between the interviewer and the interviewee. Development of rapport is essential in semi-structured interviews. If tape-recording an interview is not feasible, the use of a note-taker may be considered.

Advantages
- Provides reliable, comparable and qualitative data
- Allows subjects the freedom to express views in their own way
- Allows the interviewer to frame the questions and prepare for the interview in advance making the interviewer look competent

Disadvantages
- Costly and time-consuming
- Requires highly qualified, well trained interviewers

Unstructured Interview
(Non-directive Interview)

Unstructured interviews are informal in nature and appear like a conversation rather than an interview. The interview comprises a list of topics rather than predefined questions. They explore in-depth information from the participant's perspective and are least directive. Interview usually begins with general questions such as, "Can you tell me your experience of taking *ganja*?" and then proceed depending upon the initial response. These interviews consume more time and are difficult to manage. This approach is more commonly adopted in qualitative research studies where little previous knowledge exists or a different view point needs to be elicited.

Advantages
- Explores information in an unrestricted manner
- Suitable for eliciting sensitive information on topics like drug addiction, social discrimination, marital discord

Disadvantages
- Expensive and time-consuming
- Needs well-qualified, highly trained interviewers
- The data obtained from one interview is not comparable to the data from the next
- Require long time to transcribe and analyze

In-depth Interviews

In this method the interviewer does not follow a rigid format as he encourages more of open and verbal responses with limited set of questions. These capture the respondents' perceptions in their own words which is a much wanted feature in qualitative data collection process. This permits the researcher to meaningfully project the respondent's perspective. Though there is scope for both comprehensive coverage and an in-depth exploration by way of a narrow range of questions, it is at the cost of compensating one for the other. In-depth interviews are generally conducted with a small group of individuals.

Advantages
- Encourages free expression of participants
- Used to study the respondents opinion and emotions

- Gathers in-depth information
- Less prone to interviewer's bias

Disadvantages
- Expensive and time-consuming
- Needs well-qualified, highly trained interviewers
- The data obtained from one interview is not comparable to the data from the next
- Require long time to transcribe and analyze

Telephone Interview

Telephone interviews are used to conducted structured and semi-structured interviews and are a non-personal method of data collection. In this method the interviewer contacts the respondents on telephone itself and gathers information from them.

Advantages
- These are cheaper, require less travel and equipment
- More convenient mode of enquiry
- More flexible and quicker way of obtaining information
- Response rate is high
- Wider coverage of sample is possible

Disadvantages
- In the absence of face-to-face interaction it is difficult to establish a rapport with the respondent
- Limited to respondents having telephone facility
- Nonverbal response of the subjects cannot be observed
- Limited in their ability to detect detailed information
- Possibility of interviewer's bias is more

Focused Group Interview

Focus group interview is an in-depth qualitative interview with a small group of people (generally between 6 and 12) that have been specifically selected to represent a target audience (Brewerton & Millward, 2003).

It is a group discussion usually organized to generate collective views of the participants, wherein the moderator or the facilitator guides, monitors and records the discussion on a particular topic.

Concepts
- Focus groups tend to be less structured allowing participants to elaborate on an answer through the give and take of group discussion, i.e. the participants have an opportunity to express their own opinions and simultaneously react to the idea of others.
- The main feature of focus group discussion is to generate information through group interaction which otherwise would not emerge.
- These interviews allow the moderator to observe group dynamics, conversations, and primary perception of the respondents' behaviors, attitudes, language, etc.
- This interaction among focus group participants provides a powerful dynamics that may be missing from individual interviews.
- Focus groups interviews are a fine mix of both interviewing and observatory skills.
- Focus groups are designed to be non-threatening allowing the participants to express and clarify their views in ways that are less likely to occur one-on-one. Table 8.5 describes when to and when not to use a focus group.

Table 8.5: When to and when not to use a focus group

When to use focus groups	When not to use focus groups
• To generate information on collective views and the meanings that lie behind those views • To generate a rich understanding of participants' experiences and beliefs • To clarify, extend or challenge data collected through other methods	• If the participants are uncomfortable in the presence of each other they may not share their feelings and opinions openly • If the topic is not of much interest to the participants • Though focus groups provide depth and insight they cannot produce useful numerical results where statistical data is required

Group Composition and Size
- Group composition refers to the various characteristics of individuals that form a group. The individual or group characteristic can have an influence on others. This group composition will have impact on generation of data.
- Group interaction (how the group members may interact among themselves) is the key to a successful focus group.
- The group can be a combination of various ages, genders, levels of intelligence, and occupational statuses of the participants.
- It consists of 6–12 members homogeneous in terms of demographic and socio-economic characteristics.
- Small groups run the risk of limited discussion which may not reveal sufficient information.
- A large group tends to be chaotic making it hard for the moderator to manage. It also leads to frustration among the group members as they may not get an adequate opportunity to share their views.

Conducting focus group interview
- *Selection of members*: The use of purposive sampling is most often employed when individuals known to have a desired expertise are sought.
- *Preparing an interview schedule*: In focus group interviews the interview schedule is often semi-structured. The questions move from general to more specific and the order is in accordance with the research agenda. Usually the researcher proceeds with a set of predetermined questions and also probes and expands on issues according to the discussion.
- *Moderating:* Moderating a focus group requires a complex set of skills. The moderator should facilitate group discussion and keep the attention focused on a particular aspect of a problem without leading it. It is a carefully planned discussion where the moderator guides the conversation as per the fixed interview schedule. The moderator should be capable of preventing the discussion from being dominated by a single or few participants and ensure that all participants have ample opportunity to contribute, allow differences of opinion to be discussed fairly and, if required, encourage reserved participants. The duration of the interview is generally limited to 1–2 hours.
- *Venue*: The venue for a focus group should be accessible and comfortable for the participants and free from distractions.
- *Recording*: Focus group discussions are recorded either manually (by having someone take notes) or taped. While beginning the focus group interview, the moderator should intimate all the participants about the presence of audio or video recording equipment for the session and assure them of confidentiality and also provide a chance to quit if they are uneasy being taped. The presence of observers should be intimated to the participants and clarified that they are present only for observation and will be sitting away from the discussion. The contribution of each participant in the backdrop of group dynamics should be recorded along with observational notes. Usually all the information including facial expressions and body language is recorded.
- *Analysis*: The recorded information should be transcribed into written verbatim while acknowledging the contribution of each participant. Observational notes also need to be depicted to make the transcript purposeful. The analysis of focus group data should also take account of the group dynamics that have generated the remarks.

Advantages
- The facilitator can observe and note nonverbal behavior, reactions and interactions of group members
- Misunderstanding can be clarified immediately

- Unanticipated but related topics can be explored and results of the interview are immediate
- In-depth information can be generated along with new ideas and creative concepts

Disadvantages
- Time consuming and expensive to conduct
- Requires a skillful facilitator and often the presence of two individuals—one to facilitate the discussion and the other to record observations and nonverbal behaviors
- The quality of data is influenced by the skills and motivation of the facilitator
- Focus groups may not elicit accurate information if the facilitator is inexperienced or introduces his or her bias into the discussion
- Recording of the group session may seem intrusive to participants and inhibit them from sharing their opinion freely

Differences between Questionnaire and Interview Schedule

In research surveys, questionnaire and interview schedule are the two commonly used methods for collecting data. The differences between questionnaire and interview schedule are presented in Table 8.6.

Table 8.6: Differences between questionnaire and interview schedule

Questionnaire	Interview schedule
Questionnaire refers to a technique of data collection which consists of a series of written questions along with alternative answers.	Schedule is a formalized set of questions, statements and spaces for answers provided to the data collectors who ask questions to the respondents and note down the answers.
Questionnaire is generally sent through mail along with a covering letter containing instructions to answer the same. However no further assistance is provided by the sender.	The schedule is usually filled by the data collector and clarification provided where necessary.
Data collection is economical as only the cost of printing and dispatching the questionnaire is involved.	Data collection is very expensive as money has to be spent on hiring and training the data collector and preparing the necessary schedules.
This method is employed only when the respondents are literate and cooperative.	This method can be employed for both literate and illiterate respondents.
If questionnaires are sent by mail or post personal contact is not possible.	Direct personal contact is established.
When the respondents are unable to comprehend the questions properly, the risk of receiving incomplete or inaccurate information is fairly high.	As the data collectors are present throughout the interview process any difficulties in comprehending the questions faced by the respondents can be resolved immediately. As the schedule is filled by data collectors, the chance of collecting incomplete information is remote.
The quality and physical appearance of questionnaire is one of the contributing factors in achieving a high response rate.	Honesty and competence of data collectors is a contributing factor in collecting complete information as per the schedule.
Non-response is usually high as most respondents do not respond or answer all questions.	Non-response is quite low as the schedule is filled by data collectors themselves who elicit answers to all questions.

OBSERVATION

Meaning

- Research observation deals with systematic selection, observation, and recording of physical characteristics, behaviors, events, and settings relevant to a problem under study.
- It is a deliberate process of concentration and attention on the subject that one wants to investigate further and analyze.

Under the observation method the information is recorded by way of investigators own direct observation. Data can be observed through senses with or without mechanical devices. In this process the observer receives the information passively through his senses, verifies this information actively through self-interrogation followed by validation and interpretation of his perception.

Observation is a two part process which includes the observer (one that is observing) and the observed (one that is being observed). Observation is based on four broad questions:

1. What is to be observed?
2. How to record the observation?
3. How to ensure accuracy of observation?
4. What relationship should exist between the observer and observed and how should such relationship be established?

A lot of information about individual characteristics, behavior, activities, skills, verbal and nonverbal communication and the environment can be gathered by direct observation. Conditions amenable for observation are presented in Table 8.7.

When to use Observation Method

Observation method is commonly used in behavioral sciences (psychology, nursing and medical setting) and social sciences (anthropology). This method is particularly well suited to nursing research. Several situations that require the nurses to use the observation method for data collection include behavior and characteristics of patients and their family members and hospital staff, etc.

1. *To understand an ongoing program or treatment:* An observational method, especially participant observation permits the researcher to evaluate the effectiveness of a program or treatment. For example, the researcher can evaluate the effectiveness of a program by observing how many people attended a program or patient progress after a specified treatment.
2. *To gather data on individual behaviors or interactions between people*: Through direct observation the researcher can observe behaviors and interactions of subjects and the outcome. For example, a nurse can observe the violent behavior of a patient and his interactions with other patients and its effect on ward environment.

Table 8.7: Conditions amenable for observation

Amenable conditions	Characteristics
Individual's characteristics	Physical, physiological conditions (rashes, alopecia, wound status, edema, etc.)
Activities and behavior	People's actions, roles, number of visits the patient made to the hospital, eating habits, aggressive behavior, etc.
Verbal and nonverbal communication	The content and structure of participant's conversation, emotions, facial expressions, gestures, body movement, etc.
Skills	Job performance, decision making, skill attainment in a particular procedure, etc.
Environmental characteristics	Noise level, safety measures, cleanliness, etc.

3. *To know about a physical setting*: Examining a physical set up where any activities or events are taking place can give the researcher a better understanding of the activity or event. For example, through observation the nurse can identify the environmental factors which are influencing violent behavior among agitated patients. These may be overcrowded wards, structured interventions in the ward, nurse interaction with the agitated patients and administration of medication and use of restraints, etc.
4. *Data collection by alternate methods is not feasible*: When respondents are incapable of giving verbal reports of their feelings (e.g. young children or mentally-ill people), are unaware of their own feelings (e.g. preoperative anxiety), are uncomfortable to report their activities (e.g. displays of aggressive behavior), are emotionally loaded (e.g. grieving behavior after the loss of a loved one).

Steps in Observation Process

The four steps in observation process are presented in Figure 8.12.

1. *Determine the area of focus*: The researcher determines what is to be observed and collected, i.e. observing specific situations, incidents, and activities for collecting the required data. For example, in an observational study to identify infant and nurse behaviors during the bathing process, the first step for the researcher will be to specify which behavior of the infant needs to be assessed, i.e. sudden movements, facial grimaces, grasping movement, etc.
2. *Design a system for data collection*: In this process the researcher specifies the operational definition for each variable chosen. The setting, subjects, list of interactions, processes or behaviors to be observed, timing, mode of observation, instruments to be used and recording method are to be specified. In this process the researcher also specifies recording sheets, field notes and checklists to be used for data collection. In the above example, the researcher should specify the number of infants that need to be observed, list of behavioral activities, duration of recording, and the use of mechanical devices like video tapes.
3. *Select observers and provide training*: The selection of observers' should be based on their levels of concentration, memory, and unobtrusive nature. The observer should be imparted both theoretical and practical training so as to enable collection of quality and consistent data.
4. *Implement observation*: The researcher should schedule the observations and ensure the functioning of the mechanical devices. The observation must cover an adequate number of representative case samples and be recorded accurately.

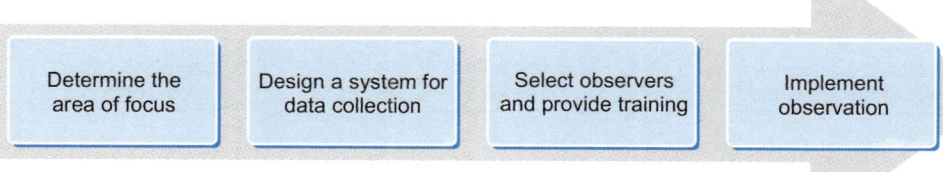

Fig. 8.12: Steps in observation process

Types of Observation Method

Observation may be classified in different ways depending upon the type of data being collected (Fig. 8.13).

Structured Observation

In this method the researcher describes what is to be observed and how the observations are to be made and recorded. For observations to be structured the researcher develops a category system for organizing and sorting the behaviors or incidents being observed. The structured observation is generally carried out using checklists and rating scales which are coded in the form of numbers (Box 8.2). This method indicates the presence or absence of prespecified behavior/attribute. Through this method more subjects can be observed in less time.

Rating scale is a device having questions to evaluate respondent's judgment or opinion along an ordered dimension. Rating questions are typically bipolar with the end points indicating opposite extremes on a continuum. The number of markings on the rating scale can differ but should necessarily be an odd number such as 3, 5 or 7 points. These are used to evaluate the attitudes, interests, personal characteristics, performance, and product outcomes. Rating scales can be graphic, descriptive or numerical in nature.

In graphic rating scale, the performance is printed horizontally at various points from lowest to highest. It is anchored by two extremes and presented to respondents or observed for evaluation of a concept or object. For example, a scale to measure the extent to which a staff nurse participates in a clinical conference (Fig. 8.14).

A descriptive rating scale divides the verbal or observed assessment into a series of verbal phrases to indicate the level of performance. For example, a scale to measure the amount of pain a person is having (Fig. 8.15).

A numeric rating scale divides the evaluation criteria into a fixed number of points and defines only numbers at the extremes. For example, a scale to measure the intensity of pain (Fig. 8.16).

Box 8.2	Tools used for structured observation

- *Rating scale*: It is a tool to assess or rate the performance of a task, skill level, quality of a trait or attribute of the participant based on predetermined criteria. Unlike a checklist it indicates the level of accomplishment rather than a simple yes or no.
- *Checklist*: It is a tool to recognize the presence or absence of behavior, conceptual knowledge or skills. The researcher observes, verifies, and marks whether the subject demonstrates them.

Advantages

- Rating scales compare different objects, people or things in a structured fashion
- Easy to construct, administer and score the measured attributes
- Requires little time for administration

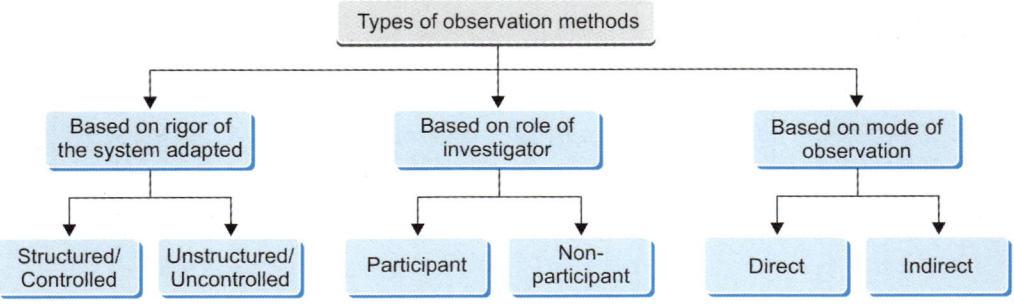

Fig. 8.13: Types of observation method

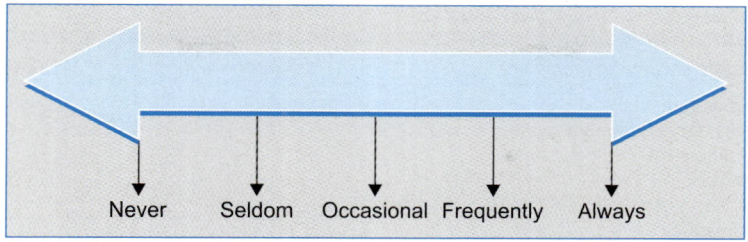

Fig. 8.14: Graphic rating scale

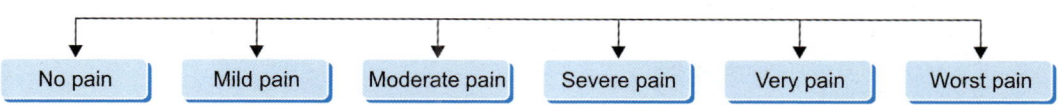

Fig. 8.15: Descriptive rating scale

- Easily used for large group and more flexible
- May also be used to evaluate skills, activities, attitudes, and personal characteristics

Disadvantages
- Chances of subjective evaluation
- Difficult to fix up rating for many aspects of an individual. Also some aspects of an individual cannot be rated.
- Chance that the rater may under or overestimate the qualities.

Checklist: A checklist contains list of items related to performance or characteristics which are evaluated by the researcher for their presence or absence. It is a two-column arrangement with one column containing a series of questions or task descriptions and the adjoining column providing the response alternatives to check off the task completion.

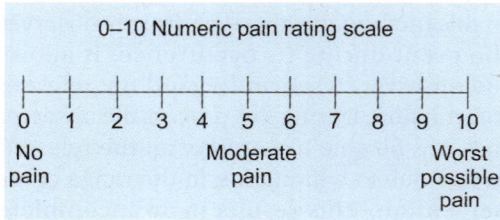

Fig. 8.16: Numeric pain rating scale

Where the questions are related to activities or behavior, the observer observes and records whether the particular behavior is present or not, the incident happened or not. It enables the observer to only note the presence or absence of a trait. Example of a checklist is presented in Table 8.8.

Advantages
- Easy to construct and use
- Efficient and easy for respondents to understand
- It allows interindividual comparisons
- Simple method to record observations
- Useful in evaluating learning activities, skills and particular behaviors

Disadvantages
- Provides limited information
- Through checklist quality of performance cannot be assessed (degree of accuracy of performance)

Unstructured Observation

It involves spontaneous observation and recording of what is seen in words. It is commonly used in qualitative studies. This method is carried out by using logs, field notes, anecdotes, and mechanical devices (Box 8.3). Unstructured observation provides rich and deep understanding of human

Table 8.8: Checklist to evaluate student's performance during surgical dressing		
Parameter/Steps in procedure	Yes (performed)	No (not performed)
1. Explains procedure 2. Collects necessary equipment 3. Arranges equipment 4. Prepares patient 5. Washes hands 6. Removes dressing 7. Observes condition of wound 8. Cleans wound 9. Follows aseptic techniques 10. Applies dressing 11. Removes equipment 12. Places patient in comfortable position 13. Records procedure 14. Care of equipment		

> **Box 8.3 Tools used for unstructured observation**
>
> - *Logs:* It is a record of events and conversation maintained on a daily basis.
> - *Field notes:* It is a means to document the continuous observation of participant's behavior, location or event for a certain length of time. The observer attempts to record factual data, description of setting, participant's behavior, conversations and actions including his own thoughts, ideas and concerns in context.
> - *Anecdotes:* It is a written record of a directly observed incident which is typically short, concise and nonjudgmental.
> - *Mechanical devices:* These are cameras, tape recorders, video tapes, microscopes, one way mirrors, closed circuit television, etc.

behavior. Observer bias, influence and memory distortions are limitations of this method.

Participant Observation

In this method the observer plays the role of an observer and a participant, where he is a part of the phenomenon or group. This method is commonly used by anthropologists. There are three types of participant observation: the *"observer as participant"* may undertake intermittent observation along with interviewing and their role is known; *"participant as observer"* undertakes prolonged observation and is involved in all the organization's activities and makes their role known (nonconcealed observation); *"complete participant"* role where the researcher interacts in the situation but their role is concealed (concealed observation). During participant observation unstructured tools are used to collect the data. Since he is a part of the phenomenon he can better understand the emotional responses and get a deeper insight of their experiences. However, if the observer participates emotionally, the objectivity is lost.

Non-participant observation

In this method the observer stands apart and does not participate in the event or phenomenon observed but simply views the situation. In this method subjects are not aware that they are being observed. This method possesses ethical problems as it involves observation of people without their consent.

Direct observation

In this method the observer directly observes the event during its occurrence. It allows the observer to see and record the relevant information. During this process the observer may not be able to perceive all the relevant events due to a limitation in the range of his perception. This results in an incomplete observation.

Indirect observation

In this method observer is not physically present and recording is done by mechanical devices which is a source of permanent record. This method is less biasing and is a source for analyzing various aspects of the incident. It is less flexible compared to direct observation.

Observation Sampling Techniques

Long periods of observation are tedious and generally associated with exhaustion and boredom. To overcome these difficulties, time sampling and event sampling methods are used.

Time sampling involves collection of data using specific time periods. The researcher randomly selects a place and time and then records what participants are doing when they are first seen and before they respond to the researcher's presence. For example, observation of ICU nurse activities for several minutes during an 8-hour shift. The time period can either be randomly selected or predetermined according to the daily routine of the ICU.

Event sampling includes selection of the particular event or activity. For example, observing the sterile technique during dressing procedure by a student nurse.

Validation of Observational Data

The data can be validated by inter-rater reliability and intrarater reliability. In an inter-rater reliability the observation is done by two observers/raters and there is 85% agreement between the two. In intrarater reliability same rater observes the same behavior/event on two or more occasions and compares the observations. It involves multiple observations extending over days and weeks.

Advantages of Observation Method

- Directness is the main feature of this method. It allows the study of human behavior especially when interventions are involved.
- It allows a view of complete situation first hand and includes sequence of events. It provides not only an in-depth but also a variety of information.
- All the data obtained by an observation are usable unlike in a questionnaire where irrelevant information may be included because respondents may misunderstand the questions posed to them.
- It is most open to use of recording devices such as tape-recorders and cameras.
- One can make use of assistants to carry out observations.
- Provides ample opportunity to recognize unexpected outcomes.
- Conducted in natural, unstructured, and flexible setting.

Disadvantages of Observation Method

- Observation and interpretation is a challenging and demanding task which requires the full attention and concentration of the observer.
- Lack of consent to being observed.
- Time and duration of an event cannot be predicted. Also the observer has to wait until the event actually takes place. Therefore it is difficult to know when to be present to observe key events.
- Behavior or set of behaviors observed may be atypical.
- Data obtained is vulnerable to many distortions and biases.
- Observed events are subjected to researcher's cultural background and personal interpretations.
- Use of recording devices is expensive.
- Extensive training is necessary if assistant observers are hired.
- Observers may get involved in a situation which can cause threat to the objectivity of the data collected.
- Rating scales are especially susceptible to various errors such as Halo effect, Hawthrone effect, error of leniency and error of severity.

- Halo effect: Tendency of the rater to be influenced by a single characteristic of the participant that impacts the evaluation of his specific traits. Overall impression of a person colors the observer's judgment of that person's character.
- Hawthrone effect: Tendency of the people to perform better when being observed. This can be overcome by indirect observation.
- Error of leniency: Tendency of the observer to rate everything positively.
- Error of severity: Tendency of the observer to rate too harshly.

ETHICS

Ethical implications involving the rights and willingness to be observed are a few concerns that need to be addressed while observing human beings. The three ethical requirements that need to be considered are: voluntary participation, freedom from physical or psychological harm and distress, and anonymity. Observation in the absence of participant's permission does not presume to be subject's voluntary participation. A sudden disclosure of being observed may result in distress and mental trauma to some participants. As it is difficult to maintain anonymity in an observation, it is appropriate to inform the participants that they will be observed even if they do not know the particulars of where and when.

BIOPHYSIOLOGICAL MEASURES

Presently many nurses are involving themselves in clinical and patient-centered research activities. This trend has led to the use of biophysiological measurements to assess the status of subject's biological and physiological variables.

Biophysiologic measurement involves the collection of biological and physiological data from the subjects and assigning a number or value to the individual's biological and physiological functioning. These measures can be used on an all alone basis or along with other methods. These variables require specialized equipment and trained personnel to measure and interpret the results. The measures can be:

- Directly observed (e.g. vomiting, delirium, edema, cyanosis and wound status can be observed for presence or absence and intensity)
- Self-reported (e.g. fatigue, pain, nausea, discomfort, dizziness, etc.)
- Directly measured (e.g. temperature, blood pressure, etc.)
- Indirectly measured (e.g. blood count, hormone levels, etc.)
- Electronically monitored (e.g. EEG, ECG, pulse oxymeter)
- Diagnostic tests (e.g. X-ray, CT scan, ultrasonography, etc.).

Characteristics of Biophysiological Measures

The biophysiological measures should be accurate, precise and sensitive and consistent (Fig. 8.17).

- Accurate: It refers to the proximity of a measured value to a standard or known value. For example, if a measured weight of a person is 50 kg, while his actual known weight is 50.2 kg, then the measurement is said to be accurate.

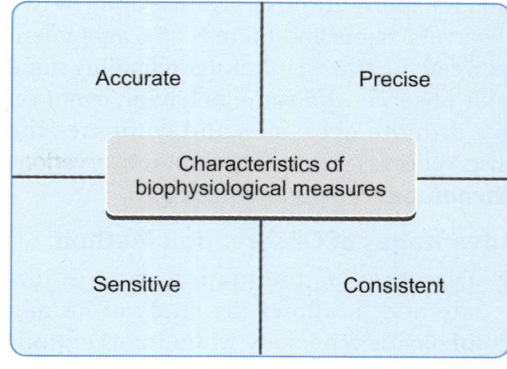

Fig. 8.17: Characteristics of biophysiological measures

- **Precise:** It refers to the nearness of two or more measurements to each other. In the above example, if the person is weighed multiple times and records 50 kg each time then the measurement is said to be very precise.
- **Sensitive:** It is the ability of the test to correctly identify those with the disease so as to provide valid measures for variables related to physical functions.
- **Consistent:** It refers to the data being collected from each participant in exactly the same way. For example, if the research involves measuring the temperature of all the study participants, the researcher should ensure that all temperatures were taken with the same type of instrument and in exactly the same way. An undesirable situation is one in which one data collector obtains temperature using an oral thermometer while another data collector obtains the temperature using an anal thermometer. The researcher's goal is to have minimal variability in the data collection procedure.

Types of Biophysiological Measures

Physiological measurements can be classified into, in vivo and in vitro. In-vivo measurements refer to those measurements that are carried out directly within or on living organisms themselves. Example: blood flow determination through radiography, cholecystography, angiogram, etc. An in-vitro measurement by contrast is carried outside the organism's body. Example: serum, Na^+, K^+, blood urea, X-ray, CT scan, bacterial count, etc. (Table 8.9).

Advantages
- Objectivity, precision and sensitivity are the major advantages of this measurement
- Provides exceptionally high quality data

Disadvantages
- Need for calibration of the equipment

Table 8.9: Commonly used biophysiological measures

Measurement	Example
Physical	Temperature, blood pressure
Chemical	Hormone levels, blood sugar, blood urea
Microbiological	Identification of organisms and their count
Anatomical and cytological	X-rays, tissue, biopsies, tomography, CT scan

- Some instruments are expensive and require significant amount of knowledge, training and experience
- Use of these measures may cause fear and anxiety among participants
- Some measures may have harmful effects on participants, e.g. repeated exposure to X-rays

PSYCHOLOGICAL MEASURES

Psychological measures mainly make use of psychological tests. These tests are designed to collect subjective information directly from subjects in order to measure a sample of certain aspects of human behavior. These tests yield objective and standardized descriptions of behavior which are quantified in numerical scores. Various scales are used to quantify the feelings, attitudes, and opinion of individuals.

Scales

Scales have been constructed to differentiate people based on their attitudes, fears, motives, perceptions, personality traits, and needs. Just as a thermometer is a scale that permits a quantitative differentiation between two different temperatures, a scale that measures attitudes attempts to distinguish between individuals who are more or less favorable towards some concept. Most scales measure psychosocial and physiological variables like attitudes, fears, motives, personality traits, pain, nausea or functional capacity.

Meaning

- Scaling is a method of changing attributes (a series of qualitative facts) into variables (a quantitative series).
- A scale is a device designed to assign a numerical score in order to place subjects along a continuum with respect to the attribute being measured.
- Scale is a self report measure that consists of a series of items designed to measure the attributes being investigated. The subject is presented with the items and responds to each item on the scale provided.
- Scales ask the respondents to rank some trait or ability on a continuum of possible responses. The individual entries on the scale correspond to variations in the strength of the response.

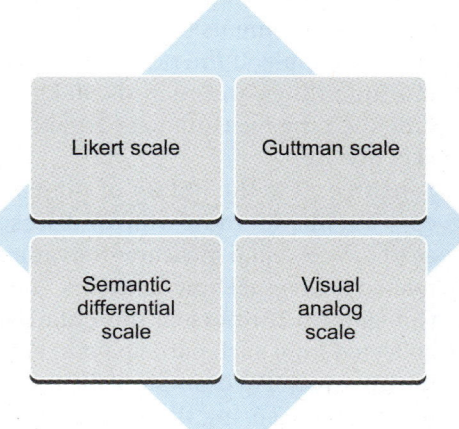

Fig. 8.18: Types of scales

Types of Scales

The most common types of scales are discussed here (Fig. 8.18).

Likert (summated) scale

It was originally developed by the psychologist Rensis Likert in 1932. It was designed to measure the opinion or attitude of a subject. It contains a number of declarative statements (some are positive and some negative) which express a viewpoint on a topic. Respondents are asked to express agreement or disagreement on a 5-point or 7-point scale. Each degree of agreement or disagreement is given a numeric value. Thus a total numeric value can be calculated from all the responses.

An example of 5-point Likert's scale to assess the educational stress among students is presented in Table 8.10.

Advantages

- Easy and takes less time to construct, fairly easy to interpret
- Highly reliable, adopted for measuring different kinds of attitudes
- Useful to measure attitudes before and after program

Table 8.10: Educational stress scale

[Kindly read the following sentences and indicate "√ mark" against the item (1–5) found most suitable. 1—indicates strongly disagree (SD), 2—indicates disagree (D), 3—indicates uncertain (U), 4—indicates agree (A) and 5—indicates strongly agree (SA)]

Sl. No.	Items	1 (SD)	2 (D)	3 (U)	4 (A)	5 (SA)
1.	I feel a lot of pressure in my daily studying					
2.	There is too much competition among classmates which brings me a lot of academic pressure					
3.	Future education and employment brings me a lot of academic pressure					
4.	My parents care about my academic grades too much which brings me a lot of pressure					

- Frequently used for opinion research
- Easy to administer since respondents only have to tick in space provided against each statement.

Disadvantages
- Cannot tell how much more or less respondents are favorable to a topic
- No basis for the assumption that five points are at equal distance on the scale
- Yields ordinal data which can lead to several limitations in subsequent analysis, e.g. use of statistical techniques that do not rely on arithmetic mean.

Guttman (cumulative) scale
Guttman scale is a set of items on a continuum or statement ranging from one extreme to another. It was developed by Louis Guttman in 1944. The purpose of Guttman scaling is to establish a one-dimensional continuum for a concept we wish to measure. This scale follows a cumulative hierarchy, i.e. if a person agreed to the fourth item, then it indicates that he agrees to the first three items too. Each item on the scale is worth a point and the total score is cumulative. So if a respondent's score is five, it means that the respondent is in agreement with all the statements from 1 through 5. In other words the responses are progressive and cumulative.

Example
1. A nursing research course at the undergraduate level should be available to students.
2. Students would very likely benefit from taking an undergraduate nursing research course.
3. A nursing research course would be in the best interest of undergraduate students.
4. A course in nursing research should be mandatory for all undergraduate nursing students.

Advantages
- Does not allow subjective judgment of researcher
- Easy to administer as it requires few items
- Possible to use in personal, telephone or a mail survey

Disadvantages
- Not reliable to assess attitude towards complex objects
- Construction is tedious and complex and requires lot of time and effort

Semantic differential scale
Semantic differential (SD) scale is a type of graphic rating scale designed to measure the connotative meaning of objects, events, and concepts. These connotations are used to derive the respondent's attitude towards the given objects, events or concepts. It was developed by Osgood, Suci and Tannenbaum in 1957.

The scale consists of bipolar rating with appropriate adjectives (such as good, bad; important, unimportant; strong, weak; beautiful, ugly; and so forth) representing extreme points and in between categories having blank space or numbers on a 7 point scale. The scale is assigned a score from 1 to 7. The respondent is asked to rate the given concept on a series of bipolar rating scales.

Example: Nurse Practitioner
Kind __ __ __ __ __ __ __ Cruel
Biased __ __ __ __ __ __ __ Unbiased
Patient __ __ __ __ __ __ __ Impatient
Pleasant __ __ __ __ __ __ __ Unpleasant
Serious __ __ __ __ __ __ __ Friendly
Passive __ __ __ __ __ __ __ Active

Advantages
- Highly flexible and easy to construct
- Any concept can be rated, related to person, place, situation and abstract ideas
- Concept can be a single word, a phrase or a sentence
- Produce large quantity of information with relatively little effort
- Attitudes are measured both in direction and intensity

Disadvantages
- Only useful for questions involving bipolar opposites

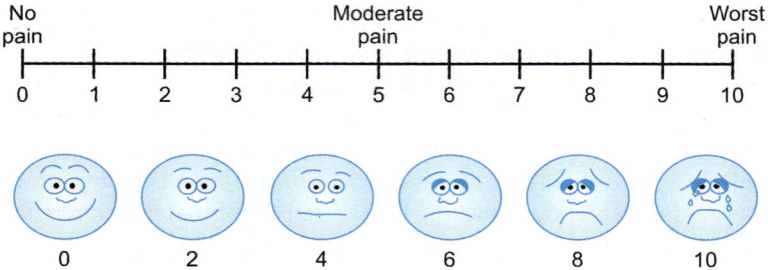

Fig. 8.19: Visual analog pain scale

* Clear instructions and examples are necessary, otherwise it can be confusing to respondents

Visual analog scale

The visual analog scale (VAS) is one of the most commonly used scales in healthcare for measuring perceptual measures such as pain, anxiety, fatigue, shortness of breath or nausea. It is a self-report measure consisting of a 10 cm (100 mm) line with a statement at each end representing one extreme of the dimension being measured. Example: "no pain" at one end and "worst pain" at the other end. Subjects are asked to mark a point on the line indicating the severity of the phenomenon experienced at that time. The intensity of the phenomenon is scored by measuring the millimeters from the low end of the scale to the subjects mark. The scale is uni-dimensional, quantifying intensity only (Fig. 8.19).

Advantages
* Easy to administer
* It is a reliable and valid measure for assessing subjective patient experiences
* Simple for participants to understand
* Language is uncomplicated
* Takes little time to complete

Disadvantages
* Cannot be used for visual impairment patients
* Psychomotor disability patients may find it difficult to mark on the line

Measurement of Personality

Personality is the individual's disposition to act to its environment/situation. Personality includes attitudes and other non-intellectual aspects of behavior such as values, motives, and interests. Personality is measured by personality inventories, projective techniques, vignettes, and Q-sort procedures (Fig. 8.20).

Personality Inventory

In an inventory the respondents are typically presented with a number of descriptive statements which they rate as either characteristic or uncharacteristic of them. Example: A tense individual is likely to score yes/agree to a statement like "I often worry about what the future holds for me." The individuals score is usually calculated by

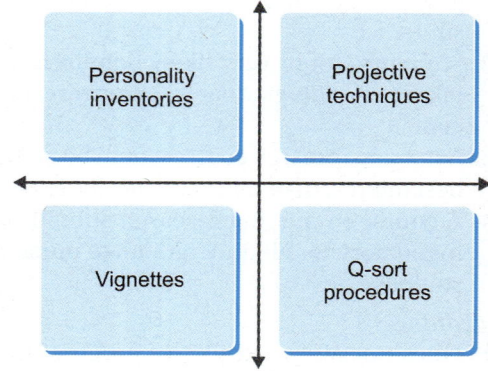

Fig. 8.20: Measurement of personality

summing the number of affirmative responses. Examples for personality inventories are California Psychological Inventory, Sixteen personality factor questionnaire, Minnesota Multiphasic Personality Inventory (MMPT), IPAT Anxiety Scale/Self Concept Scale, etc.

Projective Techniques

Projective techniques are methods for measuring psychological attributes like values, attitudes, and personality. These are based on the principle that responses to unstructured stimuli reveal a subject's underlying motives, attitudes, fears, and aspirations. In projective tests the subjects are presented with unstructured, vague, ambiguous stimuli in the form of objects or situations which permit a range of interpretations by the subject. The subject's interpretation of the task "projects" his or her personality, opinions, emotions, and desires enabling the investigator to understand the finer aspects of his or her personality. These techniques are more useful in the case of children, adolescents, low literates, and people in the face of natural disasters.

The most commonly used projective techniques are:
- Pictorial Projective Device: Rorschach Inkblot Test, Thematic Apperception Test (TAT) (Figs. 8.21A and B).
- Verbal Projective Techniques: Word Association Method, Sentence Completion Techniques
- Expressive methods: Play techniques, role playing

Vignettes

In order to explore people's believes, perceptions and meanings of certain situations, vignettes act as a valuable technique. These involve brief description of events or situations to which subjects are asked to react. Descriptions can be either fictitious or factual and used to elicit subjects perceptions, opinions or knowledge about certain phenomenon under study. Vignettes are mostly presented in written form but videotapes or audiotapes are also used. Questions posed to subjects after the exposure to vignettes may be open ended or closed. The number of vignettes included in a study usually ranges from 4 to 10.

Example: Mr. B is a 48-year-old male having a B.A. degree, diagnosed with chronic schizophrenia. You find him lying on the bed, refusing to follow instructions and participate in any ward activities. He refuses to take bath and opposes every instruction.

1. Which of the following is most effective in getting a patient to take bath?
    a. Associate bathing with occurrence of positive reward

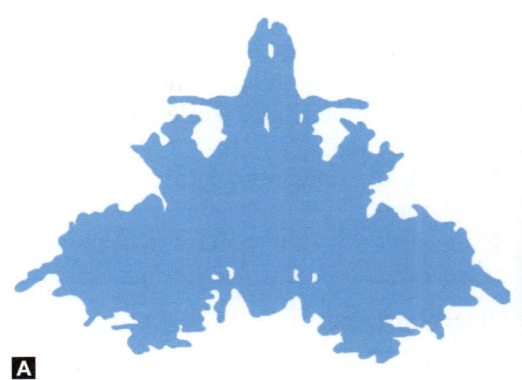
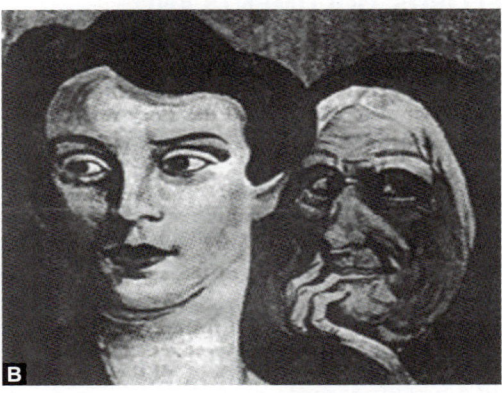

Figs. 8.21A and B: Pictorial projective device. (A) A Sample picture from Rorschach Inkblot Test and (B) Thematic apperception test

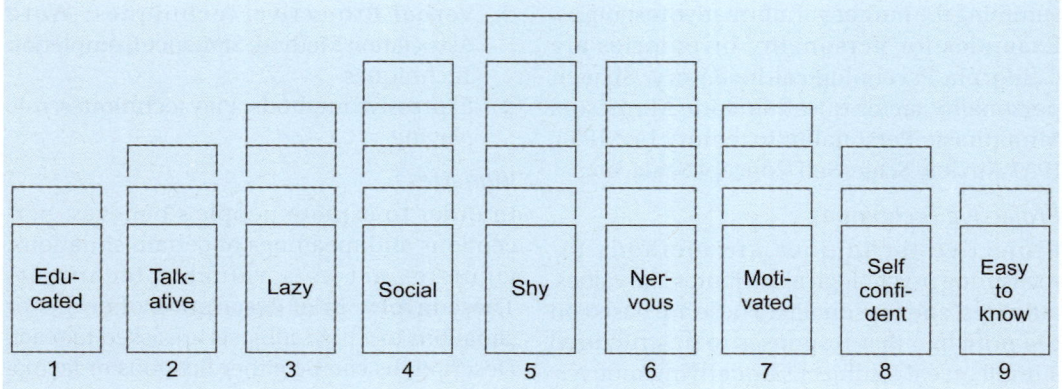

Fig. 8.22: Example of a Q-sort

b. Punish him for refusal to take bath
c. Persuade by gentle words to take bath
d. Explain to the patient how to take bath

Q-Sort Procedures

In a Q-sort measurement the participants are provided a set of cards with words, statements or other messages written on them. Participants are asked to sort the cards along a particular dimension such as approve or disapprove, most likely or least likely or highest priority or lowest priority. An analysis of this sorting helps the researcher to get an insight into the attitude and personality of the participant (Fig. 8.22).

RECORDS, DOCUMENTS AND AVAILABLE DATA

Records are a compilation of writings and figures that individuals have collected. These are a valuable and beneficial source for nursing research data. Nurse researchers can find records in hospitals (care plans, patient charts, shift reports, physician orders and other medical records), educational institutions (student's records, health records, academic records, etc.) and Government organizations (birth and death records, census, morbidity and mortality records, etc.)

Narrative documents in addition to quantified institutional records serve as a potential data source for qualitative researchers. These include personal documents such as diaries and letters, organizational policy statements, etc.

Advantages

- More economical
- By collecting information repeatedly from pre-existing records researcher can study trends over time
- Records available in their pure form that are compiled in a neat and orderly fashion save a lot of time during the data collection process
- Researcher cannot introduce bias in the data collection process as the records have already been collected
- Existence of large quantity of information in the records gives the researcher a considerable choice while culling out the data
- Data are obtained by an unobtrusive method
- Records do not rely on recall as they were recorded as and when they occurred

Disadvantages

- Amount of information in the records is limited to what is available as the subjects are not present. If a record is incomplete there is no way to complete it

❖ No one is sure under which conditions the data were collected
❖ There is no assurance of accuracy of the records
❖ Search for very old records and extracting information from them may be very time consuming
❖ Requesting people who are not involved in the research work to provide records may be an intrusion into their work schedule

Problems

❖ Permission to access records has to be sought from concerned authorities
❖ Difficult to trace if not kept in a well organized manner.
❖ Authorities/concerned people/officers may not like their records to be disturbed for the fear of misplacement or loss of documents.
❖ Organization/institution may not prefer anyone other than the selected individuals to go through their private files.
❖ While retrieving information anonymity, privacy, truth and accuracy have to be taken care of.

VALIDITY AND RELIABILITY OF THE MEASURING INSTRUMENT

Measurement is the assigning of numbers to the characteristic of an object or event in order to quantify the phenomena. In nursing, many of these phenomena such as quality of life, wellbeing of the patient, adherence to medication, symptom experience and care effectiveness are abstract concepts. Measurement involves the operationalization of these concepts/variables, application of instruments or tests to quantify these variables. For example, wellbeing may be operationalized as subjective feelings of contentment, happiness, satisfaction with life's experiences and of one's role in the world of work, sense of achievement, belongingness and no distress or worry. The wellbeing is assessed using wellbeing inventory.

A good instrument is essential if research results are to be useful. The usefulness of the data collection instruments depends on the extent to which researchers can rely on data as accurate and meaningful. Assessing quality of an instrument is done by evaluating the properties of reliability and validity in relation to the instrument being used. This process is called psychometric evaluation.

Characteristics of Research Tool

An ideal measuring instrument is one which results in relevant, accurate, objective, sensitive, and efficient measures. Physiological or physical measurements have a greater chance of having these characteristics than psychological measurements. Scales developed to measure these psychological variables are often imperfect and error prone. A number of techniques are available to evaluate the quality of these measuring tools to minimize error. These techniques estimate reliability, validity, objectivity, sensitivity, specificity, and appropriateness. Thus if the measuring tools are reliable, valid, objective, sensitive, specific and appropriate it will improve accuracy and enhance scientific quality of the research (Fig. 8.23).

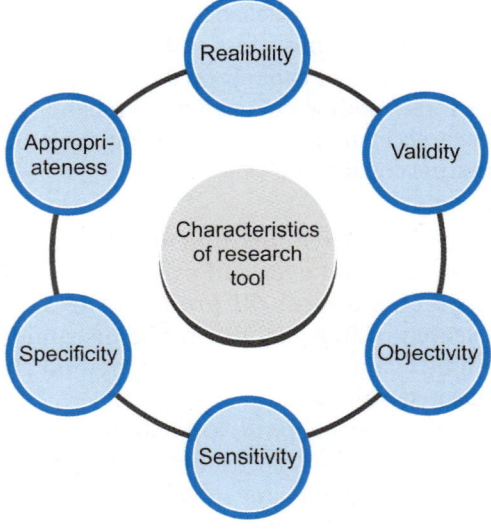

Fig. 8.23: Characteristics of a research tool

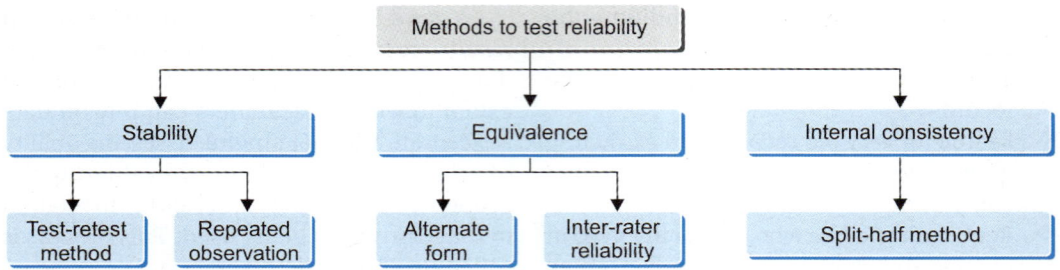

Fig. 8.24: Methods to test reliability

Reliability

At the heart of all measurements is reliability. It is the degree to which an assessment tool produces stable and consistent results. Instruments are considered reliable if they consistently measure a given trait with precision, i.e. the degree of reproducibility or the generation of consistent values every time an instrument is used.

Meaning
- Reliability refers to the consistency with which an instrument or test measures what it is supposed to measure.
- Reliability is the extent to which a measurement or instrument or test yields the same results on repeated administration.

Methods of Testing Reliability

The more reliable a test or instrument, the more researcher can rely on the scores. There are three methods of testing the reliability of research instrument: Stability, equivalence, internal consistency (Fig. 8.24).

Stability

A stable research instrument is one which when repeated over and over on the same research subject will produce the same research results. Stability of the instrument can be evaluated by test-retest method and repeated observations.

  a. *Test-retest method*: Repeated measurements over time using the same instrument on same subjects is expected to produce the same results. In this method the researcher administers the same test twice over a period of time to a group of individuals. The scores from time 1 and time 2 can then be correlated in order to evaluate the stability of the test. If the test or instrument is reliable, individual scores will be very similar at both tests (Fig. 8.25). For example, a test is developed to measure the knowledge of psychopharmacology among nursing students. The test is given to a group of nursing students and repeated 2 weeks later. Assuming that the students have had no additional classes regarding the topic during the 2-week period between the tests, results from the first testing can be correlated with the second testing. The obtained correlated coefficient would indicate the stability of the test. Karl Pearson's correlation coefficient is used to estimate reliability. Reliability coefficient ranges from 0.00 to

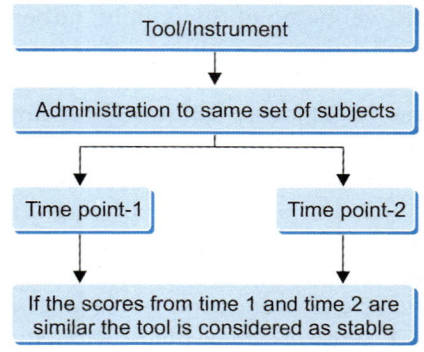

Fig. 8.25: Assessing stability of the instrument

1.00 with higher coefficients indicating higher levels of reliability. A completely reliable test has a reliability coefficient of 1.00 and a completely unreliable test has a reliability coefficient 0.00. A score above 0.80 indicates an acceptable level of reliability of the tool.
- A concern with this type of reliability is how to determine the amount of time that should elapse between the two testings. Knapp and Brown say that test-retest reliabilities are generally higher when the time lapse between the testing is short, usually no longer than 4 weeks. If the intervals are too short, memory of the responses given during the first session may influence responses during the second session.
- A reliable questionnaire will give consistent results overtime. If the results are not consistent the test is not considered reliable and will need to be revised until it does measure consistently.
- Test retest is used primarily with questionnaires but the concept of repeated measurement to establish stability can also be used with tools like thermometer and hemodynamic monitors and in instances where the variable being measured is not expected to fluctuate.
- The main limitation is that the test for stability can be performed only when the measuring trait remains constant over time. An example for a stable concept is intelligence. It should be possible to measure intelligence repeatedly at regular intervals and obtain the same score. An unstable concept such as pain is changeable and subject to frequent fluctuations even for a person with chronic pain. Repeated measures of pain in a subject would result in widely different scores. These differences would not mean that the instrument is unstable but rather that the individual's pain was changing (variable being measured was changing).

b. *Repeated observations*: When using observational methods of data collection the test of stability of the instrument is called repeated observation. The measurement of the variable is repeated overtime and the results at each measurement time are expected to be very similar. For example, if the researcher develops an observational scale to rate the nurse's behavior during the process of counting narcotics 3 days in a row, it would have similar rating each day. If the ratings are different each day, question arises regarding the reliability of rating, whether or not the trait or character being measured is stable and whether or not the observation is done the same way every day, i.e. whether or not the observer is consistent (Fig. 8.26).

Equivalence
When the variable being measured is not a stable one the reliability of an instrument cannot be tested by repeated measures. Test of equivalence attempts to determine if similar tests administered at the same time yield the same results or if different observers, observing same phenomena at the same time report similar results.

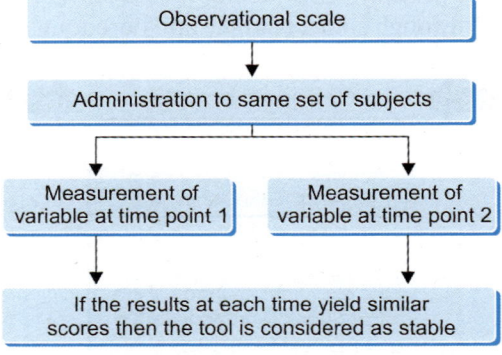

Fig. 8.26: Assessing stability of the observation scale

Equivalence is based on the idea of using alternate forms of measurement of the same trait at the same time and comparing the results. Test of equivalence are of two categories: Alternate form and inter-rater reliability.

a. *Alternate form:* The test of equivalence using alternate forms of paper and pencil tests consisting of two sets of similar questions designed to measure the same trait is called alternate form testing. The two tests are based on similar content but the individual items are different. When these two tests are administered to subjects at the same time, the results can be compared just as in test/retest method. Obtaining similar results on the two alternate forms of the instrument gives support for the reliability of both forms of the instrument. For example, the instructor develops two tests with the same content but different questions are administered to same subjects. If one student were to take two forms of the test, the result should reflect the same level of knowledge if the tests are reliable (Fig. 8.27).

The major problem with alternate form of questions is that they tend to be boring for the subject. When the questionnaire and interview is very long the addition of another questionnaire with the same length may be too tiring for the subjects. This may introduce new source of error through subject fatigue and boredom.

b. *Inter-rater reliability (interobserver agreement):* If a measurement process involves rating by observers, a reliable measurement will require consistency between different ratings. It is used to determine whether two observers using the same instrument at the same time will obtain similar results. A reliable instrument should produce the same results if both observers are using it the same way. Inter-rater reliability requires completely independent ratings of the same event by more than one rater. No discussion or collaboration can occur when reliability is being tested. Reliability is determined by the correlation of the scores from two or more independent raters. Inter-rater reliability is often assessed using Cronbach's α when the judgments are quantitative or Cohen's Kappa when judgments are categorical. For example, in an observational tool designed to measure the assertiveness of an individual, two researchers observe the interaction together and rate the assertiveness of the subjects using the same scale separately. These ratings are then compared for equivalence. The extent to which they agree serves as a measure of the reliability of the tool. This method is also useful to test the reliability of interpreting the physiological tools. For example, to test the inter-rater reliability of a blood pressure reading, a double stethoscope is used which enables two people to listen and agree on blood pressure reading at the same time (Fig. 8.28).

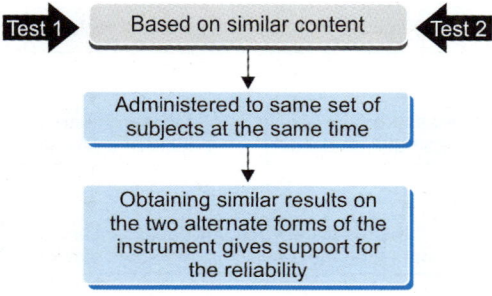

Fig. 8.27: Assessing equivalence of the instrument

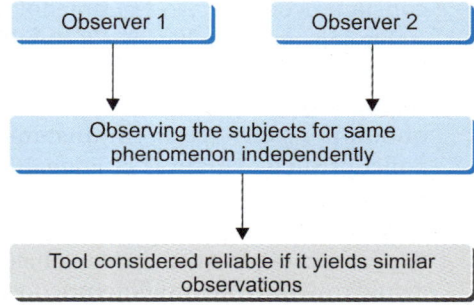

Fig. 8.28: Assessing inter-rater reliability

Internal consistency or scale homogeneity

Internal consistency refers to the extent to which all parts of the measurement technique are measuring the same concept. It gives an estimate of the equivalence of set of items from the same test. It is based on the assumption that items measuring the same construct or concept should correlate. For example, in a questionnaire to measure depression each question should provide a measure of depression consistent with the overall results of the test. In laboratory tests this concept includes the idea that the results obtained from counting the red blood cells in one drop of blood from a specimen should be the same as though obtained from another drop of blood from the same specimen. To ensure internal consistency, all the questions in the structured questionnaire should be able to measure a single trait or characteristic or phenomena contributing to the overall measure of the concept.

- If the variable being measured is a changeable one, test-retest method cannot be used. If alternate form of questions is not possible because the length of the questionnaires would prohibit asking the subjects to complete two at the same time then equivalence is not an option. Only internal consistency will provide useful measure of reliability in these cases.
- Split half correlation is used to test the internal consistency in which the items on the instrument are divided into two halves, and the correlation between the scores on the two parts is computed. The halves may be divided by obtaining the scores on the first half of the test and comparing them with the scores on the second half of the test or by comparing odd numbered items with even-numbered items. If all the items are consistently measuring the overall concept then the scores on the two halves of the test should be correlated (Fig. 8.29).
- To get a good measure of reliability, the test is divided into two halves in an unbiased manner and Cronbach's alpha coefficient calculated to establish internal consistency (when items of an instrument are scored on summated scales like Likert-type scale such as quality of life instrument, depression scale, etc.).
- Another statistical procedure used to assess internal consistency is Kuder–Richardson 20 when the items of an instrument are scored dichotomously. Example: 1 = yes, 0 = no.
- Internal consistency is a useful device for establishing reliability in a highly structured quantitative data collection instrument. It is not useful in open-ended questionnaires or interviews, unstructured observations, projective tests or other qualitative data collection methods and instruments.

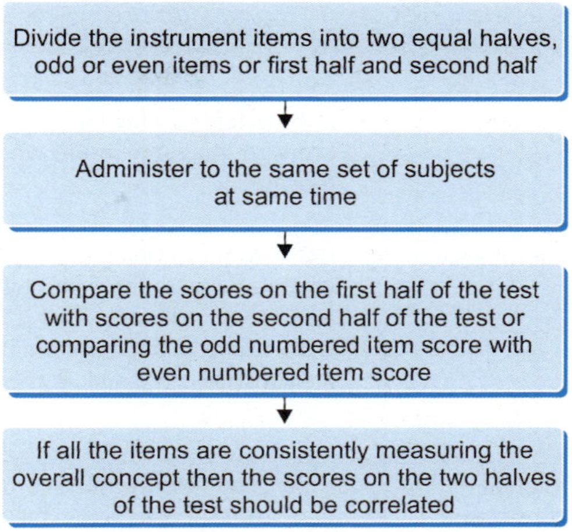

A brief summary of methods of testing reliability is presented in Table 8.11.

Fig. 8.29: Assessing internal consistency

Flowchart:
1. Divide the instrument items into two equal halves, odd or even items or first half and second half
2. Administer to the same set of subjects at same time
3. Compare the scores on the first half of the test with scores on the second half of the test or comparing the odd numbered item score with even numbered item score
4. If all the items are consistently measuring the overall concept then the scores on the two halves of the test should be correlated

Validity

Validity is the second important criterion for evaluating a quantitative instrument. It is defined as the extent to which a concept is accurately measured. It also refers to the degree or extent to which an instrument measures what it is supposed to measure.

Table 8.11: Methods of testing reliability		
Method	Meaning	Evaluation
Stability	• Is the extent to which the measure produces the same results when used repeatedly	How stable is it over time? Determined by: • Test-retest method • Repeated observation method
Equivalence	• Is the extent to which the measure produces consistent results by similar tests • Is the extent to which different observers are consistent in their judgments	How consistent are the results by similar tests? How consistent are observers in their judgments? Determined by: • Alternate form • Inter-rater reliability
Internal consistency	• Is the extent to which the consistency of people's responses across the items on a multiple-item measure	How consistent are people's responses across the items? Determined by: • Split-half method

Reliability and validity are not independent qualities of an instrument. Although validity is an important characteristic of an instrument, reliability is necessary before validity can be considered. An instrument that is not reliable cannot be valid. However, an instrument can be reliable without being valid. A few examples which underline the concepts of reliability and validity are:

❖ An alarm clock which rings at 6 am while it is actually set for 5.30 am. Here the clock is very reliable as it regularly rings at the same time every morning, i.e. 6 am. However, it is not valid as it is not ringing at the preferred time, i.e. 5.30 am. In the said scenario if the clock rings at various times every morning then it is not considered reliable too.

❖ A researcher constructed a multiple choice questionnaire to assess the drug knowledge among nursing students. It is found that the questionnaire was yielding same scores when it was repeatedly administered. However, it was found to be assessing the arithmetic skills instead of the drug knowledge. Though this questionnaire is reliable it is not valid.

❖ An instrument may consistently measure anxiety each time the instrument is administered. However, if the concept to be measured is depression, the instrument is not considered valid.

The accuracy and meaningfulness of the data depend on validity and reliability of the instrument. While high reliability of an instrument provides no evidence of its validity; low reliability of a measurement is evidence of low validity. It is essential to consider validity and reliability of the data collection instrument while conducting or critiquing research.

Types of validity

There are three major types of validity—content, construct and criterion-related validity (Fig. 8.30).

Content validity

Content validity involves a subjective judgment about whether a measurement makes sense or not.

❖ It is the extent to which an instrument has an appropriate sample of items for the construct being measured.

❖ It is the extent to which an instrument adequately covers all the contents with respect to the variable being measured.

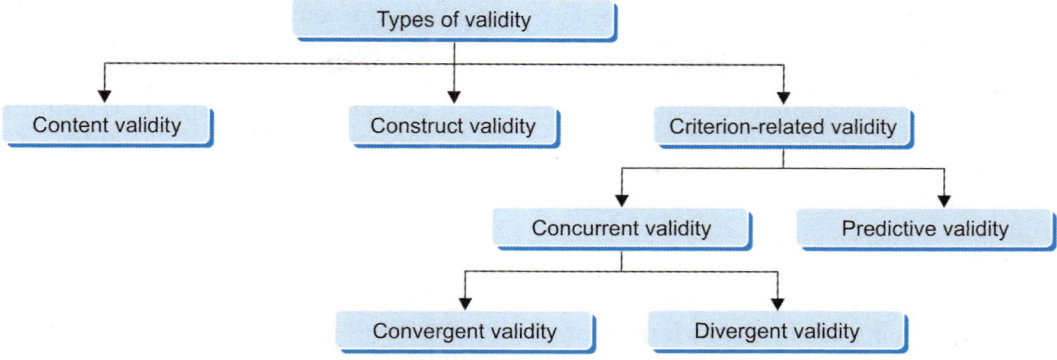

Fig. 8.30: Types of validity

- A subset of content validity is face validity. It is the extent to which an instrument measures the concept intended.
- Usually content validity is used in the development of a questionnaire or interview schedule. For example, in an undergraduate nursing course with nursing research as one of its subjects, the questionnaire with content validity would cover the entire course content with greater focus on themes or topics that have been dealt with at more depth.
- One of the ways to ensure adequacy of content coverage of an instrument is through a panel of experts. The panel is comprised of at least three experts, the number of which may increase if the construct is complex. The panel of experts evaluates each item of the questionnaire for relevance and appropriateness on a five-point scale (from 1 = not relevant to 5 = very relevant) in respect to all dimensions of the construct being measured. Based on their evaluation content validity is calculated.

Construct validity
Construct validity is the extent to which an instrument measures an intended concept or construct.
- What is this instrument really measuring? Does it adequately measure the abstract concept of interest?
- Construct validity refers to whether the researcher can draw inferences about test scores related to the concept being studied. For example, if a student scores high on a survey that measures depression, does this student actually have a high degree of depression?
- Construct validity is useful mainly for measures of feelings or traits such as grief, quality of life; satisfaction, etc. Through construct validity theoretical base for the concept is tested.
- Construct validity can be determined using known group technique and multitrait-multimethod approach.
  ○ In the known group approach, the instrument is administered to two different groups which are expected to differ on the concept. For example, if quality of life questionnaire is administered to two different groups viz., chronic ill patients and healthy individuals, it would be expected that the healthy individuals would score higher on quality of life when compared to the chronic ill patients. Correlations that fit the expected pattern contribute to evidence of construct validity.
  ○ In the multitrait-multimethod approach the researcher measures the concept

by using two or more methods. For example, anxiety concept can be measured by self-report method and observational checklist. If high correlation exists between the tools measuring the same construct then it substantiates good construct validity.

Criterion-related validity

Criterion-related validity involves determining the relationship of an instrument to some criterion. It is the extent to which the scores on the new measure correlate with other measures of the same concept. Correlations can be conducted to determine the extent to which the different instruments measure the same variable. For example, if the researcher developed a tool to measure the professionalism scores among nurses, it would be valid if the scores correlated with alternative criterion such as number of research articles published, conferences attended and papers presented. It assesses the ability of the instrument to determine a subject's response at the present time or predict a subject's response in the future.

The two types of criterion related validity measures are *concurrent validity* and *predictive validity*.

- ❖ Concurrent validity refers to the degree of correlation of two measures of the same concept administered at the same time. For example, if a researcher developed a behavioral checklist to measure nurse's job satisfaction, to validate this test the researcher would need to compare it with the results of a standardized job satisfaction instrument shown to be valid for nurses. A high correlation between the results of the two tests would indicate concurrent validity for the checklist. It can be measured in the following two ways:
  - ○ *Convergent validity:* It shows a high correlation among instruments measuring similar variables. For example, there should be a high correlation between an instrument that measures aptitude and one that measures performance.
  - ○ *Divergent validity:* It shows a poor correlation among instruments measuring different variables. For example, there should be a low correlation between an instrument that measures motivation and one that measures hopelessness.
- ❖ Predictive validity refers to the adequacy of an instrument in predicting performance or behavior of individuals at some point in future. It is the degree of correlation between the present scores of a concept with future performance. Differently put it is a judgment of the degree to which an instrument can accurately forecast the future. For example, how well do the entrance test scores predict the future performance of the student? This can be done by correlating the entrance test scores with achievements in subsequent years, i.e. 1st, 2nd, 3rd and 4th year test scores. In another example, a score on high efficiency related to performing a task should predict the likelihood of a participant completing the task.

The difference between predictive and concurrent validity is the difference in the timing of obtaining measurements on a criterion. The brief summary of types of validity is presented in Table 8.12.

Objectivity

Objectivity means the yielding of a correct test score independent of personal judgment or bias.

Sensitivity

Sensitivity and specificity are measures of validity used in biomedical sciences because they measure characteristics of diagnostic tools used to detect disease. Sensitivity is the capacity of an instrument to detect disease if it is present. Instrument sensitivity is its rate of yielding "true positives" which helps the researcher avoid false negatives. For example,

Table 8.12: Brief summary of types of validity

Types of validity	Meaning	Evaluation
Content validity	The extent to which a research instrument accurately measures all aspects of a construct	Is the domain adequately covered? • Determined by panel of experts
Construct validity	The extent to which a research instrument measures the intended construct	Does it conform to existing theory? • Determined by multitrait-multimethod approach
Criterion related validity	The extent to which a research instrument is related to other instruments that measure the same variable	Does it measure what it is supposed to measure? • Determined by comparing against a gold standard
Concurrent validity	It refers to the degree of correlation of two measures of the same concept administered at the same time	Does it highly correlate with instruments measuring similar variables? • Determined by comparing with similar standard tool
Predictive validity	The adequacy of an instrument in predicting performance or behavior of individuals on some future criteria	Does it accurately forecast the future? • Determined by measuring the criterion at some point in the future

a diagnostic tool such as a mammography must be sensitive enough to detect breast cancer if it is present.

Specificity

Specificity is the capacity of an instrument to differentiate when the disease is not present. A diagnostic tool is specific if it can definitively conclude that the disease is not present when it is not. Instrument specificity is its rate of yielding "true negatives" which helps the researcher avoid false positives.

Both sensitivity and specificity are needed to be confident that results accurately represent the distribution of the disease in the sample (Dawson and Trapp, 2004).

Appropriateness

Appropriateness is the degree to which an instrument is suitable to a particular subject, position or event. It also refers to the extent to which the study subjects can meet the demands of the instrument such as understanding the questions and directions, possess strength and motivation to complete the instrument. Other characteristics are:

❖ Economy (test should take short period of time to complete and be less expensive)
❖ Practicability (simplicity of administration, scoring and interpretation) refers to how suitable the instrument is for a particular individual.

ITEM ANALYSIS

An item is a single question on a test or questionnaire or a single statement on a scale. Item analysis is an integral part of test development and deals with the process of determining the effectiveness of each test item by analyzing the sample's response to the item.

Purposes of Item Analysis

❖ To observe the characteristics of a particular question and ensure appropriateness of each item
❖ To select items for test inclusion
❖ To differentiate difficult items from easy items
❖ To know the effectiveness of distracters

- To identify how well the item discriminates between high and low achievers
- To help identify poor quality questions that were too difficult for the subjects or sample

Steps in Item Analysis
- Frame items
- Assign score for each item
- Rank the answer papers in order from the highest to the lowest score
- Divide these papers approximately one-third into three groups
   - The top scores one-third according to the rank
   - The low scores one-third according to the rank
   - The middle scores one-third according to the rank
- Estimate difficulty of each item (percentage of people who got the item right)
- Estimate the discriminating power of each item. This is the difference between the number of samples in the upper and lower groups who got the item right. Discrimination refers to how well the question separates participants of similar abilities.
- Evaluate the effectiveness of distracters in each item.

Calculation of Item Analysis

Let us suppose that we have corrected 40 papers of a test. Rank the papers in order from the highest to the lowest score. Select the 13 papers with the highest score and 13 papers with lowest score. For each test item tabulate the number of subjects in the upper and lower groups who selected each alternative. Estimate difficulty and discrimination indices.

Estimation of Difficulty Index

It is estimated by calculating number of subjects who answered correctly divided by the total number of persons responding to them. Item difficulty of a test is indicated by the percentage of subjects who got the item right. Difficulty index (D) = (R/t) × 100 where "R" is the number of subjects who got the item right and "t" is the number of subjects who tried the item.

Another formula to estimate difficulty index (D) = [(H+L)/N] × 100
where,
H—correct responses in the higher group
L—correct responses in the lower group
N—total number of subjects

For example, out of a total 30 subjects, if a question is answered correctly by 15 higher group subjects and 5 lower group subjects the difficulty index would be calculated as follows:

Difficulty index = [(15+5)/30] × 100 = 66.7

If the value of difficulty index is between 30 and 70 then the question is accepted. The higher the value the better the item and easier the question.

Estimation of Discrimination Index

This index shows how significantly a question discriminates between high score and low score students. It varies from –1 to +1.
Discrimination Index

$$D = \frac{2(H-L)}{N} = \frac{2(15-5)}{30} = \frac{2 \times 10}{30} = 0.67$$

If the value is "zero" it can be concluded that there is no discrimination and that either the question is too easy that all have answered it or it is too difficult that nobody could answer it. Higher the index the more a question will distinguish between high score and low score students. Guilbert suggested the following index to judge the questions.
- 0.35 and above—excellent question
- 0.25 to 0.34—good question
- 0.15 to 0.24—marginal questions to be revised
- Below 0.15—poor questions need to be discarded

Evaluating the Effectiveness of Distracters

In multiple choice questions, stem is the statement of the problem in the form of a question or incomplete sentence. The distracters are alternative responses for the question (incorrect responses) while key is the correct response. A good distracter is the one that attracts more subjects from the lower group than the upper group. When a distracter attracts more subjects from upper group and less from the lower group the distracter is a poor one. Example:

Stem	Distracters
The Indian Mental Health Acts was passed in the year	<ul><li>1947</li><li>1967</li><li>1977</li><li>1987</li></ul>

CRITIQUING DATA COLLECTION METHODS

- Did the research report provide information on what data were collected, how it were collected, who collected it, where and when it was collected?
- Was an appropriate instrument used to measure the research variables?
- Had the instrument been tested for reliability and validity?
- Were the same instruments used for the pilot study?
- Were the items in the instrument appropriate to collect adequate data?
- Did the items adequately cover the range of content?
- Did the order of the items influence subjects' responses?
- Were the items and the directions for completing items clear?
- Was the instrument administered to all the subjects in the same manner?
- Was the data collected for all the subjects at the same setting?

IMPLEMENTING RESEARCH PLAN

Implementation of a research plan refers to the process of putting a research plan into action. It involves the following steps:

- Preparation of data collection material
- Data collection
- Data analysis and
- Interpretation of the findings

Preparation of Data Collection Material

- In this step the researcher selects data collection material which depends on the research approach and the variables being assessed. Researcher needs to select the method of gathering data, i.e. questionnaire, interview schedule or an observation technique.
- Before starting the study the researcher needs to obtain ethical clearance from the institutional ethics committee or institutional review board to safeguard the dignity, rights, safety, and well-being of the research participants.
- The researcher also obtains permission for conducting the study from the concerned authorities.
- The researcher must develop a plan for gathering and recording the data.
- The researcher needs to decide the nature of setting, proximity, and number of settings.
- If the sample is large and the settings are more than one, time schedules need to be prepared.
- In case of explorative study using self report questionnaire, it needs to be decided whether the questionnaire will be distributed and collected directly from the respondents or will be sent by mail or collected through email. In case of experimental study, duration of intervention and the person providing the intervention should be specified.

Data Collection Procedure

- The process of data collection begins even before the data is collected from the first subject and ends with the data collection from the last subject.

- In quantitative research various instruments, surveys, and measurements are used to collect numerical data. In qualitative research, questionnaires are used to collect language based data.
- The researcher needs to prepare procedures for data collection which will facilitate consistency in data collection across study participants and data collectors.
- The quality of data collected is the basis for validity of study findings. This quality data collection requires a systematic approach and includes training data collectors, monitoring completeness and accuracy of raw data.
- During data collection, variables may be measured by observation, interview, questionnaires, scales or physiological measurements or methods. The data collectors need to be trained on how to administer these measurements. They also require training on how questions are asked (interview method), questionnaires are administered (self-report method), variables are observed (observation method) and participant's responses are recorded.
- The researcher may be required to complete training or certification related to data collection.
- The researcher needs to approach the potential subjects who meet the sampling criteria and collect the data systematically for each subject.
- The procedure for data collection is usually described in the methods section of a study report. A step by step procedure of how exactly the data were collected should be given. In case of an experimental study the duration of intervention and the person providing the intervention is specified. It gives a clear picture of the data collection.
- The collected data are recorded systematically in the computer for each subject to facilitate retrieval and analysis.
- Data collectors are required to verify if responses have been recorded against each item before completing the interview. The researcher should review the data collection instruments for completeness and accuracy for a second or even a third time.
- After all the checks of raw data are completed, the individual items are assigned a code name, consistent rules used for coding variables, after which data collection instruments are ready for data entry.
- Early data collection efforts are closely supervised to ensure compliance with procedures.
- Sometimes during the data collection process accidental discovery of something useful or valuable may happen. Such discoveries should not be ignored. These could be used as additional findings of the study and should be included in the study while writing the final report. These would enrich the study and may even open the doors for further research concerning the issue at hand.

Guidelines for Evaluating the Data Collection Procedure

- If a questionnaire is used in a study, adequate information should be provided to decide whether it was appropriate. The manner in which the questionnaire was developed, the reliability and validity of the instrument, the number of questions, how the instrument was scored, and the range of possible scores should be addressed.
- When an interview has been used, information about how long the interviews took, who conducted the interviews, and how the interviewers were trained need to be mentioned. Means of ensuring confidentiality should be presented.
- When observation technique is used information about how observations were made, who made the observations,

- and how data were recorded and whether subjects were being observed need to be mentioned.
- ❖ If physiological instruments are used, the accuracy of these data collection measures needs to be addressed. Whether the researcher has the expertise to use these instruments needs to be confirmed.
- ❖ Before the researcher uses a psychological data-collection method, such as an attitude scale or a personality test, the appropriateness of these instruments and the qualifications of the researcher to use them need to be determined.

Data Analysis

Data analysis in quantitative studies is the reduction, organization, and statistical testing of information obtained during the data collection phase. In quantitative research, statistical test is employed depending upon the research question. It may either be descriptive or inferential in nature. The tests are predetermined before data collection takes place. Various computer software programs are available for conducting statistical analysis. Description of data analysis is detailed in Unit 9.

Interpretation of Findings

The results obtained from data analysis require interpretation to be meaningful. Interpretation of research outcome involves examining the results of data analysis, explaining what the results mean in the light of current practice and previous research, identifying study limitations, forming conclusions in consideration of study limitations, deciding on the appropriate recommendation for generalization of findings, considering the implications for nursing's body of knowledge and suggesting directions for further research. Description of interpretation of findings is detailed in Unit 9.

An example of data collection procedure in an intervention study is described in Box 8.4.

Box 8.4 — **Data collection procedure in an intervention study**

Title of the study: "Effectiveness of Body-Mind-Spirit Intervention on wellbeing, functional impairment and quality of life among depressive patients- A randomized controlled trial"

Data collection procedure

Recruitment of subjects took place at a psychiatric outpatient department of the District Hospital in Kolar, India. Data were collected from July 2011 to Jan 2013. The investigator initially identified patients who had a diagnosis of mild or moderate depression and were on antidepressant treatment.

Each patient was contacted and a personal interview was arranged in a psychiatric counseling room for baseline assessment. They were informed that they would be randomly assigned to either the BMS or TAU groups and also about the kind of participation required from them.

The subjects responded to the Beck Depression Inventory II, Body-Mind-Spirit Well-being Inventory, Quality of Life, and Work and Social Adjustment Scale at the outpatient department.

Following baseline assessment, all participants were randomly assigned by the investigator to either the BMS or TAU groups.

Participants in BMS group underwent the BMS intervention spread over 4 weeks, along with routine treatment in the hospital. Intervention was given as a group approach by the investigator, who received Body-Mind-Spirit practitioner training at Centre on Behavioral Health, the University of Hong Kong, Hong Kong, and is a certified practitioner. Each group consisted of 3 to 4 participants. The intervention consisted of a weekly 3-hour session for 4 weeks. A total of 15 groups completed the 4 week intervention.

Participants in the TAU group received (a) antidepressants (tricyclic antidepressants or specific serotonin reuptake inhibitors); (b)structured psycho-education (education about causes, signs and symptoms of depression, side effects of medication, early signs of relapse, importance of medication compliance and follow-up); (c) brief counseling for any emotional/interpersonal issues for 15 minutes duration by psychiatrist.

The outcome measures were assessed at baseline and at four follow-up assessments in the 1st, 2nd, 3rd, and 6th months.

AVOIDING BIAS—COLLECTING RELIABLE DATA (BIAS IN RESEARCH)

In research the goal is to understand the true relationship between variables (a predictor and an outcome). In designing a research project the researcher's goal should be to control other factors which will influence true relationship between variables (controlling bias), so that the researcher can have a clearer picture of the true relationship between variables (predictor and outcome).

Bias in research is anything that produces systematic variation in research findings and that can threaten the study validity and trustworthiness. These variations in research findings can lead to serious consequences in clinical practice. Hence the researcher should understand that bias can occur at any stage of research process irrespective of the design and is difficult to eliminate.

Bias can occur while designing research, selection of participants, during data collection process, analysis process, interpretation of results, reporting the results and publication. Various measures to control bias are:
- Select an appropriate research design based on study purpose
- Random selection of participants, and in the case of clinical trials random assignment of participants into comparison groups
- Choose an adequate sample size
- Have a well-designed research protocol clearly outlining data collection and analysis process
- Use objective and validated questionnaire
- Prepare questionnaires that will be finished in a reasonable amount of time (say around 30 minutes)
- Ensure clarity in questions
- Read reliable references on how to prepare questionnaires objectively
- Once the questionnaire is ready, validate it to a non-respondent group
- Do not provide the choices to respondents in personal interviews
- Train study personnel for data collection
- Undertake pilot study to refine protocols and procedures
- Use blinding, i.e. having different examiners measure the outcome than those who implemented the treatment/intervention
- Use matching, masking, and random allocation as needed
- Monitor each stage of research, including periodic check of the data
- Minimize non-response and partial response. Double check the data and cleanse it of errors in recording, entries, etc.
- Use appropriate statistical methods
- Interpret the results in an objective manner based on evidence
- Exercise extreme care in drafting the report and keep comments or opinions separate from the results.

PILOT STUDY

Pilot study is the study carried out at the end of the planning phase of research. It is often developed on similar lines to the proposed study, using similar subjects, setting, data collection tools, and same intervention procedures and data analysis techniques.

Definitions
- Pilot study is defined as a small sample study conducted as a prelude to a large-scale sample study.
- Pilot study is a trial, small scale study carried out before final research. It is conducted to test, refine or modify research methodology and help in preparing a larger and more comprehensive investigation.

Reasons for Conducting Pilot Study
- Determine feasibility and practicability of proposed research in terms of availability of subjects, time and money
- Identify problems with design
- Determine whether sample is representative of the population or whether the sampling technique is effective

- Examine the reliability and validity of the research instruments
- Refine the methodology of the research proposal, data collection procedures and analysis plan
- To get an experience of the subjects, settings, methodology and measurements and implementation of intervention
- Determine the resources required for research
- Identify potential problems
- Convincing funding bodies that the main study is worth funding and feasible
- To evaluate the feasibility of recruitment, randomization, assessment procedures and implementation of novel interventions. The elements which are not feasible or unsatisfactory can be modified in the subsequent trial.

Pilot study is the pre-research activity to refine research methodology and a plan for appropriate use of resources with adequate beforehand information about the main study parameters.

BIBLIOGRAPHY

1. Brewerton, P., & Millward, L. (2003). *Organizational research methods*. Thousand Oaks, CA: Sage.
2. Burns, N., & Grove, S.K. (2004). Th*e practice of nursing research*. Philadelphia: W.B. Saunders Company.
3. Burn^s, N., and Grove, S.K. (2001). The practices of nursing research: conduct, *critique and utilization* (4th ed.). Philadelphia, WB Saunders Company.
4. Cohen, J. (1988). Statistical power *analysis for the behavioral scien*ces (2nd ed.). Hillsdale, NJ: Lawrence Eribaum.
5. Creswell, J.W. (1994). Research design: Qualitative and quantitative app *oaches. Thousand Oaks,* CA: SAGE Publications.
6. Dawson, B., Trapp, R.G. (2004). Basic and clinical biostatics (4th ed). New York: McGraw-Hill Education.
7. Kerlinger, F.N., & Lee, H.B. (2000). Found*ations of behavioral research. New York: Harcourt Brace.*
8. Knapp, T.R., and Brown, J.K. (1995). Ten measurement commandments that often should be broken. Research Nursing Health, 18(5), 465-9.
9. Polit, D.F., Beck, C.T., & Hungler, B.P. (2001). *Essentials of Nursing Research: Methods, Appraisal, and Utilization* (5th ed.). Philadelphia: Lippincott Williams & Wilkins.
10. Polit, D.F., Beck, C.T., & Hungler, B.P. (2006). Essentials of nursing *research: Methods, appraisal* and utilization (6th ed.). Philadelphia: Lippincott Will*iams & Wilkins.*
11. Schotfetdt, R.M. (1977). *Nursing Rese*arch: Reflection of values. Nursing Research, 26(1), 4-8.
12. Treece, E.W., and Treece, J.H. (1989). *Elements of Research in Nursing*, C.V. Mosby Co., St. Louis.

REVIEW QUESTIONS

I. Long Essays

1. Define data collection. Write about the concept of data collection in nursing research.
2. Define research tool. Explain the characteristics of research instruments.
3. List out the types of data collection methods. Explain any one method briefly.
4. Discuss the construction of questionnaires and interview schedule.
5. Explain about observation method in detail.
6. Discuss in detail about focus group interview.
7. Explain various approaches to conduct interview.
8. Explain in detail about validity and reliability of an instrument.

II. Short Essays

1. What are the types of data collection sources? Explain briefly.
2. Differentiate between questionnaire and interview methods of data collection in nursing research.
3. What is survey method and explain types of tools used in survey method?
4. Explain types of questionnaires and discuss advantages and disadvantages of questionnaire method of data collection.
5. Detail the steps in designing questionnaire.
6. Advantages and disadvantages of Interview method.
7. Explain rating scales.
8. Item analysis.
9. Pilot study.

III. Short Answers

1. Give examples of open-ended questions.
2. What are the conditions amenable for observation?
3. List commonly used biophysiological measures in nursing research.
4. Visual analog scale.
5. Likert scale.
6. Stability.
7. Construct validity.
8. Content validity.

IV. Multiple Choice Questions

1. Data collection is a process of _____.
   a. gathering and measuring information
   b. gathering and interpreting information
   c. gathering and analyzing information
   d. gathering and reporting information
2. Data collected directly from the subjects by the researcher for the purpose of research study is called
   a. Primary data collection
   b. Secondary data collection
   c. Both a and b
   d. Mixed data collection
3. Following are the purposes of data collection, *except*
   a. to get answer to the research question
   b. to test the hypothesis
   c. to identify and measure phenomena
   d. to explain need for the study
4. _____ is a common data collecting instrument in nursing research.
   a. Interview
   b. Questionnaire
   c. Critical incident
   d. Anecdotal record
5. Which of the following are types of rating scale, *except*
   a. Graphic
   b. Numerical
   c. Descriptive
   d. Alphabetic
6. The structured observation is carried out by using which of the following tools
   a. Rating scale
   b. Check list
   c. Both a and b
   d. Q-Sorts
7. Which of the following involves use of data that were collected for another purpose but used in the current research study?
   a. Primary data collection
   b. Secondary data collection
   c. Tertiary data collection
   d. Both a and b
8. Researchers use open-ended questions to collect data. Which of the following statements is true?
   a. Open-ended questions directly provide quantitative data based on the researcher's predetermined response categories
   b. Open-ended questions provide quantitative data in participant's own words
   c. Open-ended questions provide qualitative data in participant's own words
   d. Open-ended questions directly provide qualitative data in researcher's own words

9. Open-ended questions primarily provide _____ data.
   a. Confirmatory data
   b. Qualitative data
   c. Predictive data
   d. None of the above
10. Which of the following is true concerning observation?
    a. It takes less time than self-report approaches
    b. It costs less money than self-report approaches
    c. Provides good opportunity for identifying unanticipated outcomes
    d. Can be carried out without assistance
11. Which of the following method takes less time for data collection?
    a. Mail survey
    b. Face to face interview
    c. Telephonic interview
    d. In-depth interview
12. Which of the following questions is an open ended question?
    a. Describe status of a nurse in the society
    b. Have been admitted in the hospital
    c. Have attended any similar program in the past
    d. Have ever visited a patient in a psychiatric hospital
13. Following are the examples of closed ended questions, *except*
    a. Describe status of a nurse in the society.
    b. Have you been admitted in the hospital?
    c. Have you attended any similar program in the past?
    d. Have you ever visited a patient in the psychiatric hospital?
14. Which of the following question is a dichotomous question?
    a. To which gender do you belong?
    b. To which community do you belong?
    c. To which state do you belong?
    d. To which country do you belong?
15. Which of the following is an example of a rating scale?
    a. How satisfied are you with the care provided by the nurses in the hospital?
    b. Describe status of nurse in society.
    c. Have you been admitted in the hospital?
    d. Have you attended any similar program in the past?
16. It is the extent to which an instrument measures an intended concept or construct or refers to whether researcher can draw inferences about test scores related to the concept being studied. This phenomena is known as
    a. Construct validity
    b. Face validity
    c. Stability
    d. Concurrent validity
17. It refers to people usually performing better when they know they are being observed. It is termed as
    a. Hawthorne effect
    b. Halo effect
    c. Error of leniency
    d. Anonymity
18. Which of the following is a typical example for semantic differential scale_____
    a. Kind..........cruel
    b. Emotion.......aloof
    c. Depression.....dull
    d. None of these
19. Which of the following is an expansion of VAS?
    a. Visual analog scale
    b. Visual analysis scale
    c. Video assessment scale
    d. None of the above
20. It refers to the consistency with which an instrument or test measures what it is supposed to measure. This phenomena is known as
    a. Validity
    b. Reliability
    c. Stability
    d. Equivalence
21. It is the extent to which an instrument measures what it is supposed to measure

a. Reliability
   b. Stability
   c. Equivalence
   d. Validity
22. Pilot study is also known as _____
   a. Large scale study
   b. Small scale study
   c. Repetition of the same study
   d. Replication study
23. It refers to the degree of correlation of two measures of the same concept administered at the same time. This phenomena is known as
   a. Criterion validity
   b. Construct validity
   c. Reliability
   d. Stability
24. Which of the following is a self-report data collection instrument that asks respondents to report their attitudes or feelings on a continuum?
   a. Visual analog scale
   b. Attitude scale
   c. Q-sort
   d. Delphi technique
25. Which of the following is an advantage of an interview method of data collection versus a questionnaire?
   a. Data are less costly to obtain
   b. Less time is required to collect the data
   c. The collected data tends to be more complete
   d. Data can be collected from a widespread geographical area
26. Which of the following data-collection methods is most likely to obtain objective data?
   a. Observational method
   b. Questionnaire method
   c. Physiological measures
   d. Interview method
27. The researchers want to collect the data about the evaluation process of staff nurses on a unit. Which of the following measurement tool is best suited to gather the data?
   a. Interview
   b. Focus group
   c. Experiment
   d. Questionnaires

ANSWER KEY

1. a	2. a	3. d	4. b	5. d	6. c
7. b	8. c	9. b	10. c	11. b	12. a
13. a	14. a	15. a	16. a	17. a	18. a
19. a	20. b	21. d	22. b	23. a	24. b
26. c	27. d				

UNIT 9

Plan for Data Analysis and Interpretation

Planning for data analysis is the most significant part of any research process. Even before initiating the study the researcher should select suitable statistics to analyze the data. The researcher should also identify the data entry method and the data analysis software that will be used for the study. Enough time should also be spent in the initial phases of the project to familiarize with the software being used.

To plan for data analysis a table may be prepared. The first column of the table should include the research question or hypothesis; the second, all related variables; and the third, the suitable statistical tests to be used.

This process ensures that suitable variables and statistical tests are selected for each hypothesis. A few examples are presented in Table 9.1. The services of a statistician may be utilized where necessary. The necessary computer commands can be written well in advance before the data collection is completed.

ADVANTAGES OF PLANNING FOR DATA ANALYSIS

The various advantages of planning for data analysis before commencing a study are:
- ❖ The researcher is exactly aware of how the collected data should be handled.

Table 9.1: The plan for data analysis

Hypothesis	Variables	Statistical test
• There will be significant decrease in spirometric values among smokers compared to nonsmokers.	• Spirometric values • Smoking habit	Independent t-test to compare spirometric values between smokers and nonsmokers.
• There will be no significant improvement in quality of life among experimental group cancer patients compared to control group cancer patients.	Independent variable: • Selected nursing intervention Dependent variables: • Health-related quality of life • Activities of daily living	Independent t-test to compare quality of life scores between experimental and control group cancer patients.
• There will be no significant improvement in activities of daily living among experimental group cancer patients compared to control group.		Independent t-test to compare activities of daily living scores between experimental and control group cancer patients.

- The definite plan quickens the data analysis process.
- Writing the computer commands in advance enables the running of predetermined computer program immediately after the data is entered. This enables ready interpretation of the analysis.
- Designing the statistical analysis in advance increases the scientific integrity.
- Planning ahead of time leaves little room for the researcher to redesign the analysis to go with their purpose.

The two fundamental types of research analysis are: quantitative and qualitative. These differ in the collecting and processing of data.

PHASES OF QUANTITATIVE DATA ANALYSIS

The collected raw data is in the form of digits or words. It may contain errors, omissions, and inconsistencies. Thus processing of collected data should invariably precede data analysis. This processing of data is crucial for a scientific study as it ensures the relevance of such data for proposed comparison and analysis.

The data analysis process differs from one study to another. There are three phases in analysis of quantitative data: pre-analysis phase, analysis phase, and interpretive phase (Fig. 9.1).

Pre-analysis Phase (Preparing Data for Computer Analysis and Presentation)

It involves various clerical and administrative tasks that include reviewing data forms for completeness and legibility, identifying missing information and taking steps, assigning identification numbers, and selecting software packages for doing data analysis. This also includes coding the data and entering them into computer files to generate a data set for analysis. The steps involved in pre-analysis phase are presented in Flowchart 9.1.

1. *Editing of data:* It is the process of inspecting the collected raw data to detect errors and omissions and correct them. It involves careful scrutiny of the completed questionnaires or schedules. Editing ensures that the data are accurate, consistent with other facts gathered, uniformly entered, as completed as possible, and well-arranged to facilitate coding and tabulation. It can be done at two stages, *viz.* field and post-field editing.

   The field editing is done during data collection process by editing abbreviated form of interview information collected from respondents for completeness. It should be done immediately after the interview, preferably on the same day.

   The post-field (central) editing is carried out when all the schedules or questionnaires have been completed

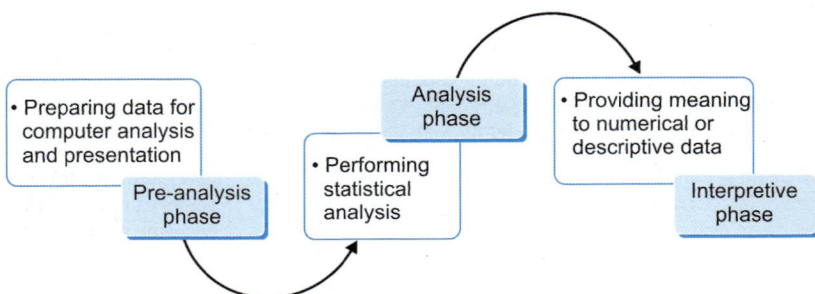

Fig. 9.1: Phases of quantitative data analysis

Flowchart 9.1: Steps in pre-analysis phase

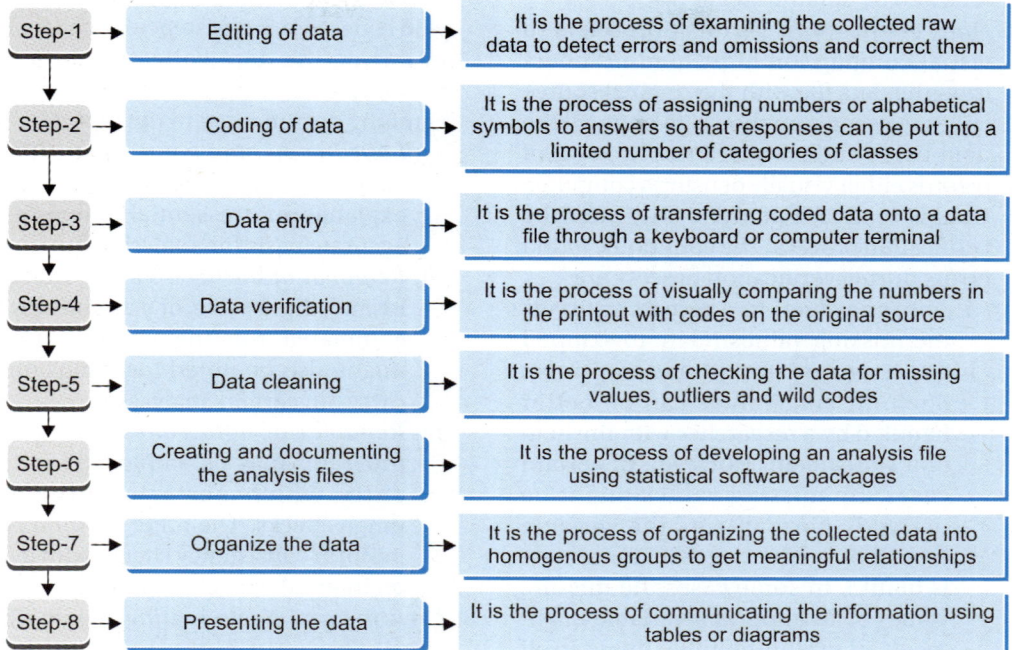

and collected. It includes reviewing of all schedules or questionnaires thoroughly for noticeable errors such as an entry in the wrong place, units such as entry recorded in months while it should have been recorded in days, etc.

2. *Coding of data:* It is the process of assigning numbers or alphabetical symbols to subject's responses so as to put them into a limited number of categories or classes. It simplifies the transfer of data from questionnaire to the master chart enabling easier and quicker calculations. They must have the following characteristics:
   i. *Exhaustiveness*: There must be a class for every data item. For example, the classes should cater to all the possible qualifications of nurses.
   ii. *Mutually exclusive*: Specific answer can be allocated to only one of the cells in a given category. For example, in a question relating to educational qualification of nurses, the alternative choices given are: Diploma in nursing, BSc (N), MSc (N), PhD (N). The numerical codes assigned to these alternatives could be 1, 2, 3, and 4, respectively. The answer to above question can only be one of the above options.
   iii. *Unidimensional*: Every class is defined in terms of a single variable. For example, the classes should refer to only the educational qualification of nurses and not any other parameter such as experience, occupation etc.

3. *Data entry:* Once the data is coded, it is transferred to a data file using a keyboard or computer terminal. Data entry is a tiresome and monotonous process prone to errors which can be simplified using various computer programs. The errors in data entry can occur due to coding problem, wrong entry or misreporting

of information. The data entry process is followed by data verification.

4. *Data verification:* Verification refers to visual comparison of printed numbers from the data file with the original source codes. A second method is to enter all the data twice and compare the two sets of records either visually or using a computer. Data is ready for analysis only after the verification process. The commonly found errors during verification process are:

   i. *Missing values:* In a research survey, the missing values relate to skipped questions or unendorsed options. Such missing values can be better handled by a researcher with the help of a statistician. However, in certain cases the missing values might be perfectly normal (e.g., the variable "result of pregnancy test" for a male is blank). In some cases the missing values of an important variable might result in excluding the subject itself from certain analyses. At times, it is suitable to put normalized values in the place of missing values.

   ii. *Outliers:* "Unusually" large or small scores that are significantly separated from the rest of the data might be: "out-of-range" or physically impossible values that are a result of improper entry or processing error. Merely "peculiar" values might be on account of an entry error, random fluctuation, or data from another study. Example, the monthly income of INR 20,000 for a participant in a distribution where all other incomes are below INR 2,000 is an outlier.

   iii. *Wild code:* It refers to a code that is not permissible. For example, the variable "gender" might have the four defined codes—1: male, 2: female, 3: transgender and 9: not responded. If a code of 7 is discovered in the data, it would indicate an error.

5. *Data cleaning:* Data cleaning involves checking for missing values, outliers, and wild codes. As inconsistencies might creep in during the data collection process, the data cleansing procedure must be carefully documented in the report.

   i. *Labeling missing values:* Labeling of each missing value with a suitable explanation is essential to assure an accurate basis for analysis.

   ii. *Removal of outliers:* Values that are invalid, impossible, or extreme may be eliminated from the dataset. Outliers might also be noted for exclusion to carry out certain analyses.

   iii. *Removal of wild codes:* Computer programs may be employed for data entry which perform automatic range checks. The other method is to perform consistency checks with focus on internal data consistency.

6. *Creating and documenting the analysis files:* The data cleaning process is followed by developing an analysis file using a statistical software package. The researcher needs to keep a code book which essentially lists each variable along with necessary information, codes linked with the values of the variable and other basic information.

7. *Organization of data:* The collected data from various sources should be organized into homogenous groups to get meaningful relationships. This organization can be done by way of classification. The first task in classification of data is developing a master chart. For example, while classifying the demographic details of the patients, the researcher records the ID numbers of the patients in rows and the corresponding demographic details such as age, gender, occupation, qualification, etc. in columns. The information thus arranged is termed as an array of data. The set of information related to the specific demographic entity is termed as the field.

Classification of data: The collected raw data must be grouped to enable easy retrieval of essential data. The process of categorizing data into groups, types or distinct classes according to certain similarities or resemblances is called classification of data. Data is grouped into classes based on their common characteristics making comparison among them easier. Classification can be according to attributes or numerical characteristics.

- *Classification according to attributes:* In this the data are categorized according to descriptive characteristics such as gender, type of family, marital status, religion, etc. These descriptive characteristics cannot be measured numerically but only the presence or absence of the characteristic can be observed.
- *Classification according to numerical characteristics:* Numerical characteristics are referred to as quantitative phenomenon which can be measured objectively. For example, data relating to income, height, temperature, etc. Numerical data can further be classified into discrete and continuous. Discrete data represents items that can be listed making it possible to count. For example, count of marks in an examination which can go from 0 to 100. Continuous data, on the other hand, represents measurements which cannot possibly be counted but can only be described using class intervals. For example, monthly income up to INR 5,000 may form continuous data from INR 1 to INR 5,000, represented by the class interval (1–5,000), inclusive. Subsequently, an income group (5,000–10,000) can be formed and so on. The respondents reporting income against each class form the frequency of the class. Every class has a lower and an upper limit and the difference between them is known as the range of the class. The class intervals are usually kept equal.

8. *Presentation of data:* Once the data has been classified the researcher needs to summarize, organize, and communicate the information using tables or diagrams which is termed as presentation of data. The presentation of data could be in tabular or graphical form. In tabular form of presentation, the researcher summarizes the raw data and displays the same in columns and rows for further analysis. In graphic form of presentation, data are presented in the form of graphs, diagrams or maps.

   i. *Tabular presentation:* The main purpose of this presentation is to summarize or present the data in an informative and meaningful manner. It should facilitate interpretation and subsequent analysis. Tabulation may be classified as simple or complex. Simple tabulation is used to present a single characteristic of the data whereas complex tabulation is used to present several interrelated characteristics.

   ii. *Graphical presentation:* It is an advanced technique which provides complete picture of the data at a single glance. It is more effective than presenting data in tabular form. With the help of computer software packages, data can be graphically presented in many different ways, *viz.* bar chart, pie chart, histogram, frequency polygon, frequency curve, and line diagram.

Analysis Phase (Statistical Analysis)

The researcher can proceed with data analysis once the problems relating to missing data are resolved and other necessary transformations made. During the analytical phase, analysis of data is carried out to make the raw data meaningful or draw results from it after proper statistical treatment. Thus, the purpose of analyzing the data is to describe the data in meaningful terms, test hypothesis, test statistical significance of the data, draw inferences, make generalization, and test parameters.

Meaning of Analysis
- Analysis is the process of organizing and synthesizing the data to answer the research questions and test hypothesis.
- Analysis is a process of systematically applying statistical techniques to describe, summarize, and compare data.

Quantitative analysis is a highly systematic and organized process. It deals with analyzing numerical values using statistical techniques for describing and explaining the research outcome. In other words, quantitative analysis uses numerical data to describe and interpret the results.

As data for quantitative analysis are numerically represented, reliability of data collection, accuracy of data entry, and appropriateness of analytical process assume significance for drawing accurate conclusions. Quantitative analyses are classified as descriptive and inferential based on the aim of the study. Descriptive analyses deal with an accurate description of sample characteristics. Inferential analyses are used to determine if results found in a sample can be applied to a population.

TYPES OF QUANTITATIVE ANALYSIS

There are many types of quantitative analysis. These can be categorized in several ways based on the goals of the analysis or assumptions made about the data or the number of variables involved (Flowchart 9.2).

Classification Based on Goals of Analysis

Quantitative analyses are categorized into descriptive and inferential statistics based on the goals and aims of the study.
- *Descriptive statistics:* Descriptive analyses are concerned with accurately organizing, describing, and summarizing the numerical data gathered from samples such as range of values and their averages. These allow the researcher to examine

Flowchart 9.2: Types of quantitative analysis

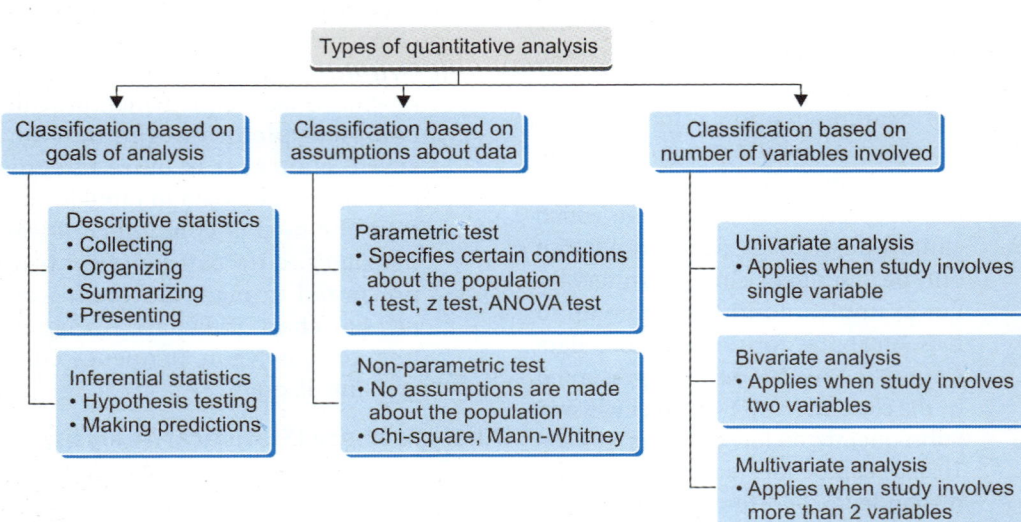

the characteristics, behaviors, and experiences of study participants (Polit, 1996). The main purpose of descriptive statistics is to provide in as much detail as possible the characteristics of the study sample. Through descriptive statistics, hypotheses cannot be tested.

Descriptive statistics can be categorized in many ways—(1) measures to organize the data; (2) measures of central tendency; (3) measures of variability; and (4) measures of relationship.

- Measures to organize the data: When the researcher deals with a huge volume of data, it needs to be condensed into a more understandable form. Data can be organized by frequency distributions, graphic presentations, and percentages. These topics are detailed in Part B-Biostatistics.
- Measures of central tendency: These statistics describe the average, typical or most common values for a group of data. Center here refers to the middle or average value and tendency refers to the inclination of the values to cluster in a certain way. A measure of central tendency thus summarizes a frequency distribution using a single number and represents the way the data tend towards the center. These are appropriate for summarizing interval or ratio data. The most common measures of central tendency are the arithmetic mean, the median, and the mode. These topics are detailed in Part B-Biostatistics.
- Measures of variability: Two important features of a data set include the center of the data and the spread of the data. While the center can be measured using mean, median, and mode, the spread of data set can be measured using range, variance, standard deviation, and coefficient of variation. These topics are detailed in Part B-Biostatistics.
- Measures of relationship: It measures the relationship between two or more variables or sets of data, i.e. the degree to which the value of variable X is related to the value of variable Y. The various ways to examine such relationships include correlation coefficients, scatter plots, and contingency tables. These topics are detailed in Part B-Biostatistics.

❖ *Inferential statistics*: Inferential statistics is a statistical method used to infer results of sample (statistic) to population (parameters). It is a process of inductive reasoning based on the mathematical theory of probability (Fowler J, Jarvis P, 2002). These statistics measure the difference between two variables or subgroups of a variable. It also allows the researcher to make predictions about a specific population based on sample information that is representative of the population. It also allows the researcher to test hypothesis concerning a population using data obtained from study samples. Example, inferential statistics helps in finding the differences, relationships, and associations between two or more variables with the help of parametric and nonparametric tests. Thus inferential statistics not only helps the researcher to describe the mere study results but also provides a platform for further clinical practice and research.

Components of inferential statistics:
- Estimation: Estimation denotes calculating a single parameter like a "mean" from the given data. It can be point or interval. Point estimation involves calculation of a single value such as mean from random samples of the population through which the researcher estimates the population parameter. Interval estimation involves calculation of an interval or a range of values from a sample data through

which the researcher estimates the range of values within which the population parameter has the probability of lying.
- ○ Hypotheses testing: It involves testing an assumption or hypothesis about a population parameter using a sample data through which the researcher decides whether the hypotheses are supported by empirical evidence or not.

Classification Based on Assumptions of Data

Quantitative analyses are generally grouped into two large categories based on assumptions about the data. These are parametric and nonparametric.

Parametric Test

Parametric test is one that makes assumptions about population parameters and the distribution from which the data is drawn. If the information on population parameters is completely known then a parametric test can be carried out. The various characteristics of parametric tests are:
- ❖ These are based on the assumptions that the data fall into a normal or bell-shaped distribution
- ❖ This can be assumed only when interval or ratio level measures are collected
- ❖ When samples are large enough to achieve normality
- ❖ These tests are more powerful than non-parametric tests. In other words, a parametric test is more able to lead to a rejection of H_0. Example, t-test, F-test, z-test, and one-way analysis of variance (ANOVA)

Non-parametric Test

Even if there is no knowledge about the population or parameters, but yet the hypothesis of the population is required to be tested, the resulting statistical test is called a non-parametric test. Example, Chi-square test, Mann–Whitney test, Rank sum test, and Kruskal–Wallis test. The various characteristics of nonparametric tests are:
- ❖ Simple and easy to understand
- ❖ No assumptions are made regarding the population
- ❖ They do not rely on normal distribution
- ❖ Data is on nominal or ordinal level and does not involve complicated sampling theory
- ❖ It is not as powerful as the parametric test

In the field of health sciences and nursing, the nonparametric tests are increasingly used as the observations are presented in numerical figures and also the researchers may not be aware of the nature of population distribution and other parameters. In addition, the sample may be too small to test the hypothesis and generalize the findings for the population from which the sample is drawn. In other words, the nonparametric tests are valid in a broader range of situations, e.g. grading bed sores, assessing pain, effectiveness of drug action, etc.

Classification Based on Number of Variables in the Analyses

Quantitative analyses can be classified in terms of the number of variables that are to be considered. These tests are classified both by the number and type of variables involved. These are univariate, bivariate, and multivariate analyses.

Univariate Analysis

It deals with examination of the distribution of cases on only one variable at a time. This analysis is applied when the study involves single dependent variable or only one group is included, e.g. height of school children. The main purpose is to describe the variables.

Bivariate Analysis

It deals with examination of two variables simultaneously. The most common is the correlation, e.g. the relation between gender and height of school children. This analysis is also used to determine if a single variable can predict a specified outcome. The main purpose is to determine the relationship between the two variables.

Multivariate Analysis

It deals with examination of more than two variables simultaneously, e.g. relationship between gender, race, and height of school children. The purpose is to determine the relationship between multiple variables.

Interpretive Phase

Collection and analysis of data is followed by interpretation of the results. Data interpretation provides meaning to numerical or descriptive data that has been collected, analyzed, and presented. Interpreting the research results includes discussion of findings, examining the meaning of results, considering the significance of the findings, generalizing the findings, drawing conclusions and suggesting implications for practice and further study (Burns & Grove, 2001). The components of interpretive phase are presented in Figure 9.2.

Interpretation of results forecasts the study usefulness based on the objectives of the study, its theoretical basis, existing body of knowledge, and limitations of the adapted research methods. Interpretation of findings is usually found towards the end of a research report under the discussion heading.

1. *Discussion of findings:* Discussion of a study report allows the researcher to explain the study results in light of the existing body of knowledge and the new understanding of the research problem that has been generated. The discussion should connect to the research question, hypothesis, and the review of literature. In the discussion section, the researcher discusses aspects of the results which are either in agreement or not with previous research and theoretical explanations. The

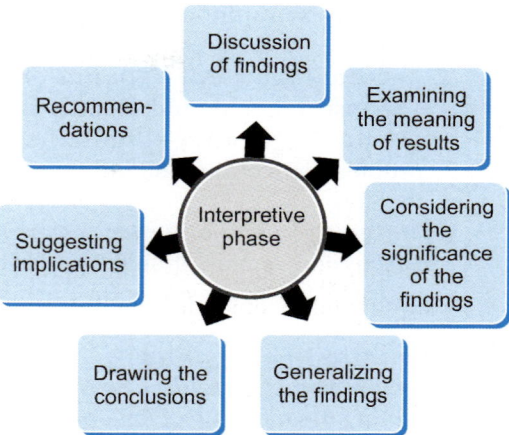

Fig. 9.2: Components of interpretive phase

general rules for writing discussion are presented in Box 9.1. The following should be considered while discussing the study findings:

   i. *Restate the research problem and major findings:* Briefly explain research problem, methods used, and major findings of the study.
   ii. *Detail the meaning and importance of each finding:* The underlying meaning and significance of each finding may be systematically explained. First explain unanticipated findings or most significant finding followed by systematic review of each finding.
   iii. *Relate the findings to similar studies:* Discussion should involve comparing and contrasting the present study findings with that of other studies. While comparison supports and highlights the present study results, contrast explains how the present study findings differ from other similar studies.
   iv. *Consider alternative explanations of the findings:* While writing the discussion section, the researcher should reflect on all plausible explanations pertaining to the study results and not limit to those concerning the

hypothesis or prior assumptions and biases.
  v. *Acknowledge study's limitations:* The researcher should identify and acknowledge study's limitations, problems encountered, and reasons thereof.
  vi. *Make suggestions for further research:* Discussion section should conclude with making suggestions for further research.
2. *Examining the meaning of results (interpretation of results):* It involves explaining the meaning of data based on the objectives of the study also termed as interpretation of results. To be useful, the evidence from data analysis must be carefully examined, organized, and given meaning. The interpretation differs in quantitative and qualitative studies.

In quantitative studies, statistical results are included to support the statement of results. These results are in the form of test statistics and probability levels which may include calculated values, degrees of freedom, and the significance level to which researchers need to attach a meaning.

  i. *Interpreting the results of descriptive statistics:* The researcher initially describes the data using descriptive statistics. These describe the basic features of the data in a study by summarizing and organizing data including measures of central tendency and variability. The output includes N, mean, median, standard deviation and graphs. "N" describes size of the sample. The mean and median describe the sample with a single value that represents the center of the data. These both measure central tendency. These indicate whether the data are symmetric or not. Standard deviation determines how spread out the data is from the mean. A higher value indicates greater spread in the data. Graphs explain shape and spread of data distribution and identify outliers. In a normal distribution, the graph appears as a bell-shaped curve. The mean, mode, and median have the same value. Histogram is used to detect skewness or distortedness. Skewness is asymmetry in a statistical distribution in which the curve appears distorted either to the right or left. The skewness can be quantified to define the extent to which a distribution differs from a normal distribution. Plot diagrams determine the spread of the points and how much the sample varies. The more the points are spread out from the center of the data, the greater the variation in sample. Outliers can also be easily identified using plot diagrams.

  ii. *Interpreting the results of inferential statistics:* Inferential statistics makes inferences about a population using a sample data. These help the researcher to conclude if the difference found between two groups (e.g. experimental and control groups) is indeed a real one or one that occurred by a chance due to an unrepresentative sample being chosen from the population. Hypotheses' testing is used in this inferential process. While a null hypothesis indicates that there are no differences in the groups or relationships among variables, the alternative hypotheses indicate a difference in the groups or a relationship in variables (Gravetter & Wallnau, 2012). For example, a researcher wants to investigate if holistic intervention on school children would decrease examination anxiety. Here null hypothesis would be that holistic intervention does not alter the examination anxiety among school children while alternative hypothesis would be that holistic intervention for school children reduces examination anxiety.

iii. *Interpretation of p-value and effect size:* A *p*-value or significance level indicates the probability that a result is obtained by chance. In nursing research, the most common significance levels are 0.05 or 0.01, which indicate a 5% or 1% chance, respectively of rejecting the null hypothesis when it is true. A smaller *p*-value of 0.01 as compared to a *p*-value of 0.05 will decrease the chances of rejecting the null hypothesis when it is true. When a *p*-value is less than or equal to the significance level designated by the researcher, he should have rejected the null hypothesis and reported a difference in the groups or a relationship among the variables (Gravetter & Wallnau, 2012). While a significant *p*-value indicates statistical significance, effect size denotes the relative magnitude of the differences or the relationship (Gravetter & Wallnau, 2012). Effect size is more useful for clinical practice as it indicates clinical significance and importance. In the above example, if the calculated *p*-value is 0.03 which is lesser than the common significance level of 0.05 then the researcher can reject the null hypothesis and report that holistic intervention for school children reduces examination anxiety.

iv. *Interpretation of independent samples t-test:* The independent samples *t*-test can be employed when comparing two independent groups on a continuous dependent variable. In these tests, the groups must be independent with different participants in each group and the dependent variable must be continuous (Gravetter & Wallnau, 2012). Example, if the researcher hypothesizes that there are significant differences in mean somatic symptoms for men and women, the dependent variable is somatic symptoms and the designated significance level is *p*-value less than 0.05. Differences were noted in mean somatic symptoms of female depressive patients (M = 19.61, SD = 10.3) and male depressive patients (M = 13.42, SD = 10.3) with a value of t = 3.53, p = 0.007. The significance (*p*-value) of 0.007 indicates that the difference in the mean somatic symptoms between male and female depressive patients is statistically significant.

v. *Interpretation of paired samples t-test:* A paired samples *t*-test compares two sets of data from one group of people on a continuous dependent variable (Gravetter & Wallnau, 2012). This test is used in pre and post-intervention. If the researcher hypothesizes that there is a significant change in participant's level of anxiety following holistic intervention, a statistically significant decrease from pre-test anxiety level (M = 15.60, SD = 2.55) to post-test anxiety level (M = 13.10, SD = 3.55) is found (t = −5.83, p = 0.0001). A *p*-value of 0.0001 signifies statistical significance.

vi. *Interpretation of one-way analysis of variance:* ANOVA compares two or more independent groups on a continuous dependent variable to investigate the differences between groups (Gravetter & Wallnau, 2012). A researcher hypothesizes the difference in mean anxiety scores across three treatment groups of: (1) progressive muscle relaxation, (2) meditation, and (3) holistic intervention. The researcher fixed a significance level of $p<0.05$. In this study the results showed that there is a statistically significant difference in mean anxiety scores for three treatment groups: $F_{2, 432} = 4.36$, $p = 0.002$. Though these results indicate different anxiety scores for all the three groups, they do not explain which group is having higher anxiety scores. This can be resolved using a post hoc comparison test.

vii. *Interpretation of Pearson product-moment correlation*: The Pearson product-moment correlation coefficient measures the relationship between two continuous variables. It is reported as the statistic r and the values range from -1.00 to 1.00. Negative r values indicate an inverse (negative) relationship, i.e. as the value of variable "x" increases the corresponding value "y" decreases. Positive r values indicate a direct (positive) relationship, i.e. as the value of variable "x" increases the corresponding value "y" increases. The strength of the relationship can be described with reference to r value, weak (± 0.00 to <0.30), moderate (± 0.30 to 0.50), and strong ($> \pm 0.50$) (Gravetter & Wallnau, 2012). In a study to assess the relationship between depression and fatigue among depressive patients the variables examined are depressive scores and fatigue scores. The study results showed that $r = 0.58$, $p < 0.001$, i.e. perception of fatigue is strongly related to depression.

viii. *Interpretation of Chi-square test*: A chi-square test ($\chi 2$) is used to examine the relationship between categorical level variables. The $\chi 2$ test compares the observed and expected frequencies of the data (Gravetter & Wallnau, 2012). In a study to assess the relationship between gender and medication drop out among depressive patients, the results showed that $\chi 2 = 0.37$, $p = 0.56$, i.e. there is no significant relationship between gender and dropping out of medications.

ix. *Interpretation of hypothesis testing:* The results of hypothesis testing fall into one of three categories: (1) the null hypothesis is not rejected, (2) the null hypothesis is rejected and the research hypothesis is supported, (3) the null hypothesis is rejected and the results are in the opposite direction from the prediction of the research hypothesis.
   a. When hypothesis is supported, describing the results is relatively easy as the researcher might have given a relevant explanation with previous research results in review of literature and theoretical framework sections.
   b. Interpreting results is difficult when hypothesis is not supported. The researcher should identify the cause for nonsignificant results that could be due to small sample size or use of inadequate instruments. Nonsignificant results may also be in contrast with previous research results. The researcher in that situation should provide some meaning to the findings and give tentative explanation for the result. Recommendations for further research may be made based on explanations. Researchers must be objective when considering the nonsignificant results. Negative results are equally important as positive results as both results still advance scientific knowledge.

3. *Considering the significance of the findings:* Statistical significance and clinical significance are two important factors that need to be considered while interpreting research findings. Statistical significance indicates that findings from an analysis are true and unlikely to be the result of chance. Research findings that are meaningful for patient care in the absence or presence of statistical significance are

termed as being clinically significant. It is a subjective interpretation of the research result that is practical or meaningful for the patient. It often depends on the magnitude of the effect being studied and has little to do with statistics. However, achieving statistical significance does not automatically mean that study findings are valuable for nursing profession.

i. *Statistical significance:*
   a. Statistical significance refers to the probability of findings due to chance. Significance testing relies on *p*-values and only provides whether the hypothesis is accepted or rejected or difference exists or not exists between the groups.
   b. Statistically significant differences are determined using a certain level of probability (the "*p*-level", or α) that the researcher chooses so that one does not wrongly reject the null hypothesis due to chance, when the null hypothesis is in fact accepted (Type I error).
   c. The generally accepted *p*-level of $\alpha = 0.05$ suggests that there is a 95% probability that the researcher correctly rejects the null hypothesis when there is no difference between groups. Therefore the *p*-value is only the chance that the researcher makes the correct "yes" or "no" decision regarding a hypothesis.
   d. Significance testing relies on *p*-values and only provides whether the hypothesis is accepted or rejected or difference exists or not exists between the groups.
   e. The statistical significance by itself does not provide any information on clinical applicability of the findings. Large studies can be significant without being clinically important and small studies may be important without being significant (Effective Clinical Practice, July/August 2001, ACP).
   f. Statistically significant differences do not provide clinical insight into important variables such as treatment effect size, magnitude of change, or direction of the outcome. In addition, whether results achieve statistically significant differences is influenced by factors such as the number and variability of subjects, as well as the magnitude of effect. Therefore, *p*-values should be considered along with effect size, sample size, and study design (Sainani, 2009).
   g. Evidence-based practitioners should examine research outcomes for their clinical significance rather than just statistical significance. Several measures can be used to determine clinical relevance including clinical significance, effect sizes, confidence intervals, and magnitude-based inferences.

ii. *Clinical significance:*
   a. Clinical significance is a decision based on the practical importance or relevance of a particular intervention or treatment. This may or may not involve statistical significances.
   b. For determining the clinical significance, the nurse should evaluate research findings for internal and external validity.
   c. Internal validity reveals the amount of bias within a study that may influence the research results. The factors that are influenced in internal validity include proper study design, recruitment of sample, randomization, blinding, standardized tools, etc. and statistical analysis.

d. External validity reveals the ability of a study to be generalized to other population and settings. The factors that are influenced in external validity include complexities of the protocol and cost effectiveness of the intervention. A repeatable protocol enables reproduction of study results in alternate settings. If an intervention is not cost-effective, it may not be feasible in clinical practice. Studies with the highest internal validity may still lack external validity thereby limiting their applicability in clinical setting.
e. The most common question regarding clinical significance is whether the treatment is effective and whether or not it will change clinical practice. Some studies use the term efficacy and effectiveness. While efficacy refers to the benefit of an intervention compared to control or standard treatment under ideal conditions, effectiveness refers to the benefit of an intervention to the greater population, including noncompliant subjects. Treatment efficacy is evaluated using compliant subjects, while treatment effectiveness includes an intent-to-treat analysis of all patients enrolled in the trial. This can be done by including subjects who dropped out in the final analysis thus providing more clinically relevant outcomes.
f. Effect size and confidence intervals (CI) are ways for a researcher to decide if a particular statistical result is of relevance to practice or not. Effect size indicates the magnitude of the difference in outcomes between groups. A high effect size indicates a larger difference between experimental and control groups. The CI provides information about the magnitude and direction of an effect, offering more clinical value than answering a hypothesis-based question.

4. *Generalizing the findings*: Generalizing the findings means the extent to which the research findings can be generalized beyond the given research situation to other settings and subjects. For example, if a new intervention is found to be successful, will it be applicable to other settings? This is termed as external validity. The nurse researchers should assess the generalizability of the findings by considering the research design, sample representativeness, and size of the sample.
   i. If the study used true experimental design, results can be applied to target population.
   ii. If the sample characteristics are representative to the population characteristics, the results can be applied to the entire target population.
   iii. If the sample size is small, it is less likely to be representative. Including larger samples will generalize the results to the target population.
   iv. When interpreting the findings of the study, the researcher examines the risk to validity that may have been introduced at various stages of the research process. These are sample selection process and sample size. If the sample is representative and adequate in number, the obtained results can be applied to the entire target population.

5. *Drawing conclusions*: Study conclusions explain what knowledge has been gained from the present study. They are derived from research findings. While formulating conclusions, the researcher must interpret the results within the

context of the study by considering sample size and characteristics of the sample. In writing conclusions, the researcher returns to the study problem, purpose, hypothesis, and theoretical framework. The researcher attempts to answer the following questions: Was the study problem answered? Was the research purpose met? Was the research hypothesis supported? Was the theoretical framework supported? The researcher should clearly explain to the readers what the study has demonstrated in these areas.

i. The findings of a study are very specific and related to the study data whereas conclusions are more abstract and involve the use of more general terms.

ii. Conclusions are not just a restatement of the findings. Consider the statement: "There is a significant increase in the exercise performance of senior citizens who have used mental practice to increase their performance." This is a finding and not a conclusion. The conclusions should go beyond the findings. A conclusion based on this finding would be: "Mental practice appears to be an effective means of increasing exercise performance in the elderly." Though both seem similar, findings address the difference in exercise performance of senior citizens from the pretest to the posttest, while conclusion is an attempt to generalize the result to other senior citizens and to other points in time. Phrases such as "results of the study indicate" and "study findings demonstrate" link both the summary and meaning of those results.

iii. While forming conclusions it is important to remember that research provides support for a position rather than prove anything.

6. *Suggesting implications for practice and further study:* Once conclusions are drawn, the researcher states the research implications. Research implications are basically conclusions that are taken from results and explain how the findings may affect nursing practice, education, administration and research. In other words, a research implication refers to the impact that research results might have on future prospects in the subject area of research. The research implications are always supported by a strong statistical significance and correlation of results from other research keeping in view the limitations of the study. For every conclusion of a study, there should be at least one implication. Implications may be directed to practitioners, educators, researchers, administrators, etc. The commonly used statements in the implication section of research report include: nurses should..... or nurse educators should..... For example, a study concluded that guided imagery is an effective means of controlling anxiety in preoperative patients. An implication of this conclusion might be nurses should consider using guided imagery technique with preoperative patients. Another implication for nurse educators might be that nurse educators should teach nursing students about the usefulness of guided imagery techniques

7. *Recommendations:* Once researchers have drawn conclusions, they are better placed to make recommendations for future studies. Recommendations urge specific actions to be taken with regard to policy, practice, theory or subsequent research. These are specific suggestions that the researcher makes with regard to logical extension of the present research study by considering the limitations. These recommendations should be presented in the last section of the research report.

i. The researcher should have a broad knowledge of the topic being addressed.

He should combine facts and values while stating the recommendations.

ii. Recommendations are based on the results of research and indicate the specific measures or directions that can be taken. For example, a clinical study might have implications for cancer research and might recommend against the use of a particular hazardous drug. While implications signify the impact of research, recommendations propose concrete steps that need to be taken.

iii. When making a recommendation, the researcher can firmly state what the next steps are to be taken to address a problem, the immediate actions that need to be implemented to solve a particular question, what needs to be corrected and avoided to solve a problem. However, the recommendations should be strongly supported by research findings.

iv. Replication of a research study refers to conducting a study similar to one that has previously been conducted. In replication studies, same hypothesis are tested repeatedly on different samples in different settings to build confidence in research results. Junior researchers conduct replication studies to gain research experience while experienced researchers conduct them to verify previous research results. Overall, the body of nursing knowledge needs to be based on replication studies.

v. Recommendations are not an automatic extension of the results. When recommending future research studies, delimitations and limitations of the present study should invariably be considered. A few examples of frequently made recommendations considering the study limitations are:

   a. Select different characteristics of sample. For example, various age groups, both male and female or subjects with different educational level.
   b. Select a random sample instead of using a convenience sample.
   c. Modify the existing tool or use another tool.
   d. Use interview technique while collecting data from participants rather than using self-report measures.
   e. Implement the intervention for an extended period of 6 weeks instead of 4 weeks.

Common errors while stating conclusions and recommendations are:
- Generalizing the findings beyond the research question, population and interventions that were actually studied.
- Not considering important limitations of the study.
- Falsely interpreting statistical significance.
- Selectively focusing on some results while ignoring others.
- Stating conclusions without having any evidence.

Thus each research report should contain findings, discussion on findings, generalizations, conclusions, implications and recommendations for future research. Table 9.2 differentiates meaning of findings, interpretations, generalizations, conclusions, implications and recommendations.

QUALITATIVE DATA ANALYSIS

Analysis and interpretation of qualitative data is different from quantitative data. It is the process of analyzing raw data to provide explanations, understanding and interpretation of the phenomena, people and situations. The main aim of analyzing

Table 9.2: Meaning of findings, discussion, interpretation, generalization, conclusions, implications and recommendations

Concept	Meaning
Findings	Presentation of the study results in the form of empirical data
Discussion	Interpreting study findings in the light of previous literature review and theoretical context. It also includes problems occurred while conducting the study.
Interpretation	Indicates what the results mean within the study and the context of prior research on the topic
Generalization	Extension of research results beyond study sample
Conclusions	Explains what knowledge has been gained from the study
Implications	Suggests how the findings may be important for practice, theory, administration and subsequent research
Recommendations	Stating specific actions in respect to practice, theory, policy and research

qualitative data is to discover the meaning of abstract or concept. Qualitative findings contribute a great deal of knowledge to nursing science and theory development.

Qualitative data analysis (QDA) involves the identification, examination, and interpretation of patterns and themes in textual data and describes how these patterns and themes answer the research questions (Lewins, Taylor & Gibbs, 2010).

Qualitative research studies are based on broad range of philosophical underpinnings which use various methodological approaches to answer the research question. The questions may concern patient experience, thoughts and feelings of people regarding an incident or event and also why it occurred. The collected data in qualitative studies is in the form of words or text messages.

Purposes

1. To explore, describe, understand, and gain an insight about a particular phenomenon or group of individuals.
2. It helps to search the data and discover underlying themes, core pattern and concepts that become the basis for inferences, interpretation
, and generating hypothetical statements about the meaning of the phenomenon.
3. Analysis can be furthered to construct an explanatory scheme, model or substantive grounded theory.

Qualitative Data Analysis Process

Various approaches to qualitative research analysis are analytical induction, thematic content analysis, phenomenological analysis, narrative analysis, constant comparison, and matrix analysis. The process of analysis includes transformation and interpretation. In qualitative studies, data for analysis is obtained in various forms:

- ❖ Interview transcript from open ended, focused and exploratory interviews
- ❖ Field notes
- ❖ Recorded observations—both audio and video
- ❖ Texts and documents, meeting minutes, E-mails
- ❖ Multimedia or public domain sources, photographs and autobiographical information.

Irrespective of the purpose of the qualitative study and the form in which it is obtained, the researcher ends up with volumes of written text that needs to be analyzed. The common steps involved in qualitative analysis are planning, organizing, transcribing, coding, developing themes, interpreting results, and verifying the data and reporting data (Fig. 9.3).

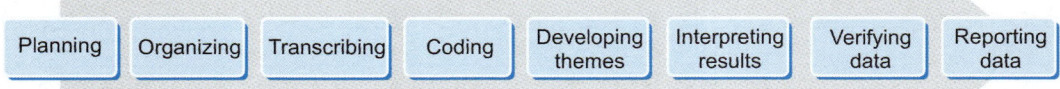

Fig. 9.3: Steps in qualitative analysis

- *Planning*: Data analysis plans differ with specific qualitative type of study undertaken. For example, researchers conducting grounded theory studies use constant comparative process by comparing concepts and themes identified through analysis with those identified in subsequent data. In grounded theory, analysis begins with first participant interview so that ideas from that participant can be integrated into questions and probes in subsequent interviews. In phenomenological studies, this engagement in the data is referred to as dwelling with the data. This phase is used to indicate the considerable time the researcher spent in reading and reflecting on the data.

  In qualitative research studies, the data analysis and data collection go hand in hand. The researcher attempts to collect, handle, and interpret the growing volume of data simultaneously. This requires the researcher to meticulously plan the naming of files and storing the data for retrieval. Computer Assisted Qualitative Data Analysis Software (CAQDAS) programs are available for data management.

- *Organizing:* Gathered data needs to be arranged into a format that is useful for analysis. Data pertaining to each subject (which may be an individual interview or observation note) needs to be placed in a separate file, using a word processing package. All files may be placed in a folder and labeled in a systematic manner. The researcher should read, re-read, and analyze the data over time to maintain a close link with data being analyzed. The software allows the researcher to add thoughts and comments as and when they emerge. This creates an audit trail for the study.

- *Transcribing*: Many qualitative studies collect audio or video data (e.g. recordings of interviews or focus groups), which are usually transcribed into written form for closer study. Transcripts are prepared by typing the recording verbatim (word for word). Voice activated computer programs may also be used for producing a written document of the recording. Verbatim transcript captures participants own words, language and expressions and allows the researcher to decode behavior and cultural meanings attached to participant's viewpoint. The transcripts from such recordings can result in voluminous data for analysis.

- *Coding:* The researcher has to read the transcript again and again and identify words and phrases that occur frequently and organize them into codes or categories. In this phase, researcher moves from raw data to meaningful concepts or themes by coding, categorizing, and developing concepts.
  - Coding is a process of reading the data, breaking down text into subparts and labeling them. These labels help the researcher to identify patterns in

- the data which in turn are used for comparing similarities and differences.
- A code is a symbol or abbreviation used to classify words or phrases in the data. In a word-processing program or CAQDAS, researcher highlights the codes by a section of text and making a comment in the margin or sidebar.
- Codes may result in themes, processes, or exemplars of the phenomenon being studied. When coding data for a phenomenological study, the researcher first labels the emergent meaning in the flow of the transcript (Liamputtong, 2009). A grounded theory researcher first labels statements using open codes to compare the data. In a qualitative study on exploring factors influencing medication adherence, the participants mentioned words like clocks, schedules, and hours. The researcher codes these words as "time". In another explorative descriptive study on pain experiences of surgical patients, codes like type of pain, activities that resulted in pain, and strategies for pain relief emerged. The three stages of coding are presented in Box 9.1.
- Grouping of all concepts belonging to a similar topic into sub-categories is called categorization. From codes, categories can be formed, which in turn can be integrated into one main theme. These themes have thick narrated descriptions of original data. Memos are used to explain categories and themes. These memos are usually in the form of researcher's notes jotted during the research process. The intention is to elaborate on the related thoughts and coded categories. It is an opportunity for the researcher to explore his hunches, thoughts, and ideas and then space them out so as to find broader explanations for them.

❖ *Developing themes*: Themes emerge as codes that are combined into more abstract phrases or terms. Sometimes there are several layers of themes, with each layer further away from the initial codes. Generating links between these themes and the original data may become more complicated as the themes become more abstract. The rigor and clarity in linking are of great importance, and it is the researcher who must remain rigorous in showing the links from the themes back to the original data.

❖ "Identifying salient themes, recurring ideas or language, and patterns of belief that link people and settings together is the most intellectually challenging phase of the analysis and one that can integrate the entire endeavor"(Marshall and Ross, 1995).

Box 9.1	Three stages of coding	
	Open coding:	• Coding original data line-by-line into codes that the researcher determines to be valuable. It is extremely subjective in nature.
	Axial coding:	• Combining original codes into major categories and defining subcategories and their relations to the majors.
	Restricted coding:	• Identifying relationships among codes and categories.

- *Interpreting results:* During interpretation, the researcher should place the findings in a larger context and link different themes or factors in the findings to each other. Interpretation may focus on the usefulness of the findings for clinical practice or used for theorizing. Qualitative research methods include the interpretation of textual material derived from in-depth interviews or observations. While interpreting qualitative findings, the researcher should evaluate for credibility, dependability, confirmability, and transferability.
    - Credibility simply means whether the results are accurate or not. The accuracy can be ascertained based on one's own observation and not on hearsay, circumstances and biases that have gone into reporting of an observation or reliability of the subjects. This explains how consistent the explanations are with the data collected. Negative findings should be effectively dealt with by providing all potentially competing explanations of the results. While interpreting the qualitative results, possible sources of bias should be checked. Bias can be eliminated by the process of reflexivity. Reflexivity involves self-examining one's "conceptual baggage", assumptions and preconceptions, and how these affect research decisions, particularly, the selection and wording of questions. These should be explained adequately while reporting limitations and strengths of the study.
    - Dependability refers to the extent to which a study could be repeated by other researchers with the findings being consistent. In other words, if a replication study needs to be carried out, the research report should provide adequate information on research process so as to arrive at similar results.
    - Confirmability is the degree of neutrality in the study findings. It suggests that the study findings are a result of participants' responses and not associated with researcher's personal bias or motivations. This process ensures that the interpretation of participant's narrative is not distorted by the researcher bias. To establish neutrality of study findings, the researchers highlight every step of data analysis using audit trail to provide a rationale for the decisions made. It helps depict the participant's responses in research findings.
    - Transferability refers to using the findings to make inferences to other similar populations, situations or phenomena. In qualitative research, findings are presented using thick descriptions to convey that the study findings are applicable to other settings, contexts, and situations.
- *Verifying the data*: In qualitative research, the data can be verified by identifying outliers, checking the researcher effect, using triangulation method, obtaining feedback from participants, and external verification of coding strategies.
    - As the researcher peruses the emerged themes and patterns, he should look for negative instances (outliers) which are not fitting to any of the patterns and themes. The researcher should carefully examine and write possible explanations for these negative patterns.
    - Many factors relating to interviewer and the interviewee play an important role in the interaction process during data collection. For example, age, gender, education, cultural background, and language will have an effect on the outcome of the interview. These factors need to be recognized and taken into consideration when doing the analysis. The researcher effects can be reduced

- by selecting the researcher from the same community as he will be seen less of an outsider.
- Accuracy of the research findings can be verified using triangulation. Triangulation means crosschecking research findings using multiple data sources, methods or researchers. For example, the validation of concepts of pain using triangulation method are illustrated below:
  - Using more than one instrument to measure the same concept (the concept of pain is assessed by using self-report method and observation method).
  - Collecting information from multiple sources (interviewing various patients who are suffering with various types of pain to get different perspectives on pain).
  - Using different methods (information on pain is collected by conducting individual interviews or focus groups).
  - Data is collected by different researchers (information on pain is collected by two different researchers).
- The best way for the researcher to assess the validity of the research findings is to seek feedback from study participants and confirm if the interpretation is similar to what they expressed.
- External verification of coding strategies can be done by selecting few passages from qualitative data for developing codes, categories and themes. The same passages are then again given to a colleague for developing codes, categories, and themes which are then compared with the former. This process ensures validity of the data analysis process and the research findings.
- The researcher should acknowledge factors beyond his/her control that may influence the participant's response, *viz*. time of the interview conducted, presence of other people within range during the interview process.

❖ *Reporting data:* The qualitative data report should begin with a brief explanation of data collection process. The result findings should include the process of data coding, various ways of categorizing and sub-categorizing the data, and how individual concepts were used to develop themes and how these themes were put together to build an integrated explanation. The researcher should also refine the concepts, and explain how the concepts were linked together to create a clear description of main theme under study. These themes need to be explained in the light of literature and theoretical framework. This process allows for the emergence of some over-arching themes that can be helpful in binding the individual pieces of the data together (Rubin & Rubin, 1995). This entire method helps the reader to understand the connection between qualitative data, coding structure, and developing themes.

BIBLIOGRAPHY

1. Burns, N. & Grove, S.K. (2001). *The practice of nursing research: Conduct, critique & utilization* (4th ed.). Philadelphia: WB Saunders.
2. Burns, N., & Grove, S.K. (2004). *The practice of nursing research*. Philadelphia: W.B. Saunders Company.
3. Chinn, P.L., & Kramer, M.K. (1995). *Theory and nursing: A systematic approach* (4th ed.). St. Louis: Mosby Yearbook.
4. David, C. Goodman, Elliott, S. Fisher, George, A. Little, Thérèse, A. Stukel, Chiang-hua, Chang et al. (2001). Effective Clinical Practice: the uneven landscape of newborn intensive care services: variation in the neonatology workforce. *American college of physicians*. Philadelphia: WB Saunders, 2(4), 143-9.
5. Fowler, J. & Jarvis, P. (2002). *Practical statistics for field biology* (2nd ed.). Chichester; New York: Wiley.

6. Gravetter, F.J. & Wallnau, L.B. (2012). *Statistics for the behavioral health sciences* (9th ed.). Belmont, CA: Wadsworth.
7. Kerlinger, F.N., & Lee, H.B. (2000). *Foundations of behavioral research*. New York: Harcourt Brace.
8. Lewins, A., Taylor, C., & Gibbs, G. (2010). *What is Qualitative Data Analysis* (QDA)? Retrieved 31/08/2014, from http://onlineqda.hud.ac.uk/Intro_QDA/what_is_qda.php.
9. Liamputtong, P. (2009). *Qualitative research methods*. Australia: Oxford University.
10. Marshall, C., & Rossman, G. (1995). *Designing Qualitative Research*. Thousand Oaks California: Sage Publications.
11. Polit, D.F. (1996). *Data analysis & statistics for nursing research*. Stamford, CT: Appleton and Lange.
12. Polit, D.F., Beck, C.T., & Hungler, B.P. (2001). *Essentials of Nursing Research: Methods, Appraisal, and Utilization* (5th ed.). Philadelphia: Lippincott Williams & Wilkins.
13. Rubin, A., & Rubin, L. (1995). *Qualitative interviewing: the art of hearing data*. London: Sage Publications.
14. Sainani, K. (2010). *Clinical versus statistical significance*. Physical Medicine and Rehabilitation. USA, Stanford University, 4 (6), 442-445.
15. Sainani, K. (2010). *Problem of multiple testing*. Physical Medicine and Rehabilitation, USA, Stanford University, 1(12):1098-103 DOI:10.1016/j.pmrj.2009.10.004.
16. Treece, E.W., & Treece, J.H. (1989). *Elements of Research in Nursing*, The C.V. Mosby Co., St. Louis.

REVIEW QUESTIONS

I. Long Essays
1. Describe in detail the phases of quantitative data analysis.
2. Describe qualitative data analysis process.

II. Short Essays
1. Describe in detail the levels of measurement.
2. What is data verification? How will you organize the data in quantitative research studies?
3. Write on different ways of presentation of data.
4. Describe how to interpret the descriptive statistics?
5. Explain interpretation of independent samples t-test.
6. Explain statistical and clinical significance.

III. Short Notes
1. Outliers
2. Wild code
3. Data cleaning
4. Univariate analysis

IV. Multiple Choice Questions
1. Which of the following methods is appropriate for the presentation of research findings?
   a. Tables
   b. Figures
   c. Both a and b
   d. Only Figures
2. Consider the following conclusion: "There is a positive relationship between children's anxiety levels and their failure to cooperate with physical examinations". Determine appropriate implications derived from this conclusion.
   a. Nurses must discover why high anxiety levels cause children to be uncooperative during physical examinations
   b. Nurses should try to assess the anxiety levels of children before physical examinations
   c. Physical examinations for small children should be conducted less frequently

d. A parent should be instructed to remain in the room with the child during a physical examination
3. The recommendations of a study might contain which of the following?
   a. A discussion of the study findings
   b. Suggestions for extension of the study
   c. Comparisons of results with previous research findings
   d. Comparison of results with similar studies
4. Interpretation of quantitative study results is useful to:
   a. Determine the statistical significance of the findings
   b. Give a reason for the study
   c. Perform action oriented activities
   d. Determine the usefulness of the findings for practice
5. Data analyses are conducted to reduce, organize, and give meaning to the data. Data analyses are used to produce which of the following?
   a. Conclusions
   b. Results
   c. Implications
   d. All of the above
6. The test that specifies certain condition about the parameter of the population from which a sample is taken is known as:
   a. Parametric test
   b. Non-parametric test
   c. Chi-square test
   d. Mann–Whitney test
7. If there is no knowledge about the population or parameters, but still is required to test the hypothesis of the population then the statistical test is called:
   a. Parametric test
   b. Nonparametric test
   c. F-test
   d. t-test
8. Bivariate analysis means:
   a. Examination of one variable
   b. Examination of two variables
   c. Examination of three variables
   d. Examination of many variables
9. The following are characteristics of a parametric test, *except*:
   a. When samples are large enough to achieve normality
   b. It has more statistical power than the nonparametric test
   c. They do not rely on normal distribution
   d. Assumptions that the data fall into a normal or bell-shaped distribution
10. Nonparametric test examples involve:
    a. Mann–Whitney & chi-square test
    b. "t" test and "F" test
    c. "Z" test and ANOVA test
    d. Only b and c
11. Levels of measurement in ascending order are:
    a. Nominal, ordinal, ratio, interval
    b. Nominal, ordinal, interval, ratio
    c. Interval, ordinal, nominal, ratio
    d. Ordinal, nominal, ratio, interval

ANSWER KEY

1. c	2. d	3. b	4. d	5. d	6. a
7. b	8. b	9. c	10. a	11. b	

UNIT 10

Dissemination (Communication) and Utilization of Research Findings

Communicating research findings is the concluding stage in the research process. A research project cannot be considered complete until the research results are effectively communicated to its users and consumers. Communication of the research findings is carried out through dissemination process.

MEANING OF DISSEMINATION

The word dissemination denotes communication or flow of information from a source. It includes a series of activities designed to transfer generated empirical research evidence (research findings/knowledge) to a target audience (users and consumers) either by written or oral means.

It is the process of obtaining important or key information from research results and communicating it to the intended subjects or the decision makers so as to encourage the implementation of the research findings into their work.

Dissemination means "to distribute or scatter about" (Collins English Dictionary, 3rd ed. 1994).

Dissemination is the process by which target group become aware of, receive and utilize information (Freemantle and Watt, 1994)

FEATURES OF DISSEMINATION

- ❖ It is an integral part of the research process.
- ❖ In dissemination information is specific to the intended audience.
- ❖ Dissemination of research findings is much more than formal publication in journals or books and can include non-refereed publications, web pages, other media and digital repositories.
- ❖ For effective dissemination the researcher should have adequate knowledge, creativity, clinical judgment, and skills.

The growth of and support for nursing research are reflected by the impressive number of journals dedicated to the publication of nursing research studies.

PURPOSES OF DISSEMINATION (IMPORTANCE OF COMMUNICATING RESEARCH FINDINGS)

Regardless of how innovative research is, it will not make an impact unless it is communicated in a timely manner to the audiences that can directly benefit from it. If the research findings are not communicated and used by other nurses, the conduct of research becomes an unproductive effort. The various purposes of dissemination are presented in Figure 10.1.

- ❖ Effective dissemination leads to increased awareness of the research results and maximizes the impact the research can

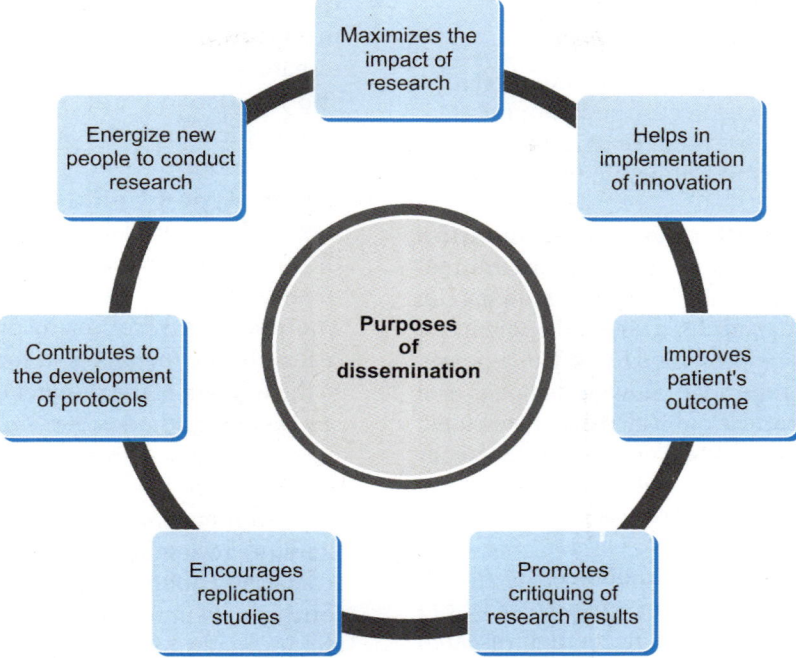

Fig. 10.1: Purposes of dissemination

have in improving the health outcomes of the patients
- Effective dissemination can support the staff in sharing information on the progress in healthcare practices and simultaneously adopt and implement the innovations where necessary.
- Dissemination ultimately leads to improved patient outcomes and advances the body of knowledge unique to the nursing discipline
- It promotes the critiquing of research results and encourages replication studies. Replication means repeating the same study on different samples. When the study has been replicated multiple times with similar results, the evidence can be used with more confidence.
- Quality nursing care can be provided only if the results are communicated by the researchers.
- Dissemination is a key process in evidence-based practice. To have an impact on clinical practice the research findings should be implemented into clinical practice, which can happen only through dissemination.
- If the researcher disseminates research activity effectively it will contribute to the development of effective protocols and policies.
- Effective dissemination can bring marked changes in clinical practice and motivate the passive nurse to conduct or participate in research.

A greater amount of effort needs to be exercised by the nurse in implementing research findings as compared to the effort put in while conducting research. This can only be achieved by effective dissemination.

CRITERIA FOR EFFECTIVE DISSEMINATION

Once the statistical analysis and interpretation is done, the findings need to be communicated. In order to report the research findings the researcher has to follow the below criteria (Fig. 10.2).

- **Select an effective communication channel**: Research can be communicated orally or in writing. Oral presentations can be a formal talk for a targeted audience. It can also be presented by way of a poster. Written report can however appear as a research article published in a professional journal or website. The student researcher selects outlets like thesis and dissertation or publishes in professional journals, books.
- **Knowing the target audience**: The researcher should know in advance to whom they want to communicate their research findings. For example, to bedside nurses, nurse educators, nurse administrators, health care professionals or to the general public. This will help in choosing the right method of communication.
- **Develop a plan**: Before beginning the preparation of research reports the researcher should develop a plan which should also include decision about communication outlets and the audience for the report.
- **Decide type of publication**: Nurse Researchers publish research not only in nursing journals but also in several medical, health or clinical based journals. The decision whether to publish in a research or clinical based journal is left to the wisdom of the researcher. Research studies and methodologies are most suited for scholarly research journals. Clinical and evidence based guidelines, quality improvement, program evaluation and literature review are most often published in specialty publications or clinical based journals. Depending upon the focus of the journal a researcher may expand a specific section of the research report. For example, the researcher may write more on discussion of findings in relation to nursing practice in clinical journals. On the other hand if journals are research based

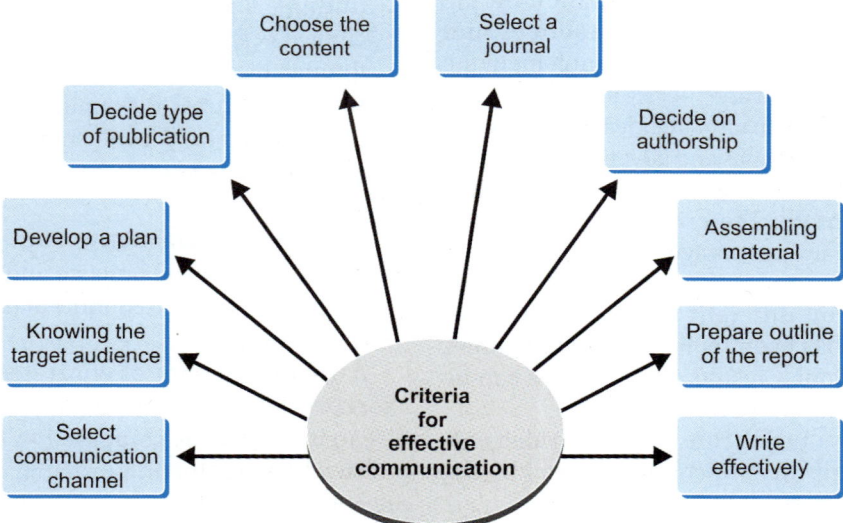

Fig. 10.2: Criteria for effective dissemination

the researcher might write more on the methodology section of the manuscript.

- **Choose the content**: It includes decision on how many pages are required to communicate the findings effectively and what aspect of the study to write on in a given paper. Most of the journals limit the manuscript to 15-20 double spaced typed pages. Researchers who collect both qualitative and quantitative data often report on each separately. Each paper from a study should independently make a contribution to the subject knowledge. Unnecessary duplication or overlap should be avoided. It is also considered unethical to submit essentially the same or similar paper to two journals simultaneously.

- **Select a journal for publication**: For selecting a suitable journal some important factors to be considered are, the journal's goal, audience, frequency of publication, citation details and acceptance procedure.

- **Deciding on authorship**: On completion of the study by a team of member, deciding on authorship is important. The international committee of medical journal editors (ICMJE) advises that authorship credit should only be given to those who have made a substantial contribution to the conception and design of the study or to data analysis and interpretation, drafting or revising the manuscript and approving the final version of the manuscript. The lead author is usually the first named author. The lead author and co-authors should segregate the roles and responsibilities in preparation of manuscript well in advance. While doing so the order of authors also needs to be finalized. However, when the contributions are comparable, the names of co-authors are listed alphabetically.

- **Assembling material**: The researcher should read the guidelines for journals manuscript and clearly understand them before the actual writing begins. The researcher should also assemble the relevant literature and references, description of the study sample, output of the computer analysis, figures, photographs and permissions to use copy right material if any.

- **Prepare outline of the report**: Written outlines are very useful to organize the material. An outline provides the direction for inclusion of content to be covered in the manuscript and also includes headings and sub-headings. The outline should also include the timeline for completing the manuscript. Journal guidelines need to be followed for publishing a research article in a journal while the university guidelines need to be followed for submission of thesis or dissertation.

- **Write effectively**: Writing well is a key component which is supported by resources that suggest on how to frame sentences, select appropriate words and organize the thoughts effectively. It is better to prepare the entire draft and then review for incomplete sentences, spelling mistakes and grammatical errors followed by reorganization of sentences.

On the whole research findings provide guidelines for establishing care standards, framing policies and support effective patient care delivery. If the researcher is not competent enough to share and spread the research findings or results, the above developments cannot be achieved. Research findings can be communicated through research report which can take many forms. Nursing research is of little value if the results are never communicated to other nurses.

RESEARCH REPORT

A research report is complete only when the research findings have been disseminated through a research report. Writing a report is the last step in research study and requires special skills. To complete this task the researcher needs assistance and guidance from experts. Preparing a research report is not only an important component but also an integral part of the research process.

Meaning of Research Report

❖ Research report is a brief description of the research work done by the researcher.
❖ A research report summarizes key aspects of the study and includes the following elements: title, introduction, methods, results, discussion and conclusions.

Characteristics of Research Report

❖ *Focus:* An effective report should center on important information.
❖ *Accuracy*: An effective report emphasizes on accurate information and does not mislead the reader.
❖ *Clarity:* An effective report should be clear and not confuse the reader.
❖ *Conciseness:* A report should concise the information and not waste the reader's time.

Guidelines for Preparing Research Report

A well written research report is one which effectively, efficiently and widely disseminates the research information to its users. A good research report should follow certain guidelines (Box 10.1).

Steps in Writing Research Report

Preparing an effective research report is very different from composing a regular essay or a report. The skills required are incredibly distinct and must be practiced in order to be fully mastered. Though not taught as frequently or in as much depth as they should be, they are nevertheless essential skills. Scientific writing requires modesty, objectivity, and openness to new possibilities. They should be composed in clear English using short and direct sentences avoiding jargon. The research report should give attention to all the details and be mindful of the underlying scientific theories that are related to the empirical work.

Box 10.1	Guidelines for preparing research report

- Be objective
- Minimize the use of technical language
- Treat the data confidentially
- Revise and rewrite
- Use visual aids
- Show originality
- Use appropriate layout in accordance with the objective
- Free from grammatical mistakes
- Subject matter should be presented in a logical sequence
- Index must be prepared, attractive in appearance, neat and clear
- Use headings and sub-headings to attract the reader's attention
- The methodology and findings in the final report are written in past tense
- Have peer review of the research report if possible
- Bibliography of sources consulted is a must for a good report
- Appendices should enlist all the technical data in the report

The steps involved in writing research report are presented in Figure 10.3.

❖ *Assembling and arranging the subject-matter:* Assembling and arranging often consists of developing the material from the simplest possible to the most complex structures. These are based on a connection or sequence and generally follow the chronological order.
❖ *Preparing the layout*: It is the next important step where in a faint outline is prepared which serves as the framework upon which the whole report is built. This preparation of layout helps in logical organization of the material and prompts on the points to be stressed in the report.
❖ *Preparing a preliminary draft*: This is in furtherance to the previous step wherein the researcher actually writes down what he has done. It includes the procedure adopted for conducting the study, limitations, analysis techniques adopted, broad findings and generalizations.

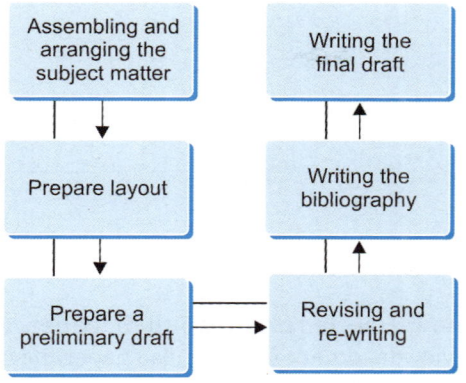

Fig. 10.3: Steps in writing research report

Remember to cite all sources even in the draft.
- *Revising and rewriting*: This step involves careful revision of the preliminary draft to overcome the flaws in logical development and presentation. The researchers should emphasize on cohesion, distinct pattern and consistency. Due focus should also be given to grammar, spelling and usage.
- *Writing the bibliography*: It should include the list of books and works that have contributed or been consulted in preparation of the research report.
- *Writing the final draft*: This constitutes the last step. The final draft should have very few errors, be clearly organized and formatted correctly. Brevity and objective style of presentation should be the main feature. Use of simple language and avoiding vague expressions should be encouraged. The final report must motivate the reader and generate interest. Last but not the least every report should in a way contribute to the solution of the problem and must add knowledge to the profession.

Types of Research Report

Research reports are written for different purposes. Accordingly they comprise of different information and structure, including headings and subheadings. A report is prepared for publishing in journals, presenting in the conferences (oral and poster presentation), writing dissertations or thesis (Fig. 10.4).

Publication in Journals

One method of communicating research findings is through publication. The main purpose of nursing research is to build knowledge and disseminate it through publications. The preparation of a research report or manuscript for publication differs little among journals. The following are the steps in preparing manuscript for publication (Fig. 10.5).

Select a journal: Before selecting a journal for publishing the researcher should consider the following factors which will greatly reduce the chances of rejection:
- Select a journal that will match the subject focus of the article and reach the target audience

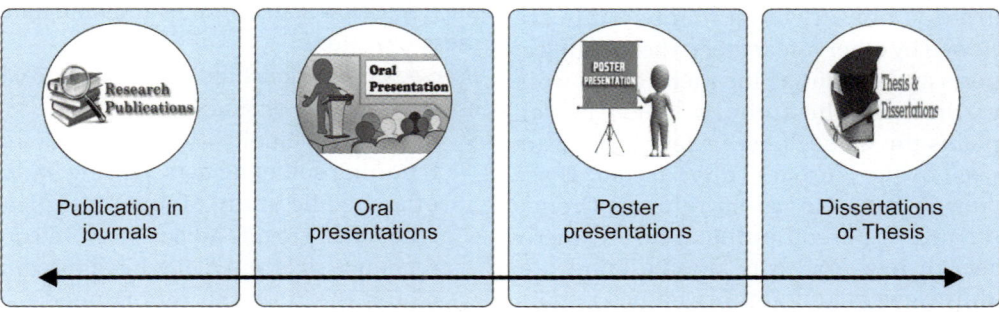

Fig. 10.4: Types of research report

Fig. 10.5: Steps in preparing manuscript for publication

- Ensure the appropriateness of the proposed article to the journal's scope and aims
- Determine the impact factor/journal rank/article influence/H-index which are generally linked to citation rate of articles
- Check for journal requirements like word count, publication charges, style of writing, peer review period, publication timeline, publication mode (online/print) and frequency of publication

The journal can be chosen either before or after the manuscript is ready. If the manuscript has already been prepared, the author can search for a journal which best suits the proposed article. On the other hand an appropriate journal can be selected based on the content of the article and manuscript prepared in accordance with the journal guidelines. If the manuscript does not suit the journal's scope the acceptance of the publication is minimal.

The author must in advance decide whether to publish the manuscript in a refereed or a non-refereed journal. A refereed journal is one in which manuscripts are reviewed by other researchers who are subject experts and can judge the merit of the work (i.e., these are the author's "peers", which explains the name "peer review"). They are chosen by the journal's editorial staff. These reviewers are also called referees (hence the name "refereed publication"). Mostly a peer review process is "double-blind" i.e. both reviewers and authors names remain anonymous to each other (authors do not know who is reviewing their paper, and reviewers do not know whose paper they are reviewing). Non-refereed journal is one that publishes articles that have not gone through a formal peer review process.

Send query letter: A query letter is written to an editor to determine the level of interest the editor has regarding publishing a research report. A query letter contains a brief description of the title, purpose of the study, methods, results, implications of the study, names and credentials of investigators. Most journals do not require it, but these letters can save the researcher a lot of time. If an editor is interested in the manuscript, he or she will ask the researcher to submit the entire manuscript.

Locate and read author guidelines: Most professional publications give author guidelines to instruct authors about page limit, specific instructions on preparing tables and figures, type of referencing, types of articles accepted, formatting, the review and submission process. It is essential that the researcher reads, understands and follows these directions.

Prepare publication: Prepare outline and write effectively based on guidelines.

- Researcher should also follow a standard reporting guideline for reporting findings of a specific study (Table 10.1). These guidelines provide advice on word count, reference style and major headings under which the research report need to be written.

Table 10.1: Guidelines for reporting findings of a research study

Type of research study	Guidelines	Description
Randomized control study	CONSORT (Consolidated Standards of Reporting Trials)—Appendices 12 and 13	It suggests strategies for authors to prepare complete and transparent RCT reports and aid their critical appraisal and interpretation.
Observational study	STROBE (Strengthening the Reporting of Observational Studies in Epidemiology)—Appendix 14	It offers a checklist of items that should be included in articles reporting observational studies.
Case report	CARE (Reporting Guidelines for Case Reports)—Appendix 15	It offers a standard way for authors to systematically report data and evaluate submissions for medical journals. These guidelines help reduce bias and increase transparency.
Systematic reviews and meta-analysis	PRISMA (Preferred Reporting Items for Systematic Reviews and Meta-Analyses)—Appendices 16 and 17	It is useful for critical appraisal of published systematic reviews and helps authors improve the reporting of systematic reviews and meta-analysis.
Non-randomized studies	TREND (Transparent Reporting of Evaluations with Non-randomized Designs)—Appendices 18 and 19	It promotes transparent reporting of intervention studies, improve research synthesis and advance evidence-based recommendations for best practices and policies.

❖ *Organize the content*: Most of the journal guidelines instruct the authors to organize the manuscript under the following headings. • Title Page • Abstract • Introduction • Methods • Results • Discussion • Conclusions • Acknowledgments • References • Tables and Table Captions • Figures and Figure Captions.
  ○ Title Page: This page should include the title of the manuscript, authors and author affiliations, key words, short or running title and complete contact information of the corresponding author.
  ○ Abstract: An abstract concisely summarizes the article and is usually a paragraph in length. It is a prospect to grab the reader's attention and promote their curiosity to continue read the complete article. The method for writing the abstract, particularly regarding headings and word limits is usually provided in the 'guidelines for authors' section. The abstract ought to be regarded as an independent document, wherein both the content of the abstract and the body of the report do not depend on each other. The abstract should start with the objectives or aims of the study followed by a brief description of how the investigation was carried out and the study results. It should conclude with a description of the significance of the results and its impact in the field of study. Care must be taken that the descriptions are as precise as possible without being verbose.
  ○ Introduction: This section should include background of the problem in a manner that the significance of the study is evident early in the paper. It calls for a brief literature review pertaining to the research study so as to blend the ideas and point the gaps in literature. Beginning with a broad

topic, the introduction should narrow down to the area of the study. It can begin with small opening sentences familiarizing the reader with the area of research. Conceptual or theoretical framework should find a place in this section. The final paragraph is critical which should focus on the hypotheses, questions or aims that shall be answered by the present study. Next, a brief description of the approach that was taken to test the hypothesis can be given. Finally, a summary remark at the end stating how the answer to the research problem will contribute to the overall field of the study may be included.

- Methods: This section describes the methods employed in the study enabling others to replicate it. The content in this section and the title may vary depending on what is being reported. This section includes design, setting, sampling procedure, population, protection of human subjects, data collection instrument and procedures, and data analysis techniques. A description of the statistical methods used to analyze the results may be included in the closing remarks of the section. Explanations may be kept brief and concise.
- Results: Often presented using tables and figures, this section includes the research findings or evaluation of what one did. Discussion or interpretation of the data should be avoided in this section. Each table and figure needs to be introduced in a separate paragraph and cited in the text. For experimental studies, key statistics such as the number of samples (n), the index of central tendency (mean, median or mode), the index of dispersion (SD, SEM), type of statistical test performed and p-values should be included. Descriptions should invariably be brief.
- Discussion: It is a place where the researcher would like to point out what he did and what new knowledge he discovered. The discussion section may begin with a brief overview to the work followed by identification of notable and significant findings presented in the results section and compare these with existing literature, conceptual or theoretical framework. The inferred results should further be interpreted so as to elicit suggestions in the direction of practice and research. This should ease the construction of logical arguments for supporting or rejecting the hypothesis and finally aid in making recommendations that may be made for the future study and development. Other relevant literature that addresses the topic and how the present work contributed to the overall field of study may be included at the end of the discussion section. Limitations should be discussed but not focused upon. Over generalizations may be avoided.
- Conclusions: The work may first be introduced followed by a brief statement of the major results. Major points of the discussion may be mentioned, ending it with a statement on how the study contributed to the profession in a major way.
- Acknowledgments: It is a brief statement recognizing the contributing role of participants or consultants who do not meet the requirements for authorship but have provided a valuable contribution to the work. Source of funding for the study may be stated ensuring that the statement adheres to the guidelines provided by the funding institution.

- References: All references quoted in the text should invariably be included in this section. The references should be well compiled to include all the key sources and previous studies that support or inspire the present work. However, extraneous references should not be included in an effort to simply cite particular authors or journals. While submitting the manuscript, reference format mandated by the journal should be used. Organizing and formatting of references be done using reference managers.
- Tables and Table Captions: Tables are usually placed in a separate section after references. Each table should have a title in bold (i.e., Table 1: Socio-demographic characteristics), followed by a presentation of data which should comply with the content in the main text. The table should be formatted so as to clearly present the data and be easily interpreted by the reviewer. Ensure that each table is referred to in the manuscript text.
- Figures and Figure Captions: Like tables, figures are also placed in a separate section after references. Appropriateness and clarity are the key factors while demonstrating the data using graphs and figures. As in the case of tables, both graphs and figures should comply with the content of the text. All figures should include accurate scale bars and explanatory notes to help the readers understand the meaning without referring to the main text. In graphs the data points and axis labels should be in a large font. Legends can be included within the graph or in the caption. All figures should have a brief title in bold and present the significant results.
- Originality: Plagiarism needs to be considered while submitting for publication. It refers to the use of another person's ideas or statements with no due credit to the original author. As plagiarism is a major concern, the author should ensure proper citation where an original research paper contains any form of previously published data. Many anti-plagiarism software are available to detect plagiarism of words and phrases.
- Authorship: The three criteria for authorship include those who provide substantial contribution to the formulation of the study design or analysis and interpretation of data, those who draft or revise the article and those who take up the responsibility for the published version (Benos et al., 2005; Graf et al., 2007).
- There should be a consensus on the order of authorship among all the authors and any other personnel who are a part of the study but not included as an author.
- Duplicate publication / submission: It refers to submitting the same article around the same time to more than one journal or revising a previously published article and submitting it to an alternate journal for publication. It not only dissipates the valuable resources but also violates international copyright laws. It results in double-counting of research work and leads to distortion of evidence-based medicine. While artificially enlarging one's scientific work such duplication also gives unfair advantage in career growth and contention for research funds.

❖ *Submit manuscript*: Once the manuscript is ready for journal submission, it has to be uploaded in the portal along with a covering letter. The covering letter should include title of the paper, details of all the authors and contact information of the corresponding author. Undertakings as regards the originality of the paper, non-submission of the article to other journals, approval of the authors and no-conflict of interest need to be given.

❖ *Review, Revision, Rejection and Re-submission process*
  ○ Review: Peer reviewed journal usually assigns the articles to two to four reviewers to critique the manuscript. In most cases the author is blinded to the reviewers of the manuscript. Along with the reviewers the editorial staff may also critique the manuscript based on its originality, timeliness of the problem, objectivity, honesty, completeness, readability and rigor of the study. Finally, the editor takes a decision regarding acceptance with revision, revision with a second review or rejection. Most journals specify the probable review time when they receive a manuscript.
  ○ Revision: The researcher needs to address the reviewer's comments point by point. Resubmission should include a covering letter mentioning how the corrections were handled. If the researcher chooses not to accept some of the comments, a clear rationale should be provided. Directions and timeline for resubmission may vary based on the journal.
  ○ Rejection: A poorly written manuscript or inaccuracies in the content are the most common reasons for rejection. The other reasons for rejection may include methodology problems, clinically not applicable or statistical problems. While rejecting the article, most editors provide the author with reasons for rejection along with reviewer's comments. The researcher needs to take an objective look at the constructive criticism. The comments should be used to redraft the article and submit to another journal, but not to the original journal. Rejection of an article is not an indicator of the quality of the article. It may not probably be appropriate for that particular journal or the journal may have recently published a similar article.

Other publication opportunities include book reviews, electronic journals, evidence-based guidelines, policy briefs and quality improvement articles. The advantages and disadvantages of publication are presented in Table 10.2.

Table 10.2: Advantages and disadvantages of publication

Advantages	Disadvantages
• Can reach a larger audience based on the circulation of the particular journal. • Dissemination can occur more rapidly through electronic means. • The articles found in many scholarly journals go through a peer review process and therefore the information is reliable. • Many journals include comprehensive information of the research study.	• Likelihood of delay in actual publication of the report and poor feedback from target group. • E-journals are not always referred. • Increased potential for plagiarism.

Oral Presentation

In an oral presentation also referred to as a paper presentation, the report of the study is presented to the group of professionals at conferences. It is another method of communicating a research report. Presentations can be done formally at local, national or international level and informally among peers. Before the conference the authors are invited to submit a research abstract based on the conference theme in a given format. In an oral presentation the **IMRAD** (**I**ntroduction, **M**ethodology, **R**esults, **a**nd **D**iscussion) format is followed similar to a journal article. If the submission is accepted the researcher needs to attend the conference and present the paper. During such conferences the researcher is given about 15–30 minutes to present the findings and another 5 minutes to interact with the audience and clarify their doubts. This interaction enables the researcher to not only get an early feedback but also expand on the various aspects of the study. This can be helpful in writing manuscript for journal submission. Some of the important suggestions for oral presentation are:

- Oral presentations are appropriate when the research study has a limited scope.
- Informal or conversational delivery makes the presentations more effective rather than being read verbatim.
- The researcher should rehearse the presentation several times to familiarize himself with the script and keep a check on the allotted time.
- Dress appropriately and make eye contact with the audience during the presentation
- Check presentation hall before hand to become familiar with the environment.
- The challenge for the researcher is to limit the report to only the essential points of the study.
- Researchers often use slides, overheads or handouts to further communicate their findings at presentations.
- The text slides should preferably contain no more than six lines per slide and seven words per line.
- Bullet statements should be presented.
- Use of simple language and minimal technical jargon is suggested.
- Choose the right font such as Times New Roman or Arial. Text written in all capital letters may be avoided.
- The recommended font sizes for title lines is 44, major text is 32 and minor text is 24 with a 1.5 line spacing so that the lines are easier to follow.
- Use contrasting colors but at the same time restrict the use of many colors.
- Use schematic diagrams in methodology section and graphs in the results section. Let each graph make one specific point, and plan to put just one graph on each slide. Be sure to clearly state the axes when discussing each graph.
- Photos can be used effectively to break up the monotony of text and graphs and also keep the audience's attention.
- If one must provide a table, not more than four columns and three rows may be included for effective reception by audience. Another way of dealing with this is to highlight the column or row under discussion.
- Encourage questions and discussion after presentation. Answer the questions and end the presentation by thanking the audience for attending the session.
- Ensure that the closing is natural, provide contact information and inform the audience that the questions are welcome over email.

The advantages and disadvantages of the oral presentation are presented in Table 10.3.

Table 10.3: Advantage and disadvantages of oral presentation

Advantages	Disadvantages
• Ability to disseminate findings much more quickly. • Ability to get feedback from participants during or after the presentation. This helps the researcher to rethink on the research findings.	• Information is transmitted to limited number of people. • Very little time to establish context of research. • Little opportunity for in-depth discussion on results. • Uncomforting for those who dislike presenting to larger groups.

Poster Presentation

- Poster presentation is another method of communicating a research report wherein the researcher summarizes the highlights of the study using visual graphic presentation. Here the study results are examined by the audience with or without the active interaction of the investigator.
- Research conferences usually include poster sessions for which 1–2 hours are allotted. During these sessions several researchers display their posters in a specified area. The conference attendees go around this exhibit area and examine the displays. This provides the attendees an ample opportunity to focus on topics of interest, interact with the particular researcher and avoid posters of little interest.
- The researcher should be present at the poster location all through the session and ensure effective communication. Presenter interacts with the audience one-on-one and answers questions as they arise.
- The poster size varies as per the specifications indicated in the research conference. Most researchers supplement the poster presentation with written handouts.
- This visual method of presentation can reach a greater audience in a short period.

The main purpose of poster presentation is educating others about research findings and getting feedback from peers before submitting a manuscript for publication.

Points to be focused upon while preparing a poster are:

- The poster should be to the point and must be presented in a way that is easily understood.
- The major titles should preferably be of large size, at least 1 inch high enabling the viewers to see these letters from about 3 feet away.
- Typed material should be set with minimum 16 font size. Avoid using ALL CAPS.
- Use correct grammar and spelling.
- Use of phrases instead of sentences may be encouraged as much as possible.
- Avoid background graphics that make the text difficult to read.
- Use of color is encouraged but it is ideal to limit their number. Light colored background with black or dark colored text print is preferred.
- Graphs and photographs may be used to highlight the results. Technical assistance of a graphic artist may be sought where necessary.
- Diagrams, graphs and tables must be effectively used to present certain aspects of the study.
- Give citations on a poster when paraphrasing other's work. Use appropriate style when citing.
- Posters should contain the following information (Fig. 10.6):
  - Heading: Title of the poster, authors of the poster with affiliations.
  - Introduction: Should be concise and visually pleasing.
  - Research problem statement and hypothesis.
  - Methodology: Research design, sample characteristics, sample size, variables, measurements and methods of data collection.
  - Results: Findings can be presented using easy to read table(s) or concise bullets. Explain only interesting findings.
  - Implications: Provide information on how the findings can help practitioners, educators and administrators.
  - Acknowledgments: Briefly acknowledge the individuals who assisted with the project and funding sources.

Points to be focused upon while presenting a poster are:

- Attire should be professional, wear name tag
- Smile and make eye contact with people who pass the poster

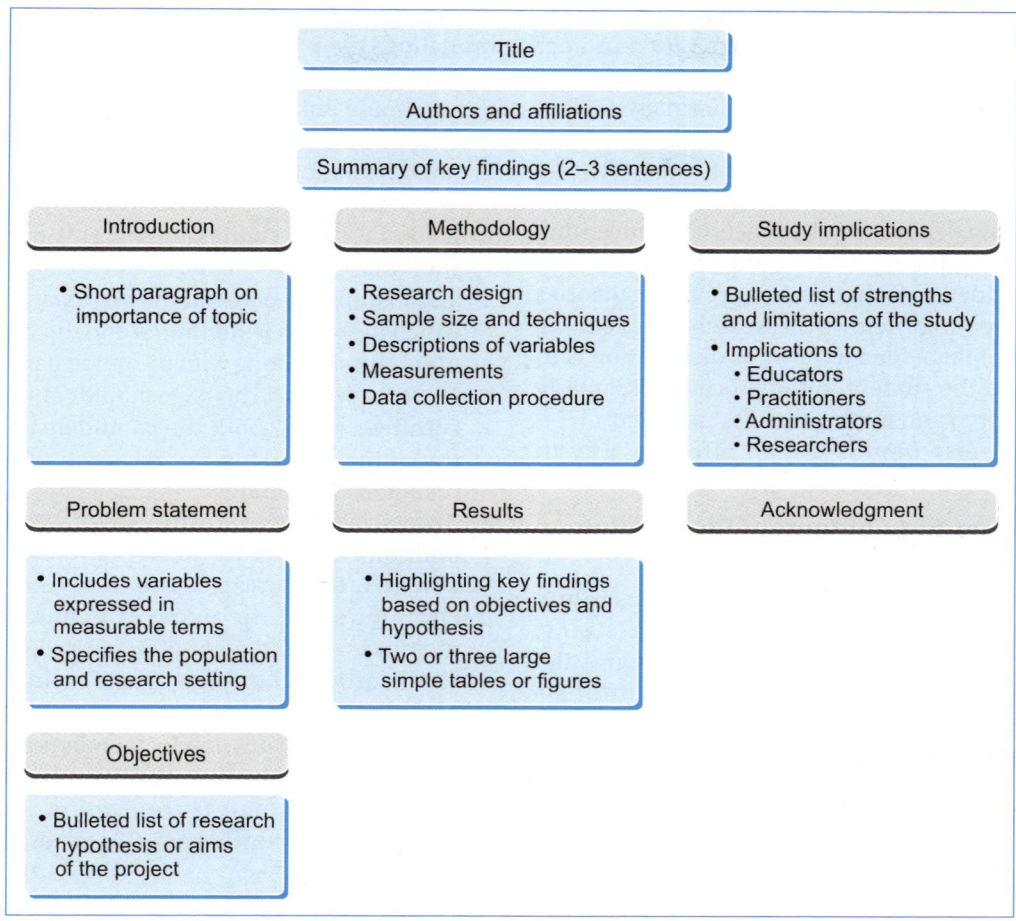

Fig. 10.6: Poster layout

- Allow the viewers time to read the poster without interruption
- Greet viewers with a hello and offer to answer any questions they may have
- Do not take criticism personally

The advantages and disadvantages of the poster presentation are presented in Table 10.4.

Table 10.4: Advantages and disadvantages of poster presentation

Advantages	Disadvantages
• A poster session has the potential to reach a larger number of people than a typical oral presentation • It allows one-to-one interaction with people interested on particular research • Poster sessions make it possible for a huge number of researchers to present their findings at conferences	• Once a poster is printed it is difficult to make corrections, thus less flexible when compared to a presentation • Limited number read the poster • Limited amount of information can be presented

DISSERTATION OR THESIS

A dissertation or thesis contains author's research findings that are submitted in partial fulfillment of attaining a professional qualification. Though used interchangeably, the words 'thesis' and 'dissertation' represent two different types of academic papers. The word 'thesis' refers to the final project submitted as a part of the bachelor's or master's course, while 'dissertation' is normally applied to a doctoral degree. A dissertation contains more in-depth investigation than a thesis and offers new knowledge for the profession. While a thesis is usually concerned with testing existing theory, a dissertation requires the candidate to focus on refining existing theories or creating their own research. The leading principle behind a thesis or dissertation is to guide the student in the process of scholarly research and writing the research report.

These papers are an effective way to communicate the research findings.

Format and Contents of Dissertation or Thesis

Universities generally have a prescribed format for their thesis and dissertations; however basic content mainly remains the same. The commonly used format consists of preliminary material, main body and end report (Table 10.5).

Preliminary Material

The pages in the preliminary material are numbered using small roman numerals (e.g. ii. iii, iv, etc.) while the main body papers are numbered using Arabic numerals. A 1½ inch left margin is allowed to provide enough space to bind the final copies. One inch top (about one inch to the first line of text), bottom, and right margins are allowed throughout the paper including preliminary pages and appendices. The text, tables and figures should remain within the margins.

- *Title page:* The title page should include the title of the study. It should be concise and indicate the purpose of the study. It should be in capital letters. This page should also include name of the researcher and institution, name of the university to which the report is submitted and the year of submission along with the guide name.
- *Declaration page:* This page should contain certificates from both the candidate and the guide declaring the research work bonafide and genuine.
- *Acknowledgments:* It expresses gratitude and appreciation to those people who contributed towards the successful completion of the work. It generally includes the guide, co-guide, principal/HOD, other faculty members, ethical committee members, statistician, study participants, friends, family members and other people. If the research is funded by organizations, their patronization also needs to be acknowledged. It is generally 1–2 pages long.
- *Table of contents:* This should include the sequence of the contents placed in the thesis/dissertation with respective page numbers. This facilitates easy location of information for the reader.

Table 10.5: Format of thesis or dissertation

Preliminary material	Main body	End report
• Title page • Declaration page • Acknowledgments • Table of contents • List of tables • List of figures • List of appendices • Abbreviations • Abstract	Chapters 1. Introduction 2. Review of literature 3. Methodology 4. Results 5. Discussion 6. Summary and conclusions	• References • Appendix/Annexure

- *List of tables, figures, appendices:* This includes a list of table and figure headings, appendices in a sequence as they have been placed in the thesis/dissertation with corresponding page numbers.
- *Abbreviations:* It includes description of the abbreviations used in the thesis/dissertation for facilitating smooth reading.
- *Abstract:* It is a concise summary of research report which includes introduction, objectives, methodology, results and implications for clinical practice and recommendations. It should be written in 150–300 words. A well written abstract provides the reader with an overview of the remaining sections of the report.

Main Body

Until recently most universities used **IMRAD** format (**I**ntroduction, **M**ethodology, **R**esults, **a**nd **D**iscussion) for presenting the main body. The content of the main body can be divided into the following six chapters:

Chapter 1: Introduction

- The first chapter introduces the study and begins with background information on the research problem under investigation. Introduction provides the readers a short summary of literature and leads up to the statement of the problem. It generally begins with a broader perspective of the problem and narrows down as the text proceeds further.
- This section includes current literature, the study's conceptual framework, the problem statement, operational definitions, research questions, assumptions, hypotheses, conceptual or theoretical framework and rationale for conducting the study (why this study is important, what studies have already been done, how this study differs from other study findings, what new knowledge it will bring to nursing knowledge) which may run from three to six pages.
- The purpose of the study is usually included at the beginning of the chapter. It should also contain the objectives of the study which need to be numbered and presented in a sequential order. It forms the basis for data analysis and discussion. The scope should be mentioned so as to identify the population for which the results of the study can be generalized (delimitations).
- The final section of this chapter summarizes the contents of the subsequent chapters that constitute the study. It provides a bird view and facilitates finding specific information without actually leafing through all the pages.

Chapter 2: Review of Selected/Related Literature

- This chapter provides the reader with a comprehensive review of the literature related to the problem under investigation.
- It includes existing theories and models, a historical overview, current trends and significant research data relevant to the problem.
- The first section of this chapter provides a description of the organization and an explanation of the subsections in the chapter.
- As the chapter is lengthy and contains between 15 and 30 pages, the researcher needs to logically organize the information into as many sections and subsections required.
- Citations should be used extensively throughout the chapter as the information and conclusions are drawn by other researchers. Overuse of direct quotations may be avoided to maintain transition and flow, and make it easy to read. The chapter ends with a short summary of the review presented.

Chapter 3: Methodology

- The methods section of the research report informs the reader about the

- research design, sampling procedure, setting (physical location and prevailing conditions during data collection), data collection procedures and tools used to measure outcome variables.
- The design is often described in detail in experimental and quasi-experimental studies than in non-experimental studies.
- In experimental studies the researcher should indicate the specific design adopted, variables manipulated, assigning of subjects to groups, number of times data were collected, who collected the data, who implemented the intervention, beginning and ending dates for data collection. It is also important to mention how extraneous variables have been controlled.
- This section includes a description of sample, sampling technique, sample size, inclusion and exclusion criteria and information about response rates.
- This section provides information on various phases of data collection and ethical principles followed to protect human subjects.
- The researcher should describe any untoward events occurred during data collection that could have affected the findings.
- The report should also include study instruments, a rationale for their use, methods used for pretesting, scoring procedures and interpretation details along with information on reliability and validity of instruments.
- This section ends with a summary of statistical methods used to analyze the data.

Chapter 4: Results
- This chapter focuses on significant findings and answers the research question or tests hypotheses.
- Data are presented objectively with little discussion. Tables, graphs and figures are usually used to present the data.
- The tables should have suitable headings and titles. They should be numbered in sequential order.
- Results should be reported using appropriate statistical symbols. Based on the objectives, results need to be presented.
- The researcher must ensure an accurate and complete reporting of results regardless of whether the hypotheses were supported or not.
- Where both descriptive and inferential statistics have been used, the descriptive statistics are usually explained first so as to provide an overview of study variables followed by description of inferential statistics.
- Where the research question involves comparing the groups on dependent variables the initial section of the results should provide information on comparability of the groups with regard to extraneous variables.
- Reports should include the values of calculated statistics, degrees of freedom and significance level.

Chapter 5: Discussion
- The discussion section begins with a brief summary of introduction, hypothesis, aims or research questions and the main findings.
- The findings of the study should be discussed in line with the study objectives and hypothesis. Under each objective, data analysis and interpretation should be discussed with supporting literature.
- In this section the researcher explains what the results mean in relation to the purpose of the study and compares the research results to that of other studies on the same topic.
- In this section the researcher should provide justification for the results, simultaneously commenting on why alternative explanations have been ruled out.

- Where the findings are conflicting with the previous studies, suitable explanations may be offered.

Chapter 6: Summary and Conclusions
- It includes brief summary of research steps, major findings and importance of study.
- This section includes conclusions from each finding, test of hypothesis and generalizations. It also describes how far the objectives of the study have been attained along with the chief strengths of the present study.
- Limitations of the study are also addressed in this section.
- Implications are mentioned to identify possible application of the results in terms of nursing practice, education, administration and research.
- This section should include recommendations for further studies in relation to the present research findings. These recommendations help other researchers to test similar hypothesis.

End Report
The end report usually includes references and appendices.

References: The reference list is very important to the research report and provides references related to the research study. It should be current. They may be written based on the institution/university guidelines. Commonly used reference styles are American Psychological Association (APA) or Vancouver or Harvard style. Details of these reference styles are presented separately in this chapter.

Appendix/Annexure: Appendices should be placed towards the end of the report. It should include tools with scoring details, consent form, ethical clearance certificate, permission letter, modules, panel of experts consulted for content validity of modules or tools, coding sheet and master data sheet.

REFERENCES
Referencing is the act of mentioning or alluding to something. It is a standard format for presenting the sources of information used in the written work. It properly credits the originators of ideas, theories, and research findings and allows the reader to trace them to create a solid argument.

Terminology
- A *citation* is a way of giving credit to the original author for his creative and intellectual work that has been used to support the research without plagiarizing. It helps to identify particular sources, reduce plagiarism and know the amount of research done. In includes information on the author, study title, year and month of publication, location of the publishing company, journal title, or DOI (Digital Object Identifer).
- *Footnote* is a reference or an explanation or an acknowledgment of the source mentioned at the bottom of the same page where the citation occurs. These are indicated by a number or a symbol in the text and again at the bottom in front of the footnote. It is used when references are very few.
- *Reference* is the act of acknowledging the sources of data, research or ideas of others on which the work has been drawn.
- A *reference list* is the list of sources cited in the written work arranged in the order they appeared within the text. It is placed either as a footnote (at the bottom of the page) or an end note (at the end of the chapter or book). This list allows the reader to trace the sources and give credit to authors for their ideas.
- A *bibliography* is a list of all the sources used during research process and background reading not just the ones cited in the writing. It includes books, articles and papers. It is listed alphabetically by the author's surname.

- An *annotated bibliography* is a list of research sources with a brief description and evaluation of the research on a particular topic. It is usually about 150 words in length. The main purpose is to inform the reader of the relevance and accuracy of the cited sources.
- A *referencing style* is a specific format on how to acknowledge thoughts and works of others for citing in-text references, footnotes and bibliography. It also includes rules regarding punctuations, order of information and other formatting details. These are important for writing scientific work.

Purposes of Reference
- Is crucial to successful research
- Indicates origin of material and is a source for further reading
- Gives credit to other people's work
- Required to support all significant statements
- Establishes that substantial research has been carried out and adds authenticity to the argument
- Avoids plagiarism
- Improves writing skills

Types of Information to be Cited
Printed books are not the only sources that require acknowledgment. Any words, ideas or information taken from the journal articles, books, magazines, newspapers, electronic sources, online discussion forums, personal interviews, reprinting of diagrams, illustrations, charts and pictures, etc.

When and How to Use Quotation
- It is good to use a quotation when it needs to be analyzed or challenged or if it is felt that the quotation supports the argument or point of view.
- When it is required to add interest or impact to an introduction or conclusion
- When directly quoting from a work, the author, year of publication and page number of the reference need to be included in the citation. Example, According to Jones (1998), "Students often had difficulty using APA style, especially when it was their first time" (p. 199).

Reference is not Required
- When writing about own observations, experiences or experiment results (for example, a report on a field trip)
- When writing personal opinions, remarks or conclusions
- When presenting own evaluation
- When using facts or information of common knowledge

Errors in Reference
- Spelling mistakes in quoting author or journal names
- Incorrect title name, year, volume number and page number
- Omission of citations in text and bibliography

Types and Elements of Reference
The common types of reference include journals, books and internet sources. The elements of reference include authors name, article title, journal name, year, volume, page numbers.

Different Styles of Writing Reference
Scholarly reference styles are divided into three main categories based on the recording style of the sources: documentary note style, parenthetical (or author-date) style, and numbered styles.

1. *Documentary note style*: In this the references are provided either as a footnote or an endnote. In the text, they are identified by a numeral, usually in superscript. The numeral is placed after the concluding punctuation or full stop ending the sentence to which the reference belongs. Oxford referencing style and Chicago referencing style are examples of

documentary note style primarily used in History, Philosophy and Classics.
2. *Parenthetical style or author date style*: In this the in-text references are given within parentheses before the sentence full stop. American Psychological Association reference style and Harvard referencing style are examples of parenthetical style primarily used in the sciences and social sciences. It is listed alphabetically by the author's surname.
3. *Numbered style*: In this the sources are indicated using Arabic numbers within square brackets or in superscript, and the references are listed in a numbered reference list after the text. References are listed chronologically in the order of their appearance in the text. Vancouver referencing style is an example of numbered style and widely used in health sciences.

Vancouver Style of Writing References

It was developed in Vancouver in 1978 by editors of medical journals. Over 500 medical journals use this style of reference.

Citation within the text: In the text, references are sequentially numbered. A number should be given in superscript format e.g.[5] or enclosed in bracket e.g. (5). Citations are sequential numbers in the order of their appearance in the text. Each citation corresponds to a numbered reference which contains information on the source of publication in the reference list at the end of the publication. Once a source has been cited and the same is repeated, the same original number should be assigned to it. While citing multiple sources for any text, all the reference numbers are cited sequentially separated by a comma between each of them, for example.[3,4,6] The detailed description of Vancouver style of writing references is presented in Table 10.6.

Table 10.6: Vancouver style of writing reference

Type of references	Description	Examples
Book	**Book by a single author:** Author's Surname with Initial. Title of the book. Edition if later than 1st. Place of publication: Publisher Name; Year of publication.	Riyaz S. Difficult cases in primary care: women's health. London: Radcliffe Publishing; 2012.
	Book by two authors: First Author's Surname with Initial, Second Author's Surname with Initial. Title of book. Edition if later than 1st. Place of publication: Publisher Name; Year of publication.	Marcdante KJ, Kliegman RM. Nelson essentials of paediatrics. 7th ed. Philadelphia, PA: Elsevier Saunders; 2015.
	Book by a corporate author Name of the corporate author. Title of book. Place of publication: Publisher Name; Year of publication.	NHS Institute for Innovation and Improvement. Improvement leaders' guide: general improvement skills: improvement knowledge and skills. Coventry: NHS Institute for Innovation and Improvement; 2007.
Edited book	Editor's Surname with Initial(s), editor. Title of book/dictionary/encyclopedia etc. Edition if later than 1st. Place of publication: Publisher Name; Year of publication.	Lally F, Roffe C, editors. Geriatric medicine: an evidence-based approach. Oxford: Oxford University Press; 2014. Wilson W, Tom L, editors. Oxford English dictionary. 4th ed. Oxford: Oxford University Press; 2002.

Contd...

Contd...

Type of references	Description	Examples
Journal articles	Author's Surname with Initial. Title of journal article. Abbreviated journal title. Year; volume number (issue number if there is one): page numbers.	Cooper C, Sommerlad A, Lyketsos CG, Livingston G. Modifiable Predictors of Dementia in Mild Cognitive Impairment: A Systematic Review and Meta-Analysis. Am J Psychiatry. 2015;172(4):323-334.
Newspapers	**Article in a printed newspaper:** Author's Surname with Initial. Title of article. Title of Newspaper. Year Month Day; Location in newspaper.	Clarkson M. Outreach studies in the community. The Guardian. 1998 Jun 16; Sect. A:3 (col.4).
	Article in an online newspaper: Author's Surname with Initial. Title of article. Title of Newspaper [Internet]. Year Month Day [cited Year Month Day]. Available from: URL.	Boseley S. NHS cancer guide for GPs and patients could save 5,000 lives a year, says Nice. The Guardian [Internet]. 2015 Jun 23 [cited 2015 Jun 24]. Available from: http://www.theguardian.com/society/2015/jun/23/nhs-cancer-guide-gps-patients-could-save-5000-lives-a-year-nice.
Government Documents	Name of the Government Department. Title of paper/report, Cm number – also called the Series number. Place of publication: Name of Publisher; Year of publication.	Department of Health. Healthy lives, healthy people: our strategy for public health in England, Cm7985. London: Stationery Office; 2010.
Conference proceedings	Editor's Surname with Initial, editor. Title of publication if there is one. Conference; date; location. Place of publication: Publisher Name; Year of publication.	Holland-Elliott K, editor. What about the workers? Proceedings of a symposium held at the Royal Society of Medicine; 2004 Mar 30; London, UK. London: Royal Society of Medicine Press; 2004.
Theses and dissertations	Author's Surname with Initial. Title of dissertation/thesis etc [dissertation/thesis etc]. Place of publication: Publisher Name (generally the University that the student attended); Year of Publication.	Yates MT. Effect of ESC/EACTS guidelines on myocardial revascularization on heart team discussion of patients with severe coronary artery disease in the United Kingdom [thesis]. London: St Georges, University of London; 2015.
Patent	Name(s) of inventor(s), inventor; Name of assignee., assignee. Title of the patent (italics). Country or region of patent, patent number. Date of patent.	Pagedas AC, inventor; Ancel Surgical R&D Inc., assignee. *Flexible endoscopic grasping and cutting device and positioning tool assembly*. United States patent 20020103498. 2002 Aug 1.

American Psychological Association Style of Writing References

American Psychological Association (APA) style is most frequently used within the social sciences, in order to cite various sources. APA Style was first developed in 1929. The sixth edition of APA manual is the most current one released in July 2009.

Citation within the text

❖ APA uses the author date method of citation. When referencing or summarizing a source, provide the author and year. For example, in one experimental study (Singh, 2001), Children learned.... Or in the study by Singh (2001), children learned....

Unit 10: Dissemination (Communication) and Utilization of Research Findings

- When quoting or summarizing a particular passage, include the specific page or paragraph number as well. For example, one study found that "the listener's familiarity with the topic of discourse greatly facilitates the interpretation of the entire message" (Gass & Varonis, 1984, p. 85).
- When quoting in text, if a direct quote is less than 40 words, incorporate it into text and use quotation marks. If a direct quote is more than 40 words, make the quotation a freestanding indented block of text and DO NOT use quotation marks. For example: This suggests that familiarity with nonnative speech in general, although it is clearly not as important a variable as topic familiarity, may indeed have some effect. That is, prior experience with nonnative speech, such as that gained by listening to the reading, facilitates comprehension. (Gass & Varonis, 1984, p. 77).
- Everything cited in text appears in the reference list. The list should be written in an alphabetical order. The detailed description of APA style of writing references is presented in Table 10.7.

Table 10.7: American Psychological Association style of writing references

Type of references	Description	Examples
Book	Author(s) of book – family name, initials. use & for multiple authors. (Year of publication). Title of book – italicized. Place of publication: Publisher.	Single author Berkman, R. I. (1994). *Find it fast: How to uncover expert information*. New York, NY: Harper Perrenial.
		Moir, A., & Jessel, D. (1991). *Brain sex: The real difference between men and women*. London: Mandarin.
		Three to five authors O'Keefe, J. H., Bell, D. S. H., & Wyne, K.L. (2009). *Diabetes essentials*. Sudbury, MA: Jones and Bartlett Publishers.
		Six or more authors John, T., Levon, P., Peter, S., Harris, Y., Morgan, G., Morrrison, B., . . . Smith, P. (2002). *How far is far?* London: McMillan.
		No author *The CCH Macquarie dictionary of business*. (1993). North Ryde, NSW: CCH Australia.
Chapter in a book	Author(s) of chapter – family name, initials. use & for multiple authors. (Year of publication). Title of chapter. In Editor(s) – initials and family name - of book (Eds), Title of book – italicized, (pp. Page numbers). Place of publication: Publisher.	Baker, F. M., & Lightfoot, O. B. (1993). Psychiatric care of ethnic elders. In A. C. Gaw (Ed.), *Culture, ethnicity, and mental illness* (pp. 517-552). Washington, DC: American Psychiatric Press.
Dictionary or Encyclopedia	Author(s) of work – family name, initials. use & for multiple authors. (Year of publication). Title – italicized. Place of publication: Publisher.	Wolman, B.B. (Ed.). (1989). *Dictionary of behavioral science* (2nd ed.). San Diego, CA: Academic Press.
Journal article	With DOI: Author(s) of journal article – family name, initials. use & for multiple authors.	Rentala, S., Lau, P.H.B., & Chan, L.W.C. (2017). Association Between Spirituality and

Contd...

Contd...

Type of references	Description	Examples
	multiple authors. (Year of publication). Title of journal article. Journal name – italicized, Volume – italicized (Issue or number), Page number(s). doi:xx.xxxxxxxxx	Depression Among Depressive Disorder Patients in India, Journal of Spirituality in Mental Health, 19(4): 318-33. DOI: 10.1080/19349637.2017.1286962.
	Without DOI: Author(s) of journal article – family name, initials. use & for multiple authors. (Year of publication). Title of journal article. Journal name – italicised, Volume – italicised(Issue or number), Page number(s). Retrieved from http://www.xxxxxx	Rentala, S., Fong, T.C.T., Nattala, P., Chan C.L.W., & Konduru, R. (2015). Effectiveness of body-mind-spirit intervention on well-being, functional impairment and quality of life among depressive patients - a randomized controlled trial. Journal of Advanced Nursing, 71(9): 2153-2163.
Conference proceedings	Author(s) of paper – family name, initials. use & for multiple authors. (Year of publication). Title of paper. Title of published proceeding –italicized. Place of Publication: Publisher.	Stephen, S. (2017). Improving teaching and educational policy. In M. O'Keets, E. Webb, & K. Hoad (Eds.), Learning and teaching, 12-14. Melbourne, Australia: Australian Council for Educational Research.
Newspaper	Author(s) of article – family name, initials. use & for multiple authors. (Year of publication, month day). Title of article. Title of newspaper – italicized, p. page number(s).	With author: Cook, D. (2002, January 28). All in the mind. The Age, p. 8. No author: Meeting the needs of counsellors. (2001, May 5). The Courier Mail, p. 22.
Magazine article		Marano, H.E. (2008, March-April). Making of a perfectionist. Psychology Today, 41, 80-86.
Government publications	Author(s) of report – person or organization. use & for multiple authors. (Year of Publication). Title of report – italicized. Place of publication: Publisher.	Queensland Health. (2005). Health systems review. Final report. Brisbane, Australia: Queensland Government.
Theses and dissertations	Author. (Year of preparation of thesis). Title of thesis – italicised (Doctoral dissertation or master's thesis, Institution, Location). Retrieved from institutional or personal website.	Thesis- retrieved from institutional or personal website Rentala S. (2013). Body-Mind-Spirit intervention on wellbeing and process of recovery among depressive patients. (Doctoral dissertation, RGUHS, Karnataka, India). Retrieved from http://espace.library.uq.edu.au/view/UQ:158747
		Thesis – retrieved from database Rentala S. (2013). Body-Mind-Spirit intervention on wellbeing and process of recovery among depressive patients. (Doctoral dissertation, Retrieved from Proquest Digital Dissertations. (AAT NR25719)
Patent	Author or authors—family name, initials. use & for multiple authors. Year (in round brackets). Patent number (in italics).Place of publication. Publisher.	Bryant, S.J. (1998). European Patent No. EP GB2322334. Munich, Germany: European Patent Office.

Difference between Bibliography and Reference

A reference list and a bibliography look a lot similar and appear at the end of a document. They both contain the same basic information and are arranged alphabetically. However some differences do exist. They are presented in Table 10.8.

Table 10.8: Differences between references and bibliography

References	Bibliography
A reference list generally contains only sources cited in-text.	Bibliography generally is a list of all the sources used i.e. in addition to listing the sources cited in-text, the list of resources read or referred to generate ideas about the topic are also included.
References are cited directly in the text.	Bibliography is not cited directly in the text.
References help in supporting and adding credibility to a statement or argument. These help the reader to evaluate the correctness of a statement.	Bibliography does not support or add credibility to a statement or argument but merely refers them in a personal way.
Reference list comes before the bibliography.	Bibliography comes after the reference list.
References are listed in numerical order according to their appearance in the text. They can also be arranged in alphabetical order.	Bibliography is arranged only in alphabetical order.

RESEARCH CRITIQUE

When a critical question in nursing practice arises, nurses usually look to published research literature with the assumption that the printed words are factual. However, not all published research is scientifically sound. Thus it is essential for a nurse to be able to critically assess a report and decide the appropriateness and adequacy of research findings for use in practice. Deciding on the overall usefulness of a research report requires systematic review and critical appraisal. Failing to critique a research report adequately may adversely affect the patient outcomes.

Definition

"Systematic, unbiased, careful examination of all aspects of a study to judge the merits, limitations, meaning and significance based on previous research experience and knowledge of the topic."
—**Burns, N. & Grove, S., 2005**

"Critiquing is a systematic method of appraising the strengths and limitations of a piece of research in order to determine its credibility and/or its applicability to practice."
— **Valente, 2003**

Research reports are evaluated using specific criteria and guidelines to assess how well the research process was executed. In critiquing process the evaluator makes precise and objective judgments about the research study, weighing its strengths and weaknesses. For a nurse to critique a research report she requires critical thinking and intellectual skills.

Importance of Critiquing a Research Report

- To broaden understanding for use in practice
- For implementing an evidence-based nursing practice
- To provide feedback for improvement
- Nurses with an ability to critically review contribute to the body of nursing knowledge

Purposes of Critiquing

- Highlights strengths and weaknesses of the research study
- Helps in deciding whether to publish the study or not
- Points out methodological flaws in the research study

Process for Conducting a Research Critique

The critiquing process should begin with reading the entire study to get an overview and appreciate its contribution to knowledge development. This should be followed by an examination of the organization and presentation to understand the complexity of the material and compare it with the rules for ideal study. The strengths and weakness of the study may be identified objectively followed by modifications for future studies.

- Begin with considering the author(s) credentials
- Assess the title of the study for its clarity and conciseness
- Examine whether the abstract imparts a condensation of the main points from the research project
- Determine whether the design and methodology are consistent with the research purpose and problem
- Verify if the methodology is applied logically
- Assess if the research results and conclusions are plausible and supported by previous research findings
- Reflect on the overall quality, strengths, limitations, missing elements and suggestions for further research

While critiquing, focused examination needs to be conducted to evaluate each aspect of the research article with rules of ideal study (Table 10.9).

Research is critiqued to improve practice, broaden understanding, and provide a base for the conduct of a study. Thus nursing students, practicing nurses, nurse educators and nurse researchers perform research critique.

Guidelines for Critiquing a Research Report

Critique guidelines are key components to be considered when evaluating research reports. A few important guidelines are as follows:

- Critiquing is a process of reviewing and evaluating the strengths and limitations of a research report. It should not be used to belittle the researcher's ability. It is the creation and not the creator that is being evaluated.
- The reviewer maintains objectivity right through the critiquing process and does not express any personal views.
- While critiquing, a balanced approach needs to be maintained by presenting both strong and weak points of the report.
- The use of personal pronouns is avoided in order that objectivity can be maintained.
- When pointing out a study's weakness provide explanations justifying the comments.
- Choose clear and concise statements to communicate observations.
- Include supportive and encouraging comments where essential.

Generally research studies comprise of both strong and weak components. A critical evaluation of all these components is important in determining the usefulness of these research results for knowledge development.

RESEARCH UTILIZATION

The main goal of conducting nursing research is to promote evidence-based nursing practice. This movement has brought implementation of empirically based interventions within the domain of nursing practice. This justifies the decisions the nurses make and the care they provide. Thus, the study findings should find a way into nursing practice so as to be useful for the profession. Going beyond the artificial research setting to the actual practice setting, i.e. use of research findings in real practice setting is called research utilization.

Definitions

Research utilization is the process of synthesizing, disseminating and using research generated knowledge to make an impact on or modify existing nursing practice (Burns and Groove 2005).

Table 10.9: Process for conducting a research critique

Components of the research article	Rules of ideal study	Questions for critiquing a research report
Writing style and logical consistency	• Should be written concisely without any grammatical mistakes • Steps should flow logically	• Is the report well written-concise, grammatically correct, avoid the use of jargon? • Is it well laid out and organized? • Does the research report follow various steps in research process?
Author Credentials Who conducted the research including their job title(s) and qualifications	• Author should have adequate knowledge and skill in conducting the research study	• Is researcher having the necessary knowledge and skills to do the research? • Is researcher qualified to undertake the research?
Research Title Clearly indicates what the research is about	• Should be between 10 and 15 words long • Should be clear, accurate and identify the purpose of the study	• Is the title clear, accurate and unambiguous?
Abstract Provides a brief summary of the contents of the article	• Should include information regarding purpose of the study, method, sample size, main findings, conclusions and recommendations.	• Does the abstract offer a clear overview of the study including the research problem, sample, methodology, finding and recommendations? • Does it explain why the research was carried out?
Research Problem/Purpose States relevant background information and justifies the study	• Should emphasize significance of the problem • Should state aim of study unambiguously • Should be practical	• Is the problem clearly stated with pertinent background information? • Is there justification for the study? • Is the study purpose clearly identified? • Is problem researchable?
Review of Literature Gives an overview of the available literature which provides a context for the study. Establishes what is known and not known about the research problem	• Should organize review logically and offer balanced critical analysis of the literature • Should provide rationale and direction for the present study. • Should mainly include empirical literature • Most literature reviews should include articles published within the last 3 to 5 years	• Is the literature review clearly organized, logically developed and concisely written? • Are the most recent and relevant studies are included? • Is the literature mainly from primary sources and of an empirical nature? • Is the current knowledge about the research problem described? • Does the literature review identify the gap in the knowledge? • Does it offer an unbiased analysis of the literature? • Does the literature review provide the basis for study conducted? • Are the references cited accurately?

Contd...

Contd...

Components of the research article	Rules of ideal study	Questions for critiquing a research report
Theoretical Framework Guides the study by providing themes, frameworks and sets boundaries	• Should explain clear link between theoretical frame work and research question or purpose • Should present model or map logically	• Has a conceptual or theoretical framework been identified? • Is the conceptual or theoretical framework applicable to the research? • Is the framework clearly developed and adequately described?
Aims, Objectives, Research Question and Research Hypothesis Form a link between the initially stated purpose of the study and how the study will be undertaken	• Should express aims, objectives, research question and hypothesis appropriately and clearly • Should logically relate to the research purpose, aim and theory	• Have aims and objectives, a research question or hypothesis been identified? If so are they clearly stated?
Variable It is the measurable characteristic that varies among the subjects being studied	• Should identify concepts within the theoretical framework • Should define variables operationally • Conceptual definition should be consistent with operational definition of each variable	• Are relevant variables defined operationally? • Are variables expressed in measurable terms?
Research Methodology/ Research Design Clearly states what a researcher did and how it was done. This section includes description of participants, the materials and the procedures	• Protocol should be clearly evident for conducting research study • Methodology should minimize threats to internal validity • Methodology should be logically connected to sampling method and statistics applied	• Is the type of research design identified? • Does the research design fit appropriately according to the variables studied and purpose of the study? • If it is an experimental design what methods are used to control internal and external threats to validity? • Is the research design adequately designed to infer the cause and effect relationship between the variables? • Was a pilot study undertaken?
Ethical Considerations Describes process of obtaining ethical clearance and how ethical standards were maintained	• Should protect human rights • Should obtain ethical clearance • Should maintain ethical standards	• Were the participants well informed about the nature of the research and their amount of involvement? • Are the subjects assured of their anonymity and confidentiality of data? • Are the participants free from harm? • Has the researcher obtained ethical permission for the study?

Contd...

Contd...

Components of the research article	Rules of ideal study	Questions for critiquing a research report
Sampling Method Describes number and characteristics of participants and their selection process	• Should use appropriate sampling technique • Should identify biases • Should describe setting and be appropriate for target population	• Is the sample representative of the population? • Have the target and accessible population been clearly identified? • Did the researcher select the suitable sampling method to answer the research question? • Did the researcher select the adequate number of sample to obtain valid results? • Is the sampling method described? • Was the method of choosing the sample (probability vs non-probability) appropriate? • Are potential sampling biases identified? • Is subject dropout discussed? • Are the inclusion/exclusion criteria clearly identified?
Data Collection Describes data collection procedure in a step-by-step manner	• Should clearly describe techniques for collecting data • Should clearly describe the data collection process	• Did the report describe what, how, who and when of data collection?
Measurements Describes details of measurements, instructions to participants, mode of administration, validity, reliability and scoring details	• Should use suitable instruments to measure the study variables • Should check validity and reliability levels of the instruments • Should clearly describe instruments scoring techniques	• Were the research variables measured using a suitable instrument? • Had the instrument been tested for reliability and validity? • Was there enough evidence on validity and reliability of the instruments? • Was the pilot study conducted using same instruments? • Were the items in instrument appropriate to collect adequate data? • Were the subject's responses influenced by the order of questionnaire items? • Were the instructions clear and adequate to complete the questionnaire? • Were all the subjects administered the instrument uniformly? • Was data collected for all subjects in the same location?

Contd...

Contd...

Components of the research article	Rules of ideal study	Questions for critiquing a research report
Data Analysis Contains main results and findings with tables and figures	• Should use suitable analysis procedures • Should appropriately analyze outcome variables	• Is the choice of statistical procedures suitable for the methodology proposed? • Are the sample characteristics described? • Are table or graphs used to present data? If so, are they labeled clearly and discussed in the text?
Discussion Evaluates and interprets the implications of the research results in relation to the research question. Contains a clear statement of supporting or not supporting hypothesis. Includes results of the present study and those of other studies with suggestions for improvements or further research	• Should interpret the results in relation to research question • The discussion of the findings should logically flow from the data and place the study in the context of previous literature • Should highlight the most important results • Should highlight the relevance and usefulness of the results to the practice	• Are the findings related to the previous literature? • Is the identified hypothesis supported or not? • Are generalizations made beyond the sample identified in the study? • Are suggestions, recommendations made by the researcher for nursing practice, education or for further research? • Were the strengths and limitations, generalizability of the study discussed? • Did the discussion on strengths and limitations of the study include generalizability?
Conclusion Summarizes the main points and indicates the usefulness of research.	• Should draw out the main points • Should demonstrate new insights on the topic • Should make recommendations based on the research • Should make suggestions for future research	• Were the main points drawn out? • Were insights on the topic demonstrated? • Were there any suggestions for future research?
Bibliography/References Contains a list of all sources referred or actually accessed in preparation for the article.	• Should provide all sources cited clearly with full bibliography	• Were all referred books and journals for the study referenced accurately?

Research utilization is a multistage process which involves analysis and synthesis of various study findings, their application in bringing a change in nursing practice, and a measure of its outcome.

Through research utilization process research based knowledge is implemented in practice.

Elements of Research Utilization

Research utilization deals with the application of research evidence to practice, program and policies to improve outcome. The main elements of research utilization include:

❖ Summarizing the research generated knowledge

❖ Communicating the research knowledge to nurses and other health care professionals, policy makers, consumers of health care
❖ Achieving desired outcomes for patients and health care agencies

Steps in Research Utilization Process

Research utilization is a step-by-step process that involves recognizing a clinical problem which requires a scientific basis through formulation and evaluation of a research-based innovation in the practice setting. The steps in research utilization process are presented in Figure 10.7.

Types of Research Utilization

The concept of utilization is generally defined as putting research into practice. Five types of research utilization defined by Reid and Fortune (1992) are presented in Table 10.10.

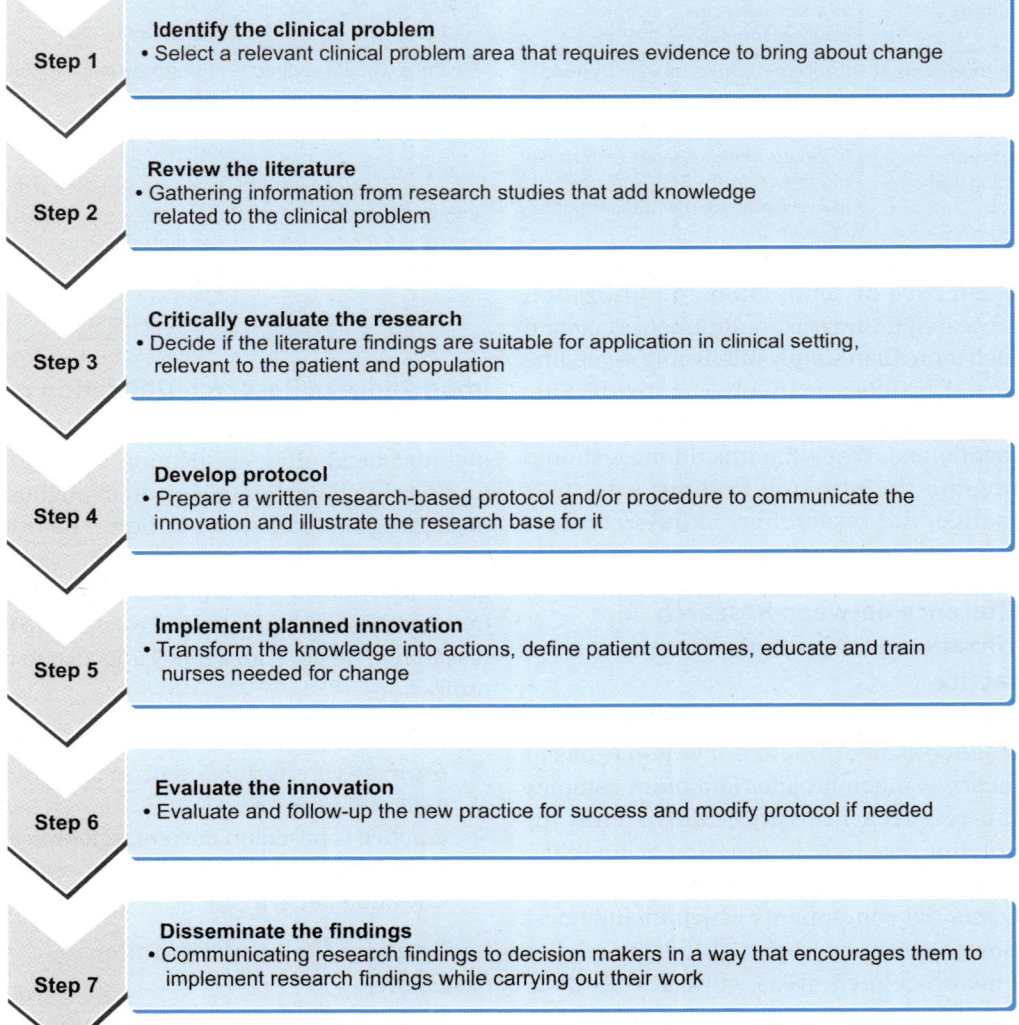

Fig. 10.7: Steps in research utilization process

Table 10.10: Types of research utilization

Types of research utilization	Description
Instrumental utilization	It occurs when research is used to make decisions or alter practices
Conceptual utilization	It takes place when research is used to enhance insight about an issue without actually influencing the practice or decision
Persuasive utilization	It involves use of research findings as a persuasive tool to legitimate a position or practice
Methodological utilization	It occurs when specific research or assessment tools are used to improve practice
Indirect utilization	It occurs when theories, practice models or procedures are used to improve practice that is the result to research

Effective dissemination and utilization of research findings is multidimensional and much more than simply publishing or reading journal articles. It involves considerable collaboration between researchers and practitioners. While the practitioners should integrate the research findings into their practice, the researchers should conduct studies in natural settings.

Difference between Research Utilization and Evidence-based Practice

Research utilization has a lesser focus than evidence-based practice. Evidence-based practice is much broader and more complex than research utilization but is vital for applying research to practice at bedside. Evidence-based practice involves integration of essential components which include best research evidence from high-quality studies in health-related areas, clinical expertise, patient values and cost-effective health care (Table 10.11).

Table 10.11: Comparison of research utilization and evidence-based practice

Research utilization	Evidence-based practice
Identification of clinical problem	Identification of clinical problem
Solving the problem using research already conducted	Using research already conducted
Uses various steps of the research utilization process	Combines all the evidence and integrates it with expert opinion and patient input
Findings usually applied at the organizational level	Findings usually applied at the bedside and customized to the individual patient
Uses research generated knowledge to influence or change the existing practice	Evidence based practice encompasses evidence generated from scientific findings, expert clinical opinion and patient and family preferences

Importance of Research Utilization

The ultimate goal of research utilization includes facilitating application of research findings in clinical practice and changing or improving the patient condition. The other goals include developing clinical practice guidelines, protocols and dissemination of findings. Research utilization is of value to the researcher, health care agency and also to the profession.

Importance of Research Utilization to Patients
- Innovative changes lead to improved patient outcomes.
- Practice is based on current, scientifically sound knowledge. It ensures provision of safe and effective care.

Importance of Research Utilization to Researcher
- Helps to discover new clinical problems for investigation

- Validates the efforts of the researcher
- Motivates the researchers to continue discovering new knowledge

Importance of Research Utilization to Health Care Agency
- Nurses can provide cost-effective and high quality nursing care
- Improved patient outcomes
- Professionally satisfied and stimulated nursing staff, improves retention

Importance of Research Utilization to Nursing Profession
- Expands scientific knowledge base in the field of nursing
- Enhanced autonomy of practice
- Positive professional image
- Strengthens professional status
- Validates the existing nursing knowledge or procedures or interventions
- Promotes critical thinking and reflective practice
- Enhances professional self-concept and reinforces professional accountability
- Enhances self-confidence of the nurse

Though the nurses have the benefit of using research-based approach for providing nursing care, it is not optimally utilized. As a result the patients are devoid of best possible care.

BRIDGING GAP BETWEEN RESEARCH AND PRACTICE

Since long there has been a considerable gap between research and practice in the field of nursing. This inequality between the availability of research evidence and its use in practice is referred to as research practice gap i.e. gap between knowledge production and knowledge application. Research utilization constantly examines whether clinical practice is utilizing the best available research evidence.

Various models of research utilization (RU) have been applied to integrate new knowledge into nursing practice. The widely known projects that have promoted research utilization are the Conduct and Utilization of Research in Nursing (CURN) project, Stetler Model of research utilization and Roger's Innovative Diffusion Model.

Conduct and Utilization of Research in Nursing (CURN) Project

The Conduct and Utilization of Research in Nursing (CURN) project was developed during 1975-1980 by the Michigan State Nurses Association. This project was designed with an aim to implement research based knowledge in real clinical practice setting. In this project, research utilization is viewed as an organizational process wherein planned change is integrated throughout the research utilization process. This change is essential to establishing research-based practice on a large scale.

Here research utilization was viewed as an organizational process.

The steps to be carried out to incorporate research into clinical practice are:
1. Identify a patient care problem (practice problem).
2. Examine the existing knowledge related to the practice problem.
3. Based on the existing body of knowledge design a nursing practice innovation.
4. Implement nursing practice innovation.
5. Evaluate the innovation for adoption, alteration or rejection.
6. Based on the evaluation develop strategies to extend innovation to other settings.
7. Prepare mechanisms to monitor the implementation of innovation over a period of time (Fig. 10.8).

Stetler Model of Research Utilization

It was first described in 1976 by Stetler and Marram. This model formulated a series of critical thinking and decision making steps designed to facilitate safe and effective use of research findings. The revised Stetler model (2001) of research utilization which applies

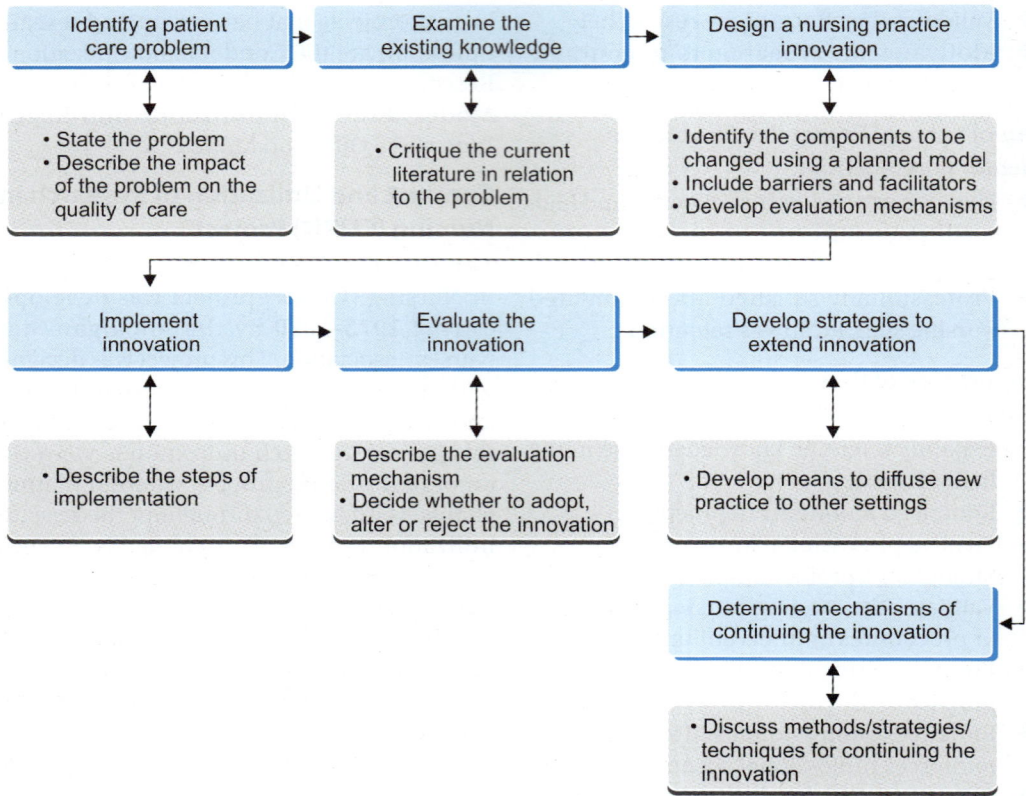

Fig. 10.8: Conduct and utilization of research in nursing model of research utilization

research findings at the individual practitioner level has five phases (Fig. 10.9): preparation, validation, comparative evaluation/decision making, translation/application and evaluation.

Phase I: Preparation

It involves establishing the purpose and potential outcomes of making evidence based change in a clinical organization. It involves examining the internal and external factors of organization that could influence the proposed practice change. Once the committee approves the purpose of the evidence based project, a detailed literature review is conducted to sort and select sources of research evidence.

Phase II: Validation

In this phase the research reports are critically appraised to determine their scientific evidence. If the research evidence base is strong in a selected area, the organization must take a decision regarding priority of using the evidence in practice.

Phase III: Comparative Evaluation/Decision Making

The comparative evaluation is done under four phases:
1. Substantiation of the evidence – Validation of evidence is produced by replication in which consistent, credible findings are obtained from several studies in similar practice settings.

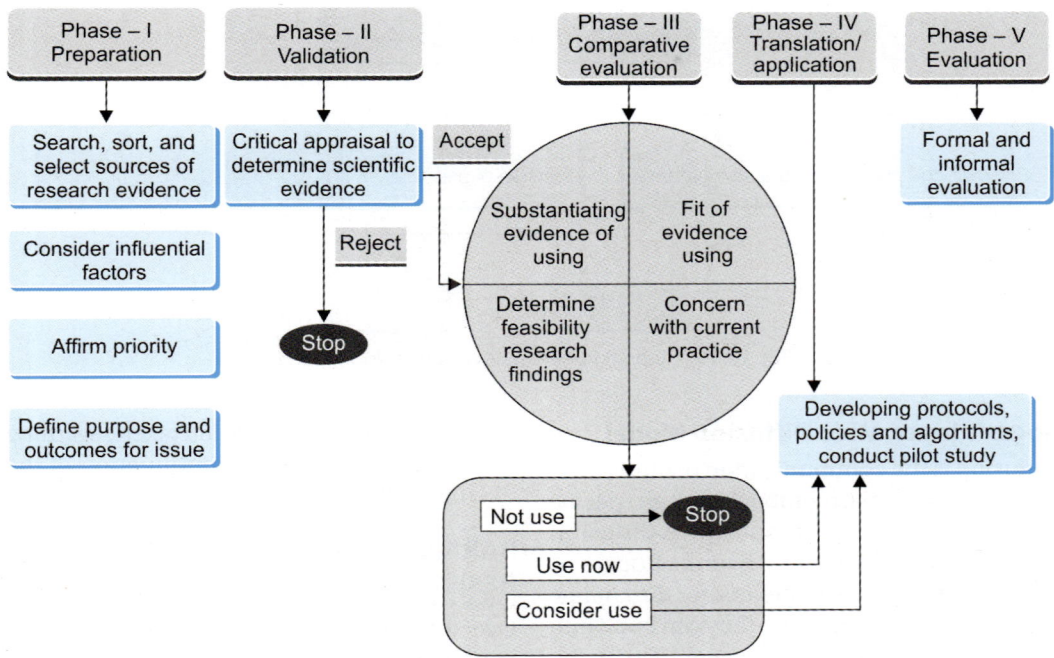

Fig. 10.9: Stetler model of research utilization

2. Determination of the fit of evidence with the health care setting – Examine the characteristic of the setting and determine the factors that will facilitate or inhibit implementation of evidence based change such as policies, protocols, etc.
3. Feasibility of using research findings – It involves examining the potential risks, resources needed and readiness of the personnel involved.
4. Concerns with current practice – Determine whether the research information provides credible, empirical evidence for making changes in the current practice. During this phase decide to use or not use based on the benefits and risks to the individual or organization or both.

Phase IV: Translation/Application

This phase describes how to implement findings or recommendations. The translation phase involves determining exactly what knowledge will be used and how that knowledge will be applied to practice. The application phase includes the situation to be changed, development of a plan for change and its implementation. During this phase the protocols, policies or algorithms are developed to implement research knowledge into practice. The organization may conduct a pilot study to evaluate the results of this project to determine if the change should be extended throughout the health care agency.

Phase V: Evaluation

The evaluation process can include formal and informal activities conducted by nurse clinicians, administrators and other health care personnel. Informal evaluation includes discussion with patients, families, peers and other professionals. Formal evaluation can include audits, case studies, quality improvement or outcome research projects. After the evaluation process evidence is integrated into practice.

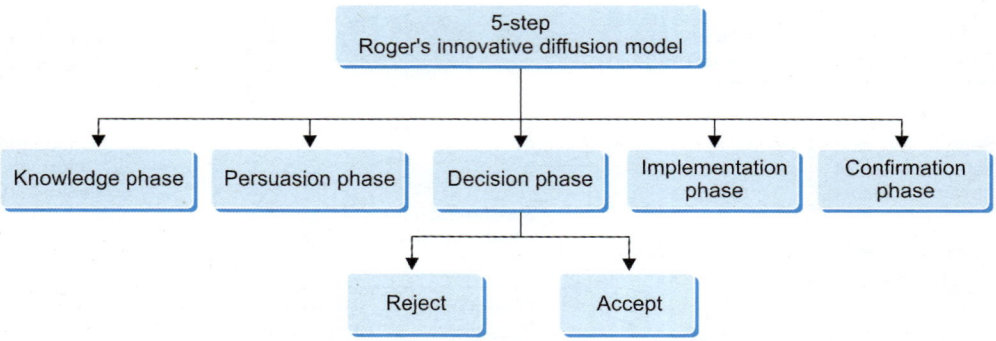

Fig. 10.10: Steps in Roger's innovative diffusion model

Roger's Innovative Diffusion Model

Diffusion is the communication of innovation among professional members through specific channels. The Roger's innovative diffusion model was developed by Everett Rogers in 1995. It provides the guidelines for the change agents about what qualities they can build into innovation to facilitate its acceptance by the intended adopter. It follows a 5-step process (Fig. 10.10):

1. *Knowledge phase*: In this phase the nurse obtains knowledge by attending conferences, reading journal articles and discussing with colleagues leading to an understanding of the research based nursing intervention and developing some idea of how it functions.
2. *Persuasion phase*: During this phase the nurse forms a favorable or unfavorable attitude towards the intervention. If she has a positive attitude she actively seeks related information and details.
3. *Decision phase*: It is a decisive phase where the nurse must weigh up the pros and cons of adoption and decide on whether to accept the new intervention or reject it.
4. *Implementation phase*: In this phase the nurse puts the intervention into practice exactly the way it was described in research studies.
5. *Confirmation phase*: This phase deals with evaluation of intervention for its effectiveness and decision taken regarding continuation and discontinuation of the intervention.

BARRIERS IN UTILIZATION OF RESEARCH FINDINGS

Over the last 25 years though there is a dramatic growth in nursing research and development of nursing theories, nurses frequently fail to base their practice on the findings of research. Through research, nurses can generate new knowledge which can improve care in clinical practice. Even though such new knowledge is generated its dissemination remains low on account of barriers in clinical practice. In order to address this problem the researchers and area experts examine the reasons for non-utilization and propose suitable strategies to overcome it. A common strategy to bridge the gap is to identify the barriers and practice the necessary change to overcome it.

Roger (2003) developed the framework for understanding the multiple factors related to barriers and facilitators in utilization of nursing research (Table 10.12).

When barriers to research utilization are identified nurse clinicians, educators, administrators and researchers can design and implement specific strategies to overcome these barriers. They can play the following roles:

Unit 10: Dissemination (Communication) and Utilization of Research Findings

Table 10.12: Factors related to barriers and facilitators in utilization of nursing research

Individual factors	
Barriers	**Facilitators**
• Inadequate educational preparation with limited exposure to research utilization • Negative attitude towards research among nurses • Inadequate knowledge of research findings among nurses • Unable to evaluate the quality of research • Lack of time and resources to keep up with colleagues conversant with research • Resistance to change	• Develop critical thinking ability • Develop positive attitude towards research • Commit to research training and continuous learning • Join professional organizations and involve in journal clubs • Pursue higher education • Stay updated with recent literature • Attend in-service trainings, pursue and participate in research activities • Collaborate with researchers to relay clinical issues and questions • Overcome risk to bring about changes and improve clinical practice
Organizational factors	
Barriers	**Facilitators**
• Insufficient time on the job to read recent literature and implement new interventions • Inadequate support from staff and management in implementation of research • Failure to motivate or reward nurses in carrying out research activities • Lack of staff to carry out research activities • Inadequate infrastructure and library facilities • Lack of requisite authority to improve practices • Insufficient funds from research granting agencies and professional organizations to support implementation of new research findings • Non-cooperation of medical personnel in implementation of new research findings • Limited communication and collaboration between educators and researchers	• The institutional setting provides an apt platform for mandating practice change. The institution must support the ongoing implementation and empower the nurses to question the current practices. • Provide scheduled time for reading research and discuss it with colleagues • Supportive leadership that prioritizes research utilization • Reward efforts for implementing research based activities • Provide research resources such as personnel, literature, funds, infrastructure, internet access, consultants etc. • Establish a research friendly culture • Promote in-service training at regular intervals • Encourage the nurses to attend and present research papers at conferences • Encourage the nurses to publish research articles • Explore for grants from Indian Council for Medical Research, Trained Nurses Association, University Grants Commission, Department of Science and Technology and Universities (Rajiv Gandhi University of Health Sciences, etc.) • Encourage collaborative research projects to create global support for organized nursing research • Collaborate with professional organizations like the Indian Nursing Council, Nursing Research Society of India for conducting research • Identify barriers

Contd...

Contd...

Research Factors	
Barriers	**Facilitators**
• Methodological flaws in research studies • Findings are not amenable for practice • Confusion about conflicting results in literature • Research results not applicable to practice context • Time lag between research and practice	• Replicate research to demonstrate applicability to local practice • Focus research activity on current clinical problems • Incorporate recommendations related to local practice setting and suggest implications • Disseminate research results as early as possible
Communication factors	
Barriers	**Facilitators**
• Lack of availability or limited access to research reports • Implications of research for practice not made clear • All relevant literature not available from a single source • Statistical analyses not comprehendible • Less research publications in clinical practice • Research findings not presented in understandable manner • The dissemination process is not intense at all levels of education	• Present results in a user-friendly and understandable manner • Provide facility to access research through databases and libraries • Enhance researcher-practitioner collaboration • Involve administrators in planning and implementation of research projects

Nurse Clinicians

❖ Nurses shall update their research skills by pursuing higher education, attending continuing nursing education programs and joining professional organizations. This will enable them to think critically about their patients and implement innovative interventions.

❖ They should cater time for reading literature in order to update themselves with new research findings.

❖ They should take initiation in conducting and participating in research studies.

❖ They should also take steps in bringing changes in clinical practice through innovative research practices.

❖ They must acknowledge the importance of nursing research for the improvement of patient care and the profession.

Nurse Educators

❖ The nurse educator should introduce research findings in nursing curriculum to emphasize the importance of nursing research among student community and facilitate its transition to clinical practice.

❖ In the teaching process the nurse educators should incorporate research related information to support lectures and teachings.

❖ They should encourage the students to incorporate research findings in their assignments and the clinical seminars should invariably include discussion on current research literature.

❖ While encouraging the students to seek the latest research findings in current practice the nurse educators should also facilitate them in carrying out research activities. Educators can thus strive to make research exciting for students.

Nurse Administrators

❖ The nurse administrator is rightly placed in a managerial position to implement research based practice. Her knowledge

and attitude will have due influence on translating research into practice.
- She should create intellectual curiosity among nursing staff for developing innovative solutions to clinical problems.
- She should periodically organize CNE programs and conferences, encourage staff to participate, present research findings and publish research articles.
- Should provide conducive environment for implementing research activities and promote it to support integration of nursing research into practice.
- Establish institutional level nursing research department having an expert consultant to provide necessary support for staff nurses.
- She should also encourage collaborative research projects and include research role in their job description.
- She should reward innovative practices and provide research resources.
- Policies and procedures should be regularly updated in accordance with the scientific updates.
- Encouraging and permitting nurses to involve in research activities increases research awareness and utilization of findings.

Nurse Researcher
- Researcher should focus their research activity on current clinical problems and perform high quality research studies to ensure valid and transferable findings.
- All the studies should suggest clinical implications.
- Nurse researcher should present research findings to the clinical nurses in a way so as to be able to replicate them in clinical practice.
- Commit to replicating studies and publishing the results as early as possible.
- Disseminate the research findings through scientific presentations at conferences and workshops and publish in journals for wider integration of research into current practice.

RESEARCH UTILIZATION STUDIES

Lee (2004) conducted qualitative study and applied Rogers Innovative Diffusion model to analyze nurses' perceptions towards use of a computerized care plan system. Twelve nurses participated in one-to-one in-depth interview. The content that emerged was compared with the model's five innovation characteristics as perceived by new users. Results indicate that Roger's model can accurately explain nurse's behavior during the process of adopting workplace innovations.

Romp and Kiehi (2009) applied Stetler model of research utilization in staff development: revitalizing a preceptor program at one hospital. This resulted in the improvement of nurses' satisfaction with their preceptors and a reduction in turnover rate.

RESEARCH PROPOSAL

A research proposal is a document that is typically written by a scientist or academic proposing an idea for an investigation on a certain topic. Proposals are prepared before the commencement of the study and outline the research process from beginning to end. It comprises a request for sponsorship of that research or an essential task before starting a dissertation/thesis.

Meaning of Research Proposal
A research proposal is a detailed description of a planned study meant to investigate a given problem (Traenkel, 2017).

Functions of Research Proposal
- It serves to communicate to an organization/committee about the research problem, its significance and methods used to investigate it.
- It helps the researchers to clarify their own thinking and guides them in carrying out the research project.
- It is intended to convince the funding organizations that the research project

is worthwhile and the researcher has the competence to complete it.
- It can also be used to seek ethical approval from the ethics committee.
- It helps the researcher to communicate to the faculty/guide what he/she proposes to study enabling them to seek suitable suggestions and support.
- The soundness and potential impact of the research is evaluated based on the proposal.

Format of a Research Proposal

Different funding organizations, universities and educational institutions have different guidelines/formats for preparing the research proposals. The principal investigator should prepare the proposal in line with those guidelines. The content and organization of a research proposal is similar to that of a research report but proposals are written in the future tense and not include results and conclusions. A research proposal usually includes the following elements:
- Title
- Abstract
- Introduction
- Methodology
- Work plan
- Budget estimation
- Method of dissemination
- References
- Appendices

Title

The title should be concise and appealing. An effective title should further evince reader's interest. It should clearly indicate the variables and population of interest.

About the investigator: It includes full names of the researchers, their qualifications and institutional/departmental affiliations. Brief up-to-date curriculum vitae of each of the investigators and co-investigators should be provided.

About the institution: In this section the institutions under whose umbrella the research project will be conducted need be mentioned.

Abstract

It is a short summary of the proposed project approximately 200-300 words in length. It should include the main research question, rationale for the study, hypothesis (if any), design, data collection procedure, sample and instruments that will be used. It should be independent in itself and not refer the reader to points in the project description.

Introduction

The researcher should use this section to evince an interest on the topic among the readers, lay the foundation for the problem that leads to the study and place the study within the larger context of the scholarly literature. It should explain about the need for research and its relevance.

The introduction should typically begin with a statement of the research problem in precise and clear terms. It mainly focuses on the need for undertaking proposed research and describes the need for the study systematically so as to reflect on the priority of the topic to the profession. It also facilitates peer review of the research proposal by the funding organizations. The introduction should include background information, significance of the problem, objectives and hypotheses.

Background information: This section is devoted to description of how the proposed research builds on an existing base of evidence. The background information orients the readers to what is already known about the problem and indicates how the proposed study will augment the body of knowledge. It should also showcase the researcher's control and authority in the field. This background information provides a rationale and lays a strong foundation for the proposed study.

It also includes critical review of existing research and relevant theory.

The problem and its significance: The problem statement should clearly point out the scope and importance of the problem, how the proposed research will contribute to knowledge and enhance evidence based practice. It sets the stage for the research question in a way to highlight its necessity and importance.

Objectives: Research objectives are goals that need to be achieved by conducting research. These should be closely related to the statement of the problem. They may be stated as 'main' and 'specific'. The main objective of the study states what the researcher expects to achieve by the study in general terms. On the other hand specific objectives systematically address various aspects of the problem. An example for main and specific objective is as below:

- Main objective
  - To assess the associated factors among diarrhea patients in a selected village.
- Specific objectives
  - To identify water purification methods
  - To determine their food habits
  - To find out excreta disposal methods

Variables: It is essential to spot the key variables in the planning stage itself. The methods of their measurement must be clearly indicated.

Hypothesis: The hypothesis gives structure and direction to research. They are tentative declarative statements that explain the relationship between two or more variables. They translate the problem statement into a well-defined, clear-cut prediction of expected outcomes.

Methodology

The methods section gives a detailed description of how the research study is conducted. It should allow the reader to verify soundness of methodology used. This section should include research design, study setting, population, sampling plan, method of data collection, data management, data analysis, ethical considerations and work plan.

Research design: It should specify the type of research study the researcher intends to carry out. For example, descriptive, experimental, comparative study etc. The selection of design is based on the research objectives.

Study setting: This specifies where the study is going to be conducted. For example, out-patient department of district hospital or in-patient department of district hospital or higher secondary schools in Bengaluru.

Population: This indicates the subjects who are to be included in the study. For example, patients suffering with chronic disorders, students studying in pre-university colleges, etc.

Sampling plan: It includes details of the sample size, method of calculating the sample size, sampling technique, inclusion and exclusion criteria and recruitment process.

Method of data collection: It outlines the general plan for collecting the data. The details included in data collection are what data needs to be collected, how it is to be collected, who will collect and when. It should also describe measurements/tools, how it will be administered and how participants will be assigned to groups. If an intervention is introduced the description must include duration of intervention, potential risks and benefits to the subjects.

Data management: It includes strategies for coding, storing and analyzing the data and details on statistical softwares, e.g. SPSS, SAS, etc.

Data analysis: It should also include the type of statistical tests that will be used. For example, student t-test, regression analysis, ANOVA test etc.

Ethical consideration: It includes methods of maintaining confidentiality, obtaining informed consent and protecting human rights. While the proposal is being submitted to the ethics committee for approval it should

Table 10.13: An example of timeline for a research proposal

Activity	Duration	Months
1. Preparation of intervention package and finalizing tools, translation of tools to local language, getting ethical clearance, preparation of setting	6 months	January 2018 to June 2018
2. Pilot study	6 months	July 2018 to December 2018
3. Modifications in Pilot study	2 months	January 2019 to February 2019
4. Final data collection process	18 months	March 2019 to August 2020
5. Data entry	1 month	September 2020
6. Statistical analysis	1 month	October 2020
7. Preparing the research report	2 months	November 2020 to December 2020

include informed consent form and ethics checklist.

Work Plan

It describes the proposed plan for managing the work flow on the project. It includes sequence of tasks to be performed, tentative time frame for each task, facilities and personnel required for their completion.

Timeline: This includes overview of proposed activities with timeframe. Weeks or months are mentioned on one side and tasks on the other side to indicate the period for which the task will be performed. An example of timeline for a research project with 36 months duration is presented in Table 10.13.

Facilities: The proposal should include facilities or equipment that are required for completion of the project. It should also mention available equipments, instruments, laboratories, clinical records, data processing equipment and special documents. The proposal should include the willingness letter from the head of the affiliated institution for utilization of space, equipment, service or data for the proposed project.

Personnel: Proposals to funding organizations should include the full details of the principal and co-investigators. Funders scrutinize the curriculum vitae for factors such as researcher's training education, publications and research experience.

Budget Estimation

A budget translates project activities into monetary terms. It is extremely important for requesting financial support. It includes a statement on how much money will be required to complete various tasks. The proposed budget should also include item wise expenditure with necessary justification. It usually includes staff, contingency and overhead charges. The researcher must indicate how money is distributed for various activities in each time period (Table 10.14)

Table 10.14: Budget proposal

(Amt in ₹)

Sl. No.	Particulars	1st year	2nd year	3rd year
1.	Staff			
2.	Contingencies			
3.	Recurring			
4.	Non-recurring (equipment)			
5.	Travel			
6.	Overhead			
	Total			

References

Related references should be included at the end of the proposal. The cited literature should be as current as possible and written as per prescribed guidelines.

Appendices

It should include informed consent form, covering letter, official letter for permission to conduct research and questionnaires with scoring details.

ROLE OF COMPUTERS IN RESEARCH PROCESS

Computers are an indispensable tool throughout the research process. They have changed the ways in which scientific research is compiled and analyzed. The researcher is able to compile vast amounts of data without an element of human error. Thus the use of computers in scientific research is immensely high and inevitable.

Importance of Computers in Scientific Research

- *Speed*: Computers can process numbers and information in an exceptionally short time. This helps the researcher to process and analyze the data quickly and utilize the remaining time for conducting further research.
- *Storage:* Computers can store and retrieve huge amounts of data when needed. It overcomes the risk of forgetting and losing the data.
- *Accuracy*: Computers are incredibly accurate which is very important in scientific research.
- *Organization*: Computers allow easy storage of large amounts of data in an organized manner using simple folders. This not only allows easy retrieval but also saves scarce resources such as time and energy. Computers are more productive and safer compared to paper filing system.
- *Consistency*: Computers are not susceptible to mistakes on account of tiredness or lack of concentration.

Research process consists of a series of steps necessary to effectively carry out research. These series of steps can be organized into five phases. A brief description of use of computers in all these phases is presented in Table 10.15.

The technological innovations have integrated the use of computers in research

Table 10.15: Use of computers in various phases of research process

Phases	Use of computers
Conceptual Phase: It involves developing a research idea and appropriate design	• They help in searching for relevant papers which allows the researcher to identify the gaps in existing literature • Their use provides a definite advantage over physical search for literature from books, journals and other newsletters in the library which is tedious and time consuming • They can be used for storing bibliographic references through World Wide Web which allows retrieval of published articles when required • Visual display softwares can be used to create conceptual maps, flowcharts or visual models of research conceptual framework
Design and Planning Phase: It comprises selecting the research design and developing study procedures	• They can be used for selection of appropriate research design and facilitate research design planning • Several softwares can be used to calculate the sample size • They help in selection of sample from the population by using computer software program known as a random number generator. This generates true random numbers which facilitates an unbiased random sample selection for experimental studies

Contd...

Contd...

Phases	Use of computers

Empirical Phase:
It deals with data collection and preparing the data for analysis
	• They help in designing research instruments
	• Computer programs and internet technology (E-mails, online surveys) can be used for collecting the data
	• Biophysical measurements are monitored through computers only
	   – Computers are also useful for conducting web video recorded interview sessions, narrative led interviews, etc.
	   – The subject related data are stored as word files or excel spread sheets in computers.
	   – Computers help in data entry, data editing and data management.
	   – Computers allow for greater flexibility in recording and analyzing the data. Data coded in excel sheets can be directly processed using statistical software for analysis.

Analytic Phase: In this phase analysis and interpretation of findings takes place	• Data analysis and interpretation can be done with the help of computer softwares which help in calculating average, percentage and correlation etc. For example, SPSS, STATA, Sysat, etc. • Examples of statistics that can easily be calculated through computers are descriptive statistics, chi-square, correlation, t-tests, ANOVA etc. • These softwares can also be used for checking the reliability of data, establishing and testing hypothesis, etc. • They can check the accuracy, authenticity and completeness of the data as they are collected. • They help in drafting tables by which a researcher can interpret the results easily. These tables give a clear proof of the interpretation made by the researcher.
Dissemination Phase: During this phase research results are shared with others	• After interpretation, computer helps is converting the results into a research article or report which can be published. It can be written in a word format or in a PDF format. • Computers can also be used for preparing posters and power point presentations for disseminating research study findings. • Articles can be stored or published on website also. • Computers help to access research papers on the internet effortlessly • International co-operation on scientific projects by forming virtual research teams, aggregating information and sharing of knowledge has been made possible by the use of high speed internet. • For performing Meta-analysis and systematic reviews, data from various studies can be retrieved using specialized softwares.
References: A researcher needs to give source of the literature studied and discussed in references	• References can be written automatically in different styles like APA, Vancouver, etc., which saves considerable time for the researcher. • Some reference managers like 'Medley' can be used to manage the references from where the literature is taken.

beyond imagination. However, it is to be noted that the computers and their applications are only a tool in the hands of the researcher and function as a resource. The researcher should thus exhibit a fine knowledge about the capabilities and limitations of the computer applications and software for their optimum use.

BIBLIOGRAPHY

1. Benos, D.J., Fabres, J., Farmer, J., Gutierrez, J.P., Hennessy, K., Kosek., & Wang, K. (2005). Ethics and scientific publication. *Advances in Physiology Education*, 29, 59-74.
2. Bincy, R. (2012). *Nursing research: building evidence for practice* (2nd ed.). New Delhi: Raj press, R-3, Inderpuri.
3. Burns, N., & Grove, S.K. (2005). *The practice of nursing research: Conduct, critique, and utilization* (5th ed.). St. Louis, MO: Elsevier.
4. Collins English Dictionary. (1991). *The free encyclopedia* (3rd ed.). Glasgow: Harper Collins Publishers.
5. Corinna, R., & Sara, H. (2007). Giving a Good Scientific Presentation: *The American Society of Primatologists,* St. Louis, MO: Elsevier.
6. Polit, F.D., & Beck, T.C. (2004). *Nursing research: principles and methods* (7th ed.). Philadelphia: Lippincott Williams & Wilkins.
7. Freemantle, & Ian, W. (1994). Dissemination: Implementing the findings of the research. *Health libraries review*.11, 133-7. DOI: 10.1046/j.1365-2532.1994.1120133.x
8. Graf, C., Wager, E., Bowman, A., Fiack, S., Scott Lichter, D., & Robinson, A. (2007). Best practice guidelines on publication ethics: A publisher's perspective. *International Journal of Clinical Practice*, 152, 1-26.
9. Kathy L.O., & Michael, A. (2008). *The dissemination and utilization of research for promoting evidence-based practice.* doi: 10.l300/J394v05n0l_ll.
10. Lee, T.T. (2004*).* Nurses' adoption of technology: application of Rogers' innovation-diffusion model. *Applied Nursing Research,* 17, 231-238.
11. Polit, D., & Beck, C. (2006). *Essentials of Nursing Care: Methods, Appraisal and Utilization* (6th ed.). Philadelphia: Lippincott Williams and Wilkins.
12. Reid, W.J ., & Fortune, A.E. (1992). Research utilization in direct social work practice. In A. J. Grasso, & I. Epstein (Eds.). *Research utilization in the social services* (pp. 97-116). New York: Hawthorne.
13. Romp, C.R., & Kiehl, E. (2009). Applying the Stetler model of research utilization in staff development: revitalizing a preceptor program. *Journal Nurses Staff Dev*, 25, 278-284;
14. Rose, M.N. (2006). *Foundation of nursing research* (5th ed.). Philadelphia: Lippincott Williams & Wilkins.
15. Ryan, F., Coughlan, M., & Cronin, P. (2007). *Step-by-step guide to critiquing research. Part 2: Qualitative research: British Journal of Nursing*, 16,738-743.
16. Siedlecki, S.L., Montague, M., & Schultz, J. (2008). Writing for publication: Avoiding common ethical pitfalls. *Journal of Wound, Ostomy, & Continence Nursing*, 35, 147-150.
17. Stockhausen, & Conrick, M. (2002). "Making sense of research" a guide for critiquing a paper: *Contempary Nurse*, 14, 38-45.
18. Suresh, K. Sharma. (2014). *Nursing research & statistics* (2nd ed.). Chennai: Elsevier India Private Limited.
19. Traenkel, J.R., & Wallen, N.E. (2017). *How to design and evaluate research in education.* On line learning center with power web. Available at www.highered.mcgraw-hill.com/sites/0072981369/student_view0/chapter24/key_terms.html Accessed June 18, 2017.
20. Valente, S. (2003). *Research dissemination and utilization: Improving care at the bedside. Journal Nursing Care Quality.* 18, 114-21.

REVIEW QUESTIONS

I. Long Essays

1. What is the meaning of research report? Explain types of research report.
2. What are the various methods of preparing references and bibliography?
3. How can you conduct a critical review on a published report?
4. What are the various steps in writing a research report?

II. Short Essays

1. Barriers to utilization of research findings.
2. Criteria for effective dissemination.
3. Explain the methods of disseminating research findings.

4. List out the characteristics of research report.
5. Advantages and disadvantages of publication.
6. Guidelines for preparing research report.
7. Difference between research utilization and evidence-based practice.
8. Role of computers in research process.
9. Various steps in writing research report.

III. Short Notes

1. Research utilization
2. References
3. Abstract
4. CURN Model of research utilization
5. Contents of thesis or dissertation
6. Poster presentation
7. Research proposal
8. Dissertation
9. List out the Steps of Roger's Innovative Diffusion Model.
10. Write the phases of Stetler Model of research utilization.

IV. Multiple Choice Questions

1. Dissemination is a term which denotes
    a. Communication
    b. Interaction
    c. Face to face meeting
    d. Seminar
2. Expand IMRAD
    a. Introduction, Methodology, Results, and Discussion
    b. Introduction, Material, Results and Discussion
    c. Introduction, Methods, Reporting and Discussion
    d. Introduction, Material, Results and Dissemination
3. Which of the following is a visual graphic presentation of study results?
    a. Poster presentation
    b. Oral presentation
    c. Publication in journal
    d. Peer presentation
4. Arabic numbers in superscript are used in which of the following styles of writing reference?
    a. Oxford referencing style
    b. APA reference style
    c. Vancouver referencing style
    d. Harvard referencing style
5. Which of the following is not a major part of a research report?
    a. Introduction
    b. Methods
    c. Results
    d. Footnote
6. Which of the following methods of disseminating research findings can reach largest percentage of target groups?
    a. Publications
    b. Oral Presentation
    c. Poster presentation
    d. Dissertation or Thesis
7. The following are the purposes of critiquing research studies, *except*
    a. Ensure adequacy of research findings for use in practice
    b. Determine the application to practice
    c. Decide whether to publish the study or not
    d. Presenting in research conferences
8. Which of the following groups of nurses deals with critiquing research study?
    a. Nurse educators
    b. Nursing students
    c. Clinical nurses
    d. All of the above
9. Which of the following should be investigated while critiquing a research study?
    a. Limitations of the study
    b. Suggestions for further research
    c. Missing elements in the study
    d. All of the above
10. When critiquing a study the reader should
    a. Focus only on the weaknesses of the study
    b. Focus only on the strengths of the study
    c. Focus mainly on the design of the study

d. Examine the strengths, weaknesses, and the logical links of the study
11. Who developed the Innovative Diffusion Model of research utilization?
    a. Roger
    b. Stetler
    c. Marram
    d. Michigan State Nurses Association
12. What is research utilization?
    a. Using research generated knowledge to change practice
    b. Synthesizing research information by critically analyzing the report
    c. Disseminating research finding to others
    d. Communicating research findings through dissemination
13. The following are the purposes of research utilization to patient, *except*
    a. Improved patient outcome
    b. Ensure safe and effective care
    c. Motivate researcher to conduct study
    d. Provide high quality cost-effective care
14. An abstract should ideally contain _____ words?
    a. 25-75
    b. 100-150
    c. 150-300
    d. 250-300
15. Which of the following chapters deals with interpretation of results?
    a. Introduction
    b. Method
    c. Results
    d. Discussion
16. The following factors are considered for selecting a journal for publication, *except*
    a. Refereed or non-refereed journal
    b. Scope of the journal
    c. Impact factor
    d. Place of publication
17. The following are the advantages of publication, *except*
    a. Dissemination can occur more rapidly
    b. E-journals are not always refered
    c. Includes comprehensive information
    d. Can reach larger audience
18. Which of the following can be considered as the best strategy to promote research utilization among nurses?
    a. Availability of nursing research resources
    b. Research collaboration among nurse researcher and nurse clinicians
    c. Motivating nurses to read, review, participate and utilize research
    d. All of the above
19. Which section of quantitative research report includes the implications of the findings for nursing practice and theory and the recommendations for further research?
    a. Discussion
    b. Introduction
    c. Methods
    d. Results
20. Which of the following are the four major parts most often included in a research report?
    a. Introduction, literature review, design, findings
    b. Introduction, methods, results, discussion
    c. Problem, framework, methods, discussion
    d. Review of literature, methods, results, findings
21. Which of the following choices includes the complete number of categories in a journal citation?
    a. Journal title, volume, page numbers, year of publication
    b. Journal title, volume, issue number, page numbers, year of publication
    c. Journal title, volume, page numbers, year and month of publication
    d. Journal title, page numbers, year of publication

ANSWER KEY

1. a	2. a	3. a	4. c	5. d	6. a
7. d	8. d	9. d	10. d	11. a	12. a
13. c	14. c	15. d	16. d	17. b	18. d
19. a	20. b	21. b			

PART B—BIOSTATISTICS

- **UNIT 11** : Introduction to Biostatistics
- **UNIT 12** : Measures of Central Tendency
- **UNIT 13** : Measures of Variability
- **UNIT 14** : Normal Probability Distribution
- **UNIT 15** : Measures of Relationship
- **UNIT 16** : Inferential Statistics and Hypothesis Testing
- **UNIT 17** : Application of Statistics in Health and Use of Computers for Data Analysis

UNIT 11

Introduction to Biostatistics

Nursing research as a discipline is widening its scope and gaining momentum in the 21st century.

The purpose of promoting excellence in nursing research as a science can only be accomplished by methodic investigation planned to build reliable evidence pertaining to nursing profession encompassing practice, education, and administration. To incorporate the findings of empirical research into nursing practice so as to further best care practices, the student and clinical nurses must inculcate capabilities to interpret research findings. This can happen only if a working knowledge of statistical tests and procedures along with their interpretation and proper use of the study results is developed.

It is important for nursing students and clinical nurses to acquire skills in reading and evaluating the results from statistical analysis (Brown, 2014; Craig and Smyth, 2012).

HISTORICAL NOTES

The word statistics is derived from the Latin word *"status"* or the Italian word *"statista,"* meaning "political state" or "Government". Shakespeare in the year 1602, for the first time, used the word statist in his drama Hamlet. In the year 1749, Gottfried Achenwall used the word *"statistic"* to mean the political science of different countries. During the 20th century, new methods, theories, and applications were actively developed by several statisticians. It received an impetus with the introduction of electronics in the field of modern day statistics.

Florence Nightingale (1820–1910) is the first known nurse statistician who applied statistics to improve healthcare. During the Crimean War, Nightingale used statistical data from British army files to show that improved sanitary conditions led to fewer military deaths. This statistical evidence persuaded the British Government to introduce field hospitals and provide nursing care to soldiers.

DEFINITIONS

Statistics consists of a body of methods for collecting and analyzing data (Agresti and Finlay, 1997).

Statistics is the study of techniques and procedures for collecting, classifying, summarizing, analyzing, and interpreting numerical data. It goes beyond mere organization and presentation of data, and is a means for designing and carrying out studies, exploring and describing data, making inferences, and generalizations about the phenomena.

Biostatistics is the application of statistical principles to questions and problems in medicine, public health or biology.

Biostatistics is a discipline which deals with science of collection, classification, analysis, quantification, and interpretation of data relating to health and illness.

Biostatistics is the branch of statistics that deals with vital events in a human population.

CHARACTERISTICS OF STATISTICS

Statistics are
* Numerically expressed
* Aggregation of facts
* Collected in a systematic manner
* Enumerated according to reasonable standard of accuracy

LIMITATIONS OF STATISTICS

* Not applicable to qualitative phenomena
* Studies a group but not an individual
* Requires large numbers to give accurate results
* Decisions are true on an average only

USES OF BIOSTATISTICS IN MEDICINE

* To design statistical procedures for resolving questions relating to medical or public health data
* To define and quantify the nature and extent of illness and deaths in the community
* To identify risk factors for disease and establish causation for existence of health problems through statistical analysis
* To establish signs and symptoms of diseases by using various statistical methods
* To design, monitor, analyze, interpret, and report results of clinical studies
* To evaluate outcome of health interventions
* To compare certain attributes of the two different populations
* To find the difference between efficacy of two drugs or vaccines or interventions
* To check the efficacy of biomedical equipment.

SIGNIFICANCE OF BIOSTATISTICS IN THE FIELD OF NURSING

* Biostatistics is a fundamental part of nursing profession which allows nurses to prioritize treatment and determine whether or not a patient requires follow-up care or immediate medical attention.
* Nurses can use statistics for describing phenomena, correlating the variables, finding the effectiveness of nursing interventions, and predicting outcomes in patients. It also helps the nurse to describe how one event or situation relates to another event or situation.
* Understanding statistical methodologies are important for a nurse to incorporate empirical findings into everyday nursing practice.
* It helps nurses identify patterns in signs and symptoms of patients thus enabling them to take informed decisions and better respond to the patient's medical status.
* It helps the nurse to determine if commonly used interventions should be changed or protocols should be revised.
* Biostatistics can also be useful while dealing with allocation of limited resources or bringing about a change in the nursing profession.
* Every nurse whether pursuing a bachelors or postgraduate degree should have the basic knowledge of statistics. This will boost their skills and confidence in delivering quality care to patients.

SCOPE OF BIOSTATISTICS

* Biostatistics can be applied in all health-related fields so as to address questions arising from medical, nursing, and pharmacy-related data.
* It helps in designing research studies and analyzing the research data.
* Biostatistics helps in sample size determination, development of data collection measures, and analysis and interpretation of research data.
* Biostatisticians also play vital role in the preparation of research material for publication.

TERMINOLOGY

- *Class interval:* It refers to the difference between the upper and lower limits of a class. They are generally mutually exclusive and have the same class width.
- *Class mid-point:* It is the middle value of each data class. It can be arrived by averaging the upper and lower class limits.

$$= \frac{\text{Upper class limit + Lower class limit}}{2}$$

- *Continuous data:* The data which can be measured in fractional values is called continuous data. For example: height, weight, body temperature, etc.
- *Cumulative frequency:* It includes the data elements in a particular class and all its preceding classes. It can be done either in an ascending or descending order.
- *Data:* Data is/are the basic building blocks of statistics and refer to the individual values presented, measured or observed.
- *Discrete data:* The data in a whole number is called discrete data. For example: pulse rate, respiratory rate, etc.
- *Frequency distribution:* It describes the data set and lists each class interval with the number of data values in the respective class. It is called the frequency of the class.
- *Lower class limit:* The least value that can belong to a class.
- *Nonparametric test:* A statistical test that does not involve assumptions about the distribution of critical values.
- *Parameter:* Any numerical value computed from the population is known as parameter.
- *Parametric test:* A statistical test that involves assumptions about the distribution of the variables and the estimation of a parameter.
- *Population:* Population is the collection of all individuals or items under consideration in a statistical study (Weiss, 1999).
- *Qualitative data:* When the collected data are non-numerical or categorical in nature, it is called qualitative data. For example: gender, religion, marital status, etc.
- *Quantitative data:* When the data is collected in numerical values, it is called quantitative data. For example: height, weight, Hb level, etc.
- *Range (of data):* It is the difference between the highest value and the lowest value.
- *Sample:* Sample is that part of the population from which information is collected (Weiss, 1999).
- *Sampling:* The process of taking a sample from the population is called sampling.
- *Statistic:* Any numerical value computed from a sample is known as a statistic.
- *Upper class limit:* It is the largest value present within the class limit.
- *Variable:* It is an attribute or a number that describes an individual or a data item. The value of the variable may vary from one entity to another.

COMMONLY USED SYMBOLS IN STATISTICS

In statistics, Roman letters are used to indicate sample statistics while Greek letters are used to indicate population statistics. The commonly used notations are presented in Table 11.1.

TYPES OF DATA AND ITS MEASUREMENT

Types of Data

Data are facts or figures from which conclusions can be drawn. Data can be classified as either numeric (quantitative) or nonnumeric (qualitative).

- Quantitative data consist of values that indicate counts or measurements. It is further classified into discrete or continuous data.
  ○ Discrete data are numeric data that have a finite number of possible values,

Table 11.1: Commonly used symbols in statistics

Symbol	Meaning	
Mathematical functions:		
Σx_i	Sum of the numbers in variable x; can be arrived by adding all the values of x	
Σx_i^2	Sum of the squared values of all numbers in variable x; can be arrived by squaring each value of x and then adding them up	
$(\Sigma x_i)^2$	Square of the summed value of numbers in variable x; can be arrived by adding up all the values of x and then squaring the total	
<	Less than	
≤	Less than or equal to	
>	Greater than	
≥	Greater than or equal to	
≈	Approximately equal to	
$|x|$	The absolute value of x (without sign)	
Statistical symbols:		
α	Alpha: The significance level set for the study	
p	The *p*-value of the computed statistic	
H_0	The null hypothesis	
H_A	The alternative hypothesis	
α (alpha) error	Type I error in hypothesis testing	
β (beta) error	Type II error in hypothesis testing	
N	Population size	
n	Sample size	
f	Frequency	
μ (mu)	Population mean	
$\bar{x}$ (x-bar)	Sample mean	
σ^2 (sigma squared)	Population variance	
σ (sigma)	Population standard deviation	
s^2	Sample variance	
s or SD	Sample standard deviation	
CI	Confidence interval	
df	Degrees of freedom	
χ^2 (chi-square)	Goodness of fit test	
ρ (rho)	Population correlation coefficient	
r	Sample correlation coefficient	
Measures	*Sample statistics*	*Population parameters*
Number of cases	n	N
Mean	$\bar{x}$ (x-bar)	μ (mu)
Standard deviation	s or SD	σ (sigma)
Variance	s^2 or SD^2	σ^2 (sigma squared)
Correlation	r	ρ (rho)
Proportion	p	π (pi)
Regression coefficient	b	β (beta)

i.e. it can take only whole number equivalents. For example, pulse rate can take only whole number values such as 72 beats/min, 80 beats/min, 95 beats/min and not fractional values.
- Continuous data have infinite number of possible values, i.e. not limited to whole number values; for example, age (1 year, 1 year and 6 months, 2 years, 2 years and 6 months), salary (₹ 11,000/-, ₹ 11,600/-, ₹ 12,700/-), weight (1.1 kg, 1.25 kg, 1.30 kg, etc.), and height (3′, 3′2″, 3′3″) are continuous variables (Flowchart 11.1).

❖ Qualitative data consists of non-numeric values that can be placed into categories, commonly termed as a categorical data.

The types of data greatly affect the choice of analysis method. To carry out an analysis, the variables have to be quantified by providing values and a suitable scale. There are four levels of measurements on a continuum of discrete and continuous scale.

Levels of Measurement

Before the researcher begins with the analysis he should familiarize himself with the various types of measurement scales. These data were classified by Stevens (1946) into four measurement scales: nominal, ordinal, interval, and ratio, each one adding more to the next. Analysis can be carried out on the data depending upon the relevant measurement scale. These four measurement scales are listed in their hierarchical order of describing results, with nominal scale being the least precise and the ratio scale being the most precise of them all. Thus ordinal data is also nominal, and so on. The acronym NOIR (French word for "black" N—nominal, O—ordinal, I—interval, R—ratio) depicts the hierarchical order.

Nominal Scale

Nominal comes from the Latin root *"nomen"* meaning "name". The nominal scale is the simplest and lowest level of measurement. Here the numbers are assigned as labels to represent categories or characteristics. When data are classified into two or more categories and there is no order or difference in size of these categories (i.e. no category is better or worse, or higher or lower, or more or less than another) they can be labeled using a nominal scale. For instance, in gender all are classified as either male or female. There is no difference in maleness compared with femaleness. The only relationship between these categories is that they are different in their attributes.

The categories are mutually exclusive and exhaustive. Mutually exclusive means that the categories must be distinct enough that no observations will fall into more than one category. Exhaustive means that there must be enough categories that all the observations will fall into some category. This scale lacks numeric order, magnitude, or size.

Flowchart 11.1: Types of data

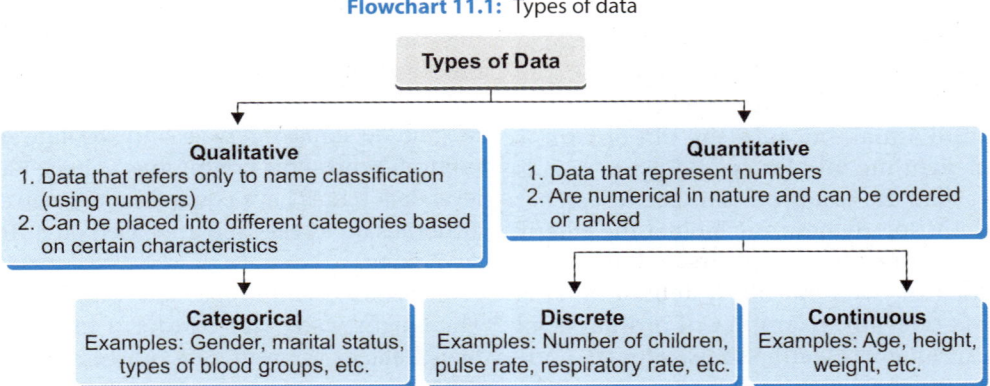

Examples of nominal scales are gender, religion, marital status, working vs non-working, etc. A scale for gender might include: Male 1, Female 2. In this scale the number is assigned for the purpose of gender identification only, and does not in any way represent magnitude, order, or size. This scale uses numerals rather than words to enable carrying out statistical analysis.

Ordinal Scale

It is the second level of measurement scale in the hierarchy. In this scale the level of measurement goes beyond mere categorization and ranks the characteristics based on certain criteria. Thus this scale is much more accurate in measuring the characteristics when compared to nominal scale. The ordinal scale classifies the data into categories as well as ranks them on a scale; for example, from poor to excellent. Though it includes ranking, it still lacks magnitude, size, equal intervals or an absolute zero point. Like the nominal scale, the ordinal scale categories must be mutually exclusive and exhaustive, i.e. an individual cannot be rated with both mild and moderate anxieties. The difference between the categories must be clearly established so that every person in the sample falls into only one category. Subjective rating scales measuring satisfaction, pain, discomfort, psychological distress, depression, opinion and all Likert scales are considered ordinal.

For example, to measure age on an ordinal scale, the researcher would develop categories such as young, middle-aged, and old. The magnitude alters with the age of the individual, because the old person is older than the middle-aged person, who is older than the young person. The researcher does not specify how much older the elderly person is than the young person. It is not the number of years but the system of ranking that is relevant. Examples of ordinal level measurement: Health status—Poor/Good/Excellent; Income status—Low/Middle/Upper.

Interval Scale

It is the third level of measurement scale in the hierarchy. In this scale the level of measurement goes beyond order and classifies data based on magnitude. It however lacks a defined size or "absolute" zero point. Its significant feature is that the numbered intervals between points are equidistant, whether those intervals are measured in centimeters or degrees. It allows for more mathematical manipulation of data.

Fahrenheit temperature scale is a good example of interval scale, where the degrees are calibrated from high to low. Each degree in the scale is equidistant from the next degree; zero point is not absolute and is arbitrary as a score below zero is actually possible (this is the reason why 80°F is not twice as hot as 40°F). The term "arbitrary zero" in the scale does not refer to a complete absence of quantity but relatively serves as an initial point.

Another example of interval level of measurement is the scholastic assessment test. A score of 500 on this test is greater than a score of 450, which in turn is greater than 400. Also the difference between 500 and 450 on the test is in all probability equivalent to the difference between 450 and 400.

Ratio Scale

In the hierarchy it is the final level of measurement scale. It allows for most manipulation of data. In this scale the level of measurement goes beyond order and magnitude and includes absolute zero point. Thus this scale has all three attributes viz. magnitude, equal intervals, and absolute zero point. It represents continuous values. Ratio level data scores have equal distance between attributes on a scale and are based on a "true zero" point.

The best example of a ratio scale is height. The height scale has an order: 1 foot is less than 2 feet. It has magnitude and the difference between 1 foot and 2 feet is the same as the difference between 2 feet and 3 feet. It also has an absolute zero point, in the sense that 0 feet is the complete lack of height. Other examples of ratio level measurement are weight, pulse, and BP.

Interval and ratio scales quantify the data and hence are quantitative. In these scales the variables can be categorized, ranked, have equal intervals, and represent a range of values. As they can be measured on a scale, they are also called *scale data*.

The characteristics and permissible statistics for four measurement scales are presented in Table 11.2 and Figure 11.1.

TYPES OF STATISTICS

The two main statistical methods used in data analysis are descriptive and inferential statistics (Flowchart 11.2).

Table 11.2: Summary of the properties for four levels of measurement

Scale	Description	Characteristics	Examples	Permissible Statistics		Graphs
				Descriptive	Inferential	
Nominal	Data is organized into categories but cannot be arranged in any specific order	Contains no magnitude, just names	Eye color (brown/black), gender (male/female)	Frequencies Percentage Mode	Chi-square, Binomial test	Bar Pie
Ordinal	Data is categorized and arranged in rank order, however the differences between data values cannot be established	Reflects only magnitude, does not contain equal intervals or an absolute zero. Have/represent rank order	Levels of depression (mild/moderate/severe), stages of cancer (1/2/3/4)	Frequencies Percentage Mode + Median	Rank-order correlation	Bar Pie
Interval	Data is categorized and ranked with meaningful intervals between measurements. No true zero point	Possesses magnitude and fixed size of interval between data points, but no absolute zero	Temperature on Centigrade scale (30°C/ 40°C/ 50°C), Intelligence Quotient Scores (70/90/100)	Frequencies (if discrete) Percentage Mode (if discrete) Median + Mean SD Skewness Kurtosis	ANOVA, Product moment, t-test	Bar (if discrete) Pie (if discrete) Histogram
Ratio	Data is categorized, ranked with meaningful intervals and has an inherent zero starting point	Possesses magnitude, equal intervals and an absolute zero (true zero point)	Height (2"/4.1"/6.3"), Weight (1 kg/2.3 kg/3.5 kg)	Mean SD Skewness Kurtosis	Coefficient of variation, t-test	Histogram

(ANOVA: Analysis of Variance; SD: Standard Deviation)

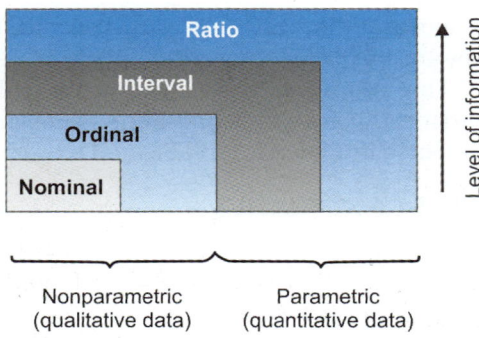

Fig. 11.1: Levels of measurement

Descriptive and inferential statistics are inter-related in the sense that methods of descriptive statistics are initially used to organize and summarize the sample information before methods of inferential statistics are used to analyze the subject under investigation.

While the descriptive statistics are initially used to organize and summarize the data, the inferential statistics are later used to estimate parameters and test the hypothesis.

ORGANIZATION AND PRESENTATION OF DATA

Descriptive statistics consist of methods for organizing and summarizing information (Weiss, 1999). These statistics summarize the data from a sample using computation of averages (mean, median, mode), measures of dispersion (variance, standard deviation, range, interquartile range), and include construction of graphs, charts, and tables.

Inferential statistics consist of techniques for measuring the reliability of conclusions about population based on information obtained from a sample (Weiss, 1999). These statistics make inferences about a population using methods like estimation (point estimation, interval estimation) and hypothesis testing based on probability theory.

The collected raw data is usually in an unorganized form. It needs to be organized to conduct statistical analysis. This organization can be done by way of *classification, tabulation,* and *graphical presentation*.

Classification of Data

The process of organizing data into groups and classes based on certain attributes is termed as classification of data. This organization eliminates irrelevant details and places data with common attributes in one class by dividing the entire data into a number of groups or classes. In this process data are combined into relatively small number of class intervals followed by an indication of number of cases in each class. This process of

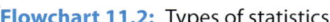

Flowchart 11.2: Types of statistics

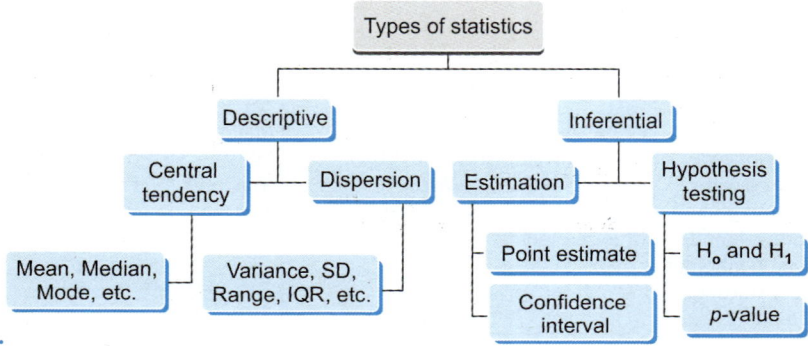

(IQR: Interquartile Range; SD: Standard Deviation)

classifying data into groups is called frequency distribution. The range of each group of data is called the class interval. Each class has a lower and an upper limit, and the difference between the two is known as class width. This process allows comparison among the categories of observations and highlights the important aspects of data. Classification can be done either according to attributes or numerical characteristics.

- *Classification according to attributes:* In this the data are classified based on descriptive characteristics such as gender, type of family, marital status, etc. These characteristics cannot be measured quantitatively but only their presence or absence in an individual item can be observed.
- *Classification according to numerical characteristics:* In this the data are classified based on numerical characteristics such as height, weight, blood pressure, etc. These characteristics are measured using some specific units.

For example in Table 3 class interval is 1–2, 2–3, 3–4.., class width is 1. The class intervals are mostly kept equal (Table 11.3).

Table 11.3: Frequency table

Height in ft	Frequency
1–2	2
2–3	5
3–4	8

(Lower class limit, Class width = 2–1 = 1, Upper class limit)

Tabulation of Data

It is the process of summarizing and presenting the data in the form of a table (rows and columns) so as to aid easy understanding. It should facilitate interpretation and subsequent analysis. Frequency distribution uses the table format to organize the data, enabling the readers to comprehend the basics of data distribution. This tabulation makes it easy to gather information about central tendency, dispersion, and outliers.

Frequency distribution: It is a table wherein the data are grouped into classes according to common attributes and the number of times each value falls into a particular class. It records the frequency of occurrence for each value of a single variable. A frequency distribution facilitates computation of various statistical measures.

Frequency distribution can be classified into two types:
1. Univariate frequency distribution: It includes values of only one variable.
2. Bivariate frequency distribution: It includes values of two variables, which can be further classified into three categories:
   i. *Series of individual observations:* It refers to listing of items of each observation. For example, well-being scores of 20 adolescents displayed individually refer to a series of individual observations:

59	59	59	15	26	59	26	15	59	48
40	33	15	26	59	40	33	26	40	26

   ii. *Discrete frequency distribution:* In this classification different values of a variable and their respective frequencies (i.e. the number of times each value occurs) are displayed side by side. This is facilitated by listing the values from highest to lowest or vice-versa, using the technique of tally bars to record the frequencies. While the first column includes all the values of the variable, the second column has vertical bars called tally bars (/) to record the frequencies indicating number of times the value occurred. For easy counting, blocks of five bars are put together with some space left in between these blocks. After placing tally bars for all the values of the data, its corresponding value is recorded in the third column. A sample discrete frequency distribution for the series mentioned earlier is constructed in Table 11.4.

Though the above discrete frequency distribution is much more compact than the individual series presentation, it is still difficult to comprehend. If there are no repeated values in the data, the frequency distribution table hardly condenses the data.

iii. **Continuous frequency distribution:** It is an arrangement of values wherein each interval of the table includes the frequency of occurrence of values within that interval. The groups into which the values of a variable are classified are known as classes and the range of values within that class is called the class interval. The size of the class interval is called the width of the class and the boundaries of the class interval (upper and lower values) are known as class limits. The arrangement of the data into continuous classes with the corresponding frequencies is known as continuous frequency distribution.

Before constructing a frequency table the number of class intervals has to be finalized. The number of class intervals should not be too many, as the data would continue to be bulky. On the other hand if the number of class intervals is less, the shape of the distribution cannot be determined. It is ideal to have 5–14 class intervals. After finalizing the number of class intervals the marking of tally bars is done to record the number of values that fall in each class interval. This is followed by recording the frequency in the adjoining column by adding the tally bars. The width (size) of the class is obtained by dividing the range of observations with the number of class intervals. In the earlier mentioned example, the range of values (wellbeing scores of 20 adolescents) is 59 – 15 = 44. This is divided by the total number of class intervals, i.e. 5 to obtain the class width, i.e. (44/5 = 8.8 ≈ 10) (Table 11.5).

Guidelines for constructing class widths
- Class widths should be of equal size. Unequal class widths should only be used to overcome large gaps in existing data
- Class intervals should be mutually exclusive and nonoverlapping
- Open-ended classes should be avoided, e.g. <100, >1,000

Two methods of classifying the data according to class intervals are
1. *Exclusive method:* When the lower limit is included and the upper limit excluded, then it is an exclusive class interval. In this method the upper limit of a particular class becomes the lower limit of the next class interval. It is called "exclusive" as the values equal to the upper limit of a class are excluded from that class and included in the next class. Exclusive type of class intervals are used in the case of continuous variate. For example, consider

Table 11.4: Discrete frequency distribution

Marks	Tally bars	Frequency
15	///	3
26	////	5
33	//	2
40	///	3
48	/	1
59	//// /	6
		20

Table 11.5: Continuous frequency distribution

Marks	Tally bars	No. of students (f)
15–25	///	3
25–35	//// //	7
35–45	///	3
45–55	/	1
55–65	//// /	6
		20

the exclusive class intervals 20–40, 40–60..., etc. In the class interval 20–40, 20 is included but 40 is excluded (40 is included in the next class interval 40–60).

2. *Inclusive method:* When both the lower and the upper class limits are included, then it is an inclusive class interval. In this method the upper class limit of a particular class is 1 less than the lower limit of the next class interval. It is called "inclusive" as the values of both the upper and lower class limits are included in the same class itself. Inclusive type of class intervals are used in the case of discrete variate. For example, 20–39, 40–59..., etc. are inclusive type of class intervals.

Guidelines for constructing a frequency distribution

- *Type of classes:* Each class should be clearly defined and not ambiguous. They should be mutually exclusive and exhaustive so that each value of a variable corresponds to only one class.
- *Number of classes:* The factors that decide the number of classes are:
  - The total frequency or number of observations in the distribution
  - The size or magnitude of the values of the variable
  - The desired accuracy
  - The ease with which the various descriptive measures can be computed, e.g. mean, variance, etc.

  The number of classes should neither be too small nor too large. With a decrease in the number of classes the intervals become broader resulting in lesser accuracy. An increase in number of classes however results in fewer class frequencies making the distribution irregular. Also, the number of class intervals should be such that the distribution is uniform and unimodal, i.e. the frequencies in the given classes increase and decrease steadily without sudden jumps and convenient for numerical computations.

- *Size of class intervals:* The size of the class interval and the number of classes in a given distribution are inversely proportional. The class intervals should be framed such that each class has a suitable mid-point around which all the observations (entire frequency) in that class are concentrated. It is always desirable to have class intervals of equal or uniform magnitude throughout the frequency distribution.
- *Class boundaries:* Class boundaries are the actual class limits (the minimum and maximum value a class interval may contain) of a class interval. In overlapping or exclusive type of classification both class boundaries and limits are the same. For example, as in 20–40, 40–60, 60–80... the upper class limits are excluded, thus the actual class limits are 20–39, 40–59, 60–79, and boundaries are also same. Whereas in nonoverlapping or mutually inclusive classification, class boundaries and limits are different. For example, as in 20–39, 40–59, 60–79 class boundaries are obtained subtracting d/2 from the lower class of each limit and adding d/2 to the upper class of each limit, where d is the gap between the upper limit of any class and lower limit of succeeding class. In the above example 20–39, 40–59, the class boundary of the class interval 20–39 can be obtained by subtracting 0.5 from the lower limit and adding 0.5 to the upper limit, i.e. 19.5–39.5.
- *Mid-value:* The mid-value can be defined as the average of the upper and lower limits of a class. It is obtained by dividing the sum of the upper and lower class limits by 2. The class limits should be so framed that the observations in any class are evenly distributed throughout the class interval. This ensures that the mid-values of the class are the true representative of the actual average of observations in that

class. In Table 5, the upper and the lower class limits of the first class 15–25 are 25 and 15, respectively. Thus the mid-value of the class would be (UCL + LCL)/2 = (25 + 15)/2, i.e. 20.

- *Open end classes:* Class intervals wherein the lower limit of the first class or the upper limit of the last class or both are not specified are termed as frequency distributions with open end classes. For example, classes such as weight less than 50 kg or height above 6 feet. As the mid-value cannot be determined accurately in such class intervals, one has to assume that the magnitude of the first class is same as that of the second class.

Table

"A statistical table is the logical listing of related quantitative data in vertical columns and horizontal rows and numbers, with sufficient explanatory and qualifying words, phrases and statements in the form of titles, heading and footnotes to make clear the full meaning of the data and their origin." —**Tuttle**

Components of table

Presenting the data in a table format though compresses the necessary information in a limited space, it should not be at the cost of clarity. Rules to be adhered to while constructing a table are given below:

- *Table number:* Each table should be suitably numbered for proper identification and future reference. The number should be quoted above the title of the table, either in the center or the left side of the table.
- *Table title:* The table title should be suitable, clear, concise and self-explanatory, and be given just above the frame of the table. The title should be brief and in itself explain the what (the data are about), where (the data are), when (the data occurred), and how (data is classified) in a concise language.
- *Caption:* It refers to the column headings, which explains what each column represents. The captions should be clearly defined and placed in the middle of the column.
- *Stub:* These define each row and are placed to the extreme left. They perform the same function for the horizontal rows as the caption performs for the vertical columns. Stubs are usually wider than column headings and kept narrow.
- *Body:* It includes the crucial part of the collected information and is numerical in nature.
- *Head note:* It is a brief explanatory note about the contents in the table not covered by the title, captions or stubs. These are generally placed in brackets immediately after the title and used to indicate units in which the data in the table are expressed.
- *Foot note:* It is written below the table and used to further clarify either the title captions or stubs. Footnotes are numbered using 1, 2, 3…or a, b, c…. or even special characters like @ or $ used to identify them.
- *Source data:* The source of the data should invariably be stated allowing the reader to cross check and gather further information if necessary.

A model of the table is presented in Table 11.6.

Requirements of a good statistical table

A well laid out statistical table does not have specific rules for preparation, but is a product of innovation and ingenuity on the part of the student or the researcher. The main idea is to economize on space and present the data clearly. To do so, one should have a clear picture of the facts being presented, the points to be stressed upon and a familiarity with the table preparation technique. Though there are no hard and fast rules for preparing a good statistical table,

Table 11.6: Components of a model table

Stub headings	Caption				Row total
	Subhead		Subhead		
	Column head	Column head	Column head	Column head	
Stub entries					
Column total					

Footnote:

Source:

the following points may nevertheless be considered in the process:

- *Purpose:* A table should suit the purpose and keep the objective of the statistical enquiry.
- *Preparation:* A table should be simple, systematic, compact, and logically organized.
- *Clarity:* A table should be readily comprehensible and complete. Overlappings and ambiguities should be avoided at all costs.
- *Size:* The table should be of manageable size. It should neither be very long and narrow nor very short and broad. It should fit into the space provided without compromising on legibility. If the space available is inadequate, the table may be split into two or more parts or appended on a separate large sheet.
- *Numbering:* In case of more number of rows and columns, they may be numbered for easy reference.
- *Approximation:* If the figures are large and contain many decimal places, they may be suitably approximated or rounded. The method for approximation or rounding may be indicated along with the units of measurement.
- *Presentation:* The table should be presented in an appealing way and grab the attention of the reader readily. Single, double or thick lines may be used to separate or highlight the rows or columns. The columns though are separated using lines, the rows may or may not be separated.
- *Units:* The units should invariably be depicted in the table below the title. However, if there are different units involved, they may be mentioned in the respective units and columns.
- *Totals and percentages:* The corresponding percentages should find a place to the right or at the bottom of the column containing the original figures. Totals and subtotals of both rows and columns may be arrived where necessary.
- *Arrangement:* The presentation of various items in the table should follow a definite pattern, i.e. the items may be arranged either alphabetically, chronologically, conventionally or in the order of magnitude (ascending or descending).
- *Font:* It is advisable to use capital and bold fonts for headings, subheadings, stubs, captions, and small letters for preparatory note, footnotes, and source. Fashionable and stylish fonts should altogether be avoided. Suitable lettering size also helps in adjusting the table within the space provided.
- *Abbreviation:* Only accepted forms of abbreviations should be used to avoid ambiguity. Footnotes may be included where necessary. Boxes or circles may be used to highlight individual items in the table. Gaps may be filled up with "NA"

indicating "not available" rather than a mere dash. The use of ditto mark (") may be avoided.

Types of tables

Tables can be classified in different ways based on the objective, nature or the elements being covered in the study. On the basis of elements covered, tables can be classified into simple or complex. The major criterion in this type of distinction is the number of characteristics being studied. Simple tabulation represents a single characteristic of the data whereas complex tabulation represents various inter-related characteristics.

- *Simple table:* Also known as one-way table, it provides information on one or more independent characteristics of the phenomenon (Table 11.7).
- *Complex table:* Provides information regarding two or more mutually dependent characteristics of a phenomenon. When two or three characteristics are depicted in a table, it is known as a two-way (double tabulation) or three-way table, respectively. A manifold tabulation depicts four or more characteristics simultaneously.
- *Two-way table:* Provides information on two inter-related characteristics of a phenomenon (Table 11.8).
- *Three-way table:* Provides information on three inter-related characteristics of a phenomenon (Table 11.9)
- *Manifold table:* Provides information on large number of inter-related characteristics for a given phenomenon—commonly used in population statistics (Table 11.10).

The main advantages of tabulation are that it simplifies the data, economizes on space, facilitates comparison and statistical analysis, saves time, depicts trends, and used as a reference. The disadvantages are that apart from being a complicated process, all kind of data cannot be tabulated and at times it lacks flexibility when changes need to be incorporated at regular intervals.

Functions of tables
- Summarizes and classifies the data systematically
- Depict the data for comparative studies
- Utilizes optimum space
- Reveals the data at a glance

Table 11.7: Simple table

Age (in years)	Number of students (in thousands)
0–10	12
10–20	15
20–30	22
30 and above	45

Table 11.8: Two-way table

Age (in years)	Number of students		Total
	Male	Female	
0–10	5	7	12
10–20	10	5	15
20–0	11	11	22
30 and above	20	25	45
Total	46	48	94

Table 11.9: Three-way table

Age (in years)	Male			Female			Total		
	Rural	Urban	Total	Rural	Urban	Total	Rural	Urban	Total
0–10									
10–20									
20–30									
30 and above									
Total									

Table 11.10: Manifold table

District	Age (in years)	Male			Female			Total		
		Rural	Urban	Total	Rural	Urban	Total	Rural	Urban	Total
1	0–10									
	10–20									
	20–30									
	30 and above									
2	0–10									
	10–20									
	20–30									
	30 and above									
	Total									

Diagrammatic or Graphic Presentations

A graphic presentation is another way of analyzing numerical data. In this the data are presented using lines or curves drawn across the coordinated points. It can also be defined as a direct or analogical representation which makes the reasoning process more natural and understandable.

❖ Graphical representation helps to quantify, sort, and present data in an easily comprehendible manner.
❖ As graphs enable the study of both time series and frequency distribution they are more suitable to provide a clear account of the problem.
❖ These display the relationship between variables by exhibiting the change in one variable corresponding to the change in the other.
❖ It provides the complete picture at a glance.
❖ It is more effective than presenting data in tabular form.
❖ Computer software packages help in presenting graphical data in a variety of ways viz. bar chart, pie chart, histogram, frequency polygon, frequency curve, and line diagram.
❖ Various graphical representations are possible depending upon the nature of the data and statistical results.

❖ A graph consists of two coordinate axes, one vertical (known as Y-axis or ordinate) and the other horizontal (known as X-axis or abscissa). These two lines are perpendicular to each other and intersect at "0" also called the origin.
❖ On the X-axis the values to the right of the origin are positive and those to the left are negative.
❖ On the Y-axis the values above the origin are positive and those below the origin are negative.
❖ The coordinate system is divided into four areas. The top right segment is called quadrant I followed by quadrants II, III and IV moving in the anticlockwise direction. The ordered pairs for each of the quadrant are (Fig. 11.2)
  ○ Quadrant I—X and Y coordinates are positive represented by (X, Y)
  ○ Quadrant II—X-coordinate is negative and the Y-coordinate is positive represented by (-X, Y)
  ○ Quadrant III—X and Y coordinates are negative represented by (-X, -Y)
  ○ Quadrant IV—X-coordinate is positive and the Y-coordinate is negative represented by (X, -Y)

Tips for constructing a graph:
❖ The graph should be properly drawn.

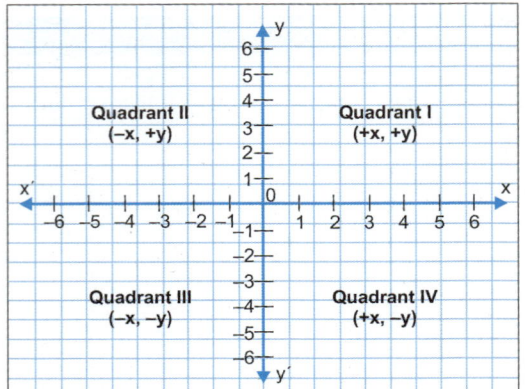

Fig. 11.2: Coordinate plane with four quadrants

❖ The size of the scale should neither be too big nor too small.
❖ The graph should convey the meaning clearly and easily. It must be self-explanatory.
❖ To make graphs easily comprehendible a combination of shades and colors can be used.
❖ Vertical graphs should be preferred over horizontal graphs.
❖ Graphs should not be made attractive or impressive at the cost of accuracy.
❖ Footnotes may be added to overcome certain ambiguities.

Types of Graphs

There are many types of graphs and charts used to indicate data. These can be divided based on the data they present: qualitative data presentation and quantitative data presentation (Fig. 11.3).

Qualitative data presentation

Qualitative data are presented in the form of bar diagram, pie diagram or pictogram.

Bar graph: This type of graph is more useful when the data is of qualitative nature. It represents frequency distribution of nominal data and ordinal data. The lengths of the bars represent the frequency of occurrence of the category. A bar graph has two axes, x and y wherein the x-axis represents the types of categories to be compared and the y-axis representing the corresponding numerical values of the data. The bars may extend in either of the horizontal or vertical directions (Fig. 11.4).

Interpreting the bar graphs could involve looking for their size and/or growth relative to another or change in bars representing the same category in different classes depending on what information one is looking for. The advantages and disadvantages of bar graph are presented in Table 11.11.

A few tips while reading the bar graphs:
❖ Look for inconsistent scales. If two or more graphs are being compared, ensure the same scale is being used. However, if different scales are being used, one should be aware of the differences and read them accordingly.
❖ Ensure all the classes are equal. For example, do not mix days and weeks.
❖ Ensure consistency in the interval between the classes. For example, if a month-on-month data for a particular period is being compared with year-on-year data of a different period, suitable steps should be taken to make the data compatible.

Types of bar graph: Commonly used bar graphs are simple, multiple, component (subdivided) and percentage subdivided bar graphs. Description of these types is presented in Table 11.12.

Pie diagram: Pie diagram is a circular representation of statistical data where the percentages are displayed as sectors of a circle; pieces of the pie. It is another way of presenting discrete data of qualitative characteristics such as gender groups, blood groups, Rh groups, types of aggression, etc. The frequencies of the group are shown in a circle wherein the degrees of angels denote the frequency and area of the sector. This aids comparison at a glance (Fig. 11.5). The advantages and disadvantages of pie diagram are presented in Table 11.13.

Unit 11: Introduction to Biostatistics

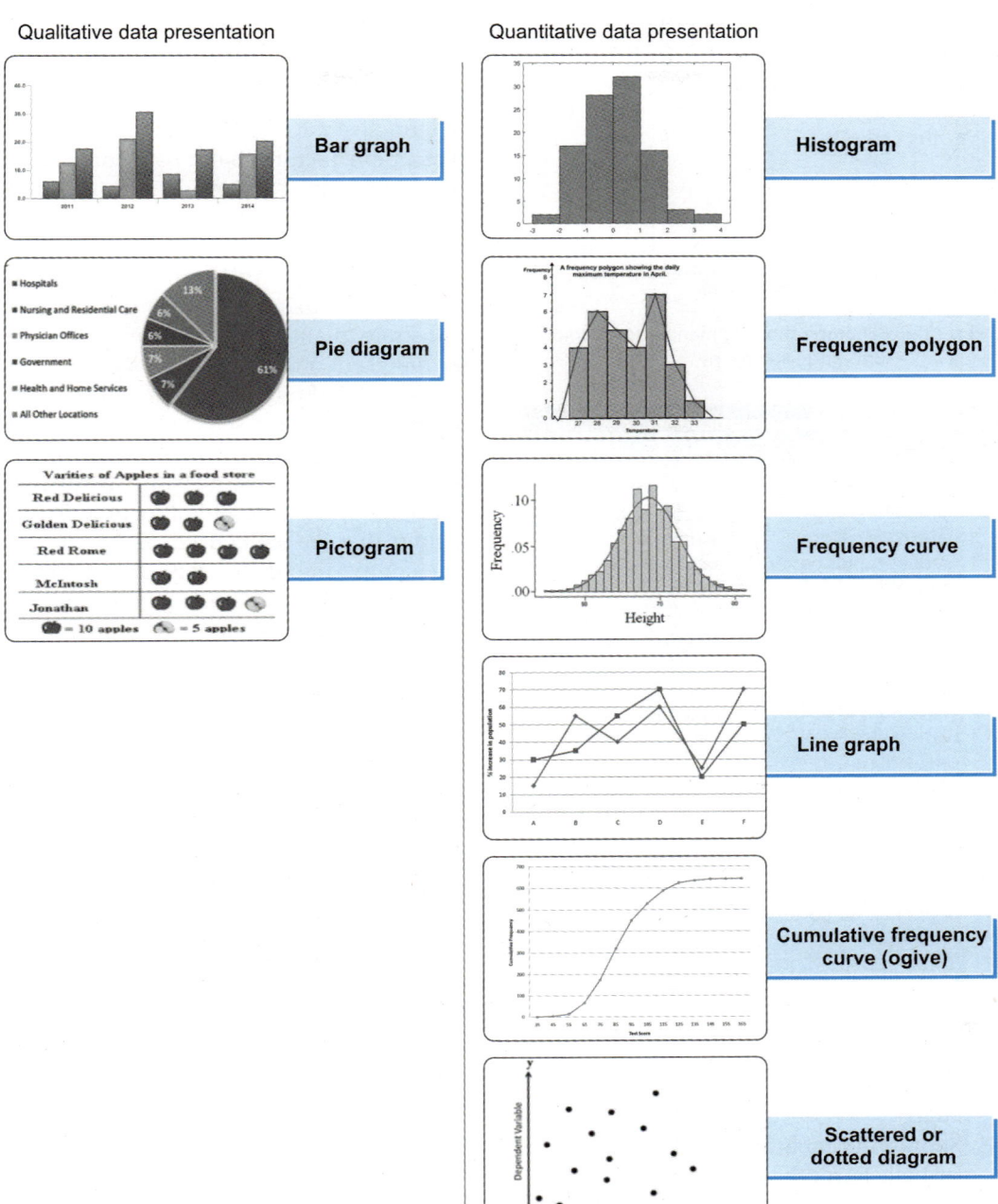

Fig. 11.3: Types of graphical presentation

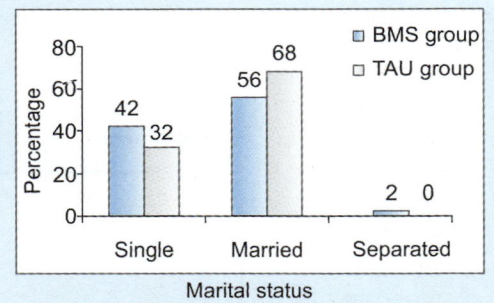

Fig. 11.4: Bar graph showing marital status among BMS and TAU groups

Table 11.11: Advantages and disadvantages of bar graph	
Advantages	Disadvantages
• Summarizes large data in visual form • Clarifies trends better than tables • Allows estimation of key values at a glance • Permits visual check of accuracy and reasonableness of calculations • Displays relative numbers or proportions of multiple categories • Shows each nominal or ordinal category in a frequency distribution	• Requires additional written or verbal explanation • Be easily manipulated to provide false impression • Fails to reveal assumptions, norms, causes, and effects

Important characteristics of a pie diagram
❖ Used only for qualitative data
❖ Only one variable can be included in the chart
❖ Should not include too many categories (usually fewer than 6 categories)
❖ Displays the division of a total quantity in the form of sectors in a circle
❖ In a circle the angle of the sector is proportional to the frequency of the data and is given by the formula:

$$\text{Angle of sector} = \frac{\text{Frequency of data}}{\text{Total frequency}} \times 360°$$

Pictogram: Pictogram is an incredibly engaging and attractive way to present data. Also called a pictograph, picture chart or an icon chart, it is a popular form of data visualization wherein statistical data is represented using symbolic figures to match the frequencies of different kinds of data. It is a variation of a bar graph, but instead of using bars they use symbols to illustrate quantity. Each picture or symbol may represent one or more units of the data. It is a simplified representation of a concept, useful in conveying a sense of large findings using icons to represent units. However, the disadvantages include possible distortions of data, the need to round off data to fit into the units that are being used, and confusion while comparing one pictogram to another. Example of a pictogram is given in Figure 11.6. The advantages and disadvantages of pictogram are presented in Table 11.14.

Quantitative data presentation
Quantitative data are presented in the form of histogram, frequency polygon, frequency curve, line graph, cumulative frequency diagram (Ogive), and scattered diagram.

Histogram: It represents frequency distribution of ordinal, interval or ratio level data using rectangles where the width of bars represents class intervals and the height represents the corresponding frequency. The data presented pertains to only one variable. In a histogram the bars are of equal width and touch each other indicating that data are being presented on a continuum. To construct a histogram, two axes are drawn: a horizontal axis (abscissa) and a vertical axis (ordinate). The abscissa represents the categories of the variable or the class intervals while the ordinate represents the frequency of the category being measured. Beginning with "0" the ordinate is divided into equal intervals so as to include the highest

Table 11.12: Types of bar graph

Type of bar graph	Description
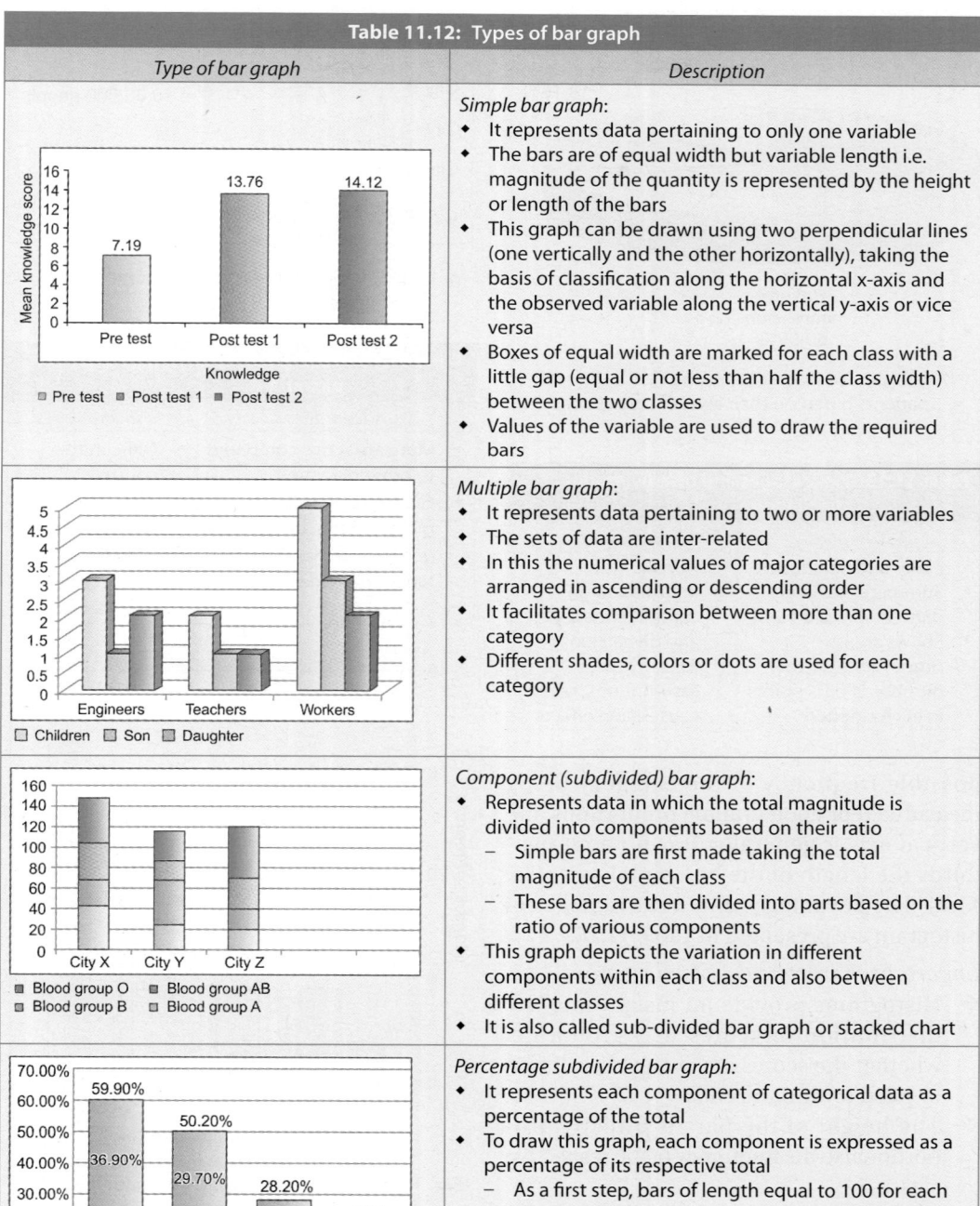	*Simple bar graph*: • It represents data pertaining to only one variable • The bars are of equal width but variable length i.e. magnitude of the quantity is represented by the height or length of the bars • This graph can be drawn using two perpendicular lines (one vertically and the other horizontally), taking the basis of classification along the horizontal x-axis and the observed variable along the vertical y-axis or vice versa • Boxes of equal width are marked for each class with a little gap (equal or not less than half the class width) between the two classes • Values of the variable are used to draw the required bars
	Multiple bar graph: • It represents data pertaining to two or more variables • The sets of data are inter-related • In this the numerical values of major categories are arranged in ascending or descending order • It facilitates comparison between more than one category • Different shades, colors or dots are used for each category

	Component (subdivided) bar graph:
	• Represents data in which the total magnitude is divided into components based on their ratio
	  – Simple bars are first made taking the total magnitude of each class
	  – These bars are then divided into parts based on the ratio of various components
	• This graph depicts the variation in different components within each class and also between different classes
	• It is also called sub-divided bar graph or stacked chart

	Percentage subdivided bar graph:
	• It represents each component of categorical data as a percentage of the total
	• To draw this graph, each component is expressed as a percentage of its respective total
	  – As a first step, bars of length equal to 100 for each class are drawn
	  – In the second step, they are sub-divided into the proportion of the percentage of their components
	• This type of a graph is useful to make comparison in components while keeping the difference in the totals constant

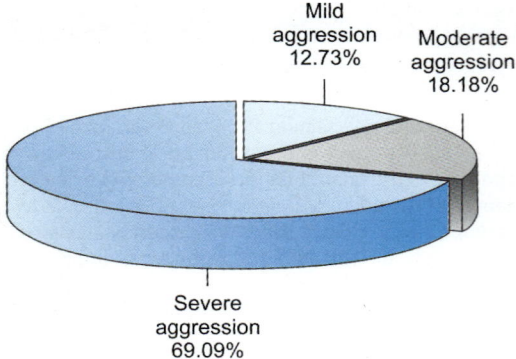

Fig. 11.5: Pie diagram showing distribution of patients based on their level of aggression

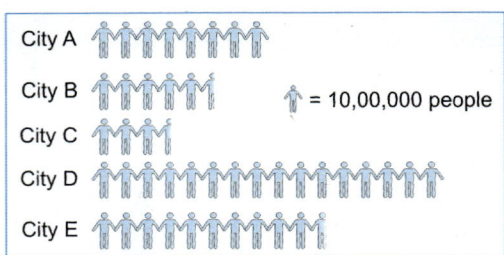

Fig. 11.6: Pictogram depicting the population of five cities

Table 11.13: Advantages and disadvantages of pie diagram

Advantages	Disadvantages
• Easily understandable • Summarizes a large data set in visual form • Shows areas proportional to the number of data points in each category	• Reveals little information on central tendency and dispersion • Fails to reveal assumptions, norms, causes, and effects

Table 11.14: Advantages and disadvantages of pictogram

Advantages	Disadvantages
• More attractive compared to other diagrams • Facts displayed in pictorial form are generally remembered longer than mere facts	• Difficult to construct • Difficult to compare • Possibility of data getting distorted

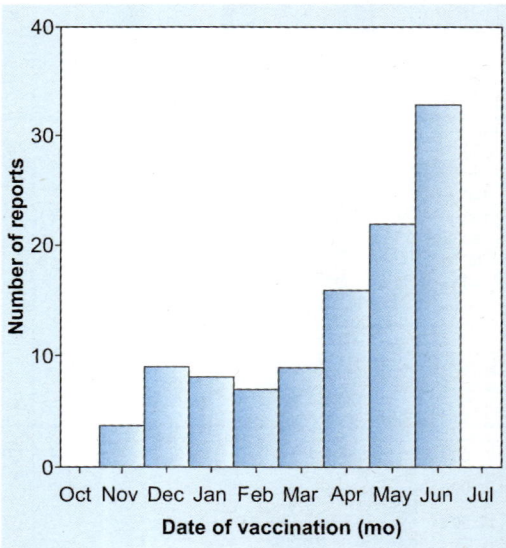

Fig. 11.7: Histogram showing vaccination statistics

possible frequency of the category being measured. For good graphic proportions, the vertical axis is generally drawn about two-thirds the length of the horizontal axis (Fig. 11.7). The advantages and disadvantages of histogram are presented in Table 11.15.

Important characteristics of a histogram
- Histograms provide an insight into the distribution of scores in a group, i.e. whether the scores are evenly distributed or piled toward the ends.
- The height of the bars is directly proportional to the frequency of the respective class.
- Though a histogram highlights the variation in the data, it can easily be manipulated.
- Histograms can be misleading if too many or too few bars are employed.
- Though a histogram does not display the individual times or the exact times a score occurs, it is still a reliable way to look at the trend of the data.

Table 11.15: Advantages and disadvantages of histograms

Advantages	Disadvantages
• Shows the central tendency and dispersion of a data set • Summarizes a large data set in visual form • Permits a visual check of the accuracy and reasonableness of calculations • Shows each interval in the frequency distribution	• Requires additional written or verbal explanation • Fails to reveal assumptions, norms, causes, and effects

Frequency polygon: It is a frequency graph that depicts the overall pattern of the frequency distribution. It is obtained by joining the top mid-points of the histogram bars. It represents the frequency distribution of ordinal, interval or ratio data. While the frequencies of the class intervals are represented on the vertical axis, the height of each dot indicates the frequency of a particular class interval. It is generally used when two or more distributions are to be compared.

In Figure 11.8, the first point indicated by "A" is on the x-axis (y = 0) and in the middle of the interval immediately preceding the first bar of the histogram. The last point indicated by "H" is also located on the x-axis and in the middle of the interval immediately following the last bar of the histogram. Interestingly, the area covered under the frequency polygon obtained by joining the mid-points of each bar and the x-axis at each end is same as the total area of the histogram. The advantages and disadvantages of frequency polygon are presented in Table 11.16.

Steps in constructing a frequency polygon
❖ Choose the class interval and mark the values on the horizontal axes. In Figure 11.8 weight of the students is marked on the horizontal axis (x-axis). The class intervals are: 25.5–30.5, 30.5–35.5, 35.5–40.5, etc.
❖ Mark the mid value of each interval on the horizontal axes. The mid-points can be arrived by averaging the upper and lower class limits of the respective class interval. In Figure 11.8, the mid values are represented by 28, 33, 38, etc.
❖ Mark the frequency of the class on the vertical axis (y-axis). In Figure 11.8, the number of students depicts the frequency.
❖ Rectangular bars with widths equal to their class-size and the lengths corresponding to the frequency of the class interval are drawn.
❖ Corresponding to the frequency of each class interval, mark a point at the top middle of the class interval. In the Figure 11.8 mid-points are indicated by B, C, D, etc.

Table 11.16: Advantages and disadvantages of frequency polygon

Advantages	Disadvantages
• Shows the central tendency and dispersion of a data set • Summarizes a large data set in visual form • Projects trends better than other graphs • Easily understandable	• Fails to delineate each interval in a frequency distribution • Requires additional written or verbal explanation • Fails to reveal assumptions, norms, causes and effects

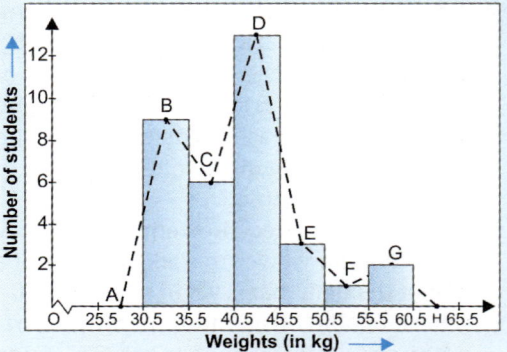

Fig. 11.8: Frequency polygon

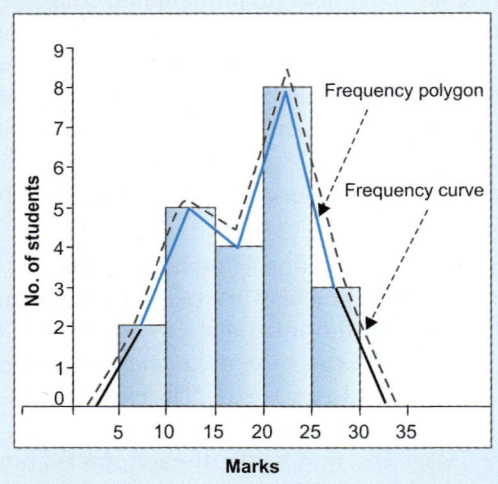

Fig. 11.9: Frequency curve

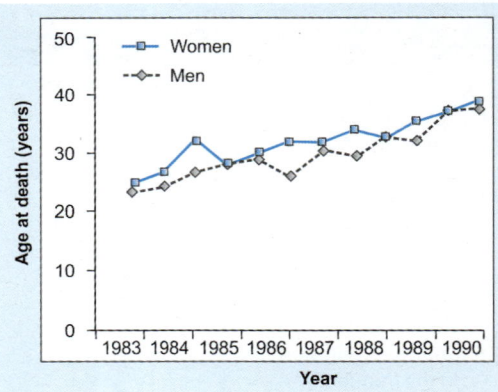

Fig. 11.10: Line graph

Table 11.17: Advantages and disadvantages of line graph	
Advantages	Disadvantages
• More simpler to construct and read than bar graphs or histogram • Projects patterns and trends over time better than other graphs • Requires minimal written or verbal explanation	• Fails to reveal assumptions, norms, causes, and effects • Does not reveal much about skew or kurtosis

❖ Connecting these points using a line segment the frequency polygon is obtained.

While a frequency polygon is obtained by connecting the top mid-points of each histogram bar by a straight line, a frequency curve is obtained by connecting those points using a free hand, i.e. by drawing a smooth curve that follows the general shape of the bars (Fig. 11.9).

Line graphs: A line graph, also called a line chart, is a graphical display of information that changes continuously over time. It has two axes. The *x*-axis (abscissa) of a line graph shows the occurrences and the categories being compared over time and the *y*-axis (ordinate) represents the scale, which is a set of numbers that represents the data and is organized into equal intervals. It is important to know that all line graphs must have a title. A line graph also includes a key that represents the event, situation, and information being measured over time. The lines in the graph can either descend or ascend based on the data (Fig. 11.10). Advantages and disadvantages of line graph are presented in Table 11.17.

Important characteristics of a line graph:
❖ These are suitable for representing the data points, i.e. given one variable the other can easily be determined.
❖ Convenient to plot time graphs along x/y axis as it clearly depicts the rise and fall of data points. By correct selection of scales for each axis (time on x-axis and the change being measured on the y-axis) the reader can easily observe the changes in one group over time.
❖ These help to detect the trends pretty early enabling the viewer to make predictions about the data that is yet to be recorded.
❖ These enable observation of both short-term and long-term changes. This aids easy comparison of two or more values.

❖ These are capable of showing the relationship between 2 or more variables and also record positive and negative values.
❖ Line graphs provide the flexibility to use various colors or different line styles such as dots or dashes.
❖ The parts of a line graph are:
  ○ *Title:* Tells what the graph is about
  ○ *Labels:* The horizontal and vertical labels describes the data on each axis
  ○ *Scales:* Show how much or how many of the data is on each axis
  ○ *Points:* Depict a specific data point on the line graph with x and y coordinates
  ○ *Lines:* These provide an estimate of the values between the points in case of a discrete function. However, in case of a continuous function, these lines provide an actual data, as opposed to an estimate.

Cumulative frequency curve (Ogive): A cumulative frequency curve, also called an ogive, is a visual representation of the cumulative frequency table which is the running total of the frequencies. It is a continuous curve which shows numbers, percentages or proportions of observations that are less than or equal/more than or equal to particular values. Unlike a histogram which uses rectangles, an ogive uses single point markings where the top right of the rectangle would be. To generate an ogive from a frequency polygon, one needs to add up the counts moving from left to right in the graph. An ogive graph plots cumulative frequency on the y-axis and class boundaries along the x-axis. Two types of cumulative frequency curves are: more than type and less than type cumulative frequency curves. Example: An ogive for the data in Table 11.18 is presented in Figure 11.11. The advantages and disadvantages of ogives are presented in Table 11.19.

From Table 11.18 the coordinates can be obtained by having upper limits on the x-axis and the respective cumulative frequencies on the y-axis (20, 4), (40, 10), (60, 17), (80, 25), (100, 34). Joining these points by a smooth curve we get an ogive.

Table 11.18: Less than cumulative frequency table

Marks	0–20	20–40	40–60	60–80	80–100
Frequency	4	6	7	8	9
Cumulative frequency	4	10	17	25	34

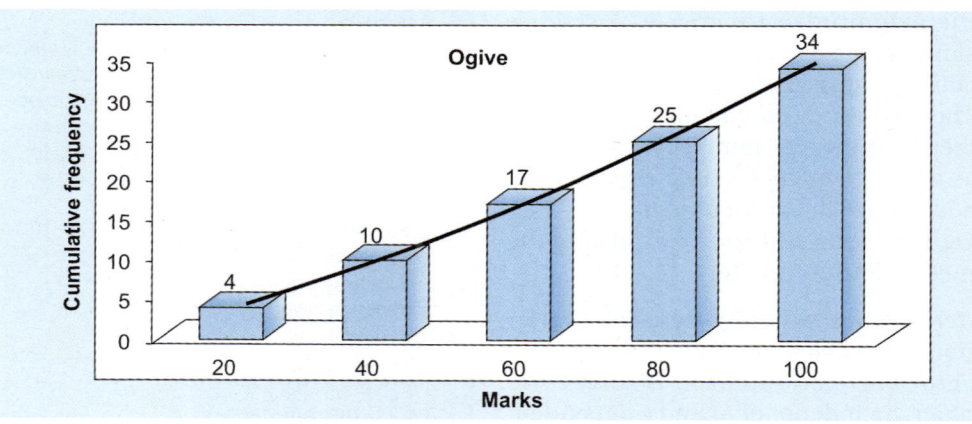

Fig. 11.11: Cumulative frequency curve (ogive)

Table 11.19: Advantages and disadvantages of ogive

Advantages	Disadvantages
• Outlines each interval in the frequency distribution • Differentiates rates of change between classes better than other graphs • Depicts proportion of data points above or below a particular value	• Complicated to prepare • Does not reflect all data points • Does not reveal much about central tendency and dispersion

Important characteristics of an ogive
❖ An ogive, also called a double curve, has the shape of an elongated "S" with one portion being concave and the other being convex.
❖ To plot an ogive it is necessary to have a frequency table, class boundaries, and cumulative frequencies. For grouped data, ogive is formed by plotting the cumulative frequency against the upper boundary of the class and for ungrouped data, cumulative frequency is plotted on the y-axis against the data which is on the x-axis.
❖ These graphs can be used to visually represent the total values that lie above or below a specified upper class boundary.
❖ The point-to-point relative slopes indicate the magnitude of increase. A steeper slope indicates a greater increase when compared to a gradual slope.
❖ The end value of the cumulative frequency is equal to the total number of data values, as all the frequencies have already been added up to the previous total.
❖ Ogives are useful for determining the median and percentiles.

Scattered or dotted diagrams: The scatter diagram, also known as scatter plot, scatter graph or correlation chart, involves two variables, an independent and a dependent variable. This diagram helps in finding the correlation between these two variables. To study the pattern of relationship, a change in the dependent variable vis-à-vis a deliberate change in the independent variable can be monitored (Fig. 11.12). The advantages and disadvantages of scatter diagram are presented in Table 11.20.

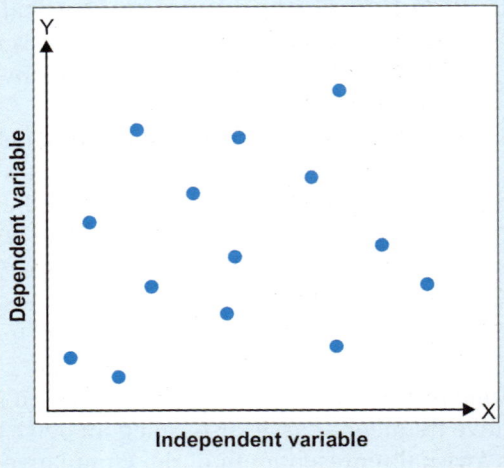

Fig. 11.12: Scattered diagram

Table 11.20: Advantages and disadvantages of scattered diagram

Advantages	Disadvantages
• Plotting the diagram is relatively simple • Easily understood and interpreted • Outliers are isolated and do affect the results • Scatter diagram helps in determining how strongly two variables are related and predicts the behavior of dependent variable as a measure of the independent variable • This diagram is especially useful when one variable is easy to measure and the other is not	• It only depicts the direction but not the degree of correlation • Useful only when data values are less • This diagram does not show the relationship for more than two variables

BIBLIOGRAPHY

1. Agresti, A. & Finlay, B. (1997). *Statistical Methods for the Social Sciences* (3th ed.). Prentice Hall.
2. Anderson, T. W. & Sclove, S. L. (1974). *Introductory Statistical Analysis*. Houghton: Mifflin Company.
3. Brown, S.J. (2014). *Evidence-based nursing: The research practice connection* (3rd ed.). Sudhbury, MA: Jones & Barlett.
4. Burns, N., & Grove, S.K. (2005). *The practice of nursing research*: Conduct, critique and utilization (5th ed.). St. Louis, MO: Elsevier Saunders.
5. Burns, N., & Grove, S.K. (2001). *The Practice of Nursing Research*: conduct, critique & utilization (4th ed.). Philadelphia: WB Saunders.
6. Craig, J.V. & Smyth, R.L. (2012). *The evidence based practice manual for nurses* (3rd ed.). Edinbergh UK: Churchill Livinsgtons.
7. Freund, J.E. (2001). *Modern elementary statistics*. Prentice-Hall, 2001.
8. Polit, D.F., & Beck, C.T. (2010). *Essentials of Nursing Research*: Appraising Evidence for Nursing Practice. Philadelphia, PA: Lippincott Williams & Wilkins.
9. Polit, D.F., & Beck, C. T. (2012). *Nursing research*: Generating and assessing evidence for nursing practice (9th ed.). Philadelphia: Lippincott Williams & Wilkins.
10. Plichta, B.S., & Garzan, S.L. (2009). *Statistics for nursing and allied health*. Philadelphia, PA: Lippincott Williams & Wilkins.
11. Stevens, S.S. (1946). On the Theory of Scales of Measurement. *Science,* 103(2684), 677-680. doi:10.1126/science.103.2684.677. PMID 17750512.
12. Weiss, N.A. (1999). *Introductory Statistics*. Addison Wesley.

REVIEW QUESTIONS

I. Long Essays

1. Define qualitative and quantitative variables with suitable illustrations. What are the different graphical representations used for these variables?
2. Draw pie diagram for the following data on distribution of blood groups among 100 persons.

Blood group	No. of persons
O	43
A	36
B	12
AB	9

3. Explain frequency distribution. Construct a frequency distribution for following set of scores.
   32, 30, 33, 22, 16, 19, 25, 26, 25, 18, 22, 30, 33, 24, 26, 27, 23, 28, 26, 21, 24, 31, 29, 25, 28, 22, 27, 26, 30, 17, 24.
4. Following scores are obtained by a group of students on a test of reasoning:
   18, 8, 30, 10, 24, 17, 26, 19, 16, 23, 11, 20, 22, 25, 16, 19, 14, 18, 13, 17, 21, 6, 22, 9
   a. Tabulate the data using a class interval of three
   b. Prepare a histogram
   c. Interpret the data

II. Short Essays

1. Define statistics? Describe scope of statistics in Nursing.
2. What are the levels of measurements? Discuss.
3. Guidelines of tabulation
4. Frequency polygon
5. Explain bar diagram
6. Why are ratio scales superior to interval scale?
7. Draw a "Pie" diagram to present the data given below.
   "Knowledge score of mothers on various temporary family planning methods"
   a. Oral contraceptive—30%

b. Intrauterine devices—45%
c. Safe periods—20%
d. Injectables—5%

III. Short Answers

1. Define statistics
2. List four characteristics of a good table
3. Define data
4. Types of statistics
5. For each of the following variables listed below, select the most appropriate measurement scale (Nominal/Ordinal/Interval/Ratio).
   - Gender
   - Temperature in celsius
   - Weight in kilograms
   - Age in years
   - Age in categories (0–6 months, 6–12 months, 12–18 months)
   - Blood type
   - Ethnic identity
   - Number of years spent in school
   - Highest educational degree obtained
   - Satisfaction with nursing care received (on a scale of 1–10)
   - Religion
   - IQ score
   - Smoking status (nonsmoker vs smoker)
   - Birth order
   - Reaction time in seconds
   - Marital status
   - Number of children
   - Score on a satisfaction scale that sums Likert items
   - Annual income in rupees

IV. Multiple Choice Questions

1. For a variable with which of the properties is nominal level of measurement used?
   a. They can be placed in meaningful order, but there is no information about the size of the interval between each value.
   b. They can be placed in meaningful order, have meaningful intervals, and have a true zero.
   c. They can be placed in meaningful order and have meaningful intervals between the times, but there is no true zero.
   d. They simply represent categories.
2. Which of the following statements about use of descriptive statistics is true?
   a. They are used in every research study, qualitative as well as quantitative
   b. They are used to identify pattern in data
   c. They are used to address objectives of some studies
   d. All of the above
3. Class intervals should be
   a. Of equal length
   b. Mutually exclusive
   c. Overlapping intervals
   d. Both a and b
4. Nominal-level data can be displayed using a
   a. Histogram
   b. Stem-and-leaf plot
   c. Bar chart
   d. Frequency table
5. Descriptive statistics have which of the following properties?
   a. They are numerical or graphical summaries of data.
   b. They are used to examine relationships between variables in a dataset.
   c. They are used to see how well sample data can be generalized to the population.
   d. Both b and c
6. Inferential statistics have which of the following properties?
   a. They are numerical or graphical summaries of data.
   b. They are used to examine relationships between variables in a dataset.
   c. They are used to see how well sample data can be generalized to the population.
   d. Both b and c
7. Which of the following is not a descriptive statistic?

a. Mean
b. Standard deviation
c. Frequency distribution
d. Correlation
8. Which of the following scale is simplest and lowest level of measurement?
   a. Nominal scale
   b. Ordinal scale
   c. Ratio scale
   d. Interval scale
9. Which of the following scale involves magnitude, equal intervals and absolute zero point?
   a. Nominal data
   b. Ordinal data
   c. Ratio data
   d. Interval data
10. Which of the following levels of measurement has a scale with an absolute zero?
    a. Ratio
    b. Nominal
    c. Interval
    d. Ordinal
11. Which of the following levels of measurement are ranked variables with unequal intervals between numbers of the scale?
    a. Nominal
    b. Ordinal
    c. Interval
    d. Ratio

ANSWER KEY

| 1. d | 2. d | 3. d | 4. c | 5. a | 6. d |
| 7. d | 8. a | 9. c | 10. a | 11. b | |

UNIT 12

Measures of Central Tendency

Measures of central tendency are statistics that attempt to describe a data set with a single value which represents the central location or position. Center here refers to the middle or average value, and tendency refers to the inclination of the numbers to come together in a certain fashion. A measure of central tendency not only summarizes a frequency distribution but also condenses the data to a single representative value. These are appropriate for summarizing interval or ratio data. It is helpful when one is working with huge amounts of data and wants to compare a piece of data with the complete data set.

For example, where age of participants in a sample is a study variable, instead of listing ages of all participants, the researcher can summarize the data using a measure of central tendency such as the average (mean) age of participants in the sample. The three most common measures of central tendency are (1) arithmetic mean, (2) median, and (3) mode (Table 12.1). When the data is normally distributed, mean, median, and mode are identical, each of which represents the most typical value in the data set.

CHARACTERISTICS OF A GOOD STATISTICAL AVERAGE

A perfect measure of central tendency has the following characteristics (Fig. 12.1).
- It should be rigidly defined
- It should be readily comprehensible and easy to calculate
- It should be based on all the observations
- It should be suitable for further statistical calculations
- It should be least susceptible to fluctuations of sampling
- It should not be affected much by extreme values

MEAN (ARITHMETIC)

The mean (or average) is the most common and extensively used measure of central tendency applicable to both discrete and continuous data, but more often used for continuous data. It is derived by adding all the values in the data and dividing the sum by the total number of values in the data set. The sample mean is indicated by the symbol $\bar{x}$ (pronounced x-bar) and the population

Table 12.1: Example on mean, median, and mode of anxiety scores of nine students viz. 6, 3, 1, 5, 9, 5, 4, 5, 7

Type	Description	Example	Result
Mean	Total sum divided by number of values	(6 + 3 + 1 + 5 + 9 + 5 + 4 + 5 + 7)/9	5
Median	Middle value (when the data are arranged in order)	1, 3, 4, 5, 5, 5, 6, 7, 9	5
Mode	Most common value	1, 3, 4, 5, 5, 5, 6, 7, 9	5

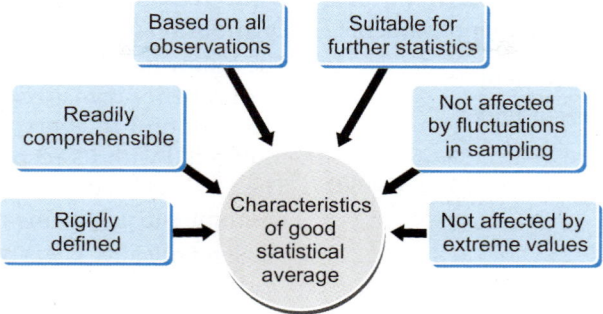

Fig. 12.1: Characteristics of a good statistical average

Table 12.2: Merits and demerits of mean	
Merits	Demerits
• Good representative of the data as it utilizes all the values in the data set • Best choice as it reflects the total of the scores • Most useful measure when further statistical computation is to be done • Applicable to both continuous and discrete numeric data • It best resists the fluctuation between different samples when drawn from the same population • As repeated samples drawn from the same population tend to have similar means, it best resists the fluctuation between different samples • Most stable measure of central tendency	• Reactive to exact position of each score in the distribution. Thus increasing or decreasing the value of any score will also change the mean • It is influenced by outliers and skewed distributions as it takes into account each value in data set, i.e. it is more responsive to the presence or absence of extreme values in the distribution • It is not suitable for categorical data, as the values cannot be totaled • May not appear in the data • Requires interval level data • It cannot be determined by inspection

mean is indicated by the Greek symbol μ (pronounced "mu"). The merits and demerits of mean are presented in Table 12.2.

Characteristics of Mean

* It includes all the data values in the calculation, i.e. it is a model of the data set, but not usually one of the observed values in the data set
* It accurately predicts the representative value of a data set
* The mean is the only measure of central tendency where the sum of the deviations of each value from the mean is always zero
* When the data is normally distributed, the mean is the best measure of central tendency.

Calculation of Mean

Calculation of Mean for Ungrouped Data

If there are n values in a data set $x_1, x_2, ..., x_n$, the sample mean is given by $\bar{x}$ is:

$$\bar{x} = \frac{(x_1 + x_2 + \cdots + x_n)}{n}$$

The above formula can also be represented using the Greek capital letter (Σ) pronounced "sigma", which means "sum of...":

$$\bar{x} = \frac{\sum x}{n}$$

Example: The anatomy marks of 10 nursing students are 54, 54, 54, 55, 56, 57, 57, 58, 58,

60. The mean marks can be arrived by dividing the total marks with the number of students.

$$\bar{x} = \frac{\text{Sum of marks of all students}}{\text{Total number of all students}}$$

$$= \frac{(54+54+54+55+56+57+57+58+58+60)}{10}$$

$$= \frac{563}{10} = 56.3$$

Calculation of Mean for Frequency Table Data

Here each frequency is multiplied by the variable, and the arrived total divided by total number of frequencies to get $\bar{x}$.

Symbolically, $\bar{x} = \Sigma fx/N$

Where f = Frequency
$\bar{x}$ = Arithmetic mean
x = Value of the variable
N = The sum of frequency or Σf

Example: The following table shows the calculation of arithmetic mean for discrete frequency table (where frequencies of a variable are given but the variable is without class intervals).

Weight (in kg)	No. of newborns
2.5	6
3	6
3.5	4
4	2

Weight in kg (X)	No. of newborns (f)	fx
2.5	6	15
3	6	18
3.5	4	14
4	2	8
	$\Sigma f = N = 18$	$\Sigma fx = 55$

As $\bar{x} = \Sigma fx/N$
$= 55/18 = 3.06$

Calculation of Mean for Group Frequency Distribution (Continuous Data)

The following example shows the calculation of arithmetic mean for continuous data. Here, the midpoint of every class interval "x" is multiplied with its respective frequency "f". The total "fx" is divided by the total number of samples to get the mean.

Symbolically, $\bar{x} = \Sigma fx/N$
Where
$\bar{x}$ = Arithmetic mean
f = Frequency
x = Midpoint
LCL = Lower class limit
UCL = Upper class limit
N = The sum of frequency or Σf

Class interval	f	x	fx
1–10	2	5.5	11
11–20	4	15.5	62
21–30	6	25.5	153
31–40	4	35.5	142
41–50	4	45.5	182
	$\Sigma f = N = 20$		$\Sigma fx = 550$

$$x = \text{Midpoint} = \frac{\text{LCL} + \text{UCL}}{2} = \frac{1+10}{2} = 5.5$$

$$\bar{x} = \frac{\Sigma fx}{N} = \frac{550}{20} = 27.5$$

MEDIAN

Median is the middle number when the data is arranged in either ascending or descending order.

It divides the distribution into upper half and lower half, i.e. there are 50% values on either side of the median. When there are odd number of values in a data set, the middle value is the median. When the number of values in the data set is even, the two most central values are averaged to obtain the median.

Characteristics of Median

- The median can be used with normal, skewed, or kurtotic distributions because it is not influenced by extreme values in the data set. Thus it is preferred over the mean when the data is skewed.
- When data is skewed, mean may not provide the best average for the data as it moves away from the central value. Under such circumstances, the median is the preferred average as it not influenced greatly by the skewed values.
- The median can be calculated for ordinal, interval, or ratio data.
- When the distribution is symmetrical as in a normal distribution, the mean and median exhibit the same value.
- If the distribution is roughly symmetrical then the mean and median will be closed together. Merits and demerits of median are presented in Table 12.3.

Calculation of Median

Calculation of Median for Ungrouped Data

- **When number of the values is odd:** The values are arranged in ascending or descending order to get the median.
  Example: Find the median for the following data: 9, 7, 2, 1, 6, 8, 5
  Arranging the values in ascending order we get: 1, 2, 5, 6, 7, 8, 9
  N—total number of items = 7
  Now $(N + 1)/2 = (7 + 1)/2 = 4$
  Thus, median is the 4th item, i.e. 6

- **When the number of values is even:** The values are arranged in ascending or descending order and the mean of the two middle values is taken to get the median.
  Example: Find the median from the following data: 18, 16, 14, 11, 13, 10
  Arranging the items in ascending order we get: 10, 11, 13, 14, 16, 18
  N—total number of items = 6
  Thus, median is $[(6 + 1)/2]$th item = size of the 3.5th item
  = (3rd item + 4th item)/2
  = $(13 + 14)/2 = 27/2 = 13.5$

Calculation of Median for Frequency Table Data

- **When number of the items is odd:** When the number of observations (N) is odd, then the median is the value at the $[(N + 1)/2]$th position.
  Example: Calculate the median for the following frequency table:

Score	Frequency
10	2
20	3
30	5
40	6
50	7

Number of scores = $2 + 3 + 5 + 6 + 7 = 23$ (odd number)
Since the number of scores is odd, the median is at the $[(N + 1)/2]$th position

Table 12.3: Merits and demerits of median

Merits	Demerits
• When compared to the mean, the median is less sensitive to extreme scores • For distributions that are positively or negatively skewed, median is the best measure as it does not give undue weightage to extreme values • Used with ordinal, interval, or ratio level data	• It does not take all values into account • Compared to mean, it is much affected by sampling fluctuations • Its calculation depends on the arrangement of the data in order of magnitudes • May not appear in data • It can be used in only a narrow range of statistical procedures

To find out the 12th position, we need to add up the frequencies as shown:

Score	Frequency	Cumulative frequency
10	2	2
20	3	2 + 3 = 5
30	5	5 + 5 = 10
40	6	10 + 6 = 16
50	7	16 + 7 = 23

The 12th position is after the 10th position but before the 16th position. So, the median is 40.

❖ **When the number of items is even**: When the number of observations (N) is even, then the median is the value at the [(N + 1)/2]th position.

Example: The following is a frequency table of the score:

Score	Frequency
10	5
20	2
30	3
40	7
50	1

Number of scores = 5 + 2 + 3 + 7 + 1 = 18 (even number)

Since the number of scores is even, the median is the value corresponding to the cumulative frequency [(N + 1)/2]th = [(18 + 1)/2]th = 9.5th position, i.e. when the values are arranged in order of magnitudes, median is the arithmetic mean of the 9th and the 10th values. To find out the 9th and 10th values, we need to add up the frequencies as shown:

Score	Frequency	Cumulative frequency
10	5	5
20	2	5 + 2 = 7
30	3	7 + 3 = 10
40	7	10 + 7 = 17
50	1	17 + 1 = 18

The score at the 9th position is 30 and the score at the 10th position is also 30. So, the median is the average of the scores at the 9th and 10th positions, i.e. (30 + 30)/2 = 30.

Calculation of Median for a Grouped Frequency Distribution (Continuous Data)

❖ The first step in calculation of median for a grouped frequency distribution involves identification of the median class, i.e. the class in which the median lies. This is done by calculating the less than type cumulative frequencies and identifying the median. The median is the value that corresponds to cumulative frequency N/2, where N is the total frequency. Once the median class is identified, the median can be calculated using the below formula:

$$\text{Median} = l_1 + \frac{(N/2) - F}{f_m} \times C$$

where,
l_1 = lower boundary of the median class
N = total frequency
F = cumulative frequency below l_1 (or sum of the frequencies of all classes lower than the median class)
f_m = frequency of the median class
C = width (size) of the median class

Example: Calculate the median of the following frequency table:

Class interval	Frequency	Cumulative frequency
2–4	3	3
4–6	4	7
6–8	2	9
8–10	1	10

Here the median is the value corresponding to cumulative frequency N/2 = 5. Here 5 is greater than cumulative frequency 3, but less than the next cumulative frequency 7. Therefore median class is 4–6 and lower boundary of the median class (l_1) is 4. The width of the median class (C) is 6–4 = 2. The median is given by:

Class interval	Frequency	Cumulative frequency
2–4	3	F = 3
4–6	$f_m = 4$	7
6–8	2	9
8–10	1	N = 10

$$\text{Median} = l_1 + \frac{(N/2) - F}{f_m} \times C$$

Here, $l_1 = 4$, $N/2 = 5$, $F = 3$, $f_m = 4$, $C = 2$

Hence, Median $= 4 + \frac{(5-3)}{4} \times 2 = 4 + 1 = 5$

MODE

Mode is the most occurring score in a data set. It can be determined by simple observation. It relates to the highest bar in a histogram. When a distribution is plotted, it appears as a peak or a hump. A single peaked distribution represents a single mode and is termed as unimodal distribution. If there are two similar peaks indicating two different modes then the distribution is called a bimodal distribution. A distribution having more than two peaks representing multiple modes is termed as a multimodal distribution. Merits and demerits of mode are presented in Table 12.4.

Characteristics of Mode

* Mode is the only measure of central tendency used with nominal variables
* Not affected by the presence of extremely large or small items

Calculation of Mode

Calculation of Mode for Simple Data

In case of individual items, the number of times each value occurs is counted and the value which is repeated the maximum number of times is the modal value.

Example: Calculate the mode for the following individual data: 14, 37, 48, 37, 99, 37

The arithmetic mode of the distribution is 37 as it is repeated maximum number of times, i.e. three times.

Calculation of Mode for Frequency Table Data

In discrete series, the arithmetic mode can be determined by inspection and finding the variable, which has the highest frequency associated with it.

Example: Calculate the mode for the following discrete data:

Score	Frequency
14	2
37	5
48	1
70	3
108	13
145	0

Table 12.4: Merits and demerits of mode

Merits	Demerits
• Easily understood • Determined by inspection of a simple frequency distribution • Used with nominal level data • Not influenced by extreme score • Suitable for both qualitative and quantitative data • It can be calculated from a group frequency distribution with open end classes provided the closed classes are of equal width	• Not suitable for further algebraic treatment • Affected by sampling fluctuations • Not based on all the values of the variable • Difficult to interpret and compare in case of bimodal or multimodal distribution • Possibility of no mode at all when all the values in the distribution are different

The arithmetic mode of the given numbers is 108 as the highest frequency, i.e. 13 is associated with 108.

Calculation of Mode for a Grouped Frequency Distribution

The following formula can be used when data is based on ranges along with their frequencies.

$$M_0 = l_1 + \frac{f_1 - f_0}{2f_1 - f_0 - f_2} \times i$$

Where
- M_0 = Mode
- l_1 = Lower boundary of the modal class
- f_1 = Frequency of modal class
- f_0 = Frequency of pre-modal class
- f_2 = Frequency of class succeeding modal class
- i = Width (size) of the class interval.

Example: Calculate the arithmetic mode for the following data:

Score	Frequency
0–5	3
5–10	7
10–15	15
15–20	30
20–25	20
25–30	10
30–35	5

Using the formula

$$M_0 = l_1 + \frac{f_1 - f_0}{2f_1 - f_0 - f_2} \times i$$

Where $l_1 = 15$, $f_1 = 30$, $f_0 = 15$, $f_2 = 20$, $i = 5$

Score	Frequency
0–5	3
5–10	7
10–15	$f_0 = 15$
(l_1) 15–20	$f_1 = 30$
20–25	$f_2 = 20$

Score	Frequency
25–30	10
30–35	5

Substituting the values we get

$$M_0 = 15 + \frac{30 - 15}{(2 \times 30) - 15 - 20} \times 5$$

$$= 15 + \frac{15}{60 - 15 - 20} \times 5$$

$$= 15 + \frac{15}{25} \times 5$$

$$= 15 + 3 = 18$$

Thus the arithmetic mode of the above range of frequencies is 18.

In case, there are two values of a variable which have equal highest frequencies, then the series is called bimodal and mode is said to be ill-defined. Then mode is calculated using the following formula:

Mode = 3 Median – 2 Mean

WHEN TO USE THE MEAN, MEDIAN, AND MODE

Comparison between mean, median, and mode and summary of all formulae for measures in central tendency are given in Tables 12.5 and 12.6, respectively.

Unit 12: Measures of Central Tendency

Table 12.5: Comparison between mean, median, and mode

Properties	Mean	Median	Mode
Average	Calculated average with balance point	Positional average with middle point	Positional average with most frequent score
Calculation	Based on all the observations	Based on middle most values	Based on most frequent score
Observations	Includes all observations	Does not include all observations	Does not include all observations
Outliers	Affects the average	Does not affect the average	Does not affect the average
Inferential statistics	Can be done	Cannot be performed	Cannot be performed
Most suitable	Normally distributed data	Skewed data	Skewed data
Results	Only one mean	Only one median	Can be more than one
Type of measurement	Interval or ratio—symmetrical data	Interval or ratio—skewed data Ordinal	Nominal

Table 12.6: Summary of all formulae for measures in central tendency

Measure of central tendency	Grouped data	Ungrouped data
Mean	$\bar{x} = \dfrac{\sum fx}{N}$ Where $\bar{x}$ = Arithmetic mean f = Frequency x = Midpoint	**Sample Mean:** $\bar{x} = \dfrac{\sum x}{n}$ **Population Mean:** $\mu = \dfrac{\sum x}{N}$ Where Σx is the sum of all data values n is the number of data items in sample N is the number of data items in population
Median	Median $= l_1 + \dfrac{(N/2) - F}{f_m} \times C$ Where l_1 = Lower boundary of the median class N = Total frequency F = Cumulative frequency below l_1 (or sum of the frequencies of all classes lower than the median class) f_m = Frequency of the median class C = Width of the median class	Median $= \left(\dfrac{N+1}{2}\right)^{th}$ term Where N = Total number of items
Mode	$M_0 = l_1 + \dfrac{f_1 - f_0}{2f_1 - f_0 - f_2}$ Where M_0 = Mode l_1 = Lower boundary of the modal class f_1 = Frequency of modal class f_0 = Frequency of pre-modal class f_2 = Frequency of class succeeding modal class i = Class interval	

BIBLIOGRAPHY

1. Agresti, A. & Finlay, B. (1997). *Statistical Methods for the Social Sciences* (3rd ed.). Prentice Hall.
2. Anderson, T.W. & Sclove, S.L. (1974). *Introductory Statistical Analysis*. Houghton: Mifflin Company.
3. Burns, N., & Grove, S.K. (2005). *The practice of nursing research: Conduct, critique and utilization* (5th ed.). St. Louis, MO: Elsevier Saunders.
4. Craig, J.V. & Smyth, R.L. (2012). *The evidence based practice manual for nurses* (3rd ed.). Edinbergh UK: Churchill Livinsgtons.
5. Polit, D.F., & Beck, C.T. (2010). *Essentials of Nursing Research: Appraising Evidence for Nursing Practice*. Philadelphia, PA: Lippincott Williams & Wilkins.
6. Polit, D.F., & Beck, C.T. (2012). *Nursing research: Generating and assessing evidence for nursing practice* (9th ed.). Philadelphia: Lippincott Williams & Wilkins.
7. Plichta, B.S., & Garzan, S.L. (2009). *Statistics for nursing and allied health*. Philadelphia, PA: Lippincott Williams & Wilkins.
8. Weiss, N.A. (1999). *Introductory Statistics*. Addison Wesley.

REVIEW QUESTIONS

I. Long Essays

1. What are the different measures of central tendency? Why are they called as measures of central tendency? Explain briefly with an illustration.
2. a. Define measures of central tendency.
   b. Calculate mean, median, and mode for the following data regarding body mass index (BMI) of 10 women.
   BMI: 23, 27, 30, 32, 20, 30, 27, 30, 25, 30.

II. Short Essays

1. Compute the mean, median, and mode for the following distribution:

Score	F
90–99	2
80–89	12
70–79	22
60–69	20
50–59	14
40–49	4
30–39	1
	N = 75

2. Describe the measures of central tendency. Calculate the median for the following test scores of 50 students.

Score	Frequency
1	4
3	6
4	8
5	14
7	8
8	6
9	4

3. List the merits and demerits of median and calculate the median for the frequency distribution:

X	F
1	8
2	10
3	11
4	16
5	20
6	25
7	15
8	9
9	6

III. Short Answers
1. Mean
2. Median
3. Mode

IV. Multiple Choice Questions

1. Number which occurs most frequently in a set of numbers is
   a. Mean
   b. Median
   c. Mode
   d. None of above

2. Distribution in which values of mean, median and mode are not equal is considered as
   a. Experimental distribution
   b. Asymmetrical distribution
   c. Symmetrical distribution
   d. Exploratory distribution

3. When the value of three measures of central tendencies mean, median and mode are equal then the distribution is considered as:
   a. Negatively skewed modal
   b. Symmetrical model
   c. Positively skewed model
   d. Bimodal

4. What is the median of the following number?
   1, 2, 2, 8, 9, 14
   a. 13
   b. 5
   c. 2
   d. 6

5. Which set of data has a mean of 15, a median of 14, and a mode of 14?
   a. 3, 14, 19, 25, 14
   b. 25, 15, 14, 3, 7
   c. 14, 22, 14, 15, 4
   d. 14, 22, 15, 15, 9

6. The following are the scores in a test: 80, 90, 90, 85, 60, 70, 75, 85, 90, 60, 80. What is the mode of these scores?
   a. 90
   b. 70
   c. 80
   d. 60

7. The following are scores in a term-end exam: 80, 90, 85, 60, 70, 80, 85, 90, 60, 80. What is the mean of these scores?
   a. 76
   b. 82
   c. 78
   d. 75

8. The mode score in a test was 94. Which of these interpretations must be correct?
   a. A score of 91 was slightly below average
   b. 99 is the highest score in the class
   c. No score is below 50
   d. More students received 94 than any other score

9. What is the mode of the following numbers: 1, 2, 2, 8, 9, 14?
   a. 14
   b. 2
   c. 9
   d. 8

10. Which of the following is not the measure of central tendency?
    a. Standard deviation
    b. Mean
    c. Mode
    d. Median

ANSWER KEY

1. c	2. b	3. b	4. b	5. a	6. a
7. c	8. d	9. b	10. a		

UNIT 13

Measures of Variability

The previous unit dealt with how statistical data in the form of a frequency distribution can be represented by a single typical value known as statistical average or simply average—Mean, Median or Mode. Though an average provides some idea about the type of data, it alone does not reveal all its characteristics. The average does not provide any information about the manner in which the values are scattered or dispersed about the average. Two series having the same number of values may have the same mean (or median), but still the values in one may be widely dispersed and the values in the other may be close to one another. Consider the following example in Table 13.1.

Figure 13.1 shows two sets of dot plots having the same mean, median, and mode,

Table 13.1: Two data sets										
Data set I	45	43	47	45	44	44	48	45	44	45
Data set II	51	42	45	38	47	41	45	52	39	50

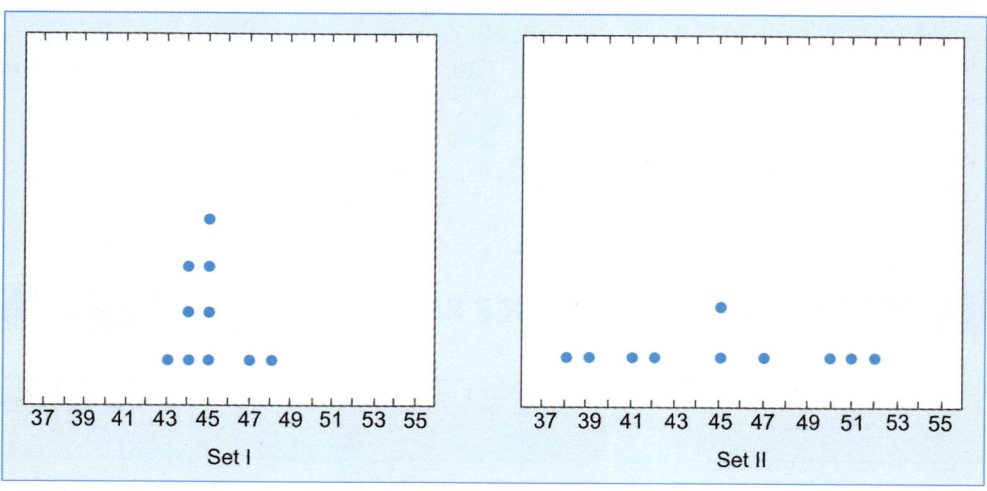

Fig. 13.1: Dot plots of data sets

i.e. 45. However, a quick look at the dot plots shows that they are remarkably different. In set I, the dot plots are clustered towards the center, while in set II the dot plots are scattered away from the center. While the measures of central tendency denote the central location and magnitude of the data set, they fail to explain quantitatively how the data is either scattered from the center or clustered around the center. This scatteredness is best explained by measures of dispersion or variation.

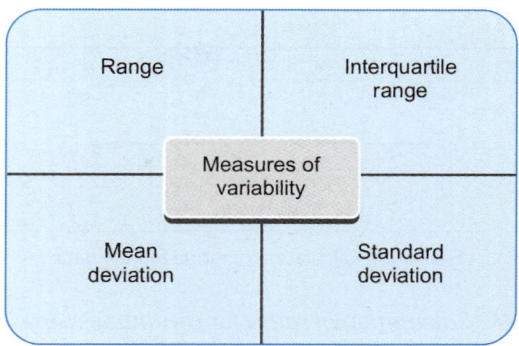

Fig. 13.2: Measures of variability

DISPERSION

The word "dispersion" indicates lack of uniformity. It could relate to either quantities or series of values in a group. Dispersion is the degree to which the values in a distribution vary from its average. In statistics the word "dispersion" connotes the variability or scatter or spread and denotes the extent to which the values in a distribution are stretched or squeezed about the central value.

Properties of a good measure of dispersion
* Easy to understand and compute
* Rigidly defined
* Take into account each value in the distribution
* Capable of further algebraic treatment
* Exhibit sampling stability
* Not be overly affected by extreme items

MEASURES OF VARIABILITY (DISPERSION)

There are four measures to quantify the extent of the variation namely: the range, interquartile range, mean deviation, and standard deviation. Range and quartile deviation measure the dispersion by calculating the spread within which the values lie. "Mean deviation" and "standard deviation" measure the degree to which the values vary from the average (Fig. 13.2).

Range

Range is the most elementary technique to study dispersion. In statistics it refers to the difference between the maximum and minimum values of a data set and is given by the formula, maximum value minus the minimum value in the data set. The difference indicates how varied the data set is. The range also provides a rough estimate of the standard deviation of a sample. Standard deviation = (Maximum value – Minimum value)/4.

Example: Range = Maximum value – Minimum value
* *Calculation of range for raw data*: For example, in the data set 3, 4, 6, 7, 9 the maximum value is 9, and the minimum value is 3. Hence, the range is 9 – 3 = 6 (Fig. 13.3).
* *Calculation of range for discrete series*

	Marks (X)	No. of students (f)
Smallest	10	6
	15	7
	20	8
Largest	25	9
	Total	30

Absolute range = Largest – Smallest
= 25 – 10 = 15 marks

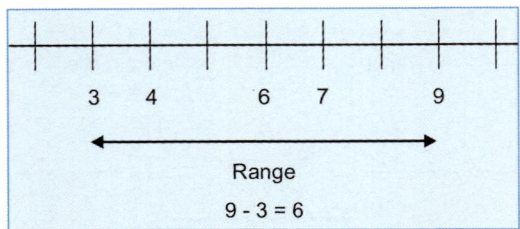

Fig. 13.3: Calculation of range for raw data

❖ *Calculation of range for continuous series*

Marks (X)	No. of students (f)
Smallest: 10 — 10–15	4
15–20	10
20–25	26
Largest: 30 — 25–30	8

Absolute range = Largest – Smallest
= 30 – 10 = 20 marks

Merits
❖ Range is easy to understand and calculate.
❖ Commonly used dispersion.

Demerits
❖ Range is an extremely crude measure of spread of data.
❖ It is unduly affected by extreme values as it takes into account only the extreme values and does not consider the middle values.
❖ So long as the extreme values remain unaltered, the other values do not influence the range.
❖ Range cannot be calculated from grouped frequency distribution with open-end class, i.e. a distribution where the classes do not have defined ends.
❖ It is highly sensitive to outliers.
❖ The range does not reveal anything about the internal characteristics of a data set. For example, in the data set 1, 2, 2, 3, 4, 5, 6, 6, 7, 9, 10 where the values are evenly spread out, the range is 10 – 1 = 9. Comparing this with the data set 1, 1, 1, 2, 2, 8, 9, 9, 9, 10 we find that the values are stretched toward the extremes but the range is yet again 9. To overcome the undue influence of extreme scores or values the interquartile range (IQR) may be reported.

Interquartile Range

It is a measure of variability that divides a rank-ordered data set into four equal parts called the quartiles. The values of the first (Q_1), second (Q_2) and the third (Q_3) quartiles divides the data set into four parts. The difference between the third and first quartiles is the IQR which contains the middle half of the values in the frequency distribution which is equal to $Q_3 - Q_1$. Q_3 is the point below which three-fourths of the distribution lies and Q_1 is the point below which one-fourth of the distribution lies (Fig. 13.4).

❖ Q_1 is the "middle" value in the first half of the rank-ordered data set
❖ Q_2 is the median value of the rank-ordered data set
❖ Q_3 is the "middle" value in the second half of the rank-ordered data set.

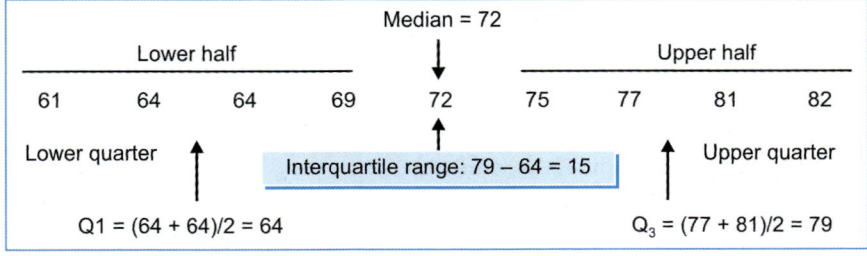

Fig. 13.4: Interquartile range (IQR)

Table 13.2: Merits and demerits of interquartile range

Merits	Demerits
Easy to calculate. Values of Q1 and Q3 are calculated and formulae of absolute and coefficient of quartile deviation applied.	Totally dependent on middle values. Irregular values are bound to generate abnormal result.
Provides better results than range method. While range considers only the extreme values, quartile deviation takes the middle 50% items into account.	All the values in the frequency distribution do not contribute to values of Q1 and Q3.
The quartile deviation is immune to the extreme items.	
It can be calculated from a grouped frequency distribution with open-end classes.	

The merits and demerits of IQR are presented in Table 13.2.

Uses of Quartiles

Quartiles are used to measure central tendency, dispersion and skewness. Second quartile Q_2 is the median which is a measure of central tendency. Quartiles Q_1 and Q_3 define quartile deviation which is a measure of dispersion. The skewness in terms of quartiles Q_1, Q_2 and Q_3 is given by the formula:

$$\text{Skewness} = \frac{(Q_3 - Q_2) - (Q_2 - Q_1)}{(Q_3 - Q_2) + (Q_2 - Q_1)}$$

$$= \frac{(Q_3 - 2Q_2 + Q_1)}{(Q_3 - Q_1)}$$

In a symmetrical frequency distribution, the values of the variable equidistant from their mean have equal frequencies which suggest:

(i) $(Q_2 - Q_1) = (Q_3 - Q_2)$

(ii) Mean = Median = Mode

❖ *Calculation of interquartile range for raw data*: For a simple series (or a simple frequency distribution) the data are first arranged in ascending order of magnitude.
Q_1 = The value of the $(N + 1)/4$th item
Q_3 = The value of the $3(N + 1)/4$th item

N = Number of values (or total frequency) Consider the following numbers: 77, 64, 64, 81, 75, 72, 61, 82, 69.

Step 1: Arrange the numbers in ascending order.

61, 64, 64, 69, 72, 75, 77, 81, 82

Step 2: Find the median.

61, 64, 64, 69, <u>72</u>, 75, 77, 81, 82

Step 3: Find Q_1 and Q_3

- Q_1 is the median (middle value) of the first half of the data set. As the number of observations in the first half of the data set is even, the middle value is the average of the two middle observations, i.e. $Q_1 = (64 + 64)/2$ or $Q_1 = 64$.
- Q_3 is the median (middle value) in the second half of the data set. Again, as the number of observations in the second half of the data set is even, the middle value is the average of the two middle observations, i.e. $Q_3 = (77 + 81)/2$ or $Q_3 = 79$.

Step 4: Subtract Q_1 from Q_3 to find the interquartile range:

The IQR is given by $Q_3 - Q_1$ (IQR = 79 − 64 = 15). Dividing the IQR by 2 we get the semi-quartile range (SQR): SQR = IQR/2.

❖ **Calculation of interquartile range for discrete series**:

Consider the below data:

Daily wages (x)	Workers (f)
80	4
100	20
110	21
130	16
150	9

In the above problem the values of Q_3 and Q_1 can be calculated as under:

Daily wages (x)	Workers (f)	Cumulative frequencies (cf)	
80	4	4	
100	20	24	Q_1 lies in this cf
110	21	45	
130	16	61	Q_3 lies in this cf
150	9	70	
	N = 70		

Calculation of Q_1:

Q_1 = the value of the $(N + 1)/4$th item
= the value of the $(70 + 1)/4$ item
= 17.75

Thus, Q_1 is the size of the 17.75th item which lies in the cumulative frequency 24, which corresponds to the value ₹ 100/-.
Thus, Q_1 = ₹ 100/-

Calculation of Q_3:

Q_3 = the value of the $3(N + 1)/4$th item
= the value of the $3(70 + 1)/4$ item
= 53.25

Thus, Q_3 is the size of the 53.25th item which lies in the cumulative frequency 61, which corresponds to the value ₹ 130/-.
Thus, Q_3 = ₹ 130/-.

Thus, interquartile range
= $Q_3 - Q_1$
= ₹130 – ₹100 = ₹ 30

❖ **Calculation of interquartile range for continuous series**:

For a grouped frequency distribution, cumulative frequencies ("less than" type) are first calculated.

While
Q_1 = the value corresponding to (i.e. opposite to) cumulative frequency N/4
Q_3 = the value corresponding to cumulative frequency 3N/4.

$$Q_1 = l_1 + \frac{(N/4) - F_1}{f_1} \times i$$

Where,
l_1—lower boundary of the Q_1 class (i.e. the class in which cumulative frequency where N/4 falls).
N—number of values (or total frequency)
F_1—cumulative frequency below l_1
f_1—frequency of the Q_1 class
i—width of the Q_1 class

$$Q_3 = l_3 + \frac{(3N/4) - F_3}{f_3} \times i$$

Where,
l_3—lower boundary of the Q_3 class (i.e. the class in which cumulative frequency where 3N/4 falls.
N—number of values (or total frequency)
F_3—cumulative frequency below l_3
f_3—frequency of the Q_3 class
i—width of the Q_3 class

Consider the below data:

Daily wages (x)	Workers (f)
Below 20	13
20–25	29
25–30	46
30–35	60
35–40	112
40–45	94
45–50	45
50 and above	21

In the above problem the quartiles can be calculated as under:

Calculation of cumulative frequency

	Age (in years)	Cumulative frequencies (less than)	
	20	13	
	25	42	
	30	88	
$Q_1 \rightarrow$		105	← N/4
	35	148	
$Q_2 \rightarrow$		210	← N/2
	40	260	
$Q_3 \rightarrow$		315	← 3N/4
	45	354	
	50	399	
	55 and above	420 = N	

Here Q_1 class is 30–35; Q_2 class is 35–40 and Q_3 class is 40–45.

N/4 = 105; N/2 = 210; 3N/4 = 315

$$Q_1 = l_1 + \frac{(N/4) - F_1}{f_1} \times i$$

$$= 30 + \frac{105 - 88}{60} \times 5 = 31.4$$

$$Q_2 = l_2 + \frac{(N/2) - F_2}{f_2} \times i$$

$$= 35 + \frac{210 - 148}{112} \times 5 = 37.8$$

$$Q_3 = l_3 + \frac{(3N/4) - F_3}{f_3} \times i$$

$$= 40 + \frac{315 - 260}{94} \times 5 = 42.9$$

Thus, interquartile range
= $Q_3 - Q_1$
= 42.9 – 31.4 = 11.5

Coefficient of Quartile Deviation

Coefficient of quartile deviation is a relative measure of dispersion based on the quartile deviation. It is a pure number without any units. It compares the dispersion in two or more sets of data and is defined by:

$$\text{Coefficient of quartile deviation} = \frac{Q_3 - Q_1}{Q_3 + Q_1}$$

Merits and demerits of coefficient of quartile deviation are presented in Table 13.3.

Table 13.3: Merits and demerits of coefficient of quartile deviation

Merits	Demerits
• Easily understood • Offers better results than coefficient of range • Mathematically simple to solve	• Sampling fluctuation • Ignorance of last 25% of data sets • Values are irregular

Percentile

Percentile is a common statistic that allows comparison of one's relative position compared to that of others. It divides the distribution of the variable into 100 groups having equal frequencies and indicates the percentage of scores that fall below the specific percentile.

For example, in a test for 50 marks, if a student Y scored 35 marks, that figure would have no real meaning unless he knows what percentile he falls into, i.e. he would have little idea how better he is compared to other students. More relevant would be the percentage of students with lower marks than his. This percentage is called a percentile. If 65% of the other students scores were below, then the Y's score would be the 65th percentile, meaning his score is better than 65% of the students who took the test. A few important percentiles are:

❖ 25th percentile also called the first quartile

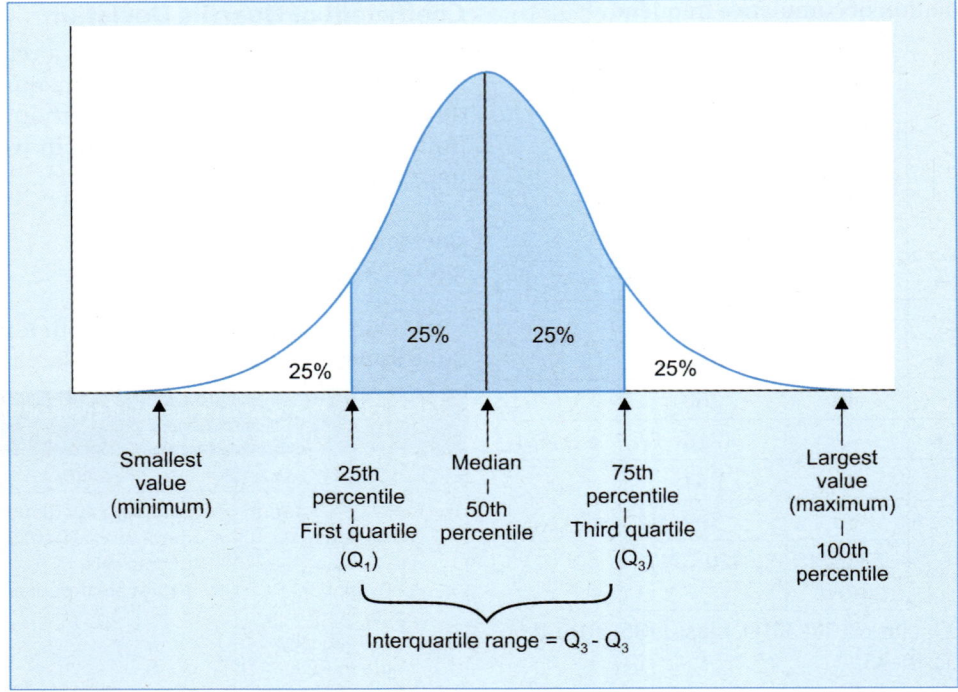

Fig. 13.5: Percentiles

- 50th percentile is generally the median
- 75th percentile also called the third quartile (Fig. 13.5).

Variance

Variance is a numerical value that indicates how widely the individuals in a group differ. It measures the spread between the observations in a data set, i.e. how far each observation in the set is from the mean. A greater fluctuation of the individual observations from the group mean indicates a bigger variance and vice-versa. It thus helps to understand how the individual values of a data set relate to each other.

Variance is calculated by initially arriving at the difference between each value in the data set and the mean followed by squaring the differences (squaring gives positive values and their sum is not equal to zero) and dividing the sum of such squares by the number of values in the data set. Thus variance can mathematically be defined as the *"average of the squared differences from the mean".* Various formulae for calculating variance are presented in Table 13.4.

Some of the features of variance are:
- Variance is widely used in probability distribution statistics. Its ability to provide information on the spread of data around the mean helps in making generalized conclusions about unknown data points.
- A variance value of zero indicates that there is no variability and that all numbers in the data set are the same
- A large variance indicates that the values in the data set are far spread out from the mean. A smaller variance indicates just the opposite.

Table 13.4: Formulae for variance

Sample variance formula	Population variance formula
Discrete data	
$s^2 = \dfrac{\sum (x_i - \bar{x})^2}{n-1}$	$\sigma^2 = \dfrac{\sum (X_i - \mu)^2}{N}$
where, s^2 = sample variance Σ = sum of... x_i = individual data values $\bar{x}$ = sample mean n = sample size	where, σ^2 = population variance Σ = sum of... X_i = individual data values μ = population mean N = population size
Frequency data	
$(s^2) = \dfrac{1}{n-1}\left[\Sigma fx^2 - \dfrac{(\Sigma fx)^2}{n}\right]$	$(\sigma^2) = \dfrac{\Sigma fx^2}{N} - \left(\dfrac{\Sigma fx}{N}\right)^2$
where, s^2 = sample variance Σ = sum of... f = class frequency n = sample size x = mid-point of class interval	where, σ^2 = population variance Σ = sum of... f = class frequency N = population size x = mid-point of class interval

❖ A range while looks at only the extreme values, the variance takes into account all the values to determine their distribution.

❖ Regardless of the direction, variance deals with all the deviations the same way. Accordingly the squaring of both positive and negative deviations to avoid their adding up to zero gives an appearance of nil variability.

❖ Though square root of variance is taken to get the standard deviation, it is not easily interpreted.

❖ Since variance involves squaring of numbers, it gives added weight to outliers skewing the data interpretation.

❖ Notations for variance of population and sample are different. Variance of a population is denoted by σ^2; the variance of a sample is denoted by s^2.

❖ The variance of a population is given by:

$$\sigma^2 = \frac{\sum (X_i - \mu)^2}{N}$$

where, σ^2 is the population variance, X is the population mean, X_i is the *i*th element from the population, and N is the number of elements in the population.

❖ The variance of a sample is given by:

$$s^2 = \frac{\sum (x_i - \bar{x})^2}{n-1}$$

where, s^2 is the sample variance, x is the sample mean, x_i is the *i*th element from the sample, and $(n - 1)$ is the number of elements in the sample.

Steps to calculate variance:

Step 1: Add each of the values and calculate the mean ($\Sigma X/N = \mu$ in the formula)

Step 2: Find the deviation score by subtracting the mean from each of the data values: $(X - \mu)$. Data values below the mean will have negative deviations, and data values above the mean will have positive deviations.

Step 3: Square each of the deviations (differences) to make it positive: $(X - \mu)^2$

Step 4: Add all the squared deviations: $\Sigma(X - \mu)^2$

Step 5: Divide the sum by total number of data values in the population to obtain variance: $\Sigma(X_i - \mu)^2/N$

Alternately, if a sample is being considered then the sum may be divided by total number of data values minus one to obtain sample variance: $\Sigma(x_i - \bar{x})^2/(n - 1)$

Example: A class has a total population of six students who have the following writing speeds: 12, 8, 10, 10, 8, 12 words/minute. The variance can be calculated using the below formula:

$$\sigma^2 = \frac{\Sigma(X-\mu)^2}{N}$$

X	$(X - \mu)$	$(X - \mu)^2$
12	2	4
8	-2	4
10	0	0
10	0	0
8	-2	4
12	2	4
$\Sigma X = 60$ $\mu = 10$		$\Sigma(X - \mu)^2 = 16$

Note: N = 6

Substituting the values in the formula for population variance above we get:

$\sigma^2 = \Sigma (X - \mu)^2/N$
  = 16/6
  ≈ 2.67

The variation is approximately 2.67.

Coefficient of Variation

The coefficient of variation (CV) is a statistical measure that shows the distribution of a set of data values around the mean. In other words, it is a measure of the variation in points from each other and the mean, and shows how regular or irregular a data pattern is. The coefficient of variation is calculated by dividing the standard deviation σ with the mean $\bar{x}$. It measures the extent of variability in relation to the mean of the population. It is also termed as relative standard deviation (RSD). Distributions with a coefficient of variation less than 1 are considered to have low-variance and high stability, thus more precise. On the other hand, a CV greater than 1 indicates high variance and less stability, thus a greater level of dispersion around the mean. Merits and demerits of coefficient of variation are presented in Table 13.5.

Formula for coefficient of variation:
  $CV = (\sigma/\bar{x}) \times 100$
where,
  CV = Coefficient of variation
  σ = Standard deviation
  $\bar{x}$ = Mean

Example: The coefficient of variation of the sample data 2, 4, 6, 8, 10 and 12 can be calculated as follows:

Step 1: Add each of the values and calculate the mean: $\Sigma x/n$
The mean of the data is $(2 + 4 + 6 + 8 + 10 + 12)/6 = 42/6 = 7$.

Step 2: Find the standard deviation using the formula $\sigma = \sqrt{[\Sigma(x_i - \bar{x})^2/n]}$
where, SD is the standard deviation, x is the population mean, x_i is the *i*th element from the population, and "n" is the number of elements in the sample.
  $\sigma = \sqrt{[\Sigma(x_i - \bar{x})^2/n]} = \sqrt{(70/6)} = 3.42$

Step 3: Find the coefficient of variation using the formula:
  $CV = (\sigma/\bar{x}) \times 100 = (3.42/7) \times 100 = 48.86\%$

| Table 13.5: Merits and demerits of coefficient of variation ||
Merits	Demerits
• Though the means of two groups are significantly different from one another, coefficient of variation aids in comparing the variation from one data series to another. • It is based on mean and standard deviation. • It is unit-less and generally expressed as a percentage. Without units, it can be run for any quantifiable data and allows for comparison between distributions whose scales of measurement are not comparable. It is this quality that separates it from standard deviation analysis. For example, though standard deviations of blood pressure and pulse rate are not comparable, the two CV values can still be compared.	• When the mean of a sample population is zero, the sum of all values above and below zero become equal to each other. Under such circumstances, CV becomes ineffective as the denominator becomes equal to zero. • Though the mean of a variable is not zero, the value of CV with a strong presence of both positive and negative values in the sample and a close zero mean can be misleading. A variable with only positive values generates a much reasonable CV.

Some of the features of coefficient of variation are:

❖ It measures the dispersion of the population data of a frequency distribution. The lower the value of the coefficient of variation, the more precise the estimate.
❖ It only uses positive numbers and is expressed in percentage terms.
❖ It is independent of the unit of measurement and is a dimensionless number. Thus, it helps in the comparison between distributions with different units/scales that are not comparable.
❖ As the mean approaches zero, the coefficient of variation approaches infinity.
❖ It is computed only for data measured on a ratio scale (as these can only take non-negative values) and not for data on an interval scale.

Mean Deviation (Average Deviation or Mean Absolute Deviation)

Mean deviation refers to the average amount of variation of a data set from any one of its averages, either the mean or the median or the mode. Such a difference is technically described as deviation. Theoretically, the deviation of values from the median is minimum when sign is ignored (absolute value). However, in practice the mean is generally used to calculate the value of average deviation. So, it is known as mean deviation. It is denoted by MD. The summary of all formulae calculating mean deviation about the mean, median and mode are presented in Table 13.6.

Example 1: Calculate the mean deviation of the following series (direct method) using arithmetic mean ($\bar{X}$), median (M) and mode (Z)—8, 11, 13, 13, 15, 20, 21, 23, 29.

(a) From arithmetic mean ($\bar{X}$):

$$\bar{X} = \frac{\Sigma X}{N} = \frac{8+11+13+13+15+20+21+23+29}{9}$$

$$= \frac{153}{9} = 17$$

Mean deviation (d_x)

$$= \frac{\Sigma X_1 - \Sigma X_2 - (N_1 - N_2)(\bar{X})}{N}$$

Table 13.6: Summary of all formulae for mean deviation

Mean deviation about the mean/median/mode	Grouped data	Ungrouped data
Mean (if deviations, $\Sigma\|X - \bar{x}\|$ are obtained from arithmetic average)	Sample Mean: $(d_{\bar{x}}) = \dfrac{\Sigma f\|x - \bar{x}\|}{\Sigma f}$ Population Mean: $(d_{\bar{x}}) = \dfrac{\Sigma f\|x - \mu\|}{\Sigma f}$ Where, d—symbol for mean deviation X—value of the variable Σf—total number of items $\bar{X}$—arithmetic average	$(d_{\bar{x}}) = \dfrac{\Sigma\|x - \bar{x}\|}{n}$ Where, d—symbol for mean deviation X—value of the variable n—number of items $\bar{X}$—arithmetic average
Median (if deviations, $\Sigma\|X - M\|$ are obtained from median)	$(d_m) = \dfrac{\Sigma f\|X - M\|}{\Sigma f}$ Where, d—symbol for mean deviation X—value of the variable Σf—total number of items M—median	$(d_m) = \dfrac{\Sigma\|X - M\|}{n}$ Where, d—symbol for mean deviation X—value of the variable n—number of items M—median
Mode (if deviations, $\Sigma\|X - Z\|$ are obtained from mode)	$(d_z) = \dfrac{\Sigma f\|X - Z\|}{\Sigma f}$ Where, d—symbol for mean deviation X—value of the variable Σf—total number of items Z—mode	$(d_z) = \dfrac{\Sigma f\|X - Z\|}{n}$ Where, d—symbol for mean deviation X—value of the variable n—number of items Z—mode
Direct method	Mean deviation $= \dfrac{\Sigma fdy}{N}$ Where, dy is the variation between middle points of class interval and values of mean ($\bar{X}$), median (M) or mode (Z)	Mean deviation (d) $= \dfrac{\Sigma X_1 - \Sigma X_2 - (N_1 - N_2)(\bar{X} \text{ or M or Z})}{N}$ ΣX_1 = sum of values greater than $\bar{X}$, M or Z ΣX_2 = sum of values less than $\bar{X}$, M or Z N_1 = number of values greater than $\bar{X}$, M or Z N_2 = number of values less than $\bar{X}$, M or Z N = total number of values $\bar{X}$ = arithmetic mean M = Median Z = Mode

Where,

ΣX_1 = is the sum of values above the actual mean
ΣX_2 = is the sum of values below the actual mean including the actual mean
N_1 = is the number of values above the actual mean
N_2 = is the number of values below the actual mean including the actual mean
$\bar{X}$ = actual mean

$\Sigma X_1 = 20 + 21 + 23 + 29 = 93;$ $N_1 = 4$

$\Sigma X_2 = 8 + 11 + 13 + 13 + 15 = 60;$ $N_2 = 5$

Substituting we get

$= \dfrac{93 - 60 - (4-5)\times(17)}{9} = \dfrac{33-17}{9} = \dfrac{50}{9} = 5.56$

From Median (M): The total number of values (N) = 9. Therefore, Median (M) = 5th term = 15

Mean deviation (d_m)

$= \dfrac{\Sigma X_1 - \Sigma X_2 - (N_1 - N_2)(M)}{N}$

Where,

ΣX_1 = is the sum of values above the median
ΣX_2 = is the sum of values below the median
N_1 = is the number of values above the median
N_2 = is the number of values below the median
M = Median

$\Sigma X_1 = 20 + 21 + 23 + 29 = 93;$ $N_1 = 4$
$\Sigma X_2 = 8 + 11 + 13 + 13 = 45;$ $N_2 = 4$

Substituting we get:

$= \dfrac{93 - 45 - (4-4)\times(15)}{9} = \dfrac{48-0}{9} = \dfrac{48}{0} = 5.33$

From Mode (Z): By inspection Z = 13; N = 9

Mean deviation (d_z)

$= \dfrac{\Sigma X_1 - \Sigma X_2 - (N_1 - N_2)(Z)}{N}$

Where,

ΣX_1 = is the sum of values above the mode
ΣX_2 = is the sum of values below the mode
N_1 = is the number of values above the mode
N_2 = is the number of values below the mode
Z = Mode

$\Sigma X_1 = 15 + 20 + 21 + 23 + 29 = 108;$ $N_1 = 5$
$\Sigma X_2 = 8 + 11 = 19;$ $N_2 = 2$

Substituting we get:

$= \dfrac{108 - 19 - (5-2)\times(13)}{9} = \dfrac{89-39}{9} = \dfrac{50}{9} = 5.56$

Example 2: Calculate the mean deviation of the following series using the arithmetic mean: 31, 35, 29, 63, 55, 72, 37

Arithmetic mean ($\bar{x}$)

$= \dfrac{31 + 35 + 29 + 63 + 55 + 72 + 37}{7} = \dfrac{322}{7} = 46$

Calculation of absolute deviations:

Value (x)	Deviation from mean $d = x - \bar{x} = x - 46$	Absolute deviation $\lvert d \rvert$
31	−15	15
35	−11	11
29	−17	17
63	17	17
55	9	9
73	26	26
37	−9	9
		$\Sigma \lvert d \rvert = 104$

Therefore, the required mean deviation using the mean is

$= \dfrac{\Sigma \lvert d \rvert}{N} = \dfrac{104}{7} = 14.86$

Example 3: Calculate the mean deviation of the following series using the median: 8, 15, 53, 49, 19, 62, 7, 15, 95, 77.

Arranging the numbers in the ascending order we get:
7, 8, 15, 15, <u>19</u>, <u>49</u>, 53, 62, 77, 95

$$\text{Median} = \frac{N+1}{2}\text{th value} = \frac{10+1}{2}\text{th value}$$
$$= 5.5\text{th value}$$
$$= \text{Mean of the 5th and 6th values}$$
$$= \frac{19+49}{2} = \frac{68}{2} = 34$$

Calculation of absolute deviations:

Value (x)	Deviation from median $d = x - M$ $= x - 34$	Absolute deviation $\|d\|$
7	−27	27
8	−26	26
15	−19	19
15	−19	19
19	−15	15
49	+15	15
53	+19	19
62	+28	28
77	+43	43
95	+61	61
		$\Sigma\|d\| = 272$

Therefore, the required mean deviation using the median is

$$= \frac{\Sigma|d|}{N} = \frac{272}{10} = 27.2$$

The merits and demerits of mean deviation are presented in Table 13.7.

Coefficient of Mean Deviation

Mean deviation can be calculated by any measure of central tendency (mean, median, and mode). A relative measure of mean deviation is required for comparing variation among different series. This relative measure based on the mean deviation is called the coefficient of mean deviation or coefficient of dispersion. It can be obtained by dividing the mean deviation with either mean, median or mode.

Mean deviation and its coefficient are used to estimate the variability making the study of central tendency of a series more precise. They are a better measure of variability than range as it considers all the values in the series. The formulae for calculating coefficient of mean deviation can be put as follows:

Mean deviation and its coefficient are a better measure of variability than range as it considers all values of the series.

$$\text{Coefficient of MD (mean)} = \frac{MD}{Mean}$$

$$\text{Coefficient of MD (median)} = \frac{MD}{Median}$$

Table 13.7: Merits and demerits of mean deviation

Merits	Demerits
• It is simple to understand and calculate. • It takes into account all the values in a series. • It depicts the dispersion or scatter of each value in the series from its central value. • It is unaffected by extreme values. • It allows comparison between different values in series. • It represents the average of deviations of values in a series accurately.	• It is not rigidly defined as it can be computed from mean, median or mode thereby producing different results. • It violates the algebraic principles as it ignores the + and − signs and takes into account the absolute deviation during calculation. • Not amicable to further algebraic treatment. • Affected by sample fluctuations. • In case of fractional or recurring decimal results, further cumbersome formulae have to be used.

Table 13.8: Merits and demerits of coefficient of mean deviation

Merits	Demerits
• More reliable than range and quartile coefficient • Least sampling fluctuation • Rigidly defined	• Less reliable than coefficient of variation • Fractional average

The merits and demerits of coefficient of mean deviation are presented in Table 13.8.

Standard Deviation

Standard deviation is a statistical term used to measure the spread or dispersion around an average. Here dispersion refers to the difference between the actual and the average value. It is the most commonly used measure of variability when interval or ratio data are involved and is represented by either "σ" (sigma) or "s". The term standard refers to "average" and the term standard deviation refers to the average deviation of all the data values from the mean value of those data.

The standard deviation of a data set can be calculated by taking the square root of the variance. Thus, standard deviation can mathematically be defined as *"the square root of the sum of the squared deviations about the mean divided by the total number of values".*

The formula used for standard deviation depends on whether the data being considered is that of an entire population, or the data is a sample representing a larger population.

* If the data being considered is that of the entire population or that of a sample of a larger population (the findings of which shall not be generalized to the entire population), it is divided by number of data values, N.
* If the data is a sample representing a larger population (the findings of which shall be generalized to the entire population), it is divided by one less than the number of data values in the sample, n – 1.

Hence, the sample standard deviation is to be used, when the researcher is presented with a sample from which he wishes to estimate (generalize) the findings and make a statement about the larger population. Confusion often arises when "sample standard deviation" is incorrectly interpreted as standard deviation of the sample (which actually refers to the population standard deviation). Merits and demerits of standard deviation are presented in Table 13.9. Formulae for standard deviation are presented in Table 13.10.

Some of the features of standard deviation are:

* All the values of a distribution are considered while calculating standard deviation.
* While a low standard deviation suggests that most of the data points are close to the average, a high standard deviation suggests that the data points are widely dispersed from the central value, i.e. mean.
* The standard deviation is always used along with the mean to summarize continuous data and not the categorical data. Also the standard deviation is appropriate when the continuous data is not significantly skewed or has outliers.

Steps to Calculate Standard Deviation (Discrete Data)

Step 1: Add each of the values and calculate the mean: ($\sum X/N = \mu$ in the formula)

Step 2: Find the deviation score by subtracting the mean from each of the data values: ($X - \mu$). Data values below the mean will have negative deviations, and data values above the mean will have positive deviations.

Table 13.9: Merits and demerits of standard deviation

Merits	Demerits
• It is the most important and widely used measures of dispersion as it possesses all the characteristics of a good measure of dispersion. • It is rigidly defined and free from any ambiguity. • It takes into account all the observations of the series and hence is representative. • It is prominently used in further statistical analysis. For example, in computing skewness, correlation, etc. • Unlike in mean deviation it gives due consideration to the + and – signs. • It is least affected by fluctuations of sampling and thus extensively used in hypotheses testing. • It enables the comparative study of two or more series and reports on their consistency (stability) through computation of coefficient of variation, variance, etc. • It enables to determine the reliability of the mean when two or more series exhibit identical means. • Though calculated using various methods it yields consistent results. • The calculation of SD can be simplified by altering the origin and the scale conveniently.	• It is more affected by extreme items. • Its calculation is difficult as it involves many mathematical models and processes. Calculation of range and quartile deviation is much easier. • It cannot be calculated accurately for a distribution with open-ended classes. • It always depends on arithmetic mean. • Not suitable for comparing dispersion of two or more series in different units.

Table 13.10: Formula for standard deviation

Sample standard deviation	Population standard deviation
Discrete data	
$s = \sqrt{\dfrac{\Sigma(X - \bar{X})^2}{n-1}}$ where, s = sample standard deviation Σ = sum of... $\bar{X}$ = sample mean n = sample size	$\sigma = \sqrt{\dfrac{\Sigma(X-\mu)^2}{N}}$ where, σ = population standard deviation Σ = sum of... μ = population mean N = population size
Frequency data	
$s = \sqrt{\dfrac{\Sigma f(X - \bar{X})^2}{n-1}}$ where, s = sample standard deviation Σ = sum of... f = class frequency n = sample size $\bar{X}$ = mean of mid points of ranges x = value of mid points of ranges	$(\sigma) = \sqrt{\dfrac{\Sigma fx^2}{N} - \left(\dfrac{\Sigma fx}{N}\right)^2}$ where, σ = population standard deviation Σ = sum of... f = class frequency N = population size

Step 3: Square each of the deviations (differences) to make it positive: $(X - \mu)^2$

Step 4: Add all the squared deviations: $\Sigma(X - \mu)^2$

Step 5: Divide the sum by total number of data values in the population to obtain variance: $\Sigma(X - \mu)^2/N$
Alternately, if a sample is being considered then the sum may be divided by total number of data values minus 1 to obtain sample variance: $\Sigma(x - \bar{x})^2/(n - 1)$

Step 6: Standard deviation of the population is obtained by taking the square root of variance: $\sigma = \sqrt{[\Sigma(X - \mu)^2/N]}$
However, if the sample standard deviation is to be calculated the formula would be:
$s = \sqrt{[\Sigma(x - \bar{x})^2/(n - 1)]}$.

Example: Calculate the standard deviation of following numbers: 6, 2, 3, 1

X	$(X - \mu)$	$(X - \mu)^2$
6	3	9
2	−1	1
3	0	0
1	−2	4
$\Sigma X = 12$ $\mu = 3$		$\Sigma(X - \mu)^2 = 14$

Note: N = 4
Substituting the values in the formula for population standard deviation above we get:
$\sigma = \sqrt{[\Sigma(X - \mu)^2/N]}$
$= \sqrt{(14/4)} = \sqrt{(3.5)} \approx 1.87$
The standard deviation is approximately 1.87.

Steps to Calculate Standard Deviation (Frequency Data)

Step 1: Locate the midpoint for each group or range of the frequency table: x

Step 2: Arrive at the total number of samples by adding up the frequencies: Σf

Step 3: Find the product of each group midpoint with its respective frequency and calculate the sum of the all such products: Σfx

Step 4: Also find the sum of the products of each frequency with its respective square of midpoint results: Σfx^2

Step 5: Estimate the standard deviation for the frequency table using the formula.

Example 1: Calculate the standard deviation for the frequency table of population data set.

Class interval (CI)	Frequency (f)
40–44	4
45–49	7
50–54	14
55–59	11
60–64	8
65–69	6

To calculate the standard deviation for the frequency table data set we draw the following table:

CI	f	x	x^2	fx	fx^2
40–44	4	42	1,764	168	7,056
45–49	7	47	2,209	329	15,463
50–54	14	52	2,704	728	37,856
55–59	11	57	3,249	627	35,739
60–64	8	62	3,844	496	30,752
65–69	6	67	4,489	402	26,934
	$\Sigma f = 50$		$\Sigma x^2 = 18,259$	$\Sigma fx = 2,750$	$\Sigma fx_2 = 153,800$

Substituting in the formula for population standard deviation (grouped data) we get:

$$\sigma = \sqrt{\dfrac{\Sigma fx^2}{N} - \left(\dfrac{\Sigma fx}{N}\right)^2}$$

Standard deviation (SD)
$= \sqrt{[(153{,}800/50) - (2{,}750/50)^2]}$
$= \sqrt{(3{,}076 - 3{,}025)} = \sqrt{51} \approx 7.14$
The standard deviation is approximately 7.14.

Example 2: Calculate the standard deviation for the frequency table of sample data set.

Class interval (CI)	0–10	10–20	20–30	30–40
Frequency (f)	4	7	14	11

To calculate the standard deviation for the frequency table we use the following formula:

$$s = \sqrt{\dfrac{\Sigma f(x - \bar{x})^2}{n-1}}$$

where,
s = sample standard deviation
Σ = sum of...
f = class frequency
n = number of scores in sample

$\bar{x}$ = mean of mid points of ranges
x = value of mid points of ranges

$$\bar{x} = \dfrac{(4 \times 5) + (7 \times 15) + (3 \times 25) + (2 \times 35)}{16}$$

$$= \dfrac{20 + 105 + 75 + 70}{16} = \dfrac{270}{16} = 16.87$$

Class interval (CI)	f	x (mid-point)	$\bar{x}$	$x - \bar{x}$	$f(x - \bar{x})^2$
0–10	4	5	16.87	–11.87	563.59
10–20	7	15	16.87	–1.87	24.48
20–30	3	25	16.87	8.13	198.29
30–40	2	35	16.87	18.13	657.39
	Σf = 16				$\Sigma f(x - \bar{x})^2$ = 1,443.75

Substituting we get:

$$s = \sqrt{\dfrac{\Sigma f(x - \bar{x})^2}{n-1}} = \sqrt{\dfrac{1{,}443.75}{16-1}}$$

$$= \sqrt{\dfrac{1{,}443.75}{15}} = \sqrt{96.25} = 9.81$$

BIBLIOGRAPHY

1. Burns, N., & Grove, S.K. (2005). *The practice of nursing research*: Conduct, critique and utilization (5th ed.). St. Louis, MO: Elsevier Saunders.
2. Craig, J.V. & Smyth, R.L. (2012). *The evidence based practice manual for nurses* (3rd ed.). Edinbergh UK: Churchill Livinsgtons.
3. Neiswiadomy, M.R. (2014). *Foundations of nursing research* (6th ed.). London: Pearson Education Limited.
4. Polit, D.F., & Beck, C.T. (2010). *Essentials of Nursing Research*: Appraising Evidence for Nursing Practice. Philadelphia, PA: Lippincott Williams & Wilkins.
5. Polit, D.F., & Beck, C.T. (2012). *Nursing research*: Generating and assessing evidence for nursing practice (9th ed.). Philadelphia: Lippincott Williams & Wilkins.
6. Plichta, B.S., & Garzan, S.L. (2009). *Statistics for nursing and allied health*. Philadelphia, PA: Lippincott Williams & Wilkins.
7. Sharma, K.S. (2014). *Nursing research and Statistics* (2nd ed.). Chennai: RR Donnelley Publishing India Pvt. Ltd.
8. Weiss, N.A. (1999). *Introductory Statistics*. Addison Wesley.

REVIEW QUESTIONS

I. Long Essays

1. Calculate the "mean deviation" for the following distribution.

Classes	Frequencies
20–40	3
40–80	6
80–100	20
100–120	12
120–140	9
Total	50

2. The anemia and worm infestation cases in 10 districts of a state is as under:

Districts	Anemia cases	Worm infestation cases
1	12	22
2	10	29
3	15	12
4	19	23
5	21	18
6	16	15
7	18	12
8	9	34
9	25	18
10	10	12

Calculate for each disease (i) Range (ii) Quartile deviation. (iii) Mean deviation and (iv) Standard deviation.

II. Short Essays

1. Compute standard deviation

Score	F
12–14	2
15–17	5
18–20	9
21–23	15
24–26	10
27–29	6
30–32	3

2. Diastolic BP of 10 patients are given below, calculate the standard deviation (SD).
130, 110, 160, 120, 170, 120, 150, 140, 160, 140

3. The sum of 10 values is 100 and the sum of their squares is 1,090. Find the coefficient of variation.

4. Meaning of interquartile range and its uses.

III. Short Answers

1. Range
2. Standard deviation

IV. Multiple Choice Questions

1. The measurement of spread or scatter of the individual values around the central point is called:
   a. Measures of dispersion
   b. Measures of central tendency
   c. Measures of skewness
   d. Measures of kurtosis

2. The scatter in a series of values about the average is called:
   a. Central tendency
   b. Dispersion
   c. Skewness
   d. Symmetry

3. The degree to which numerical data tend to spread about an average value is called:
   a. Constant
   b. Flatness
   c. Variation
   d. Skewness

4. If all the scores on examination cluster around the mean, the dispersion is said to be:
   a. Small

b. Large
  c. Symmetrical
  d. Normal
5. Given below are four sets of observations. Which set has the minimum variation?
    a. 46, 48, 50, 52, 54
    b. 30, 40, 50, 60, 70
    c. 40, 50, 60, 70, 80
    d. 48, 49, 50, 51, 52
6. The measure of dispersion which uses only two observations is called:
    a. Mean
    b. Median
    c. Range
    d. Coefficient of variation
7. If quartile range is 24 then quartile deviation is:
    a. 48
    b. 12
    c. 24
    d. 72
8. The range of the scores 29, 3, 143, 27, 99 is:
    a. 140
    b. 143
    c. 146
    d. 70

ANSWER KEY

| 1. a | 2. b | 3. c | 4. a | 5. d | 6. c |
| 7. b | 8. a | | | | |

UNIT 14

Normal Probability Distribution

In everyday life, we come across statements like, "he is probably wrong", "the chances of his winning the game are fifty-fifty". "It is very likely that it will rain tonight". These are not mathematically precise statements in the sense that we cannot form any definite idea about the occurrence or nonoccurrence of the events. In statistics, probability refers to the degree of certainty about the occurrence of a particular event. A few rules of probability are:
- All probabilities of occurrence of an event lie between 0 and 1 inclusive
- The sum of all the probabilities in a sample space is equal to 1
- The probability of an event that cannot happen is 0
- The probability of an event that is sure to happen is 1

The events can be of many types:
- *Simple event*: Also called an elementary event, which has only one outcome and cannot be broken down further. For example, the possibility of a "head" when a coin is tossed.
- *Compound event*: It is a combination of two or more simple events where there is more than one possible outcome. For example, getting two tails on tossing of two coins.
- *Certain event*: It is an event that is bound to occur. For example, rolling two dice and getting a total score more than 1.
- *Impossible event*: It is an event that cannot happen. For example, obtaining an "8" on rolling a single die.
- *Equally likely events*: Events that have equal likelihood of occurrence. For example, a "head" or a "tail" is equally likely to occur when a coin is tossed.
- *Complimentary events*: Events for which there are two possible outcomes. For example, flipping a coin to get either a head or tail. As the two options are exhaustive they are complimentary.
- *Mutually exclusive events*: Events that cannot occur simultaneously. For example, flipping a coin can result in a "head" or a "tail" but not both.

While studying probability, the following two concepts require a better understanding: sample space and probability distribution.
1. *Sample space* can be defined as the collection of all possible outcomes of an event associated with an experiment. For example, on tossing a coin, a sample space is formed with two elements in it (heads and tails).
2. *Probability distribution* is a statistical function, graph, or a table that corresponds all outcomes with the likelihood that a variable can take within a specified range. This range is bounded between minimum and maximum possible values. For example, the probability that a drug "X" will successfully treat cancer.

According to AN Kolmogorov (1956), the probability theory is based on three axioms:
1. The probability of happening of an event must be more than or equal to 0 and less than or equal to 1.
2. The sum of the probabilities of all the mutually exclusive outcomes is equal to 1.
3. The probability of occurrence of any two mutually exclusive events is the sum of their individual probabilities.

Some of the important distributions are—binomial, Poisson, uniform, normal, and exponential, of which the first two are discrete and the last three continuous.

NORMAL (GAUSSIAN) DISTRIBUTION

Normal distribution also called the Gaussian distribution after the mathematician Karl Friedrich Gauss is the most common and important continuous probability distribution (continuous frequency distribution) in statistics. Frequency distribution is described as symmetrical or nonsymmetrical according to their shape. Symmetry suggests that one-half of the distribution is a mirror image of the other half, i.e. both halves of the distribution are identical. A normal distribution is a symmetric distribution about the mean indicating that the distribution has one central peak with a bell-shaped curve and the tails on each side of the curve exact mirror images of the other. The data occurs more frequently near the mean than at the far end. It also suggests that there is no skew and the tails are exactly the same. With a sample size of minimum 30 the normal curve can be closely approximated (Roscoe, 1975; Shott, 1990).

A normal distribution graph is characterized by two parameters—(1) the mean and (2) the standard deviation (SD). These two parameters are sufficient to determine the distribution of the variable for the total population without seeking any further data. The normal distribution is very helpful as most of the natural phenomena follow it. For example, various measures related to healthcare such as age, weight, intelligence level, hemoglobin levels, etc. have a tendency to exhibit a normal distribution throughout the population. Also most of the inferential statistical techniques like t-test and analysis of variance (ANOVA) assume that the variables are normally distributed.

Characteristics of Normal Curve

❖ A normal curve is a bell-shaped curve, which is symmetrical about the mean, represented by the maximum height.
  ○ The point where the curve begins to grow faster horizontally than vertically is called the inflection point and lies 1 SD above and below the mean.
  ○ The tails of the curve never touch the base as the distribution is theoretical rather than empirical.
  ○ As most of the values are clustered around the mean than at the other extreme ends the normal distributions are denser in the center than at the tails.
  ○ The shape of the normal curve depends on the mean (μ) and SD (σ).
❖ The mean, median, and mode have the same value, i.e. mean = median = mode = μ.
  ○ In a distribution, where the mean is more than median or mode it results in a positively skewed distribution.
  ○ In a distribution where the mean is less than median or mode, it results in a negatively skewed distribution (Figs. 14.1A to C).
❖ The total area under the normal curve (above the X-axis) is equal to one square unit (Figs. 14.2A and B).
  ○ In a normal curve, 50% of the values lie on each half of the distribution. Other percentages depend on the distances of various values from the mean.
  ○ 68.26% of the distribution lies within ±1 SD from the mean.

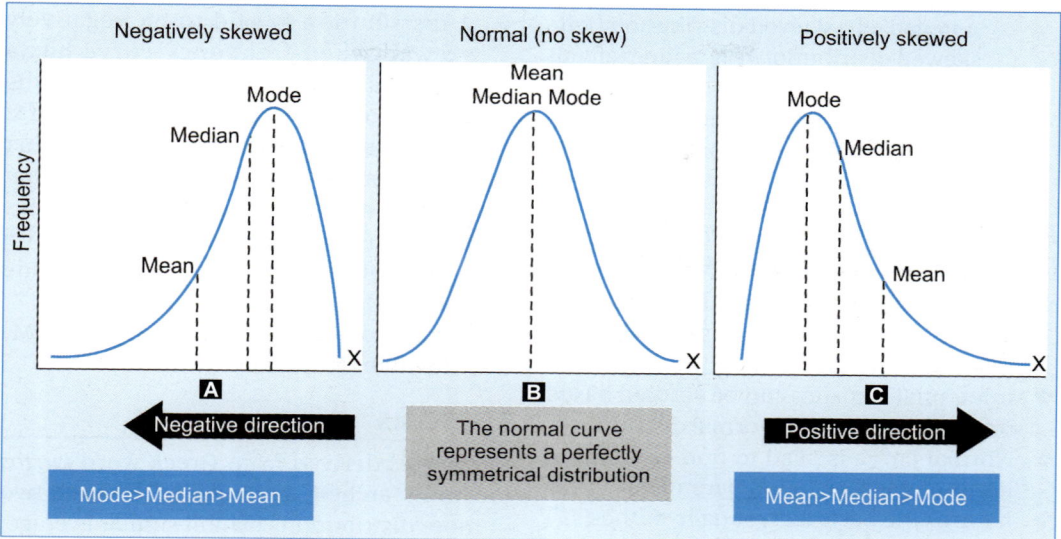

Figs. 14.1A to C: Position of mean, median, and mode in a skewed distribution

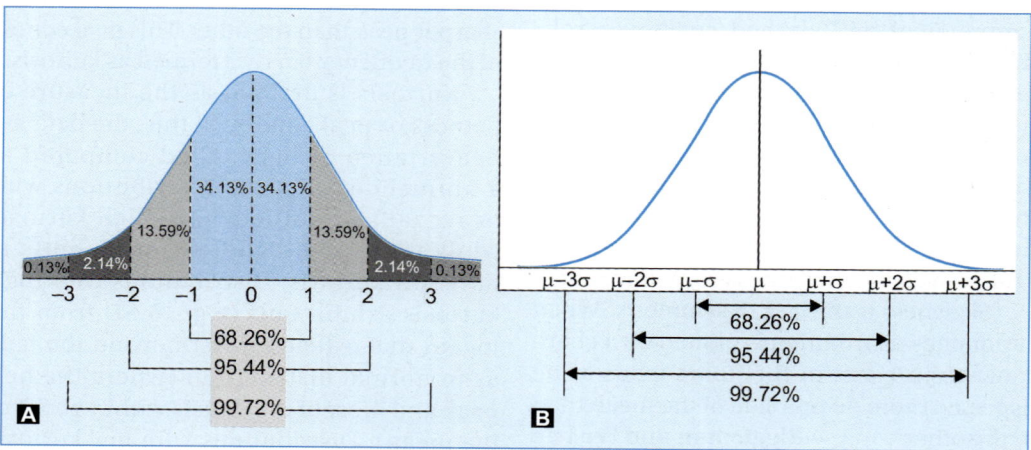

Figs. 14.2A and B: Normal curve

- 95.44% of the distribution lies within ±2 SD from the mean.
- 99.72% lies within ±3 SD and 0.1% below −3 SD.
- ❖ In nonsymmetrical distribution (also called skewed), the distribution has an off-center peak. If one tail is longer than another, the distribution is said to be skewed (Figs. 14.1A to C).
- A positive-skewed distribution (right-skewed distribution) has a long right tail in the positive direction on the number line. Accordingly, the mean also shifts to the right of the peak. For example, personal income—people with small income are more than those with large income.

- A negatively-skewed distribution (left-skewed distribution) has a long left tail in the negative direction on the number line. Accordingly, the mean also shifts to the left of the peak. For example, age of the people with chronic illness.

Application of Normal Probability Curve (Importance of Normal Distribution)
- Various physical, biological, and psychological measurements approximately follow normal distribution.
- Inferential statistics can be studied based on the assumption of normal distribution.
- Normal curve is used to find confidence limits of the population parameters.
- It forms the basis for testing hypothesis.

SKEWNESS

A normally distributed data projects a symmetrical bell-shaped curve wherein the variable values equidistant from their mean have equal frequencies. The left and the right tails of the distribution look same from the center point. Any deviation from this symmetry makes the curve appear distorted. This degree of asymmetry or distortion from the symmetrical bell curve is called skewness. It can be negative, positive, zero, or undefined.

"Skewness is the lack of symmetry. When a frequency distribution is plotted on a chart, skewness present in the items tends to be dispersed more on one side of the mean than on the other" —**Riggleman and Frisbee**

Skewness value may be positive or negative (Figs. 14.1A to C).

- A distribution is said to be positively skewed when the frequency curve has a longer tail towards the positive side or the right side of the peak, i.e. higher values of x. The mean is to the right of the peak. Another characteristic of this distribution is that there are more observations below the mean than above it. For a positively skewed distribution—Mean (M) > Median (Me) > Mode (Mo).
- A distribution is said to be negatively skewed when frequency curve has a longer tail towards the negative side or the left side of the peak, i.e. lower values of x. The mean is to the left of the peak. Another characteristic of this distribution is that there are small number of low observations and a large number of high ones. For a negatively-skewed distribution—Mode (Mo) > Median (Me) > Mean (M).
- For a symmetrical distribution: Mean (M) = Median (Me) = Mode (Mo).

KURTOSIS

Kurtosis is derived from Greek word *kurtos* meaning "arched" or "bulging". Though two or more distributions exhibit similar average, dispersion, and skewness, one might display high concentration of values near the mode, wherein the frequency curve will reflect a sharper peak than the other. This peakedness of the frequency curve is termed as kurtosis.

Kurtosis is defined as the measure of flatness or peakedness. In this, the data are heavy-tailed or light-tailed compared to a normal distribution. Distributions with heavy tails or outliers have high kurtosis while those with light tails or no outliers have low kurtosis. Distributions with high kurtosis exhibit tails (e.g. ±5 SD from the mean) that extend farther beyond the tails as in normal distribution (where the bell peak and most of the data is within ±3 SD of the mean). Distributions with low kurtosis exhibit tail data, which is less extreme than the tails in normal distribution.

"Kurtosis is the property of a distribution which expresses its relative peakedness" (Clark and Schkade).

Types of Kurtosis

The kurtosis of a distribution can be classified into any of the three categories—(1) mesokurtic (2) leptokurtic and (3) platykurtic. They are typically measured with respect to a normal distribution (Figs. 14.3A to C).

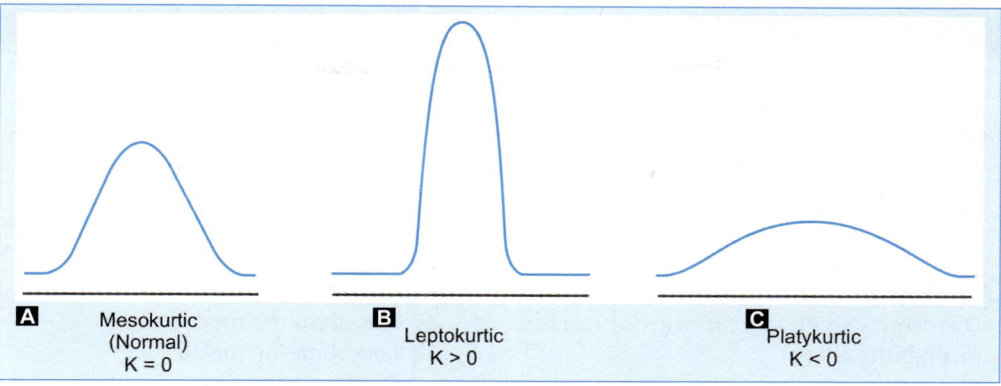

Figs. 14.3A to C: Types of kurtosis

1. *Mesokurtic:* A distribution that has tails shaped similar to any normal distribution is said to be mesokurtic. In other words, the characteristics of extreme values are similar to that of a normal distribution. In this distribution, the kurtosis is neither high nor low and is considered a baseline for the two other classifications.
2. *Leptokurtic:* A leptokurtic distribution ("lepto" meaning "skinny") displays a greater kurtosis than a mesokurtic distribution. Long tails (outliers) are a characteristic of this type of distribution, which results in the "skinniness". As a consequence, the horizontal axis of the graph is stretched making bulk of the data appear in narrow vertical fashion. These distributions are sometimes identified by peaks that are thin and tall.
3. *Platykurtic:* Platykurtic ("platy meaning "broad") distributions display short, broad looking peak with lean tails (paucity of outliers). Most times they display a peak lower than a mesokurtic distribution. All uniform distributions are platykurtic. Discrete probability distribution of a single flip of a coin is platykurtic.

BIBLIOGRAPHY

1. Burns, N., & Grove, S.K. (2005). *The practice of nursing research*: Conduct, critique and utilization (5th ed.). St. Louis, MO: Elsevier Saunders.
2. Clark, C. & Schkade, L. (1969). Statistical methods for business decisions. New York: South Western Publishing Co.
3. Kolmogorov, A.N. (1956). *Foundations of the theory of probability.* New York: Chelsea Publishing Company.
4. Neiswiadomy, M.R. (2014). *Foundations of nursing research* (6th ed.). London: Pearson Education Limited.
5. Plichta, B.S., & Garzan, S.L. (2009). *Statistics for nursing and allied health.* Philadelphia, PA: Lippincott Williams & Wilkins.
6. Polit, D.F., & Beck, C.T. (2012). *Nursing research*: Generating and assessing evidence for nursing practice (9th ed.). Philadelphia: Lippincott Williams & Wilkins.
7. Riggleman, S.& Frisbee, A. (1960). *Business Statistics.* New York: McGraw Hill Book Co.
8. Roscoe, J.T. (1975). *Fundamental Research Statistics for the Behavioral Sciences* (2nd ed.). New York: Holt Rinehart & Winston.
9. Sharma, K.S. (2014). *Nursing research and Statistics* (2nd ed.). Chennai: RR Donnelley Publishing India Pvt. Ltd.
10. Shott, S. (1990). *Statistics for health care professionals.* Philadelphia: W.B. Saunders.

REVIEW QUESTIONS

I. Long Essay
1. What is a normal probability curve? Mention its characteristics and importance. Add a note on standard normal distribution.

II. Short Essays
1. Describe the characteristics of normal probability curve
2. Skewness
3. Kurtosis
4. Normal probability curve

III. Short Answers
1. Mesokurtic distribution
2. Leptokurtic distribution
3. Platykurtic distribution

IV. Multiple Choice Questions
1. Symmetrical distributions are best described by which of the following statements?
   a. They have an equal number of data points that appear to the left and to the right of center
   b. They are normally distributed
   c. They have a U-shaped distribution
   d. They have small standard deviations
2. A normal distribution is characterized by
   a. A bell shape
   b. A mean, median, and mode that are equal
   c. A total area under the curve above the X-axis that is one square unit
   d. All of the above
3. The lack of uniformity or symmetry is called
   a. Skewness
   b. Dispersion
   c. Kurtosis
   d. Standard deviation
4. For a positively skewed distribution the mean is always
   a. Less than the median
   b. Less than the mode
   c. Greater than the mode
   d. Mean and mode are same
5. The degree of peakedness or flatness of a unimodal distribution is called
   a. Skewness
   b. Symmetry
   c. Dispersion
   d. Kurtosis
6. In which of the following distribution the peaks are thin and tall
   a. Mesokurtic
   b. Leptokurtic
   c. Platykurtic
   d. Dispersion
7. For normal distribution which property holds true?
   a. Mean = Median = Mode
   b. Mean< Mode
   c. Median< Mode
   d. Mean >Median
8. Which of the following best describes the normal curve?
   a. Bell shaped
   b. Asymmetric
   c. Positively skewed
   d. Negatively skewed

ANSWER KEY

| 1. a | 2. d | 3. a | 4. c | 5. d | 6. b |
| 7. a | 8. a | | | | |

UNIT 15

Measures of Relationship

In the previous chapters, statistical measures have been used in the context of univariate population, i.e. studying the population based on a single characteristic. However, in nursing research, data are mostly concerned with two or more variables often referred to as bivariate or multivariate population, respectively. Nurses are interested in finding whether a relationship exists between these variables or not? If so what is the nature of this relationship. Through this knowledge the nurses can accurately predict the value of one variable for an individual, when the value of the other variable is known.

CORRELATION

Correlation is a statistical technique that tests the degree (or strength) of relationship between two or more quantitative or categorical variables. The term "relationship" refers to the tendency of the variables to move together.

- If a movement (or variation) in variable X tends to generate a corresponding movement (variation) in Y, then X and Y are said to be correlated.
- The movement of variables X and Y may be in the same (i.e. both X and Y either increase or decrease) or opposite directions (i.e. if X increases then Y decreases and vice versa).
- If a change in variable X does not generate a change in Y or vice versa, then the variables X and Y are not correlated.
- Correlation may be linear or nonlinear. If both X and Y increase or decrease simultaneously at a constant rate a linear relationship exists. This linear relationship can be represented using a straight line ("linear" literally means a line). If the change in X does not generate such a systematic change in Y then the relationship is said to be nonlinear.
- The degree of linear relationship (i.e. linear correlation) between two variables is measured by correlation coefficient (r).
- Correlation can be used as a technique of analysis under the following conditions:
  - When there are two variables
  - When both the variables are related to each other
  - Sample remains the same for both the variables

CORRELATION COEFFICIENT

Correlation coefficient (r) is a statistical measure that quantifies the strength and direction of the statistical relationship and measures the degree to which a change in the value of one variable predicts a change in the other. It measures how strong a relationship is between the two variables. However, it does not indicate causation. The various methods of establishing correlation coefficient are: Pearson's correlation (also called Pearson's R) and Spearman rank order coefficient.

Features of Correlation Coefficient

- Correlation is a pure number and a unit less quantity.
- The absolute value of the correlation coefficient is an indicator of the strength of the relationship. Larger the value, stronger the relationship. For example, |−0.95| = 0.95, which has a stronger relationship than 0.75.
- Numerical value of correlation "r" ranges between −1 and +1, i.e. −1 ≤ r ≤ 1. It indicates both the strength and direction of the relationship between variables. The pattern of data is indicative of the type of relationship between variables X and Y.
- A value of "r" nearer to 0 indicates weaker relationship; nearer to 1 or −1 indicates stronger relationship. The sign of the correlation (±) only indicates the direction.
- Correlation can be influenced by outliers.
- Though the value of "r" indicates that variables X and Y are related, it does not suggest a cause and effect relationship, i.e. correlation does not imply causality. Also it does not indicate whether X influences Y or Y influences X.
- Correlation is only suitable to test the relationship between quantitative data (e.g. height) and not purely categorical data (e.g. gender and color).
- Correlational coefficient can be computed with two variables measured on the ordinal, interval, or ratio scale.

TYPES OF CORRELATION

Correlation can be classified into various types on the basis of direction, number, and the ratio of change between the variables. The researcher should familiarize himself with the correlation methods in an attempt to identify the extent to which the variables are correlated with each other. The types of correlation are presented in Flowchart 15.1.

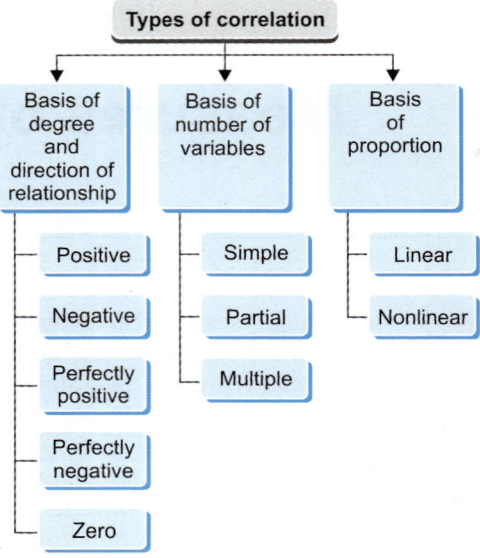

Flowchart 15.1: Types of correlation

- *On the basis of degree and direction of relationship*: On the basis of degree and direction of relationship between variables the correlation can be classified into five types. Details are presented in Table 15.1.
- *On the basis of number of variables*: Based on the number of variables studied the correlation can be classified into simple, partial, and multiple.
    - Simple correlation: In this type of correlation only two variables are studied. *Example*: A nurse researcher wants to find the correlation between stress and anxiety levels in nursing students. Here only two variables, viz stress and anxiety are being studied.
    - Partial correlation: In this type of correlation though more than two variables are studied, only two among them influencing each other are considered while controlling the effect of other influencing variables (covariates or control variables) by keeping them constant.

Table 15.1: Types of correlation based on degree and direction of relationship

Type	Characteristics	Figure
Positive correlation $0 < r < +1$	• The sign is +ve (r > 0) • The points lie close to the straight line • Direct relationship exists (an increase/decrease in one variable is associated with corresponding increase/decrease in the other variable) • The graph rises from left to right. • Example: As cigarette smoking increases, lung damage also increases	Positive correlation
Negative correlation $-1 < r < 0$	• The sign is –ve (r < 0) • The points lie close to the straight line • An inverse relationship exists (which means an increase in one variable is associated with a decrease in the other and vice versa). • The graph falls from left to right. • Example: As overweight increases, life expectancy decreases	Negative correlation
Perfectly positive $r = +1.0$	• The sign is +ve (r > 0) • The points lie on the straight line • Direct relationship exists (an increase/decrease in one variable is perfectly associated with corresponding increase/decrease in the other variable) • It is possible to predict perfectly the value of one variable by knowing the value of the second • The graph rises from left to right. • Example: As level of anxiety increases pulse rate increases	Perfectly positive correlation

Contd...

Contd...

Type	Characteristics	Figure
Perfectly negative $r = -1.0$	• The sign is –ve ($r < 0$) • The points lie on the straight line • An inverse relationship exists (which means an increase in one variable is perfectly associated with a decrease in the other and vice versa) • It is possible to predict perfectly the value of one variable by knowing the value of the second • The graph falls from left to right • Example: As level of anxiety goes up, test scores go down	Perfectly negative correlation
Zero correlation $r = 0$	• There is no pattern to the points • No linear relationship exists between variables, i.e. they are independent of each other and not related • Example: There is no relationship between amount of food intake and level of intelligence	No correlation

Example: A researcher wants to know the relationship between height and weight in males and females. As the bone and muscle structure vary according to gender, the partial correlation between height and weight are studied by removing or keeping constant the effect of gender.

○ *Multiple correlation*: In this type of correlation, three or more variables are studied simultaneously.
Example: A researcher wants to find the effect of both appearance and level of confidence on problem solving ability on school students.

❖ *On the basis of proportion*: Based on the ratio of change between the variables, correlation can be classified into linear and nonlinear correlation.

○ *Linear correlation*: The correlation is said to be linear when the ratio of change between the variables is constant.
Example:
   X: 10 15 20 25 30
   Y: 20 30 40 50 60

○ *Nonlinear correlation*: The correlation is said to be nonlinear when the ratio of change between the variables is not constant.
Example:
   X: 10 15 20 25 30
   Y: 20 40 50 55 70

NEED FOR CORRELATION

- To estimate reliability and validity of the psychological assessment measurements.
- To predict one characteristic of the patient on the basis of knowledge of the other patient characteristic.
- To ascertain which patient demographic factors are strongly correlated with primary outcome measures to develop appropriate interventions.
- The nurse can provide better counseling by knowing the correlation between various qualities of an individual.

MEASURES OF CORRELATION

In a bivariate population correlation can be studied using cross tabulation, scatter plots, Spearman's rank correlation, and Karl Pearson's coefficient of correlation. In a multivariate population, correlation can be studied with the help of coefficient of multiple and partial correlations. Cause and effect relationship between variables can be studied using multiple regression equations. The various measures of correlation are presented in Figure 15.1.

Cross Tabulation (Contingency Table)

Karl Pearson, an English mathematician who is credited with launching the study of mathematical statistics, first coined the term contingency table during the year 1904. Contingency tables also called crosstabs or two-way tables are tools used to represent data that has more than one variable. It is suitable for nominal form of data. These are statistical tables used to summarize the relationship between several categorical variables that are shown simultaneously. A contingency table allows a better understanding of the data using probability and relative frequencies.

In this method each variable is classified into two or more categories and then cross-classified into subcategories. Thus, it is basically a table of counts which displays the frequency of each data point indicating the number of times each of the two or more variables falls into different categories. It takes the form of a matrix or a grid.

Later interaction between them can be explained by symmetrical, asymmetrical, or reciprocal relationship. A symmetrical relationship is one wherein the two variables fluctuate together, though a change in one is not the result of a change in the other. A reciprocal relationship occurs when a mutual influence exists between the two variables. Asymmetrical relationship is said to exist when a change in one variable (independent variable) is responsible for change in the other variable (dependent variable). Formation of a two-way table is the first step in cross tabulation process as it indicates whether any interrelationship exists between the variables.

Example: For a study on gender differences in color of hair involving randomly sampled 100 participants, the two variables under consideration would be gender (male and female) and color of hair (black and brown). A contingency table can be drawn to exhibit the number of male and female participants with black and brown hairs. Thus a contingency table can be drawn as in Table 15.2.

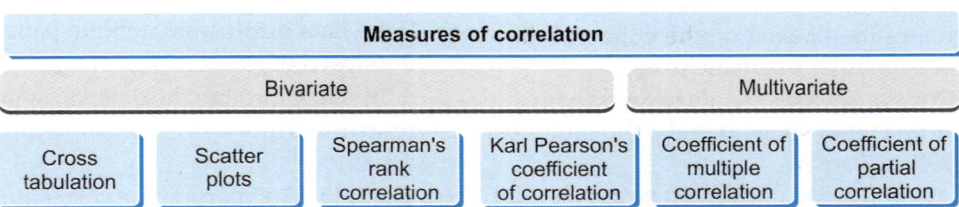

Fig. 15.1: Measures of correlation

Table 15.2: Contingency table

Gender/hair color	Black	Brown	Total
Male	34	23	57
Female	41	2	43
Total	75	25	100

The total number of the males, females, black-haired and brown-haired participants constitutes the marginal totals. The final total in the bottom corner represents the total number of participants in the contingency table.

Scatter Plots or Graphs

Scatter plots are used to plot data points on horizontal and vertical axes to show the relationship between the two variables and how much one variable is affected by another. These help to study the possible relationship between two variables associated with same "event". The relationship between two variables is called their correlation. If the markers are close to forming a straight line on the scatter plot, it signifies a high correlation among the two variables. If the markers are equally distributed in the scatter plot, the correlation is low, or zero.

Steps to Plot Scatter Diagram
- Collect paired data.
- Place the independent variable (potential cause) on the horizontal x-axis and dependent variable (effect) on the vertical y-axis.
- The range of values (minimum and maximum) for each value need to be determined based on the collected data so as to fix up a suitable scale.
- The x- and y-axes should be setup with the same length so as to make the plot look like a square.
- The values are marked on each axis with the minimum values on the lower left corner and maximum values progressing towards the other ends. Ensure the axes are divided into equal segments and labeled to enable plotting of values (paired data).
- The plotting can be done by finding the x-value on the horizontal axis and looking for the corresponding y-value vertically over the x-value in the graph. All points are plotted similarly.
- Title the graph.

Interpretation of Scatter Plot
- Tighter the plots are clustered the stronger the correlation between the variables.
- If the data displays a cluster of plots in a uphill pattern moving from lower left to upper right, there is a positive correlation between variables (if x increases or decreases, y also increases or decreases in the same direction and with same magnitude). This is the result of the y-values moving up as the x-values move towards the right on the number line.
- If the data displays a cluster of plots in a downhill pattern moving from upper left to lower right, there is a negative correlation between variables (if x increases, y decreases with the same magnitude and vice versa). This is the result of y-values moving down as the x-values move towards the right on the number line.
- If the data displays a close cluster of plots through which a straight line or a curve that "fits" well can be drawn (also called the imaginary line of best fit), it indicates a strong relationship between the two variables.
- If the data displays no definite pattern in the cluster of plots making it impossible to draw a line through the data, no apparent relationship exists between the two variables.
- The values to interpret the correlation "r" are presented in Table 15.3.

Table 15.3: Interpretation of correlation values

Size of correlation	Interpretation	Size of correlation	Interpretation
0.90 to 1.0	Very high positive correlation	−0.90 to −1.0	Very high negative correlation
0.70 to 0.90	High positive correlation	−0.70 to −0.90	High negative correlation
0.50 to 0.70	Moderate positive correlation	−0.50 to −0.70	Moderate negative correlation
0.30 to 0.50	Low positive correlation	−0.30 to −0.50	Low negative correlation
0.00 to 0.30	Negligible correlation	−0.00 to −0.30	Negligible correlation

Types of Scatter Plots

Based on the type of correlation, there are five types of scatter plots: (1) strong positive, (2) moderate positive, (3) strong negative, (4) moderate negative, and (5) no correlation. These types are described in detail in Table 15.4.

Table 15.4: Types of scatter plot

Type of scatter plot	Description	Figure
Scatter diagram with strong positive correlation	• Data points are grouped very close to each other • It shows that variables are closely related to each other • A perfect line can be drawn through them • The slope of a straight line drawn along the data points will go up • There is a clearly visible upward trend from left to right	Strong positive correlation
Scatter diagram with moderate positive correlation	• Data points are little closer together • A line drawn through them shows some kind of relationship exists between the two variables • Pattern does not closely resemble a straight line • A flat line from left to right is the weakest correlation	Moderate positive correlation

Contd…

Contd…

Type of scatter plot	Description	Figure
Scatter diagram with strong negative correlation	• Data points are grouped very close to each other • It shows that variables are closely related to each other • A perfect line can be drawn through them • The slope of a straight line drawn along the data points will go down • Clearly visible downward trend from left to right	Moderate negative correlation
Scatter diagram with moderate negative correlation	• Data points are little closer together • Line drawn through them shows some kind of relationship exists between two variables • Pattern does not closely resemble a straight line • A flat line from left to right is the weakest correlation	Strong negative correlation
Scatter diagram with weakest (or no) correlation	• Data points are spread randomly such that no line can be drawn through them • This shows no relationship between two variables	No correlation

Limitations of a Scatter Diagram
❖ Does not provide the accurate extent of correlation.
❖ Does not reflect the degree of relationship, but only expresses the direction of relationship between the variables.
❖ Does not represent the relationship for more than two variables.

Benefits of a Scatter Diagram
❖ Provides graphical representation of the relationship between two variables.
❖ Best method to show nonlinear pattern.
❖ Determines the range of data flow.
❖ Easy to plot the diagram.
❖ Not influenced by outliers.

Spearman's Rank Correlation

Some situations do not allow quantifying the magnitude of a variable as in the case of quality of life, well-being, pain, etc., where they can only be ranked in some order and measured using an ordinal scale. Spearman rank order coefficient (ρ) can be used with this kind of ordinal or ranked data and symbolized by r_s, r_{rho}, or *rho*. It is based on the rank or the order and not on the magnitude of the variable. It is a nonparametric test that measures the strength and direction of association that exists between two variables measured on an ordinal scale.

It is used less frequently than the Pearson *r* and not as powerful. Spearman's value ranges from −1 to +1, where:

- +1 refers to a perfect positive correlation between ranks
- −1 refers to a perfect negative correlation between ranks
- 0 refers to no correlation between ranks

Assumptions

- Scale of measurement is ordinal or interval or ratio.
- Data is in matched pairs.
- The association between the variables is monotonic, i.e. the two variables continue to move in the same relative direction, though not at a constant rate. For example, as the value of "x" variable increases the value of "y" either continues to increase or decrease, not necessarily at a constant rate.

Formula for Spearman's rank correlation coefficient:

$$\rho = 1 - \frac{6 \Sigma d_i^2}{n(n^2 - 1)}$$

Where,
ρ = Spearman's rank correlation coefficient
d = Difference between ranks
d² = Difference squared
n = The number of different factors in the study

Example: The depression and anxiety scores of nine patients are as under. Compute the Spearman rank correlation for the two rank order variables.

Depression scores: 35, 23, 47, 17, 10, 43, 9, 6, 28
Anxiety scores: 30, 33, 45, 23, 8, 49, 12, 4, 31

Step 1: Identify ranks for each patient by arranging the scores from highest to lowest. Assign rank 1 to the highest score and 2 to the next highest and so on.

Step 2: In the adjoining columns place "d" and "d²" for the data, where d is the difference between ranks and d² the square of the difference.

Depression	Rank	Anxiety	Rank	d	d²
35	3	30	5	2	4
23	5	33	3	2	4
47	1	45	2	1	1
17	6	23	6	0	0
10	7	8	8	1	1
43	2	49	1	1	1
9	8	12	7	1	1
6	9	4	9	0	0
28	4	31	4	0	0

Step 3: Add up all the d² values.
4+4+1+0+1+1+1+0+0 = 12

Step 4: Insert the values into the formula.

$$1 - \frac{6 \times 12}{9(81-1)}$$

$$1 - \frac{72}{720}$$

1 − 0.1 = 0.9

Thus, ρ (or r_s) = 0.90. This indicates a very high positive relationship between the ranks of depression and anxiety scores, i.e. higher the depression score, the higher is the anxiety score and vice versa. The Spearman's rank correlation for the above data set is 0.9.

Step 5: Reporting statistical significance:
The reporting of Spearman's correlation coefficient can simply be done by stating the value of the coefficient as ρ = 0.9 or r_s = 0.9. However, if the researcher wants to know whether the relationship between the variables is statistically significant or not, *p* value needs to be arrived. In the above example, ρ = 0.9, df = 7 (df = n–2) where n is the number of pair wise cases, correlation coefficient table value at 0.001 level = 0.89. As the calculated value is greater than table value we can conclude that the positive relationship between depression and anxiety is statistically significant at 0.001 level.

Merits
- Easy to calculate compared to Karl Pearson's method.
- Only measure to calculate correlation between qualitative data.
- Useful when actual data not provided, but only ranks.
- Conveniently used for irregular data as this calculation is not based on assumptions of normal distribution.

Demerits
- Cannot be used for grouped frequency distribution.
- Results are approximate as original data is not considered, but ranks.
- When the number of observations are more than 30, not convenient to use.

Karl Pearson's Correlation Coefficient (Product Moment Correlation)

The Pearson correlation coefficient referred to as the Pearson R test (product moment correlation coefficient) is generally used to calculate correlation for continuous variables and most often the precise one. It not only evaluates the linear relationship but also measures the strength between variables. To determine the strength of the relationship between two variables, one needs to find the coefficient value, which can range between –1.00 and +1.00.

Assumptions
- The variables must be either interval or ratio measurements.
- There is a linear relationship between the two variables.
- The variables must be approximately normally distributed.

Formula for Karl Pearson correlation coefficient:

$$r = \frac{n(\Sigma xy) - (\Sigma x)(\Sigma y)}{\sqrt{[n\Sigma x^2 - (\Sigma x)^2][n\Sigma y^2 - (\Sigma y)^2]}}$$

Where

n = number of pairs of scores
Σxy = sum of the products of paired scores
Σx = sum of x scores
Σy = sum of y scores
Σx^2 = sum of squared x scores
Σy^2 = sum of squared y scores

Example: Marks scored by students in Maths and Science subjects' are as under. Compute the Karl Pearson's correlation coefficient.

Maths (x)	1	3	4	4	5
Science (y)	2	5	5	8	6

To compute the Karl Pearson's correlation coefficient:

x	y	x^2	y^2	xy
1	2	1	4	2
3	5	9	25	15
4	5	16	25	20
4	8	16	64	32
5	6	25	36	30
Σx = 17 $(\Sigma x)^2$ = 289	Σy = 26 $(\Sigma y)^2$ = 676	Σx^2 = 67	Σy^2 = 154	Σxy = 99

Substituting in the above formula we get:

$$r = \frac{5(99)-(17)(26)}{\sqrt{[(5)(67)-(289)][5(154)-(676)]}} = \frac{53}{65.76} = 0.81$$

The range of the correlation coefficient is from –1 to +1. The result is 0.81, which means the variables have a high correlation. Thus coefficient of correlation measures not only the magnitude of correlation but also tells the direction. In the above example, r = +0.81 which shows correlation is positive because the sign is "+" and the magnitude is 0.81.

Merits
- Most precise method.
- It indicates the presence or absence of relationship.
- It calculates both the degree and extent of relationship between two variables.
- Helps to estimate the value of dependent variable.

Demerits
- Difficult to calculate and time consuming.
- Values of coefficient are affected by outliers.
- Cannot be computed for qualitative phenomena.

REGRESSION ANALYSIS

In medical field health professionals make many predictions. For example, a physician considers the patient's body weight to predict appropriate dose for medication. In this situation the body weight is the independent variable and the predicted medical dose is the dependent variable. This prediction is possible using regression analysis.

Regression is the quantification of a statistical relationship between two or more variables where one is the cause and the other is the effect. It is a statistical analysis used to estimate the change in dependent variable due to the change in one or more independent variables that is studying the relationship between dependent variable "Y" and one or more independent variables "X". For example, while finding the relationship between blood pressure (dependent variable-Y) and, age and weight (independent variables-X), regression analysis helps to understand how the value of dependent variable is changing, i.e. change in blood pressure with the variation in values of any one of the independent variables, i.e. age or weight.

"Regression is the measurement of the average relationship between two or more variables in terms of the original units of the data."
—MM Blair

The regression technique primarily enables:
- *Description*: Describe the relationship between the dependent variable and the independent variable statistically.
- *Estimation*: Estimate the value of dependent variable for a given value of the independent variable.
- *Prognostication*: Determine the effect of each of the independent variables on the dependent variable, controlling the effects of all other variables.

Types of Regression Analysis

The two types of regression analysis are linear regression and nonlinear regression. Linear regression analysis can be further classified into univariate or simple and multiple regression analysis. Nonlinear regression can be further classified into polynomial regression, logistic regression, power model regression, exponential regression, and Poisson regression.

Simple or univariate linear regression studies the linear relationship between one independent and one dependent variable: dependent or criterion (Y) and independent or predictor (X), i.e. Y dependents on X or Y is influenced by X. The regression line of Y on X is expressed by Y = a + bX, where "a" is the y-intercept of the line and "b" the slope.

Multiple linear regression studies the relationship between the dependent (Y) and the multiple independent variables ($X_{i=1 \text{ to } n}$).

The equation is given by $Y = a + b_1 \times X_1 + b_2 \times X_2 + b_3 \times X_3 + ... + b_n \times X_n$, where a is the y-intersect of the line and b the slope. Each of the values $b_i = 1$ to n indicates the effect of the corresponding individual independent variable X_i on Y. In this process a variable other than the independent variable in question may affect the dependent variable. This other variable is called the confounding variable. The potential influence of the confounding variables on X_i has to be eliminated as it could lead to erroneous conclusion about the relationship between the independent and the dependent variables. The two terms confounder and adjustment can be defined in this context as under:

❖ A confounder is an independent variable associated with both the dependent variable and independent variables. Its presence distorts the effect of other independent variables.
❖ Adjustment is a statistical technique employed to eliminate the influence of one or more confounders on the intervention effect.

Assumptions of Linear Regression Analysis

❖ The relation between the two variables is linear.
❖ Both the variables should be measured on interval or ratio level scale.
❖ Samples are selected randomly.
❖ Data should follow normal distribution.

REGRESSION LINE

The probable relationship between two variables can well be studied by scatter plot method as it suggests the linearity or nonlinearity of the relationship. In case of a linear relationship among the variables the points on the scatter diagram will cluster along a straight line, known as the regression line. The objective of the regression analysis is the generation of this line which best fits the observations. The best fit line for the

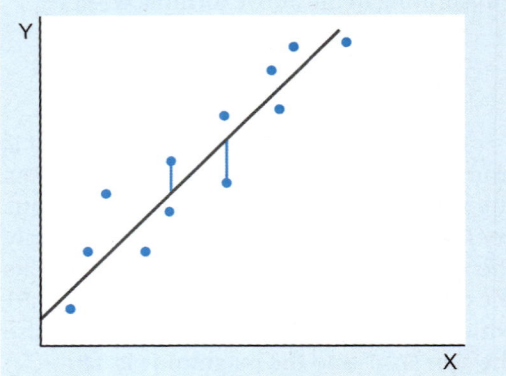

Fig. 15.2: Regression line

recorded data describes the interrelation between the dependent variable and the one or many independent variables and leaves least amount of unexplained variation in the form of dispersed points around the line. This line best fits the data, such that on a plotted graph the overall distance from the line to the variable values is the minimum. In other words regression line is the least squares line that is a plot of the expected value of the dependent variable of all values of the independent variable. This line is used to minimize the squared deviations of predictions. The greater the fit better is the predictive power (Fig. 15.2).

REGRESSION EQUATION

Regression analysis presumes a relationship between two variables that can be represented by a straight line called the regression line. The algebraic expression of this regression line is called the regression equation. It measures the extent to which the investigator can predict one variable from the other given variable. If the investigator knows that X (independent or input variable) falls on this straight line, the regression equation can be used to predict where Y (dependent or output variable) would fall on the same line. The mathematical representation of the regression model is:

$Y = a + bX + e$

Where
Y is the predicted value or the criterion
a is the Y-intercept
b is the slope and
X is the predictor
e is the error

The slope of the regression line "b" also referred to as the coefficient is defined as the rise divided by the run. The y intercept "a" also referred to as the constant is the point on the y-axis where the regression line would intercept the y-axis. The slope and y intercept are integrated into the regression equation. As the regression model is not a perfect predictor, an error term is also included in the equation "e". The distance between the line and the data point (y-value) in the Figure 15.2 represents the error.

The number of regression lines should be as many as the number of variables i.e. if there are two variables, X and Y, then there will be two regression lines:

- Regression line of Y on X provides the probable values of Y from given values of X.
- Regression line of X on Y provides the probable values of X from given values of Y.

Regression Equation of Y on X

This equation is used to predict the variations in Y from the given value of X.

$Y = a + bX$

Where
Y is the predicted value (dependent variable)
a is the Y-intercept (location where the line meets the y-axis)
b is the slope (change in the value of Y for one unit of change in X)
X is the predictor (independent variable)

The following algebraic equations can be solved to determine the values of "a" and "b".

$\Sigma Y = Na + b \Sigma X$ and
$\Sigma XY = a\Sigma X + b\Sigma X^2$

Regression Equation of X on Y

This equation is used to predict the variations in X from the given value of Y.

$X = a + bY$

where
X is the predicted value (dependent variable)
a is the Y-intercept (location where the line meets the y-axis)
b is the slope (change in the value of X for one unit change in Y)
Y is the predictor (independent variable)

The following algebraic equations can be solved to determine the values of "a" and "b".

$\Sigma X = Na + b\Sigma Y$ and
$\Sigma XY = a\Sigma Y + b\Sigma Y^2$

Merits

- Provides functional relationship between two or more variables.
- Enables the researcher to estimate the value of the dependent variable with regard to the particular value of independent variable.
- Valuable tool for measuring and estimating the cause and effect relationship among variables.

Demerits

- Calculation involves lengthy and complicated procedure.
- Cannot be used for qualitative phenomenon.

COMPARISON BETWEEN CORRELATION AND REGRESSION

Both correlation and regression describe the relationship between two variables. The correlation is used to find out whether the variables under study are related to each other or not. If the variables are related to each other through correlation, one can assess strength and direction of their relationship. The regression is used to predict the dependent variable when the independent variable is known. Correlation simply estimates strength and direction of relationship between variables, whereas regression goes beyond finding the relationship by adding prediction capabilities.

BIBLIOGRAPHY

1. Burns, N., & Grove, S.K. (2005). *The practice of nursing research*: *Conduct, critique and utilization* (5th ed.). St. Louis, MO: Elsevier Saunders.
2. Clark, C. & Schkade, L. (1969). Statistical methods for business decisions. New York: South Western Publishing Co.
3. Kolmogorov, A.N. (1956). *Foundations of the theory of probability*. New York: Chelsea Publishing Company.
4. Neiswiadomy, M.R. (2014). *Foundations of nursing research* (6th ed.). London: Pearson Education Limited.
5. Plichta, B.S., & Garzan, S.L. (2009). *Statistics for nursing and allied health*. Philadelphia, PA: Lippincott Williams & Wilkins.
6. Polit, D.F., & Beck, C.T. (2012). *Nursing research*: Generating and assessing evidence for nursing practice (9th ed.). Philadelphia: Lippincott Williams & Wilkins.
7. Riggleman, S. & Frisbee, A. (1960). *Business Statistics*. New York: McGraw Hill Book Co.
8. Roscoe, J.T. (1975). *Fundamental Research Statistics for the Behavioral Sciences* (2nd ed.). New York: Holt Rinehart & Winston.
9. Sharma, K.S. (2014). *Nursing research and Statistics* (2nd ed.). Chennai: RR Donnelley Publishing India Pvt. Ltd.
10. Shott, S. (1990). *Statistics for health care professionals*. Philadelphia: W.B. Saunders.

REVIEW QUESTIONS

I. Long Essays

1. What is correlation and correlation coefficient? Calculate the correlation coefficient for the following data.

Height of father	Height of son
70	60
68	70
65	67
71	74
75	75

2. What are the measures of correlation? Explain various measures of studying bivariate population correlation.
3. Describe correlation and liner regression in detail.
4. What do you mean by correlation? Explain scatter diagram method of ascertaining correlation between the variables.
5. Explain correlation between two sets of memory span score given below:

Test-1	Test-2
15	12
14	14
13	10
12	8
11	12
11	9
11	12
10	8
10	10
10	9
9	8
9	7
8	7
7	8
7	6

II. Short Essays

1. Describe features of correlation coefficient
2. What is Pearson's correlation?
3. What is Spearman rank order coefficient?

4. Cross tabulation
5. Features of scatter plots
6. Difference between correlation and regression
7. What are the assumptions for Pearson's coefficient of correlation?

III. Short Answers

1. Regression
2. Meaning of correlation

IV. Multiple Choice Questions

1. Correlation refers to
   a. The causal relationship between two variables
   b. The association between two variables
   c. The proportion of variance that two variables share
   d. A statistical method that can only be used with a correlational research design
2. If two variables are highly correlated, what do you know?
   a. That they always go together
   b. That high values on one variable lead to high value on the other variable
   c. That there are no other variables responsible for the relationship
   d. That changes in one variable are accompanied by predictable changes in the other
3. A coefficient of correlation computed to be −0.95 means that
   a. The relationship between two variables is weak
   b. The relationship between two variables is strong and positive
   c. The relationship between two variables is strong and but negative
   d. Correlation coefficient cannot have this value
4. Correlation coefficient values lies between
   a. −1 and +1
   b. 0 and 1
   c. −1 and 0
   d. None of these
5. If two variables oppose each other then the correlation will be
   a. Positive correlation
   b. Zero correlation
   c. Perfect correlation
   d. Negative correlation
6. A perfect negative correlation is signed by
   a. 0
   b. 1
   c. 0.5
   d. −1
7. If X and Y are independent of each other, the coefficient of correlation is
   a. −1
   b. 0
   c. +1
   d. None
8. If a scatter diagram is drawn and the scatter points lie on a straight line then it indicates
   a. No correlation
   b. Skewness
   c. Perfect correlation
   d. None of the above

ANSWER KEY

| 1. b | 2. d | 3. c | 4. a | 5. d | 6. d |
| 7. b | 8. c | | | | |

UNIT 16

Inferential Statistics and Hypothesis Testing

INFERENTIAL STATISTICS

Inferential statistics are one of the two main branches of statistics (descriptive and inferential). These are used when investigation of each member of the whole population is not convenient or possible. Thus the investigator relies on selecting a sample and uses this sample information to make generalizations and estimate the population parameters through inferential statistics.

For example, a researcher randomly selects 150 subjects with diabetes and measures changes in the blood glucose level. If the mean blood glucose level is 180 mg/dL, this represents the sample statistics. If the researcher was able to study every individual with diabetes, the average blood glucose level could be calculated. This refers to the parameter of the population. When the researchers are unable to study the entire population, inferential statistics help to draw conclusions about the larger population. In this example, the researcher conducts a study on 150 randomly selected samples with diabetes and generalizes these findings to the entire population.

PURPOSES OF INFERENTIAL STATISTICS

- ❖ Making inferences about the population using sample data
- ❖ To measure whether the difference between two or more groups on one or more variables such as experimental or control group is a real difference or only a chance difference
- ❖ Allow the researcher to make objective decision about the outcome of their study
- ❖ Enable to go beyond the immediate description of results of individual research studies so as to provide the best possible base for clinical practice or further research

TYPES OF INFERENTIAL STATISTICS

Inferential statistical procedures are divided into two types. The first involves estimation of population parameters from the sample and the second type is hypothesis testing (Flowchart 16.1).

Estimating Population Parameters

Estimation of population values can be expressed as point estimation or interval estimation.

- ❖ *Point estimation*: It estimates the population parameter with a single statistic. Here the researcher measures the sample mean, calculates a statistic, and then concludes that the value of the population mean must exactly be that number. For

Flowchart 16.1: Types of inferential statistics

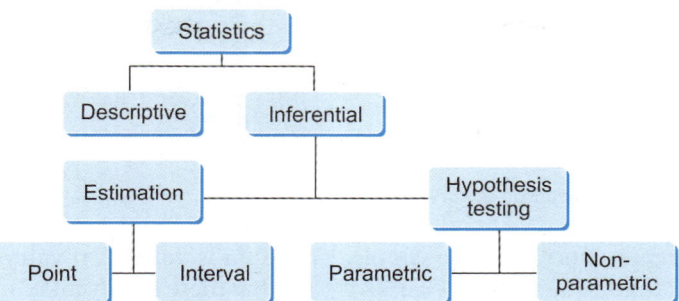

example, if the mean test score of a sample of 25 subjects was found to be 480, it would indicate the point estimate of the population mean.

* *Interval estimation*: It estimates the population parameter with a range of values within which the parameter has a specified probability of lying. In reality, sample rarely produce statistics that exactly mimic the population value. In this respect, a point estimate is less accurate than an interval estimate. In the above example, the point estimation does not detail about accuracy. The interval estimation of a parameter is a much better indicator as it deals with a range of values. With interval estimation the researcher constructs a confidence interval around the estimate. This interval is bounded by upper and lower limits called the confidence limits. These confidence limits estimate the range of values for the population mean with a certain degree of confidence. Researchers normally fix either a 95% or a 99% confidence interval. If repeated samples were taken and 99% confidence interval was computed for each sample, 99% of the intervals would contain the population mean, i.e. there is a 99% probability that the population mean is between the confidence limits.
* *Probability*: The concept of probability is vital for understanding inferential statistics. It is both a set of rules to analyze and a means to predict the outcomes. It basically refers to the likelihood that an event will occur given all possible outcomes and is represented by "p". In other words p-value is the probability that the results occurred by chance. For example, the probability of getting heads with the single flip of a coin is 1 out of 2. Therefore, the probability is expressed as 50% or $p = 0.5$. The probability of getting a 5 when a die is thrown is 1 out of 6, 1/6 or $p = 0.17$.
  ○ To estimate whether an outcome is statistically significant the researcher must set up a confidence level. A level of confidence is a probability level in which the null hypothesis can be rejected with confidence and the research hypothesis accepted with confidence
  ○ Researchers generally use 0.05 as the standard level of confidence signifying that the researchers are willing to accept a chance occurrence of five times out of 100. The 0.05 level of confidence is graphically presented in Figure 16.1. As shown, the 0.05 level of confidence is found in the small areas of the tails
  ○ These areas under the curve represent a distance of ± 1.96 SD from a mean difference of 0. A 1.96 SD in either

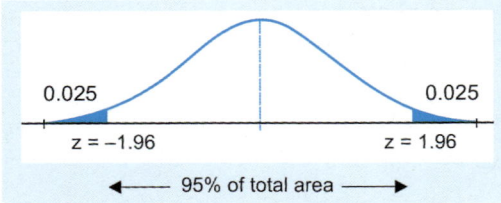

Fig. 16.1: Probability distribution curve

Table 16.1: Guidelines for statistical significance

p-value	Level of significance
p > 0.05	Statistically not significant
$0.01 \leq p < 0.05$	Statistically significant
$0.001 \leq p < 0.01$	Statistically highly significant
p < 0.001	Statistically very highly significant

direction represents 2.5% of the sample mean differences (50% – 47.5% = 2.5%)
- In other words 95% of the sample differences fall between ± 1.96 SD from a mean difference of 0
- Confidence levels can be set up for any amount of probability. For example, a more stringent confidence level is 0.01. Using this level of confidence, there is 1 chance out of 100 that the sample difference could occur by chance (1%)
- The 0.01 level of confidence is represented by the area that lies 2.58 SDs in both directions from a mean (Fig. 16.1)

❖ Once the level of significance is chosen it represents a choice that is dichotomous in nature, i.e. "yes or no", "significant or not significant". Once the decision is made, the magnitude of p reflects only the relative amount of confidence that can be placed in that decision

❖ P-value is calculated on the basis of data but level of significance is fixed in advance. P-value can be more than or less than the level of significance. If p-value is less than the level of significance it indicates a statistically significant difference between variables and H_0 is rejected. However, a p-value greater than the level of significance indicates it is not statistically significant and H_0 is accepted

❖ Low p-values indicate that the data did not occur by chance. The level of significance is usually fixed at either 5% (0.05) or 1% (0.01) or 0.1% (0.001), with 5% being the maximum desirable level to mean the data is valid. A p-value of .01 indicates that there is only a 1% probability that the results occurred by chance. Some of the crude guidelines for researchers regarding level of significance is presented in Table 16.1.

Confidence Interval

In inferential statistics the concept of confidence refers to the confidence with which the researcher can make an inference about the population based on a sample (Gardner and Altman 2000).

A confidence interval is a range of values between which a population mean is thought to lie with a particular degree usually, 95% or 99% indicating that 95% of all the calculated sample means will fall within the range of the confidence interval. If the data is distributed normally, a interval of 1.96 from the table of values corresponds to 95% confidence. Thus confidence interval is:

Confidence interval = Sample mean – (Standard error × 1.96) < Population mean < Sample mean + (Standard error × 1.96)

Example:
The mean blood glucose level of 20 sample = 100 mg

The standard deviation = 10 mg

$$\text{Standard error} = \frac{\text{Standard deviation}}{\sqrt{(N-1)}}$$

$$= \frac{10}{\sqrt{(20-1)}} = 2.29$$

where N is the number of subjects

Substituting the values in the above formula we get

Confidence interval
= 100 − (2.29 × 1.96) < population mean < 100 + (0.23 × 1.96)
= (100 − 4.49) < population mean < (100 + 4.49)
= 95.51 < population mean < 104.49

This gives a 95% confidence interval of 95.51-104.49 mg, meaning that 95% of the samples of blood glucose levels fall within the region 95.51-104.49 mmol/L.

Testing Hypothesis

One of the important objectives of research is to draw meaningful conclusions about a population based on data collected from the sample of that population. While some researchers are concerned with comparing sample statistics with that of the whole population, a few others focus on comparison between groups or on the same group over time, for example, pre and postintervention comparisons. These comparisons are made by constructing hypotheses and then testing them with inferential statistics. These statistics provide objective criteria for deciding whether hypotheses are supported by empirical evidence or not. It enables answering research questions using sample data.

HYPOTHESIS TESTING

Researchers usually arrive at decisions on population based on sample information. This involves making assumptions or guesses about the population parameters involved. Such an assumption (or statement) is called a statistical hypothesis which may or may not be true. The methodology which decides whether a hypothesis is true or not based on the sample results is called the test of hypothesis or test of significance.

It provides objective criteria for determining whether the hypotheses are supported by empirical evidence. The researcher hypothesized that cardiac patients who participated in stress management program would have lower stress levels. In this study 25 experimental group patients participated in stress management program while the other 25 control group patients did not participate in the program. All 50 patients completed a post-intervention scale of stress and, while the mean stress score for experimental group patients was 15.8, that for control group patients was 17.9. Should the researcher accept the hypothesis or not?

The results of the group mean differences though in the predicted direction might merely be on account of sampling fluctuations. The experimental and control groups might happen to be different by chance, regardless of the intervention. In this situation statistical hypothesis testing allows the researcher to make objective decisions about the study results. Through hypothesis testing the researcher can find whether the results are a consequence of sample differences or true population differences.

Hypothesis testing allows the researcher to calculate the probability that an outcome is due to something other than the intervention. It also enables the researcher to document the amount of confidence that one can have in the findings. For example, if the researcher calculates the differences in mean anxiety scores between experimental and control group patients, the researcher can express the mean difference with an identified level of confidence usually 95% or 99%. This process enables the researcher to reassure that the chances are quite low that other explanations are possible and to report findings with a documented level of confidence.

TYPES OF HYPOTHESIS

There are two types of hypothesis: (1) null hypothesis and (2) alternative hypothesis (Flowchart 16.2).

Null hypothesis states the research question in a way that suggests there will be no difference between the groups, no relationship among the variables and no effect generated from an intervention. The observed difference is merely due to fluctuations in sampling process. Null hypothesis is denoted by the symbol H_0 (H-naught). The null (or no difference) attitude on the part of a statistician before drawing any sample is the base of null hypothesis.

Alternative hypothesis is also known as research hypothesis. It states the expected relationship and usually contradicts the null hypothesis. Alternative hypothesis is denoted by the symbol H_1 (H-one).

The two hypotheses H_0 and H_1 are such that if one is true, the other is false and vice-versa. For example, if the researcher has to test whether the population mean (μ) has a specified value μ_0, then
1. The null hypothesis is $H_0: \mu = \mu_0$ and
2. The alternate hypothesis may be
   a. $H_1: \mu \neq \mu_0$ (i.e. $\mu > \mu_0$ or $\mu < \mu_0$) or
   b. $H_1: \mu > \mu_0$
   c. $H_1: \mu < \mu_0$

The alternative hypothesis in (a) is known as a two-tailed alternative and the alternative hypothesis in (b) and (c) are known as right-tailed and left-tailed alternatives respectively. The corresponding tests of hypotheses are called two-tailed (or two-sided), right-tailed (one-sided) and left-tailed (one-sided) tests respectively.

One-tailed and two-tailed tests: The word "tail" signifies the values at each end of the distribution.
- The application of a one-tailed test of significance is most appropriate when a directional research hypothesis has been stated. When this test is chosen, differences or relationships are sought in only one tail of the theoretical sampling distribution (either the left or the right tail).
- The application of a two-tailed test of significance is most appropriate when a nondirectional research hypothesis has been stated. This test is used to determine the significant values at both ends of the sampling distribution.

The selected research hypothesis determines the significance level which is needed to reject the null hypothesis. It is simpler to reject the null hypothesis when a one-tailed test is used, rather than a two-tailed test. In one-tailed test the entire area of rejection of the null hypothesis is in one end, rather than being split between the two ends, as would be necessary if a two-tailed test were used. For example, if a two-tailed test is used, and the 0.05 level of significance has been chosen, the 0.05 must be divided into 0.025 in each tail for the distribution. For a one-tailed test, as the region of rejection is all in one end of the distribution, the entire 0.05 is sought in one tail. A Z-score of 1.96 is necessary for significance at the 0.05 level for a one-tailed test. Figures 16.2A and B show the area of significant values for a one-tailed and a two-tailed test when the probability level is set at 0.05.

When designing the research model, the researcher must decide whether they will use a one or two-tailed test in determining

Flowchart 16.2: Types of hypothesis

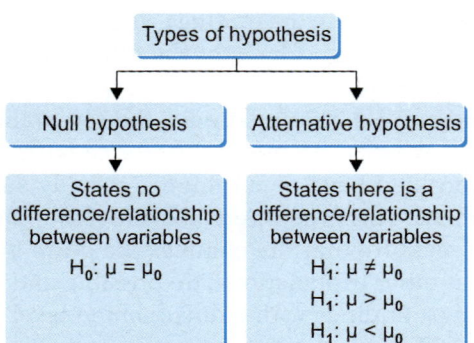

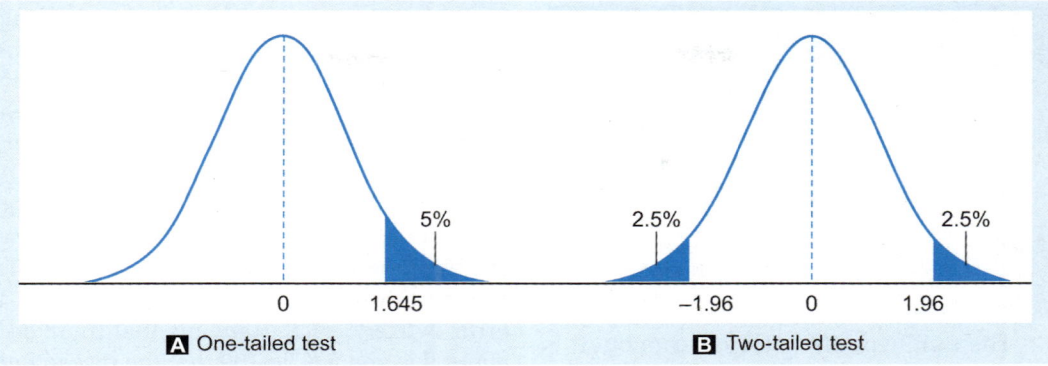

Figs. 16.2A and B: Significant values for one-tailed and two-tailed tests

the significance. If the research hypothesis predicts that the sample mean would be different from the population mean and also indicate the specific direction (directional hypothesis—$H_1: \mu > \mu_0, \mu < \mu_0$), the one-tailed test would be most appropriate. Here the region of rejection is entirely in the direction of the prediction, i.e. within one tail of the distribution.

Alternately, when a research hypothesis only predicts that one value will be different from the other without predicting the direction of the difference (nondirectional hypothesis—$\mu \neq \mu_0$), the two-tailed test would be most appropriate. Here the region of rejection (critical region) is split equally on both sides of the curve.

STEPS IN HYPOTHESIS TESTING

The five steps involved in hypothesis testing are:

- **Step 1:** *State the null and alternative hypothesis*: Null hypothesis states that there is no difference between the groups; Alternative hypothesis states that the groups are different. If the alternative hypothesis states the direction then select one-tailed test; and if it does not state the direction (greater or less) then select two-tailed test.

- **Step 2:** *Select the level of significance*: Most of the intervention studies fix significance level at 0.05 (5%) or 0.01 (1%) level.

- **Step 3:** *Identify the test statistics*: If the researcher wants to compare two groups and the sample size n > 30, select z test; if n < 30, select t-test. F test is appropriate if more than 2 means are to be compared; chi-square test is appropriate for nonparametric statistic.

- **Step 4:** *Determine the critical region*: Select appropriate distribution table for finding the critical value. For example, normal distribution table, t distribution table, chi-square distribution table and F distribution table, as appropriate.

- **Step 5:** *Perform computations*: For sample data calculate the value of the test statistic with p-value.

- **Step 6:** *Arrive at a decision*: Only one decision is possible. Either accept or reject null hypothesis.

ERRORS IN HYPOTHESIS TESTING

If a statistical hypothesis is tested, the following four cases may arise (Table 16.2).
1. The null hypothesis (H_0) is true and it is accepted by the researcher

Table 16.2: Four possible cases that may arise in any test procedure

Researcher's decision	Possible hypothesis test outcomes	
	H_0 is true	H_0 is false
Accept H_0	Correct decision (No error) Probability = $1 - \alpha$	Type II error Probability = β
Reject H_0	Type I error Probability = α	Correct decision (No error) Probability = $1-\beta$

2. The null hypothesis (H_0) is true but it is rejected by the researcher—leads to type I error (α-error)
3. The null hypothesis (H_0) is false but it is accepted by researcher—leads to type II error (β-error)
4. The null hypothesis (H_0) is false and is rejected by researcher

The errors made in situations 2 and 3 above lead to a wrong decision. The types of error in hypothesis testing are presented in Flowchart 16.3.

Flowchart 16.3: Types of errors in hypothesis testing

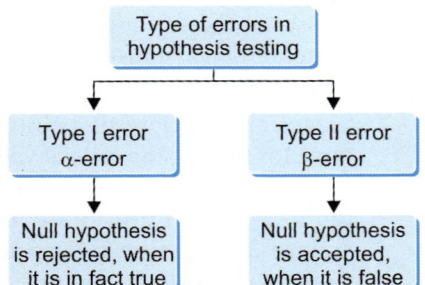

Type I error occurs when the researcher rejects the null hypothesis when it is true (incorrect rejection of a true null hypothesis). In reality there is no relationship between variables or differences between group responses to the intervention but the researcher claims there is (false positive). Thus a type I error occurs when the researcher concludes that a relationship exists while it actually does not. A common example of a type I error is a laboratory report showing a patient positive for a disease condition while he is actually not; an experiment indicating that a treatment or intervention will treat an ailment while it will actually not. This is the most serious type of error in health care which means false hope is imparted to the patient, hence is fixed at a tolerable limit.

The probability of making a type I error is called the size of the test, represented by the Greek letter α (alpha). It usually equals the significance level of the test. If type I error is fixed at 5%, it means that there are about five chances in 100 that the researcher will reject H_0, while it is actually true. Type I error is usually a design problem and has a tremendous impact on interpreting the results of quantitative studies as they do not often reveal themselves through the analytic process. It can be reduced by increasing the level of confidence.

Type II error occurs when the intervention is effective or there is a relationship among the variables and the researcher concludes there is not, i.e. the intervention works but the researcher claims it does not. Here null hypothesis is false but the researcher fails to reject it (false negative). In other words it occurs when the researcher rejects the alternative hypothesis while it actually is true. Examples of type II error would be, a laboratory investigation fails to detect a disease while the patient really has the disease; or a treatment or intervention failing to show that the treatment works when it really does.

Usually type II error occurs due to inadequate sample size. This error can be reduced by increasing the sample size. The probability of making type II error is denoted by the Greek letter β (beta) and related to the power of a test which is equal to $1-\beta$. Power is the probability of detecting a real difference. A well designed research should have a power of at least 0.80–0.90. The differences between type I and type II errors are presented in Table 16.3.

The occurrence of the above two errors is quite natural as a part of the testing process. These two errors can neither be eliminated

Table 16.3: Differences between type I and type II errors

Type I error	Type II error
Occurs when the null hypothesis (H_0) is true and the researcher rejects it	Occurs when the null hypothesis (H_0) is false and researcher fails to reject it
Erroneous rejection of true null hypothesis	Erroneous acceptance of false null hypothesis
False positive	False negative
Probability of committing error is equal to the level of significance	Probability of committing error is equal to the power of test
Denoted by α (alpha)	Denoted by β (beta)

fully nor reduced simultaneously, but can be scaled down to a prescribed level. Interestingly, reducing one type of error comes at the expense of increasing the other type of error. While one might consider using a highly restricted β (say 99%) to limit the potential for type I error, this would increase the possibility that a significant finding existed but was overlooked because of the strict standard for significance.

Level of Significance

The significance level is the maximum probability of rejecting a correct null hypothesis when it is true, i.e. the maximum probability with which the researcher is willing to risk a type I error while testing a hypothesis. It is represented by "alpha" or "α" and always indicated as a percentage (5% or 1%). The level of significance is generally specified before the commencement of the study so that the results obtained may not influence the decision. For example, a significance level of 0.05 indicates a 5% risk of concluding that a difference exists while there is no real difference. In other words, there are about 5 cases in 100 that the hypothesis would be rejected while it should have been accepted, i.e. the researcher is 95% confident that the right decision has been made. Similarly, while testing a hypothesis, if 1% level of significance is chosen then there is only 1 case in 100 that the hypothesis would be rejected while it should have been accepted, i.e. the researcher is 99% confident that the right decision has been made.

Degrees of Freedom

The notion of degrees of freedom (df) is essential while estimating population statistics. It is an essential mathematical restriction while estimating one statistic from an estimate of another. They are generally discussed in relationship to various forms of hypothesis testing in statistics.

Degrees of freedom is the number of "observations" (scores) in a distribution that are free to vary without changing the mean of the distribution. The degrees of freedom for an estimate can be arrived at by subtracting one from the number of items. In mathematical terms if "n" is the number of items in the set, then *degrees of freedom (df) = n – 1*. This number is used to determine power as greater the number of subjects, the greater is the power.

For example, consider a set of numbers that have a mean (average) of 10: (7, 13, 10) or (9, 9, 12) or (11, 7, 12). Once the first two numbers in the set are chosen, the third is fixed. In other words, there is no choice as regards the third item in the set. The only numbers that are free to vary are the first two. We can either pick 7, 13 or 9, 9 or 11, 7. But once the decision is made, the third number must be chosen to give the predetermined mean. So degree of freedom for a set of three numbers is 2. The degrees of freedom for various statistical tests are presented in Table 16.4.

Degrees of Freedom: 1-sample T-test

In 1-sample t-test, the degrees of freedom are equal to total number of observations minus number of parameter estimates. In this test, one degree of freedom is utilized in estimating the mean, and the remaining n-1 degrees of freedom to estimate variability. Thus df = n–1.

Table 16.4: Degrees of freedom for various statistical tests

Statistical test	Degrees of freedom (df)	Explanation
1-sample t-test	$n - 1$	n = sample size
Paired t-test	$n - 1$	n = sample size
Independent sample t-test	$n_1 + n_2 - 2$	n_1 and n_2 = sizes of two samples
ANOVA: Mean sum of squares within (MS_W)	$n - k$	n = total sample size in each cell, k = number of groups
ANOVA: Mean sum of squares between (MS_B)	$k - 1$	k = number of groups
χ^2 test for independence	$(r - 1)(c - 1)$	r = number of rows, c = number of columns

Degrees of Freedom: 2-sample T-test

If there are two samples, there are two "n"s to consider for each sample (n_1 and n_2), where n is number of observations. Thus degrees of freedom in this case would be $(n_1 + n_2) - 2$.

Degrees of Freedom in Analysis of Variance

In analysis of variance (ANOVA) test there are two degrees of freedom, between the groups and within the groups. Degrees of freedom for between the groups is k–1, where k is the number of groups while for within the groups it is n–k, where n is the total number of subjects in each cell and k is the number of groups.

Degrees of Freedom in Chi-Square Test of Independence

A chi-square test of independence is used to find the association between categorical variables. Here, df is the number of cells that can vary in the two-way table with the constraints of the row and column marginal totals. In a 2 × 2 table, with two categories and two levels for each category, once the row and column and marginal totals are set only one cell "x" can vary among the four cells. The value of other cells is not free to vary and predetermined by the row and column totals. So the chi-square test for independence has only one degree of freedom for a 2 × 2 Table.

	Category A		Total
Category B	x		10
			12
Total	8	14	22

Similarly, the chi-square test for independence for a 3 × 2 table has two degrees of freedom, because only two of the cells can vary for a given set of marginal totals, i.e. x and y. The value of other cells is not free to vary and predetermined by the row and column totals.

	Category A			Total
Category B	x	y		10
				12
Total	8	5	9	22

PARAMETRIC AND NONPARAMETRIC TESTS

Inferential statistics generally fall into one of the two possible categories based on assumptions of data: parametric or nonparametric. Parametric or nonparametric test is chosen depending on the level of data to be examined. Data can either be continuous, discrete, binary, or categorical. Continuous data can take any numerical value and be measured on a scale or continuum (example, height). Discrete data can take any integer value, i.e. a whole number that can be positive, negative or zero (example, number of pregnancies). Binary data are simply yes/no data: present or absent. In categorical data the attributes are different but no rank order exists (example, color or shape).

When the dependent variable is measured on a ratio or interval scale (continuous data) parametric test is used. If the dependent variable is measured on an ordinal or nominal scale (binary or discrete data) nonparametric test is used.

Parametric Test

When population parameters are completely known the researcher can use parametric tests. These tests make certain assumptions about the population parameters and assume that the data is distributed normally and follows a bell-shaped curve. These tests are more powerful and require a smaller sample compared to nonparametric tests to make solid conclusions. Since these tests are based on underlying statistical assumptions, several conditions of validity need to be met for results to be reliable. Commonly used parametric tests include t-test, z-test, ANOVA parametric test. Parametric tests often have nonparametric equivalents.

Assumptions

To carry out parametric tests the data should meet certain characteristics, generally termed as assumptions. Violation of these assumptions distorts the research results and interpretation. Thus all statistical research must follow certain assumptions for accurate interpretation (Fig. 16.3).

* *Normality*: The data should follow normal distribution, meaning all data points must follow a bell-shaped curve without data being skewed.
* *Homogeneity of variances*: Data in the different groups need to have equal variance and the same standard deviation.
* *Interval or ratio scale*: Data should be measured on interval or ratio scale and need to be continuous.
* *Independence*: Observations are independent.

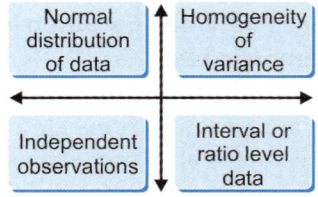

Fig. 16.3: Assumptions of parametric test

Reasons to use Parametric Tests
* *Study is represented by the mean*: If the mean is a better measure to assess the central tendency
* *Adequate sample size*: If the sample is sufficiently large
* *Presence of continuous data*: Data is measured on interval or ratio scale

Advantages
* Parametric tests provide reliable results when the groups have equal variances. Example, 2-sample t-test or one-way ANOVA
* Parametric tests have greater statistical power, i.e. if an effect actually exists, a parametric analysis can detect it. It is more able to lead to a rejection of H_0.

Disadvantages
* Not valid when the sample size is small
* Difficult to carry out the test as the size of the sample is always very big
* Results of the test are affected by the outliers of the data

Nonparametric Test

When population parameters are not known, the researcher can use nonparametric test. It is also called distribution-free test because it does not assume that the data follows a specific distribution. They can thus be applied where parametric conditions (normal distribution, equal variance, continuous, and independence) of validity are not met. Commonly used nonparametric tests include chi-square, Spearman rank coefficient, Mann–Whitney U test, Kruskal–Wallis test, etc.

In the field of health sciences and nursing the nonparametric tests are increasingly used as the observations are presented in numerical figures and also the researchers may not be aware of the nature of population distribution and other parameters. In addition the sample may be too small to test the hypothesis and generalize the findings for the population from which the sample is drawn.

In other words, the nonparametric tests are valid in a broader range of situations (fewer conditions of validity). Example, grading bed sores, assessing pain, and effectiveness of drug action, etc.

Nonparametric tests being valid for both normally and non-normally distributed data, it would be desirable to use these tests in all cases. But yet the parametric tests are preferred for the following reasons:

- Parametric tests usually have more statistical power than their nonparametric equivalents, i.e. they are more likely to detect significant differences when they truly exist.
- The researcher would not only be interested in significance of the test alone, but would also like to know about the population from which the sample originated to estimate population parameters and confidence intervals.
- Nonparametric tests are not suitable for certain statistical analysis like multiple regression.

Assumptions
1. When data do not follow any specific distribution and no assumptions about population are made
2. Data is measured on any scale

Reasons to use Nonparametric Test
1. *Study is represented by the median*: When the data is skewed the mean is adversely affected by the changes in the distribution. However, the median still continues to reflect the center of the distribution and thus a better measure. Accordingly, if the study is represented by the median a nonparametric test is appropriate.
2. *Small sample size*: For conducting a parametric test the data should be normally distributed, which in turn requires a sufficient sample. However, if the sample size is small it may not project normal distribution. In such situations nonparametric test would be a better alternative as a parametric test will not produce meaningful results.
3. *Presence of ordinal data, ranked data, and outliers*: While parametric tests require continuous data they may also be adversely affected by the presence of outliers. On the other hand, nonparametric tests can be used with ordinal and ranked data and also the results are not seriously affected by outliers.

Advantages
- Simple and easy to understand
- Does not require knowledge of the population parameters thus no assumptions are made regarding the population
- They do not rely on normal distribution
- Nonparametric tests assess the median rather than the mean which can be more suitable for some studies. Example, studies involving salaries usually present a right-skewed distribution with long tail stretching towards higher salary ranges. This long tail drags the mean away from the central median value around which the majority of the observations are clustered
- Nonparametric tests are valid when the sample size is small and the data non-normal
- While parametric tests are performed only with continuous data and adversely affected by outliers, nonparametric tests can be performed with nominal, ordinal data and outliers
- Easily applicable for attribute data

Disadvantage
- Not so powerful as a parametric test.

Differences Between Parametric and Nonparametric Test

Hypothesis testing is different between parametric and nonparametric tests. The differences between parametric and non-parametric tests are presented in Table 16.5.

Table 16.5: Differences between parametric and nonparametric tests

Basis for comparison	Parametric test	Nonparametric test
Meaning	A statistical test, in which specific assumptions are made about the population parameters	A statistical test in which no specific assumptions are made about population parameters
Basis of test statistic	Uses normal probabilistic distribution	The distribution is arbitrary
Measurement level	• Interval: Measures characteristics in terms of fixed units, e.g. IQ assessment • Ratio: Measures the characteristics with absolute zero point, e.g. pulse, weight	• Nominal: Defines a characteristic, e.g. gender, area of residence, etc. • Ordinal: Ranks the characteristics, e.g. educational level, opinion or attitude
Measure of central tendency	Uses a mean value for the central tendency	Uses the median value for central tendency
Information about population	Requires previous knowledge about the population	Does not require previous knowledge about the population
Applicability	• Measurable variables	• Variables and attributes
Related pairs of tests	*Correlation test*	
	• Pearson correlation	• Spearman correlation
	Independent measure, two groups	
	• Unpaired (independent) t-test	• Mann–Whitney U test
	Independent measure, > two groups	
	• One-way ANOVA	• Kruskal–Wallis test
	Repeated measures, two conditions	
	• Paired t-test	• Wilcoxon rank sum test
	Repeated measures, > two conditions	
	• One way repeated measures ANOVA	• Friedman's ANOVA
Statistical power	More powerful	Less powerful

The reason for selecting parametric or nonparametric test depends on whether it is the mean or the median that accurately represents the center of the data distribution. When the mean accurately represents the central tendency and the sample is large enough, the use of parametric test should be considered as it is more powerful. When the median better represents the center of the data distribution, the use of nonparametric test may be considered even though the sample size is large. If the assumptions of parametric test are met, these types of statistical tests are more powerful than nonparametric tests. However, if the assumptions are violated it is possible that a nonparametric test might be more powerful (Flowchart 16.4).

Selecting the Appropriate Quantitative Test

Selecting an appropriate statistical test is based on various factors (Fig. 16.4, Flowchart 16.5 and Table 16.6).

❖ *Research question*: The type of research question such as effectiveness of intervention or predicting the risk factors decides the appropriate statistical test.
❖ *Number of groups to be analyzed*: If the research question is to find out the differences between two groups it will

Flowchart 16.4: Determination of parametric and nonparametric test

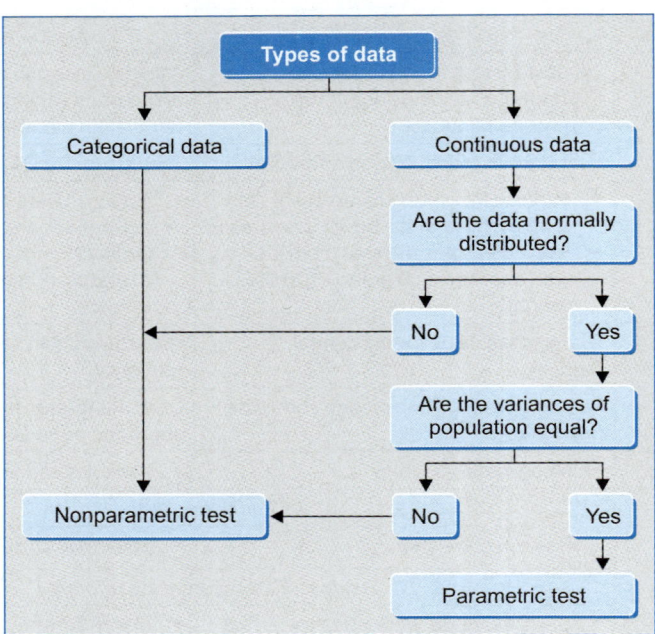

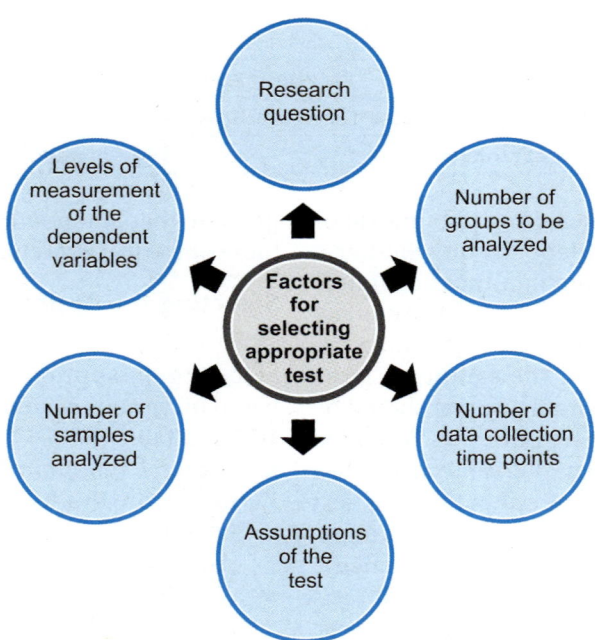

Fig. 16.4: Factors for selecting appropriate test

Flowchart 16.5: Summary of selecting appropriate statistical test

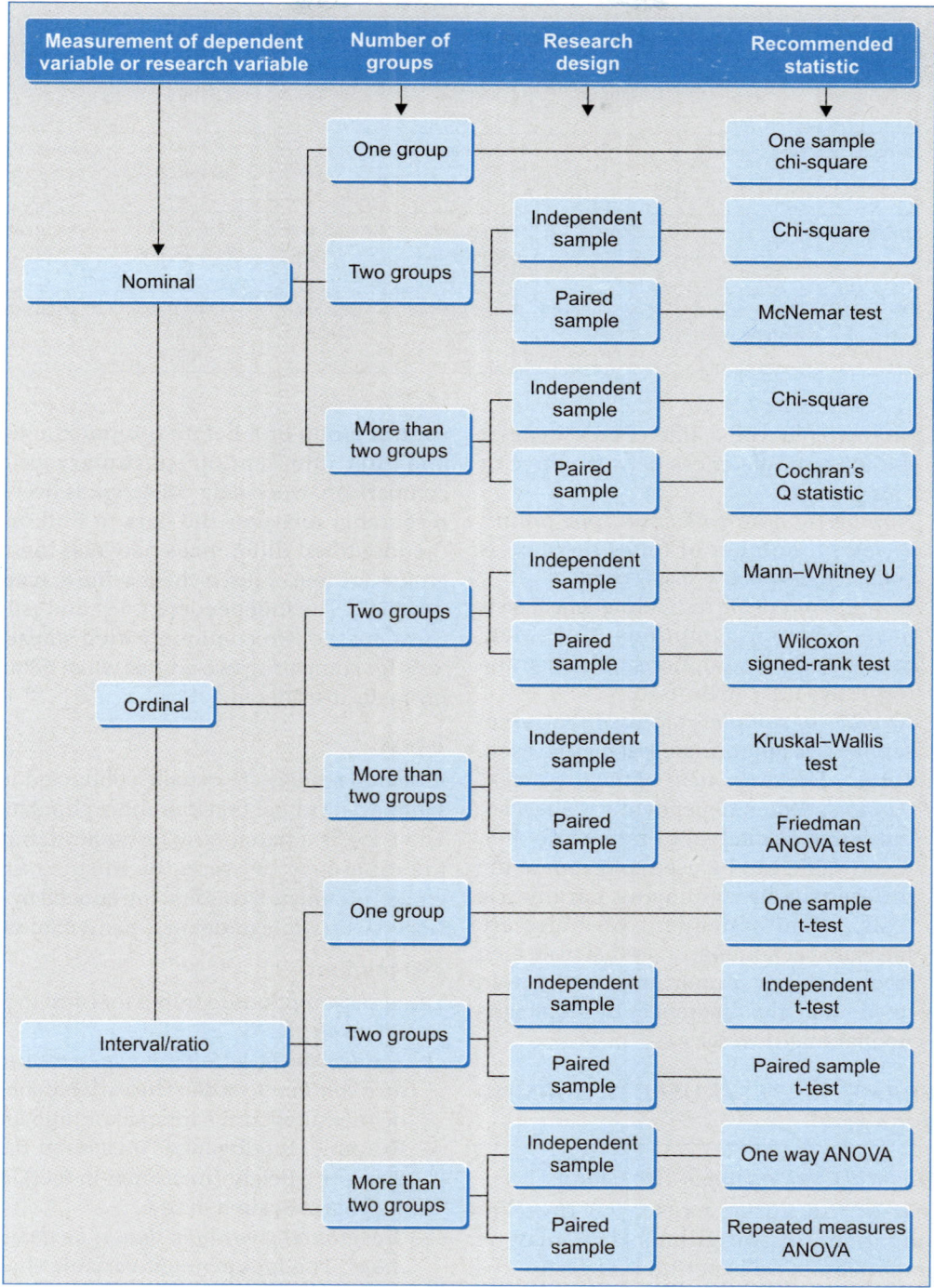

(ANOVA: Analysis of Variance)

Table 16.6: Summary table for selecting appropriate statistical test

Levels of measurement	Sample characteristics					Correlation
	One sample	Two sample		More than two samples		
		Independent sample	Dependent sample (paired)	Independent sample	Dependent sample (paired)	
Nominal	One sample χ^2	χ^2	McNemar test	χ^2	Cochran's Q statistic	Cramér's V or Cramér's phi (φ_c)
Ordinal	χ^2	Mann–Whitney U	Wilcoxon signed-rank test	Kruskal-Wallis test	Friedman ANOVA test	Spearman's rho
Interval and ratio	Z-test or one sample t-test	Independent t-test	Paired sample t-test	One way ANOVA	Repeated measures of ANOVA	Pearson's test

be answered with a different test than for finding out differences between three or four groups.
* *Number of data collection time points*: Based on number of times the data is collected, respective test is used.
* *Assumptions of the test*: All statistical tests have certain assumptions. If the data meets those assumptions only then the respective test can be used.
* *Number of samples analyzed*: Based on sample size appropriate test may be used.
* *Levels of measurement of the dependent variables*: When dependent variables are measured at interval or ratio scale then mean value can be used to compare the differences by employing parametric tests. When dependent variables are measured at nominal or ordinal scale then frequencies or proportions can be used to compare the differences by employing nonparametric tests.

PARAMETRIC TESTS USED IN NURSING RESEARCH

Statistical Comparison of Two Groups

Most of the nursing research involves comparison of two groups. This may be comparison of an experimental group to a control group or a before (preintervention) and after intervention (postintervention) comparison. Once data collection is over the researcher analyzes the data to find out if the identified differences between the two groups are real or just a chance due to natural variation. The independent t-test and paired t-test are the two commonly used statistical tests for comparing two groups when data are normally distributed.

T-test

Research studies are usually conducted with sample data rather than the entire population. The t-test is a parametric test that examines the difference between the means of two groups of values. It was first introduced by WS Gosset who wrote under pen-name "Student".

Assumptions

The six assumptions required for t-test to give a valid result are:
1. *The dependent variable should be measured on a continuous scale*: The variable should be measured at the interval or ratio level. Example, intelligence (measured using IQ score), height (measured in feet), and weight (measured in kg).
2. *The grouping variable should be dichotomous*: The independent variable should

have two categorical, independent groups. Example, gender (two groups: male or female), marital status (two groups: married or unmarried), drug addiction (two groups: yes or no), groups (two groups: experimental or control group).
3. *There should be independence of observations*: The observations in the sample are independent of each other, in the sense, measurement of each subject is no way related to the measurement of other subject. It also refers to the subjects being a part of a single group and being measured only once.
4. *The variable measuring the characteristic of interest is normally distributed*: The measuring variable data should follow normal distribution.
5. *Homogeneity of variances across groups*: Responses are close to the average values and not extensively scattered, i.e. low standard deviation.
6. *There should be no significant outliers*: Outliers are extremely large or small values that are widely scattered from the rest of the data. Example, in a study involving 100 students if the mean IQ score is 108, and if a single student has a score of 128, it will be treated as an outlier. These outlier reduce the validity of the independent t-test results.

The researcher should understand the difference between statistical significance and effect size. Statistical significance indicates whether the observed differences between two groups are real or merely due to chance. The effect size indicates whether the differences between the groups are large enough to be practically meaningful.

Types of T-tests

There are three commonly performed t-tests for different situations. They all use a test statistic that follows a t-distribution under the null hypothesis. The purpose of each t-test is presented in Table 16.7.

1-sample t-test:
One-sample t-test compares the sample mean to a hypothetically assumed value. This assumed value may be derived from either the population mean (known value) or previous data or a theoretical value. In this test the researcher initially measures the sample observations from the population of interest and estimates the population mean by calculating sample mean. The one sample t-test is commonly used to test the following:

❖ To compare the sample mean with population mean. For example, to estimate whether the mean hemoglobin level of adolescent differs from 13 (population mean).

Step-by-step computation of one sample t-test:
Example: A study to compare the sample adolescent mean hemoglobin levels with known hemoglobin value.

Table 16.7: Types of t-test		
Type of t-test	*Purpose*	*Example*
1-sample t-test	Tests whether the mean of a single population is equal to the target value	Is the mean weight of new born babies greater than 2.5 kg?
Independent sample t-test or student t-test	Tests the difference between means of two independent populations	Does the mean weight of the female newborns significantly differ from the mean weight of male newborns?
Paired t	Tests the mean of the differences between dependent or paired observations	If the weight of the newborn baby is measured prior and after a massage therapy, is the difference in the mean weight prior and after the massage therapy program significant enough to conclude that the program is effective?

Sample data: 10, 12, 13, 12, 11, 9, 8, 9.5, 10, 12
1. State the null and alternative hypothesis
   - $H_0: \mu_A = \mu_B$—there will be no difference in mean hemoglobin scores of sample and population.
   - $H_A: \mu_A \neq \mu_B$—there is a significant difference between sample hemoglobin levels with population hemoglobin levels.
2. Specify the significance level (α-level), calculate the degrees of freedom, and determine critical value
   - The degrees of freedom (n−1) = 9. Looking up the 9 degrees of freedom in the t-table at an α level of 0.05 we get 1.83. *Note*: If the α levels is not known, one can use 5% (0.05). The critical value is 1.83 (see Appendix 1).
3. Ensure the data meet all the underlying assumptions
   - Data should be normally distributed
   - Samples are selected randomly
   - Data is independent
4. Compute the one group t-test using the formula:

$$t = \frac{\bar{x} - \mu}{\frac{S}{\sqrt{n}}}$$

Where
$\bar{x}$ = sample mean
μ = population mean
S = standard deviation of sample mean
n = total number of samples
For the above sample data, the mean = 10.65. Standard deviation = 1.59. Population mean = 13.

$$t = \frac{10.65 - 13}{1.59/(\sqrt{10})} = \frac{-2.35}{0.503} = -4.67$$

The calculated t-value = −4.67
5. Determine the statistical significance and state a conclusion.
Comparing the calculated value (−4.67) with the t-table value (1.83 at 0.05 level) we find that the calculated value of 4.67 is greater than the table value of 1.83. We can conclude that there is a difference between sample and population means. The null hypothesis is rejected and the alternative hypothesis accepted.

Independent t-test (student t-test, two-sample t-test): Also called between subjects design, it is an inferential statistical test designed to compare means of two groups independent of each other, i.e. having different subjects in each group. The participants in one group do not share any relationship with those of the second group. Subjects are selected randomly from the population or randomly assigned to one of the two groups. Example, whether boys and girls have different average heights? Thus a t-test identifies whether differences between two groups' averages are real and not a random chance in sample selection.

The independent samples t-test is commonly used to test the following:
❖ Statistical differences between the subject means of two groups
Example: An independent t-test can be used to find out whether height differed on account of gender. Here the independent variable is gender having two groups: boys and girls while the dependent variable is height.
❖ Statistical differences between the subject means of two interventions
Example: An independent t-test can be used to find out there is a difference in memory scores between experimental and control group subjects (i.e. the dependent variable would be "memory scores" and the independent variable would be "intervention", which has two alternatives: treatment (experimental group) or no treatment (control group).

Step by step computation of independent t-test statistics:
Example: A study to evaluate the efficacy of memory enhancement therapy on improvement of memory scores among school going children. Memory test was administered

to two groups; group "A" received memory enhancement therapy and group "B" received no therapy. Mean memory scores of these two groups are 3.5 and 5.0 respectively. Are these differences real or are group differences the result of chance fluctuations?

To test these hypotheses, an independent sample t-test is computed.

Group A memory scores: 1, 3, 4, 6, 7, 2, 1, 1, 2, 1
Group B memory scores: 1, 2, 4, 2, 2, 1, 1, 1, 3, 4

1. State the null and alternative hypothesis:
   - $H_0: \mu_A = \mu_B$—there will be no difference in mean memory scores of the two groups.
   - $H_A: \mu_A > \mu_B$—school children in intervention group will have significantly higher memory scores than those in control group.
2. Specify the significance level (α level), calculate the degrees of freedom, and determine critical value:
   - The degrees of freedom ($n_A - 1 + n_B - 1$) = 18. Looking up the 18 degrees of freedom in the t-table at an α level of 0.05 we get 2.10. Note: If the α level is not known, one can use 5% (0.05). The critical value is 2.10 (see Appendix 1).
3. Ensure the data meet all the underlying assumptions:
   - Data points are normally distributed
   - Samples are randomly assigned to the groups
   - Data are collected independent of each other
   - Dependent variable should be measured on a continuous scale
4. Compute the independent t-test using the formula:

$$t = \frac{\bar{x}_1 - \bar{x}_2}{\sqrt{\frac{S_1^2}{n_1} + \frac{S_2^2}{n_2}}}$$

Where
$\bar{x}_1$ = Group A data mean
$\bar{x}_2$ = Group B data mean
S_1^2 = Standard deviation (SD) of Group A
S_2^2 = Standard deviation (SD) of Group B
n_1 = Total number of samples in Group A
n_2 = Total number of samples in Group B

In the above data,
Group A mean = 2.80, SD = 2.20.
Group B mean = 2.10, SD = 1.20.
Substituting the values in the above formula we get:

$$t = \frac{2.80 - 2.10}{\sqrt{(2.20^2 / 10) + (1.20^2 / 10)}}$$

$$= \frac{0.70}{\sqrt{(0.484 + 0.144)}} = \frac{0.70}{0.79} = 0.886$$

The calculated t-value = 0.886

5. Determine the statistical significance and state a conclusion.
   The calculated value is 0.886 which is lesser than t-table value of 2.10 at 0.05 level. Therefore we cannot conclude that there is a difference between means. We can now say that the memory scores of school children who have undergone memory enhancement therapy and those who have not undergone the therapy are same. The null hypothesis is accepted and the alternative hypothesis is rejected.

Paired Samples T-test
Also termed as correlated samples t-test, it is used when scores or values are associated or have some connection, i.e. two groups are related in any of the following ways. Participants in one group are same as those in the other group, i.e. same participants are repeatedly measured or participants in one group are genetically related to those in the other group.

The dependent samples t-test is commonly used to test the following:
- Statistical differences between the means of same group before or after they receive experimental treatment

Example: Paired t-test can be used to understand whether weight differed when the same subjects are measured before and after they received a nutritional intervention. The dependent variable would be "weight" and the independent variable would be "nutritional intervention", which has two values for same subjects: before intervention and after intervention.

❖ Statistical differences between the means of two genetically related groups
Example: Paired t-test can be used to understand whether anxiety scores are different among a pair of twins. A pair of twins could be divided such that one twin is assigned to the first group and the other twin to the second group.

Step-by-step computation of paired t-test statistics:
Example: A study to evaluate the effect of cognitive behavioral therapy (CBT) on wellbeing scores among cancer patients. A sample of 10 cancer patients was randomly selected and their wellbeing scores measured before CBT and again after 2 months of CBT. Are there any differences in mean wellbeing scores before and after CBT? To test this hypothesis paired t-test is used.

Before CBT wellbeing scores (Time 1):
   2, 4, 5, 7, 8, 10, 3, 3, 3, 12
After CBT wellbeing scores (Time 2):
   22, 12, 10, 20, 19, 22, 20, 23, 26, 14

1. State the null and alternative hypothesis
   ○ $H_0: \mu_A = \mu_B$—there will be no differences in mean wellbeing scores among cancer patients before and after CBT
   ○ $H_1: \mu_A \neq \mu_B$—the wellbeing scores among cancer patients will be significantly higher after participating in CBT than before participating in CBT.
2. Specify the significance level (α level), calculate the degrees of freedom, and determine critical value for the computed t-statistic.
   ○ If a specified α level is not mentioned, one can use 5% (0.05).
   ○ Subtracting 1 from the sample size we get the degrees of freedom (10 – 1) = 9.
   ○ We find the p-value in the t-table using the degrees of freedom, i.e. 9.
   ○ In the present problem, with df = 9 at 0.05 level, the t-value is 2.26 (see Appendix 1).
3. Ensure the data meet all the underlying assumptions
   ○ The two measures (before and after) of the dependent variables (wellbeing scores) are correlated
   ○ The dependent variable, "wellbeing scores" were measured by an interval scale
   ○ The wellbeing scores are normally distributed
4. Compute the paired t-statistic using the formula

$$t = \frac{\bar{d}}{s_d / \sqrt{n}}$$

Where
$\bar{d}$ = mean differences
s_d = standard deviation of the difference
n = number of sample

	Time 1	Time 2	Difference (Time 1 – Time 2)
	2	22	–20
	4	12	–8
	5	10	–5
	7	20	–13
	8	19	–11
	10	22	–12
	3	20	–17
	3	23	–20
	3	26	–23
	12	14	–2
Average	5.7	18.8	–13.1
SD	3.40	5.16	6.90
n	10	10	10

$$t = \frac{\bar{d}}{s_d/\sqrt{n}}$$

$$t = \frac{-13.1}{6.90/\sqrt{10}} = \frac{-13.1}{2.18} = -6.009$$

The calculated t-value = –6.009

5. Determine the statistical significance and state a conclusion
   - Comparing the t-table value, i.e. 2.26 with the calculated t-value (–6.009) we find that the calculated t-value is greater than the table value at an α level 0.05
   - The p-value is less than the α level: $p < 0.05$
   - Thus we can reject the null hypothesis and accept the alternative hypothesis
   - We can now say that cancer patients reported significant improvement in wellbeing scores after undergoing CBT.

Independent t-test can be performed to compare only two groups. If the means across more than two groups have to be compared, an ANOVA test may be run. When any of the assumptions of the student t-test are not met, the nonparametric Mann–Whitney U test may be used.

Statistical Comparison of More than Two Groups

The t-test is used to find the statistical significant differences between two groups. But when more than two populations or samples are meant to be compared, the appropriate statistical test is the ANOVA. It is the parametric equivalent of the Kruskal–Wallis test. ANOVA uses the F distribution.

Analysis of Variance

- ANOVA is a parametric statistical test. It examines two types of variance.
  - Variation between the means of the groups—"mean square between groups" symbolized by MS_B
  - Variation of individual scores within each of the groups—"mean square within groups" symbolized by MS_W

- To avoid rejecting a true null hypothesis, the ANOVA examines two types of variability: variability between the groups and variability within the groups. In this test each group mean is compared to the grand mean of all groups combined. Then each value within a group is compared with the mean value of the group to which it belongs. These estimates of population variation are then compared by dividing the "between" estimate by the "within" estimate. The F ratio calculated by:

$$F = \frac{MS_B \text{ (between group variance)}}{MS_W \text{ (within group variance)}}$$

- The larger the F value, the greater is the difference between the groups as compared to the differences within the groups. The significance of the F value or F ratio is determined by consulting the F-table to ascertain the critical value for F. If the F value is significant, the researcher is certain that there is a significant difference between the means of at least two of the groups. If the difference between the groups is significantly greater than the difference within the groups, the null hypothesis is rejected. In contrast, if the between groups difference is not significantly greater than the within groups variation, the null hypothesis is not rejected.
- If the F value is significant the researcher knows there is a significant difference between the means of at least two of the groups.

Assumptions

- Data are interval or ratio level.
- Independence of case: The sample should be selected randomly. There should not be any pattern in the selection of the sample.
- Normality: Distribution of each group should be normal, i.e. data have been selected from populations that are normally distributed.

- Homogeneity: Homogeneity means variance between the groups should be the same, i.e. have equal variances on the variable being measured.

Various Forms of Analysis of Variance

Various types of ANOVAs are available based on the purpose of the study.

Between-subjects ANOVA: The most commonly used forms of ANOVA is the between-subjects ANOVA. This test is used to find out the differences between independent groups on a continuous level variable. This can be categorized into one-way ANOVAs and factorial ANOVAs.

- A one-way ANOVA is used when three or more groups are being compared based on one factor variable (dependent variable). For example, a study to compare the depressive scores among rural, urban and semiurban patients. In this study there is one dependent variable (depressive scores) and one independent variable (area of residence—rural, urban, and semiurban). Here the depressive scores between rural, urban, and semiurban patients are compared.
- A factorial ANOVA also called *two-way ANOVA* is a general term applied when comparing mean differences between groups that have been split on two independent variables (called factors). A factorial ANOVA can be applied when there are three or more independent variables. This test analyses the effect of two independent variables on the dependent variable. For example, a study to compare the depressive scores among rural, urban and semiurban patients and also male and female. In this study there is only one dependent variable (depressive scores) and two independent variables (area of residence and gender). Here the depressive scores between rural men and women, urban men and women, semiurban men and women are compared.

Within-subjects ANOVA: Also called repeated measures ANOVA, it is used to examine the differences within the group over time. It is commonly used with a pretest and post-test design, with assessment at more than two time periods. For example, a study to compare depressive scores at three time intervals, measured at three time points (pretest, post-test, 3-month follow-up).

Mixed-model ANOVA: Also called *within-between ANOVA*, it is used to examine the differences within and between the groups over time. It is commonly used with quasi-experimental and true experimental designs to find out differences between experimental and control groups over time (pretest and post-test). For example, in a study to evaluate the effectiveness of CBT and holistic intervention among depressive patients at three time intervals, depression is the dependent variable and holistic and CBTs are the independent variables. The between-subjects factor is two different treatments or conditions. For example, treatment 1: CBT and treatment 2: holistic intervention. The researcher wants to find out which of the two different treatments is more effective in reducing depression levels over time.

In the above study example, 60 participants were recruited and randomly assigned to two groups with 30 participants each. While group 1 subjects received CBT, the group 2 subjects received holistic intervention for a period of 8 weeks. Both the group participants were assessed for depression at three time points, i.e. prior to intervention, at the end of the intervention and 1 month after the intervention. Mixed ANOVA test is used to find out the differences between the groups over a period of time which is the result of interaction between the type of treatment (CBT or holistic intervention) and time (within subject factor–three time points).

Analysis of covariance (ANCOVA): It is used to examine the differences between the groups while controlling the confounding variables. The "C" in ANCOVA indicates that a covariate is being introduced into the model, the examination of which can be applied to a between-subjects design, a within-subjects design, or a mixed-model design. ANCOVAs are often used in experimental studies when the researcher wants to control the effects of a pre-existing variable on the outcome variable. In the above study, the additional variables like duration of illness, family history of illness, number of previous depressive episodes, and compliance with antidepressive drugs may affect the levels of depression. These variables can be controlled statistically using ANCOVA test.

Multivariate analysis of variance (MANOVA): It is an extension on the ANOVA, used to examine the differences between the groups when multiple dependent variables are involved. For example, a researcher wants to assess the differences between two groups on reduction in depressive symptoms and drug compliance. In this example, drug compliance and depression are dependent variables. It can also be conducted with multiple independent variables, and also include covariates (i.e. MANCOVA).

One-way Analysis of Variance
The one-way analysis of variance is a parametric test used to compare the means between independent groups. It determines whether the means of three or more groups are significantly different from each other. Being an omnibus statistical test it does not reveal which specific groups are statistically significantly different from each other. This lacuna can be overcome by the post hoc test.

Assumptions
- Dependent variable should be measured at the interval or ratio level (continuous variable). Example, intelligence (measured using IQ score) and weight (measured in kg).
- Three or more categorical or independent groups are available. Example, comparing depressive scores between rural, urban, and semiurban population.
- There should be independence of observations, meaning observations of the sample are independent of each other. It also refers to the subjects being a part of a single group and being measured only once.
- No significant outliers in data, i.e. extremely large or small values that are widely scattered from the rest of the data. Outliers reduce the validity of the one-way ANOVA results.
- The values of the dependent variable should follow normal distribution
- There should be homogeneity of variance among all of the groups.

Step-by-step procedure for computing one-way analysis of variance

The research question "Are the depressive scores different among rural, urban, and semiurban population?" This question can be answered by selecting 15 depressive patients (Rural-5, Urban-5, and Semiurban-5) who are attending outpatient department of a mental hospital and computing a one-way ANOVA for data from three independent groups.

1. State the null and alternative hypothesis
   - H_0: All the groups are similar in depressive scores
   - H_1: Depressive scores differ among rural, semiurban, and urban patients
2. Specify the significance level (α level), calculate degrees of freedom, and determine the critical value for the F-test
   - α level is 0.05
   - The degrees of freedom between groups (df_b) = number of groups–1. In the above example $df_b = 3 - 1 = 2$
   - The degrees of freedom within groups (df_w) = number of participants–number of groups. In the above example $df_w = 15 - 3 = 12$

- The critical value from the F-table for $F_{2,12}$ at p = 0.05 is 3.88 (see Appendix 2)
3. Ensure the data meet all the underlying assumptions
   - Data points are normally distributed—depression scores are normally distributed
   - Dependent variable should be measured on a continuous scale—depressive scores are measured on interval scale
   - Data are collected independent of each other
   - The grouping variable should have at least three levels—area of residence is categorized as rural, urban and semiurban
   - Homogeneity of variances across groups
4. Perform the computations necessary to complete the one-way ANOVA.
   The first step in the computation is to add the scores in each column and find the sum of the squared scores. Then calculate the mean by dividing the sum by the number of scores, and compute the sum of squares (SS).

Rural (n = 5)		Urban (n = 5)		Semiurban (n = 5)		Total (n = 15)	
X	X²	X	X²	X	X²	ΣX	ΣX²
20	400	22	484	12	144	54	1,028
18	324	18	324	14	196	50	844
16	256	19	361	15	225	50	842
15	225	13	169	17	289	45	683
14	196	14	196	19	361	47	753
ΣX = 83	ΣX² = 1,401	ΣX = 86	ΣX² = 1534	ΣX = 77	ΣX² = 1,215	ΣX_t = 246	ΣX_t^2 = 4,150

The required formulae are:

$$F = \frac{MS_b}{MS_w} = \frac{\text{Mean of sum of squares between the group}}{\text{Mean of sum of squares within the groups}}$$

$$MS_b = \frac{SS_b}{k-1} = \frac{\text{Sum of squares between the groups}}{\text{df for between the groups}}$$

$$MS_w = \frac{SS_w}{n-k} = \frac{\text{Sum of squares within the groups}}{\text{df for within the groups}}$$

$$SS_b = \frac{(\Sigma x_1)^2}{n_1} + \frac{(\Sigma x_2)^2}{n_2} + \frac{(\Sigma x_3)^2}{n_3} - \frac{(\Sigma x)^2}{n}$$

$$SS_w = SS_t + SS_b$$

$$SS_t = \Sigma x_t^2 - \frac{(\Sigma x_t)^2}{n}$$

Substituting the values in the above formulae we get:

$$SS_b = \frac{(\Sigma x_1)^2}{n_1} + \frac{(\Sigma x_2)^2}{n_2} + \frac{(\Sigma x_3)^2}{n_3} - \frac{(\Sigma x)^2}{n}$$

$$= \frac{(83)^2}{5} + \frac{(86)^2}{5} + \frac{(77)^2}{5} - \frac{(246)^2}{15}$$

$$= 8.4$$

$$SS_w = SS_t + SS_b$$
$$= 116 - 8.4$$
$$= 107.6$$

$$SS_t = \Sigma x_t^2 - \frac{(\Sigma x_t)^2}{n}$$

$$= 4{,}150 - \frac{(246)^2}{15}$$

$$= 115.602$$

$$MS_b = \frac{SS_b}{k-1} = \frac{8.4}{2} = 4.2$$

$$MS_w = \frac{SS_w}{n-k} = \frac{107.6}{12} = 8.97$$

$$F = \frac{MS_b}{MS_w} = \frac{4.2}{8.97} = 0.47$$

The arrived values can be arranged as under:

Source	Degrees of freedom (df)		Sum of squares	Mean squares	F-ratio
Between Groups	k – 1	3 – 1 = 2	8.40 (SS_b)	4.20 (MS_b)	$F = \frac{MS_b}{MS_w} = 0.47$
Within the Groups	n – k	15 – 3 = 12	107.60 (SS_w)	8.97 (MS_w)	
Total	n – 1	15 – 1 = 14	115.602 (SS_t)		
	k is number of groups, n is total number of subjects				

5. Determine the statistical significance and state a conclusion

The final step is to compare the value of the F computed in this analysis with the critical value of F in the F Table. The critical value can be looked up by using the degrees of freedom. Here df_b is 2 and df_w is 12. The critical value of $F_{(2,12)}$ for an α of 0.05 is 3.88. Since the obtained F value (0.47) is lesser than this value, the null hypothesis is accepted and concluded that there is no significant difference between the groups.

One-way Repeated Measures ANOVA (within Subjects ANOVA or ANOVA for Correlated Samples)

This test is used to compare the means of three or more measures of variables taken from the same set of subjects. In this test the same set of subjects are measured at different points in time. For example, in a study to evaluate the effectiveness of cognitive therapy on depressive patients, the same set of depressive patients are measured at three different time points, viz. pretest, at 3 months and 6 months. This study utilizes one group pretest-post-test design. To find out the effectiveness of therapy from pretest to at 6 months, one-way repeated measures ANOVA is used.

Assumptions
1. Dependent variable should be measured at the interval or ratio level (continuous variable)
2. Sample are selected randomly
3. Values of the dependent variable are normally distributed

4. There should be homogeneity of variance between each measure of the characteristics
5. Same participants are repeatedly measured three or more times

Step-by-step procedure for computing repeated measures ANOVA

The researcher wants to investigate the effect of a CBT on depression and wants to measure depressive scores at three different time points (pre, 3 months, and 6 months).

1. State the null and alternative hypothesis
   - H_0: Mean depressive scores are the same at all the time points.
   - H_1: The mean depressive scores are not equal (at least one mean is different compared to another mean).
2. Specify the significance level (α level), calculate the degrees of freedom, and determine the critical value for the F-Test
   - Alpha level is 0.05
   - The degrees of freedom for time (df_t) = Number of time points − 1. In the above example $df_t = 3 - 1 = 2$
   - The degrees of freedom for error (df_e) = (n − 1)(k − 1)

   Where, n = Number of subjects, k = Number of time intervals. In the above example $df_e = (5 - 1)(3 - 1) = 4 \times 2 = 8$.
   - The critical value from the F-table for $F_{2,8}$ at p = 0.05 is 4.46 (see Appendix 2)
3. Ensure the data meet all the underlying assumptions
   - The measures constitute an independent random sample—in the above example, samples are selected randomly
   - There are at least three measures of the dependent variable—depression scores are measured at three different time points (pre, 3 months, and 6 months)
   - All the measures of dependent variable are collected from the same subjects—depression level is assessed on the same subjects at three time points
   - The dependent variable is normally distributed—depressive scores
   - The measurement scale of the dependent variable is interval or ratio level—depression is measured using interval level scale
4. Perform the computations necessary to complete the repeated measures ANOVA.

To calculate repeated measures ANOVA, consider the research study where 5 depressive patients have undergone CBT. The depressive scores are measured on three occasions: pre, 3 months, and 6 months. The depressive scores of 5 subjects given below:

Subjects	Cognitive behavior therapy			Total
	Depressive scores (x)			
	Pretest (x_1)	3 months (x_2)	6 months (x_3)	
1	20	19	12	17
2	18	16	10	14.67
3	16	14	12	14
4	15	15	12	14
5	14	13	10	12.33
Σx	83	77	56	216
$\Sigma x/n$	16.6	15.4	11.2	14.4 (Grand Mean)

One-way repeated measures ANOVA is used to find significant differences between three time points by using the following formula.

$$F = \frac{MS_{time}}{MS_{error}}$$

$MS_{time} = \dfrac{SS_{time}}{(k-1)}$	$MS_{error} = \dfrac{SS_{error}}{(n-1)(k-1)}$
$SS_{time} = SS_b$ $= n\,[(x_1-\bar{x})^2 + (x_2-\bar{x})^2 + (x_3-\bar{x})^2]$	$SS_w = SS_{subjects} + SS_{error}$ $SS_w = \sum_1 (x_{i1}-\bar{x}_1)^2 + \sum_2 (x_{i2}-\bar{x}_2)^2 + ... + \sum_k (x_{ik}-\bar{x}_k)^2$
$SS_{subjects} = k\sum (x_1-\bar{x})^2$	$SS_{error} = SS_w - SS_{subjects}$

Calculating SS_{time}

$$SS_{time} = SS_b \sum_{t=1}^{k} n_i (\bar{x}_t - \bar{x})^2$$

Where k = number of time intervals, n_i = number of subjects under each (ith) condition, $\bar{x}_i$ = mean score for each (ith) condition, $\bar{x}$ = grand mean. Substituting the values in the above formula for the example, we get:

$SS_{time} = SS_b$
$= n\,[(x_1-\bar{x})^2 + (x_2-\bar{x})^2 + (x_3-\bar{x})^2]$
$= 5\,[(16.6 - 14.4)^2 + (15.4 - 14.4)^2 + (11.2 - 14.4)^2]$
$= 5(4.84 + 1 + 10.24) = 80.4$

Calculating SS_w
Within-groups variation (SS_w) is also calculated in the same way as in an independent ANOVA, expressed as follows:

$$SS_w = \sum_1 (x_{i1}-\bar{x}_1)^2 + \sum_2 (x_{i2}-\bar{x}_2)^2 + ... + \sum_k (x_{ik}-\bar{x}_k)^2$$

Where, x_{i1} is the score of the ith subject in group 1, x_{i2} is the score of the ith subject in group 2, and x_{ik} is the score of the ith subject in group k.

Substituting the values in the above formula we get:

$SS_w = \Sigma(x_{i1}-\bar{x}_1)^2 + \Sigma(x_{i2}-\bar{x}_2)^2 + \Sigma(x_{i3}-\bar{x}_3)^2$
$= [(x_{11}-\bar{x}_1)^2 + (x_{21}-\bar{x}_1)^2 + (x_{31}-\bar{x}_1)^2] +$
$\quad [(x_{12}-\bar{x}_2)^2 + (x_{22}-\bar{x}_2)^2 + (x_{32}-\bar{x}_2)^2] +$
$\quad [(x_{13}-\bar{x}_3)^2 + (x_{23}-\bar{x}_3)^2 + (x_{33}-\bar{x}_3)^2]$
$= [(20 - 16.6)^2 + (18 - 16.6)^2 + (16 - 16.6)^2 +$
$\quad (15 - 16.6)^2 + (14 - 16.6)^2] + [(19 - 15.4)^2$
$\quad + (16 - 15.4)^2 + (14 - 15.4)^2 + (15 - 15.4)^2$
$\quad + (13 - 15.4)^2] + [(12 - 11.2)^2 + (10 - 11.2)^2$
$\quad + (12 - 11.2)^2 + (12 - 11.2)^2 + (10 - 11.2)^2]$
$= 49.2$

Calculating $SS_{subjects}$
Each subject is treated as its own block, i.e. each subject is treated as a level of an independent factor called subjects. $SS_{subjects}$ can be calculated as follows:

$$SS_{subjects} = k\sum (\bar{x}_i - \bar{x})^2$$

Where, k = number of conditions, $\bar{x}_i$ mean of i subjects, and $\bar{x}$ = grand mean.

Substituting the values in the above formula we get:

$SS_{subjects} = k\,[(\bar{x}_1 - \bar{x})^2 + (\bar{x}_2 - \bar{x})^2 + (\bar{x}_3 - \bar{x})^2]$
$= 3\,[(17 - 14.4)^2 + (14.67 - 14.4)^2 + (14 - 14.4)^2 + (14 - 14.4)^2 + (12.33 - 14.4)^2]$
$= 34.27$

Calculating SS_{error}
We know, $SS_w = SS_{subjects} + SS_{error}$
Thus, $SS_{error} = SS_w - SS_{subjects}$
$= 49.2 - 34.27$
$= 14.93$

Calculating MS_{time} and MS_{error}

$$MS_{time} = \frac{SS_{time}}{(k-1)} = \frac{80.4}{2} = 40.2$$

$$MS_{error} = \frac{SS_{error}}{(n-1)(k-1)}$$
$$= \frac{14.93}{(5-1)(3-1)} = \frac{14.93}{8} = 1.87$$

Where, n = number of subjects, k = number of time intervals, (n – 1) and (k – 1) are degrees of freedom.

Therefore, we can calculate the *F*-statistic as:

$$F = \frac{MS_{time}}{MS_{error}} = \frac{40.2}{1.87} = 21.5$$

5. Determine the statistical significance and state a conclusion.

The final step is to compare the calculated *F*-value with the critical *F*-value in the *F*-table. The critical value can be looked up using the degrees of freedom for time (df_{time}) and error (df_{error}) and decide whether the F-statistic indicates a statistically significant result.

The *F*-statistic for repeated measures ANOVA can be reported as:

$F(df_{time}, df_{error}) = F$-value, $p = p$-value

In the above example it would be: $F(2, 8) = 21.5$

Calculated $F = 21.5$, the critical value from the *F*-table for $F_{2,8}$ at p = 0.05 is 4.46 (see Appendix 2). The calculated value is higher than the table which means the null hypothesis can be rejected and the alternative hypothesis accepted. The 6 month CBT had a statistically significant effect on depressive levels.

NONPARAMETRIC TESTS USED IN NURSING

Chi-Square Test

It is a nonparametric test used to compare nominal or ordinal data. It is a popular discrete data hypothesis testing method used to compare observed data with expected data from a specific hypothesis. The hypotheses are tested for proportion of cases that fall into different categories as and when a contingency table has been created.

Chi-square test is used under following conditions:
* When data are measured on nominal or ordinal scale
* To perform a parametric test, groups should be of equal or approximately equal size. However, chi-square test can be performed even if the groups are of unequal size.

The chi-square test is conducted at both univariate and bivariate levels. At univariate level chi-square test can be used as a test of goodness of fit while at bivariate level the chi-square test can be used as a test of independence.

Test of goodness of fit

It is a single sample nonparametric test also known as the one sample goodness of fit test or Pearson's chi-square goodness-of-fit test. This test is applied when researcher has one categorical variable from a single population. It is used to determine whether observed sample frequencies differ significantly from expected frequencies specified in the null hypothesis.

Assumptions
* Sample must be selected randomly
* Variable must be measured on ordinal or nominal level (categorical data)
* The expected number of observations in each cell should atleast be 5

Example: A researcher wants to compare the sample parameters (age distribution of women in a specific district of the state of Karnataka) with population parameters (age distribution of all women in the state of Karnataka). The hypotheses are as follows:
* H_0: The age distribution of sample is same as the age distribution of State Census.
* H_1: The age distribution of sample differs from the age distribution of State Census.

Chi-Square Test of Independence

It is the most commonly used test, also called the chi-square test for contingency tables. It determines whether there is a significant association/relationship between two categorical variables. In this, the data are displayed in a contingency table with rows and columns, each row representing a category for one variable and each column representing a category for another variable. This test compares observed frequency (collected data) with the expected frequency (calculated frequency).

Assumptions
- The study participants form an independent random sample
- The level of measurement of all the variables is nominal or ordinal. Nominal variables include religion (Hindu, Muslim, and Christian), health profession (doctor, nurses, and paramedicals), etc. Ordinal variables include variables measured on Likert scale (strongly agree, agree, and strongly disagree)
- The data should be frequencies or counts rather than percentages
- Observations of the sample are independent of each other
- The groups of categorical variable must be mutually exclusive, i.e. each subject fits into only one group and each subject contributes data to only one cell
- In 2 × 2 table, each cell has at least 10 expected frequencies in each cell.

Step-by-step computation of chi-square statistic for a 2 × 2 table

A researcher wants to compare drug compliance among male and female psychiatric patients.

Below contingency table shows drug compliance among male and female patients.

Gender	Drug compliance		Total
	Yes	No	
Males	64	36	100
Females	78	22	100
Total	142	58	200

Step 1: State the null and alternative hypotheses
- H_0: There is no difference in drug compliance among male and female patients.
- H_1: There is difference in drug compliance among male and female patients.

Step 2: Ensure the data meet all the underlying assumptions
- Samples are selected randomly
- There are a minimum two measures to compare—drug compliance among males and females
- The two measures are independent of each other
- Both the measures are nominal—gender and drug compliance
- The expected cell sizes are adequate

Step 3: Specify the significance level (α level), calculate degrees of freedom, and seek the critical value for the chi-square statistic.

The degrees of freedom are (row – 1) × (column – 1), i.e. (2 – 1) × (2 – 1)=1. The critical value from the chi-square table at degrees of freedom equal to 1 and an $\alpha = .05$ is 3.84 (see Appendix 3).

Step 4: Perform the computations necessary to obtain the chi-square statistic.
- Make contingency tables

Gender	Drug compliance		Total
	Yes	No	
Males	64 (Cell 1)	36 (Cell 2)	100
Females	78 (Cell 3)	22 (Cell 4)	100
Total	142	58	200

- Determine the expected number (E) in each cell of table based on assumption of null hypothesis

$$E = \frac{\text{Column (vertical) total} \times \text{Row (horizontal) total}}{\text{Sample total}}$$

Expected values/frequencies (E)	Observed frequencies (O)	Observed frequencies – Expected frequencies (O – E)
E_1 (cell 1) = $\dfrac{142 \times 100}{200}$ = 71	O_1 (cell 1) = 64	$O_1 - E_1 = 64 - 71 = -7$
E_1 (cell 2) = $\dfrac{58 \times 100}{200}$ = 29	O_2 (cell 2) = 36	$O_2 - E_2 = 36 - 29 = 7$
E_1 (cell 3) = $\dfrac{142 \times 100}{200}$ = 71	O_3 (cell 3) = 78	$O_3 - E_3 = 78 - 71 = 7$
E_1 (cell 4) = $\dfrac{58 \times 100}{200}$ = 29	O_4 (cell 4) = 22	$O_4 - E_4 = 22 - 29 = -7$

○ Calculate the χ^2 value for each cell by the formula:

$$\chi^2 = \sum \frac{(O-E)^2}{E}$$

$$\chi_1^2 = \frac{(O_1 - E_1)^2}{E_1} = \frac{(-7)^2}{71} = \frac{49}{7} = 0.69$$

$$\chi_2^2 = \frac{(O_2 - E_2)^2}{E_2} = \frac{(7)^2}{29} = \frac{40}{29} = 1.69$$

$$\chi_3^2 = \frac{(O_3 - E_3)^2}{E_3} = \frac{(7)^2}{71} = \frac{49}{71} = 0.69$$

$$\chi_4^2 = \frac{(O_4 - E_4)^2}{E_4} = \frac{(-7)^2}{29} = \frac{49}{29} = 1.69$$

○ Sum up the χ^2 values of all the cells to get the total χ^2 value: 0.69 + 1.69 + 0.69 + 1.69 = 4.76.

Step 5: Determine the statistical significance and state a conclusion
  ○ Calculate the degrees of freedom (df): (c – 1)(r – 1) = (2 – 1)(2 – 1) = 1
  ○ Chi-square table value at 1 df under probability 0.05 is 3.84. The calculated chi-square value of 4.76 is greater than the table value (4.76 > 3.84) at 0.05 level of significance. Hence the null hypothesis is rejected and inferred that there is a significant difference in drug compliance among male and female patients.

The chi-square test only expresses whether a relationship exists or not and does not provide any information on strength of the relationship. To find out the strength of the relationship phi, Cramer's V or contingency coefficient can be used.

Yates Correction

Chi-square test can be performed only when all the cells have expected values above 10, failing which bias is introduced into the calculation. To overcome this, Yates correction can be performed. It adjusts the observed frequency in each cell of the 2 × 2 table in a way that reduces the deviation of the observed from the expected frequency for that cell by 0.5. However, this adjustment is made in all the cells without disturbing the marginal totals.

Criteria for Yates correction
❖ Both variables are dichotomous
❖ One or more of the cells has expected value of less than 5

Yates correction formula

$$\chi^2 = \frac{\Sigma(|O-E| - 0.5)^2}{E}$$

Fisher Exact Test

The Fisher exact test is a test of significance which is used to test whether the proportions of one variable are different among the values of the other variable. These variables are nominal variables. It is usually used in the place of chi-square test in 2 × 2 tables, especially in cases of small samples, when one of the expected values in a 2 × 2 table is less than 5.

Assumptions
- The study participants form an independent random sample
- The level of measurement of all the variables is nominal
- The variables are dichotomous (yes/no, cured/not cured)
- The groups of categorical variable must be mutually exclusive, i.e. each subject fits into only one level of each of the variables.

Computation of Fisher exact test

A researcher wants to compare diarrheal infections among breast fed and bottle fed infants. The below contingency table shows the distribution of diarrheal infections among infants.

Diarrheal infection	Infants		Total
	Breast fed	Bottle fed	
Yes	1 (a)	10 (b)	11 (a + b)
No	14 (c)	5 (d)	19 (c + d)
Total	15 (a + c)	15 (b + d)	30 (a+b+c+d)

The Fisher exact test uses the following formula:

$p = [(a+b)!(c+d)!(a+c)!(b+d)!]/a!b!c!d!N!$

In this formula, the "a," "b," "c", and "d" are the individual frequencies of the 2 × 2 contingency table, and "N" is the total frequency. The symbol ! indicates the factorial operator.

[Factorial symbolized by exclamation mark (!) is the product of all whole numbers from 1 to n, i.e. n! = 1 × 2 × 3 ×.....× n. For example, 5! = 1 × 2 × 3 × 4 × 5 = 120. *Note:* 0! = 1]

$$p = \frac{(1+10)!\,(14+5)!\,(1+14)!\,(10+14)!}{1!\,10!\,14!\,5!\,30!}$$

$$= \frac{11!\,19!\,15!\,24!}{1!\,10!\,14!\,5!\,30!} = 0.000824$$

The two-tailed p-value equals 0.0017.

The association between groups (rows) and outcomes (columns) is statistically significant, i.e. there is an association between type of feeding and occurrence of diarrheal infection.

McNemar Test

It is a nonparametric test used for paired nominal data. The variables can be paired either by performing repeated measures over time on the same subjects (compare before and after) or measures are taken on a case and matched control (twin studies).

Example: To compare the drug compliance status among diabetic patients before and after health education.

Assumptions
- Paired or matched data—before and after drug compliance
- There should be two variables for comparison—poor and good drug compliance
- There are sufficient observations in each cell

Step-by-step computation of McNemar test

To run a McNemar test, data must be placed into a 2 × 2 contingency table. For example, the researcher wants to compare drug compliance among diabetic patients before and after health education. A contingency table was prepared with the counts of individuals' good and poor drug compliance before and after being given the health education. The cells are labeled (a) to (d).

Before health education / Drug compliance		After health education		Total
		Good	Poor	
	Good	21 (a)	9 (b)	30
	Poor	23 (c)	151 (d)	174
	Total	44	160	204

Step 1: State the null and alternative hypotheses
- H_0: There is no difference in drug compliance before and after attending health education among diabetic patients.
- H_1: There is difference in drug compliance before and after attending health education program among diabetic patients.

Step 2: Ensure the data meet all the underlying assumptions
- The expected cell sizes are sufficient
- The variables represent paired data (i.e. same variable is measured multiple times, drug compliance is measured twice before and after health education)

Step 3: Specify the significance level (α level), calculate the degrees of freedom, and seek the critical value for the chi-square statistic.
- The degrees of freedom are $(2-1) \times (2-1)=1$. The critical value from the chi-square table at degrees of freedom equal to 1 and an $\alpha = 0.05$ is 3.84 (see Appendix 3).

Step 4: Perform the McNemar statistic.

$$\chi^2 = \frac{(b-c)^2}{b+c}$$

$$= \frac{(9-23)^2}{9+23} = \frac{(-14)^2}{32} = 6.125$$

Step 5: Determine the statistical significance and state a conclusion
- Calculate the degrees of freedom (df): $(c-1)(r-1) = (2-1)(2-1) = 1$
- Chi-square table value at 1 df under probability 0.05 is 3.84. The calculated McNemar value of 6.125 is greater than the table value $(6.125 > 3.84)$ at 0.05 level of significance. Hence, the null hypothesis is rejected and inferred that there is a significant difference in drug compliance after attending health education program among diabetic patients.

Sign Test

It is a nonparametric test used to compare the sizes of two groups. It is based on the direction of the plus and minus signs of the observation and not on their numerical magnitude. The sign test is considered the weakest test because it tests the pair value below or above the median and does not measure the pair differences. It aims to test whether the observed data is significantly different from a specific value.

Assumptions

This test does not make any assumptions about the shape of the population distribution.

Types of Sign test

Two types of sign test can be explained as follows:

1. *One sample sign test*: This test compares the median of a data set with a specific target value.
   Example: In a college the teacher states that their median class size is not greater than 25. However, the students believe that the median is greater than 25. Below given data represents randomly selected 15 class sizes in the college. Fixing 10% level of significance, what conclusions can be drawn?
   Data: {32 19 26 25 28 21 29 22 27 28 26 23 26 28 29}

In performing the sign test, each data value, t_i is compared with the target value m_0 ($m_0 = 25$), using the following conditions:

- $t_i < m_0$ replace the data value with '−'
- $t_i = m_0$ exclude the data value
- $t_i > m_0$ replace the data value with '+'

Sign test for the sample

Step 1: State the null and alternative hypothesis.
H_0: Median = 25
H_1: Median is greater than 25 (significance level—about 10%).

Step 2: Perform the sign test and attribute either a (±) sign to every observation depending on whether it is less than or greater than the specific value (m_0). Ignore the values that are equal to the specific value.

Step 3: We find N^+ = The number of observations > specific value = 10
N^- = The number of observations < specific value = 4
S = The smaller among N^+ and N^- = 4

Step 4: Determine the appropriate p-value
$P(\geq 10) = 0.089783$ (using binomial distribution table)
If the probability value is greater than the significance level, the null hypothesis is accepted. Reject the null hypothesis at the 0.089873 significance level. Thus median is greater than 25.

2. *Paired sample sign test*: This test compares the medians of two paired samples. The dependent samples should be paired or matched samples. In this test the difference between the two paired samples is arrived and the sign of the difference recorded.

No.	Class size	$t_i - m_0$	Difference
1	32	+7	+
2	19	−6	−
3	26	+1	+
4	25	0	---
5	28	+3	+
6	21	−4	−
7	29	+4	+
8	22	−3	−
9	27	+2	+
10	28	+3	+
11	26	+1	+
12	23	−2	−
13	26	+1	+
14	28	+3	+
15	29	+4	+

Mean = 25.93
Median (m_0) = 26

Distribution of data	
Data (N)	Frequency
$N^+ < 25$	10
$N = 25$	1
$N^- > 25$	4
	15

Zeroes are ignored, while the number of + and − signs are compared. If the number of + and − signs are approximately the same, the null hypothesis is accepted. However, a significant difference between the signs indicates rejection of null hypothesis.

Mann–Whitney U Test (Wilcoxon Rank-sum Test)

Mann–Whitney U test is a nonparametric test used to compare the difference between two independent groups when the dependent variable is measured on ordinal scale and the assumptions for the independent t-test are not met (example, small sample sizes, non-normally distributed data, and ordinal data). Independent t-test and the Mann–Whitney U test are used to compare averages between two independent groups with sample data. Though these two tests perform similar functions, they are used under different conditions.

Assumptions
1. Samples are selected randomly
2. Observations in the sample are independent of each other
3. Ordinal measurement scale is assumed

Example: A study designed to investigate the effectiveness of hot and cold compression in reducing pain symptoms among patients with fracture. Ten patients are randomly assigned to 2 groups of 5 patients each. One group received hot compression while the other group received a cold compression. Pain scores for both the groups were recorded after the treatment as below:

Pain scores	
Group A (cold compression) $n_1 = 5$	Group B (hot compression) $n_2 = 5$
7	3
5	6
6	4
4	2
12	1

From the above table it is clear that the participants receiving cold compression are experiencing greater pain but whether it is statistically significant? Here, the sample data do not follow a normal distribution, pain was assessed by ordinal scale and the sample size is small ($n_1 = n_2 = 5$). Thus a nonparametric test is appropriate.

If the null hypothesis is true (i.e. the two populations are equal) then participants in both groups will experience similar levels of pain. If alternate hypothesis is true then some participants would report less pain while others would report more pain in each group. To test the above hypothesis Mann–Whitney U test can be performed.

Steps for computing Mann–Whitney U test
1. State the null and alternative hypotheses
   - H_0: There will be no difference in severity of pain between participants in hot and cold compression groups.
   - H_1: Participants who received hot compression will have less pain when compared to those who received cold compression.
2. Specify the α level, calculate the degrees of freedom and determine critical value for the computed Mann–Whitney U-statistic
   - If a specified α level is not mentioned, one can use 5% (0.05)
   - There are 5 subjects in hot compression group and 5 subjects in cold compression group. The critical value can be obtained by looking at the intersection of $n_1 = 5$ and $n_2 = 5$ for 0.05 (two-tailed test). In this case the critical value is 2 (see Appendix 5)
   - To prove that the two groups are significantly different from one another the computed value of U-statistic must be smaller than the critical value. In the above example, an α-level of $p \leq 0.05$ and a two-sided test are used.
3. Ensure the data meet all the underlying assumptions

- The measurements constitute an independent random sample
- Severity of pain was assessed by ordinal scale

4. Compute the Mann-Whitney U-test statistic

To perform this test for the above data the combined or total sample (n = 10) data are arranged from smallest to largest and ranks assigned from 1 to 10.

Group	No. of episodes	Position (smallest to largest)	Rank of score
B	1	1	1
B	2	2	2
B	3	3	3
B	4	4	4.5 (tied for ranks 4 and 5)
A	4	5	4.5 (tied for ranks 4 and 5)
A	5	6	6
B	6	7	7.5 (tied for ranks 7 and 8)
A	6	8	7.5 (tied for ranks 7 and 8)
A	7	9	9
A	12	10	10

Note: When the ranks are computed, the tied scores are averaged.

- In the above table lesser ranks (e.g. 1, 2, and 3) are assigned to hot compression group while the higher ranks (e.g. 9, 10) are assigned to responses in the cold compression group.
- The sum of the ranks in Group A (cold compression group) is 37 (Ranks: 4.5 + 6 + 7.5 + 9 + 10 = 37) denoted by R_1.
- The sum of the ranks in Group B (hot compression group) is 18 (Ranks: 1 + 2 + 3 + 4.5 + 7.5 = 18) denoted by R_2.
- The sum of the ranks is equal to 55 in accordance with the formula $n(n+1)/2 = 10(11)/2 = 55$ which is equal to $37 + 18 = 55$.
- If the null hypothesis is accepted R_1 and R_2 should be similar. In the above example, lesser ranks are bunched together in the hot compression group, while the higher ranks are bunched together in the cold compression group.
- To confirm if the observed differences in R_1 and R_2 is merely due to chance, a test statistic has to be computed.
- The test statistic for the Mann–Whitney U test is denoted by "U" and is the smaller of U_1 and U_2.

$$U_1 = n_1 n_2 + \frac{n_1(n_1+1)}{2} - R_1$$

$$U_2 = n_1 n_2 + \frac{n_2(n_2+1)}{2} - R_2$$

Where, R_1 = sum of the ranks for group A and R_2 = sum of the ranks for group B.
In this example,

$$U_1 = 5(5) + \frac{5(6)}{2} - 37 = 3$$

$$U_2 = 5(5) + \frac{5(6)}{2} - 18 = 22$$

Deciding on the smallest U value can be confirmed by using the formula $U_1 = (n_1 \times n_2) - U_2 = (5 \times 5) - 22 = 3$. Thus, $U = 3$.

For any Mann–Whitney U test, the value of U ranges from 0 (H_0 most likely false and H_1 most likely true) to $n_1 \times n_2$ (little evidence in support of H_1). In every test, $U_1 + U_2 = n_1 \times n_2$. In the above example, U ranges from 0 to 25 and smaller values of U support the research hypothesis (H_0 is rejected, if U is small).

5. Determine the statistical significance and state a conclusion.

- Compare the calculated U with the critical U values to determine whether to accept or reject the null hypothesis
- If calculated U-value is larger than the critical U-value then accept H_0
- If calculated U-value is smaller than the critical U-value then reject H_0
- When the number of participants in both the groups is less than 20 (one or both groups with n < 20), the calculated value is compared with the critical value in the Mann–Whitney U-table
- When the number of participants is more than 20 (one or both groups with n > 20), the "U" value approaches a normal distribution. Thus the null hypothesis can be tested by a z-test and the z-score table is used
- In the above example the calculated/computed value U = 3 is compared with critical/table value of U, i.e. 2. The calculated value is higher than the critical value. Hence, the null hypothesis is accepted and concluded that pain scores are equal for hot and cold compression group subjects.

However, in the above example, the failure to obtain statistical significance may be due to low power, i.e. the sample sizes are too small.

Wilcoxon Signed-rank Test

It is a nonparametric test used to compare the difference between two dependent groups. In this test same participants are repeatedly measured, i.e. when changes are monitored from one time point to another. This test is the nonparametric equivalent to the paired t-test. It is used when assumptions have been violated and the use of the dependent t-test is inappropriate.

Assumptions
- Dependent variable should be measured at the ordinal or continuous level.
- Independent variable should consist of two categorical, related groups (same subjects are presented in both groups) or matched pairs.
- The distribution of the differences between the two related groups needs to be symmetrical in shape.

Example: A study is conducted to evaluate the effectiveness of yoga therapy in reducing blood sugar levels among prediabetic patients. 15 prediabetic patients participated in this study, whose blood sugar levels were measured. Each patient participated in yoga therapy 5 days a week for 4 weeks. After 4 weeks, blood sugar levels were measured again. The researcher uses the Wilcoxon signed-rank test to understand whether the participant's blood sugar level reduced after they underwent the yoga therapy. The data are as shown below:

Participants	Before	After
1	125	118
2	132	134
3	138	130
4	120	124
5	125	105
6	127	130
7	136	130
8	139	132
9	131	123
10	132	128
11	135	126
12	136	140
13	128	135
14	127	127
15	130	132

Step-by-step calculation of Wilcoxon signed-rank test

1. State the null and alternative hypothesis:
   - H_0: There will be no difference in blood sugar levels after participating in yoga therapy as compared to before.

- H_1: There will be significant difference in blood sugar levels after participating in yoga therapy as compared to before.
2. Specify the α level, calculate the degrees of freedom and determine critical value.
   The test statistic for the Wilcoxon signed-rank test is W, defined as the smaller of W^+ and W^- which are the sums of the positive and negative ranks, respectively.
   The critical value for this two-sided test with n = 15 and α = 0.05 is 25 and the decision rule is as follows: reject H_0 if W ≤ 25.
3. Ensure the data meet all the underlying assumptions.
   The dependent variable, i.e. blood sugar level is measured on a continuous scale. Same sample are measured both before and after the yoga therapy.
4. Compute the Wilcoxon signed-rank test:
   To perform the Wilcoxon signed-rank test the above data is arranged as per the following table.

- For each item in the sample obtain a difference score D between the two measurements (before and after)
- Neglect the "+" and "−" signs and obtain the set of absolute differences
- Absolute difference score of zero may be omitted from further analysis thus yielding a set of non-zero absolute difference scores, which becomes the actual sample size.
- Assign ranks 1–15 to each of the differences (D) such that the smallest absolute difference score gets rank 1 and the largest gets rank 15. In the process mean rank is assigned when there are ties (D's are equal) in the absolute values of the difference scores.
- The signs ("+" or "−") of the observed differences are then attached to each rank depending on whether D was originally positive or negative
- Add together the ranks belonging to scores with a positive sign.
  $W^+ = 5 + 7 + 9 + 9 + 11.5 + 11.5 + 13 + 14 = 80$

Participants	Before yoga therapy	After yoga therapy	Difference (D) (before-after)	Ordered absolute values of differences	Ranks	Signed ranks
1	125	118	7	0	omit	omit
2	132	134	−2	−2	1.5	−1.5
3	138	130	8	−2	1.5	−1.5
4	120	124	−4	−3	3	−3
5	125	105	20	−4	5	−5
6	127	130	−3	−4	5	−5
7	136	130	6	4	5	+5
8	139	132	7	6	7	+7
9	131	123	8	−7	9	−9
10	132	128	4	7	9	+9
11	135	126	9	7	9	+9
12	136	140	−4	8	11.5	+11.5
13	128	135	−7	8	11.5	+11.5
14	127	127	0	9	13	+13
15	130	132	−2	20	14	+14

- Add together the ranks belonging to scores with a negative sign.
  W⁻ = 1.5 + 1.5 + 3 + 5 + 5 + 9 = 25
- Whichever of these sums is the smaller, is the value of W. Hence W = 25
- The sum of the ranks (ignoring the signs) can be calculated using the formula $n(n+1)/2$ where n is the total number of participants. Here, $n(n+1)/2 = 14(15)/2 = 105$ which is equal to $80 + 25$. The test statistic W = 25.
- N is the number of differences (omitting "0" differences). In the above example the differences = 15 – 1 = 14.
  Note: This is not the same as degrees of freedom. Here, N – 1 is used because there is only 1 difference which is equal to zero.

5. Determine the statistical significance and state a conclusion.
   With the Wilcoxon test, an obtained W is significant if it is less than or equal to the critical value. In the present study the calculated test statistic is 25, while the table value is 21 (using the table of critical Wilcoxon values for a two-tailed test at the 0.05 significance level with an N of 14) (see Appendix 6).
   The observed value is greater than the table value, i.e. 25>21. It can thus be concluded that there is no significant difference in blood sugar levels after the yoga therapy as compared to before.

Friedman Test

It is a nonparametric test used to compare the differences between more than two dependent groups when the dependent variable is measured on an ordinal scale. It is the nonparametric equivalent of one-way repeated measures ANOVA and used when assumptions have been violated for one-way repeated measures ANOVA (data is not normally distributed).

Assumptions:
- One group is measured on three or more different occasions

- Subjects are randomly selected from the population
- Dependent variable should be measured at the ordinal or continuous level
- Sample do not need to be normally distributed

Example: A study to evaluate the effect of music on the perceived psychological effort required to perform aerobic exercises. Here the dependent variable is "perceived effort to perform the aerobic exercises" and the independent variable is "type of music", which is categorized into three groups: "no music", "traditional music" and "pop music". To test whether music has an effect on the perceived psychological effort required to perform the said aerobic exercises, the researcher recruited 15 members who each performed the task three times for a similar time period. The difficulty level of the aerobic exercises was maintained the same on all the three occasions. Each subject performed the aerobic exercises in a random order: (a) without music; (b) listening to traditional music; and (c) listening to pop music. At the end of each task, subjects were asked to record how hard the exercises felt on a scale of 1–10, with 1 being very easy and 10 extremely hard. A Friedman test was carried out to record the differences in perceived effort based on music type.

Kruskal-Wallis H Test

The Kruskal–Wallis H also called the "H-test", is used to compare the differences between more than two independent groups when the dependent variable is measured on an ordinal scale. It is the nonparametric equivalent of one-way ANOVA and used when assumptions have been violated for one-way ANOVA test (data is not normally distributed). This test uses ranks instead of actual data and compares medians of two or more groups. The hypothesis for this test is as follows:

❖ H_0: Sample medians are equal in all groups.
❖ H_1: Sample medians are not equal in all groups.

Assumptions
❖ Dependent variable is measured on an ordinal scale or at continuous level
❖ Three or more categorical or independent groups are available
❖ There should be independence of observations

Example: A researcher wants to identify whether there is any difference between levels of attitude towards the job based on their job position. Here, the dependent variable is attitude that is measured on a 5-point scale (from "strongly agree" to "strongly disagree") and independent variable job position which has three independent groups: top level managers, middle level managers and operational level employees. In this example, attitudes are measured on an ordinal scale.

BIBLIOGRAPHY

1. Brown, S.J. (2014). *Evidence-based nursing: The research practice connection* (3rd ed.). Sudhbury, MA: Jones & Barlett.
2. Burns, N., & Grove, S.K. (2005). *The practice of nursing research*: Conduct, critique and utilization (5th ed.). St. Louis, MO: Elsevier Saunders.
3. Burns, N., & Grove, S.K. (2001). *The Practice of Nursing Research*: conduct, critique & utilization (4th ed.). Philadelphia: WB Saunders.
4. Craig, J.V. & Smyth, R.L. (2012). *The evidence based practice manual for nurses* (3rd ed.). Edinbergh UK: Churchill Livingstons.
5. Freund, J.E. (2001). *Modern elementary statistics*. Prentice-Hall, 2001.
6. Polit, D.F., & Beck, C.T. (2010). *Essentials of Nursing Research*: Appraising Evidence for Nursing Practice. Philadelphia, PA: Lippincott Williams & Wilkins.
7. Polit, D.F., & Beck, C.T. (2012). *Nursing research*: Generating and assessing evidence for nursing practice (9th ed.). Philadelphia: Lippincott Williams & Wilkins.
8. Plichta, B.S., & Garzan, S.L. (2009). *Statistics for nursing and allied health*. Philadelphia, PA: Lippincott Williams & Wilkins.
9. Sharma, K. S. (2014). Nursing research and Statistics, (2nd ed.). Chennai:RR Donnelley Publishing India pvt. Ltd.
10. Stevens, S.S. (1946). "On the Theory of Scales of Measurement". *Science* 103 (2684): 677–680. doi:10.1126/science.103.2684.677. PMID 17750512.

REVIEW QUESTIONS

I. Long Essays

1. a. Define α-error and β-error.
   b. What are the underlying assumptions of student's t-test? If these assumptions fail which alternate test do you suggest?
   c. The pulse rate of six patients is measured before and after administering a drug. State a suitable hypothesis test to find out whether the drug has any effect on pulse rate using Wilcoxon signed-rank sum test.

Before	72	76	68	67	73	74
After	74	72	66	68	70	71

2. Distinguish between parametric and nonparametric tests.

   A researcher in her pilot study wishes to assess whether there is any significant association between the knowledge and attitude towards family planning acceptance by 10 eligible couples. By stating appropriate hypothesis compute spearman's rank correlation coefficient to assess the association between knowledge and attitude towards family planning acceptance by eligible couples. Explain with interpretation.

Knowledge	Attitude
18	64
1	21
24	85
16	49
14	55
17	69
39	98
3	20
15	88
2	39

3. Explain the procedure of testing one way analysis of variances (one way ANOVA)
4. What is chi-square test? What are the underlying assumptions of chi-square test? If these assumptions are violated, what are the correction measures?
   Using the following tabulated data find whether there is any association between gender and prevalence of cataract.
   Cataract prevalence in males and females

Gender	Yes	No	Total
Male	37	23	60
Female	30	10	40
Total	67	33	100

(With one df, the critical values of chi-square is 3.84 at 5% level of significance)

5. a. State the underlying assumptions of student 't'- test
   b. The following data are from a study on knowledge of primi antenatal mothers on breastfeeding practices after they underwent health education through two methods in two groups.

Sample size (n)		Sample mean	Sample SD
Video-assisted method	10	28.36	3.29
Lecture method	10	19.17	4.16

State suitable hypothesis to test whether video-assisted method is a better method to impart knowledge compared to lecture method at 5% level of significance and apply suitable statistical test to test this hypothesis.

6. a. What are the steps involved in testing of hypothesis?
   b. An investigator has collected the following data to compare the effectiveness of video-assisted teaching method (VATM) against conventional lecture method (CLM) in assessing the knowledge of mothers on the importance of institutional deliveries.

VATM	CLM
25	19
23	20
34	22
15	20
28	22
30	21
29	18
27	15
25	16
31	17
24	
21	

By stating suitable hypothesis, test whether the knowledge score of mothers on the importance of institutional deliveries varies significantly between VATM and CLM using unpaired t-test (critical value is 2.086).

7. What are statistical hypothesis? List out the steps in testing hypothesis. Explain type-I and type-II errors in research.
8. Analysis of data is one of the important steps in any research. Write about (a) nonparametric tests and their utilization, (b) parametric tests and their utilization, and (c) difference between parametric and nonparametric test.

9. A study on association between pregnancy complications and hypertension among 150 pregnant mothers yielded the following data:

Pregnancy complications	Mother hypertension	
	Yes	No
Present	20	40
Absent	10	80

Is there any significant association between hypertensive status of mothers and complications of pregnancy? Chi-square value for one df at 5% level is 3.84.

10. List the various statistical measures used to summarize the data.
11. Discuss the importance of t-test in testing hypothesis drawing suitable illustrations from nursing practice.
12. Explain Wilcoxon signed-rank test in detail with suitable example.

II. Short Essays

1. Various steps in testing of hypothesis
2. Types of t-test
3. Explain various forms of ANOVA
4. Describe parametric tests

III. Short Answers

1. p-value
2. One-tailed and two-tailed tests
3. Level of significance
4. Confidence interval

IV. Multiple Choice Questions

1. A type-II error is also known as a
    a. False positive
    b. False negative
    c. Double negative
    d. Positive negative
2. A chi-square test is best described as
    a. A type of correlation
    b. A parametric test
    c. A nonparametric test
    d. None of the above
3. When distribution of data is not known or cannot be considered as normal distribution, then which of the following inferential test of significance is considered to compare the difference between set of data?
    a. t-test
    b. Chi-square test
    c. ANOVA
    d. z-test
4. The mean blood pressure of a group of persons was determined and after an intervention trial, the mean BP was estimated again. The test to be applied to determine the significance of intervention is
    a. Chi-square test
    b. z-test
    c. Correlation coefficient
    d. Paired t-test
5. The ability of a test to reject the null hypothesis when it is false is known as
    a. Power of a statistical test
    b. Reason of rejection
    c. Test of significance
    d. Analysis of variance
6. Which of the following is concerned with populations using sample data to make inference about a population
    a. Descriptive statistics
    b. Inferential statistics
    c. Nonparametric statistics
    d. Parametric statistics
7. Nonparametric inferential statistics appropriate for comparing set of data that are in the form of frequencies or percentages is
    a. ANOVA
    b. Independent t-test
    c. Dependent t-test
    d. Chi-square test
8. A null hypothesis states
    a. The expected direction of the relationship between the variables
    b. There is no relationship between the variables
    c. That a relationship will be found, but does not state the direction
    d. None of the above
9. The one-sample t-test is used to compare a sample mean to a population mean when

a. The population mean is known
   b. The population SD is known
   c. The sample size is at least 30
   d. The sample size is above 30
10. A type I error occurs when the
   a. Null hypothesis is accepted when it is false
   b. Null hypothesis is rejected when it is true
   c. Sample size is too small
   d. Effect size is not defined in advance
11. A type II error occurs when the
   a. Null hypothesis is accepted when it is false
   b. Null hypothesis is rejected when it is true
   c. Sample size is too small
   d. Effect size is not defined in advance
12. Power can be increased by which of the following?
   a. Increasing the α level
   b. Increasing the sample size
   c. Increasing the effect size
   d. All of the above
13. If a statistical test is significant, it means that
   a. It has important clinical applications
   b. The study has acceptable power
   c. The null hypothesis was rejected
   d. The null hypothesis was accepted
14. The independent t-test is best described as
   a. A type of Mann–Whitney U-test
   b. A parametric test
   c. A nonparametric test
   d. It is same as paired t-test
15. The independent t-test is used to determine differences in the means of
   a. Two groups only
   b. Three groups only
   c. Four groups only
   d. Any number of groups
16. Student's independent t-test is best used when the measurement scale of the characteristic of interest is
   a. Nominal
   b. Ordinal
   c. Interval or ratio
   d. All of the above
17. Consider the following question: Do women make more visits to their physician in a year than men? Which variable is the grouping variable?
   a. Gender
   b. Number of visits to the physician
   c. Both
   d. Neither
18. Consider the following question: Do people who exercise three times a week or more have lower systolic blood pressure than people who exercise less than three times a week? Which variable should be normally distributed?
   a. Frequency of exercise
   b. Systolic blood pressure
   c. Both
   d. Either a or b
19. The Mann–Whitney U-test is best described as
   a. a special type of independent t-test
   b. a parametric test
   c. a non-parametric test
   d. A special type of ANOVA test
20. The Mann-Whitney U-test is used to determine differences in the medians of
   a. two groups only
   b. three groups only
   c. four groups only
   d. any number of groups
21. The Mann–Whitney U-test is best used when the measurement scale of the characteristic of interest is
   a. Nominal
   b. Ordinal
   c. Interval or ratio
   d. b and c
22. The Mann–Whitney U-test is best used when
   a. The total sample size is at least 8
   b. The grouping variable is ordinal level
   c. The data are paired
   d. a and b only are true
23. The paired t-test is
   a. A type of Wilcoxon matched-pairs test
   b. A parametric test

c. A nonparametric test
d. Both a and b are correct
24. The Wilcoxon matched-pairs test is best used when the measurement scale of the characteristic of interest is
   a. Nominal
   b. Ordinal
   c. Interval
   d. Ratio
25. Data are considered paired if
   a. Two measures of the same variable are taken on the same person
   b. Measures of the same variable are taken on a case and a matched control
   c. Measures of the same variable are taken on a case group and an unmatched control group
   d. Both a and b are true
26. The Kruskal–Wallis test is
   a. A type of t-test
   b. A parametric test
   c. A non-parametric test
   d. A type of chi-square test
27. The one-way ANOVA is best used when the measurement scale of the characteristic of interest is
   a. Nominal
   b. Ordinal
   c. Interval or ratio
   d. Any of the above
28. The Friedman's ANOVA test is
   a. A type of t-test
   b. A parametric test
   c. A nonparametric test
   d. a and b only
29. The repeated-measures ANOVA is a test that is used to determine if the means of which of the following are different?
   a. Two independent measures
   b. Three or more independent measures
   c. Two repeated measures from a case and a matched control
   d. Three or more repeated measures
30. The repeated-measures ANOVA is best used when the measurement scale of the characteristic of interest is
   a. Nominal
   b. Ordinal
   c. Interval or ratio
   d. Any of the above
31. A study is conducted to see if migraine headache is best treated by chiropractic interventions, medication, massage, or no intervention. The chiropractic intervention group has 24 people, the medication group has 17 people, the massage group has 14 people, and the no intervention group has 18 people. These data include
   a. Four independent measures of the same variable
   b. Four related measures taken at the same time
   c. Four repeated measures over time from the same participant
   d. Four repeated measures taken from matched patients
32. Ms. Rosy is conducting a study on patient satisfaction with nursing care, where total satisfaction score ranges between 0 and 50. If Ms. Rosy decides to statistically compare the male and female patients on the level of satisfaction i.e. highly satisfied, satisfied, dissatisfied and highly dissatisfied, she should use which of the following tests?
   a. T-test
   b. ANOVA test
   c. Correlational coefficient
   d. Chi-square test
33. Analysis of variance (ANOVA) test is used to test the difference
   a. Between two independent group means
   b. Between two related group means
   c. Among the means of more than three groups
   d. In ranks of scores of more than three groups
34. The McNemar test is used to determine if the proportions are different among
   a. A pretest measure and a posttest measure

b. A measure on a case group and a control group
   c. Two distinct groups
   d. a and b only
35. The Fisher's exact test is used when
   a. The observed frequency in a cell is < 5
   b. The expected frequency in a cell is > 5
   c. More precision in the computation is warranted
   d. None of the above is true
36. The Yates' continuity correction is used when
   a. The total sample size is at least 30
   b. The grouping variable is dichotomous
   c. The observed frequency in at least one cell is less than 10
   d. All of the above are true
37. Which of the following tests should be used to answer the question: Are men or women more likely to use seatbelts?
   a. Chi-square test
   b. McNemar test
   c. t-test
   d. a and b only
38. Which of the following tests should be used to answer the question: Are teenagers more likely to use a seatbelt after viewing a graphic highway safety video?
   a. Chi-square test
   b. McNemar test
   c. t-test
   d. a and b only
39. Kruskal–Wallis test is used to
   a. Test the difference between two independent group means
   b. Test the difference between two related group means
   c. Test the difference among the means of more than three groups
   d. Test the difference in ranks of scores of more than three groups
40. The F-statistics is calculated in
   a. ANOVA
   b. Correlation analysis
   c. Chi-square test
   d. t-test

ANSWER KEY

1. b	2. c	3. b	4. d	5. a	6. b
7. d	8. b	9. a	10. b	11. a	12. d
13. c	14. b	15. a	16. c	17. a	18. b
19. c	20. a	21. d	22. b	23. b	24. b
25. d	26. c	27. c	28. c	29. d	30. c
31. a	32. d	33. c	34. d	35. a	36. c
37. a	38. b	39. d	40. a		

UNIT 17

Application of Statistics in Health and Use of Computers for Data Analysis

Health statistics refers to data on certain aspects of health. These include both empirical data and estimates associated with health such as birth rates, death rates, mortality, morbidity, risk factors, health service coverage, and health systems. Also called vital statistics or vital events, these are an important source of demographic data. These provide quantitative information on vital events occurring in life such as birth, death, marriage, and migration in a given population. These events form essential tools in any demographic study. Public health professionals and epidemiologists use vital statistics to determine both the prevalence of a given condition at a given time point and also incidence of a new condition. Statistics are extensively used by researchers to identify disease patterns among groups so as to estimate the population at risk for certain diseases, finding means to control them and determine the preventive programs.

DEFINITIONS

Vital statistics provide cumulative summaries for successive time periods of population movements like birth, death, migration, marriage, and marital dissolution as well as demographic and other relevant characteristics of the individuals involved in these events.

Vital statistics is a branch of biometry, which deals with data and the law of human morbidity, mortality, and demography.

Vital statistics are numerical records of birth, sickness, marriage, and death by which the health and growth of a community may be studied.

NEED FOR VITAL STATISTICS

- ❖ To determine a health status of community
- ❖ To determine health problems in the community
- ❖ To determine met and unmet health needs of the community
- ❖ To decide best way for providing health services
- ❖ To plan public health program and evaluate its success or failure
- ❖ To create administrative standards for health activities
- ❖ To promote health legislation at local, state, and national level
- ❖ To demand public support for providing better health facilities

SOURCES OF VITAL STATISTICS (MECHANISMS FOR COLLECTION)

Various sources of vital statistics are presented in Figure 17.1.

Population Census

- ❖ Population census is the most important source of demographic data in India, which provides the numerical profile of the country's population at a given time.
- ❖ It is the official enumeration of the people with details of their location, age, gender, marital status, educational level, monthly

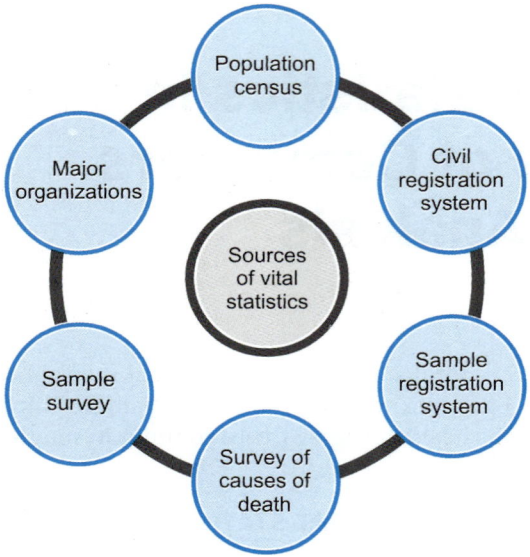

Fig. 17.1: Sources of vital statistics

- This process of registration is carried out by health, revenue, police, panchayat, and municipal bodies through grassroot health workers and local officials of the respective departments.
- Heads of the households are responsible for reporting vital events occurring in that house to the registrar within a prescribed period. The registrar records all vital events that include details such as date of occurrence of events, sex, age, cause of death, etc. The registers are maintained separately for birth, death, and stillbirth for each calendar year. The registrars send monthly reports to the chief registrar who then prepares consolidated annual statistical report for the state Government and a copy to the registrar general of India. The registrar general of India then consolidates the state reports.

income, number of children, etc. This information is collected by door-to-door visit.

- It is a regular feature and conducted once in 10 years by the Registrar General and Census Commissioner of India (RGCCI).
- These data help researchers, administrators, planners, and social organizations to suggest measures to solve various problems.

Civil Registration System

- It is a unified process of continuous, permanent, compulsory, and universal recording of vital events such as births, deaths, stillbirths, and details thereof. It is also the best source of vital statistics. The records emanating from civil registration system (CRS) provide an individual his/her legal identity and the social benefits entitled by the Government. The data thus generated has administrative and statistical use, i.e. it can be utilized for socioeconomic planning and to evaluate the effectiveness of various social sector programs.

Sample Registration System

It is an important source of vital rates in India. It was initiated to provide reliable estimates of birth rate, death rate, and infant mortality rate separately for rural and urban areas at the state and national levels. It also includes useful demographic data such as age, sex, marital status, health status, religion, etc.

Survey of Causes of Death (Model Registration Scheme)

The main objective of this survey is to identify the causes of death in rural India. The paramedical staff in the primary health center (PHC) visit households and collect information on symptoms, conditions, and duration of illness. Based on this information, main causes for death are determined. These statistics are intimated to state health quarters, either the directorate of medical services and public health or directorate of economics and statistics who compile the data at state level and in turn transmit them to the registrar general of India for consolidation and analysis.

Sample Survey

- Sample survey is an important method of collecting demographic data in India, wherein information is collected from a sample of population to find fertility, mortality, growth, etc. This is then applied to the whole population.
- In this survey, the births and deaths are continuously enumerated by a resident part time enumerator, which is then followed by an official independent survey once in 6 months.

Major Organizations

- Central Statistical Organization (CSO)
- National Sample Survey Organization (NSSO)
- Registrar General and Census Commissioner of India
- Ministry of Health and Family Welfare
- International Institute of Population Studies

Census

Population census is the entire process of collection, assessment, analysis, publication, and distribution of demographic, economic, and social data, related to a particular geographic area at a given point of time. The objective is to gather and present a true picture of the population parameters and their demographic, economic, and social attributes. This information includes age, gender, area of residence, country of origin, year of immigration, level of education, employment, monthly income, marital status, number of children, housing conditions, traveling habits, etc. This collected data is available in both public and private domains and serves as the basis for taking decisions that directly or indirectly affect the residents in various spheres of life. The statistical definition, however, suggests census to be a "survey of an entire population, as opposed to a sample survey".

Main Objectives of Population Census

- To list the households in the country.
- To acquire demographic data and estimate the population.
- To collect data and provide the information to various Governmental agencies for budgeting purpose.
- To collect socioeconomic information relating to large population samples so as to acquire data on small, unique population groups.
- To produce information that will cater to various bodies and organizations in the field of education, economy, business, research, etc.

Uses of Census

- Primary data can be utilized for administrative purposes
- Useful for calculating birth and death rates
- Estimating school going population, military, and economic manpower
- Estimating future growth of cities and requirement of food, water, housing, and health services
- Estimating number of voters—present and future
- Provides information on:
  - Trends in population structure and growth
  - Rates of fertility, mortality, migration, and urbanization
  - Changes in the national, occupational, and industrial composition
  - Levels of literacy and educational attainments
  - Analysis of economic development
  - National, local, public, and private planning

USES OF VITAL STATISTICS

Vital statistics are of much importance for the people and the nation.

- *For the individual*: A birth certificate issued by the registering authority is an important document, which records the

date, time, place, and parentage of the person. It establishes the identity as a citizen of the country.
- *Legal use*: Certificates relating to birth, death, marriage, divorce, etc. have legal importance. While a birth certificate is required for admission to a school or getting a passport, a marriage certificate records the marital status of a couple and legalizes the birth of children from that marriage. A death certificate is an important legal document for settling insurance claims or property.
- *Health and family planning programs*: The cause of deaths and the mortality rates help in assessing the health condition of individuals in different parts of the country. This data in turn can be utilized to formulate health and family planning programs of the Government and also assess their impact after implementation.
- *Study of social conditions*: The birth and death rates, divorce rates, widow remarriage, etc. reflect the social conditions as well as its customs and traditions.
- *For administrators and planners*: Trends in growth of population and various other health parameters help the planners and administrators to plan and formulate administrative standards pertaining to public health, education, housing, transport, communication, and food supplies. The administration is better prepared with measures of disease control.
- *For the nation*: Vital statistics help in analyzing the population trends at various timelines thus filling the gap between two consecutive population censuses. They include composition, size, distribution, and growth of the population. These projections provide inputs while formulating policies and procedures relating to social security, updating electoral rolls, demarcating of electoral constituencies, framing rules for immigration and emigration.
- *In research*: It is a primary tool in demographic research.

Importance of Health Statistics in the Field of Health

- They measure a wide range of health indicators in the community and in the process provide a base to evaluate the efficacy of health-related programs.
- Help the Government agencies to monitor the overall health parameters and well-being of the population.
- Assist the decision makers in identifying and controlling outbreak of emerging diseases towards improving longevity and meeting prevention targets.
- In the event of budgetary shortfalls, compiling such statistics not only sensitizes but also compels the Government agencies in mobilizing further resources to meet the healthcare goals.

BASIC FORMULAE IN VITAL STATISTICS

Disease magnitude is usually expressed as a rate, ratio or proportion. These form the basic tools of measurement in epidemiology.

Rate

A rate is defined as the number of events occurring in a population during a particular time period, which may include deaths and diseases. Here, rate refers to the measure of the speed at which new events are occurring in a community. To compute "rate", the prerequisites are a definite time period, defined population with an estimate of its size during the defined period, and the number of events taking place during the period. Rate is usually expressed per 1,000.

$$\text{Rate} = \frac{\text{Number of events}}{\text{Mid-year population}} \times 1{,}000$$

Note: Mid-year population is the population estimated as on the 1st July of a given year.

Rate is the frequency of occurrence of an event over a specific time interval. It states the risk of developing a condition. A typical example is the death rate.

$$\text{Death rate} = \frac{\text{Number of deaths in 1 year}}{\text{Mid-year population}} \times 1{,}000$$

The rates in general are of two types: crude and specific.

1. Crude rates are general rates calculated without including specific sections of the population. They measure the proportion between total events and the total population over a period of time.

$$\text{Crude rate} = \frac{\text{Total number of events that occurred in a given geographical area during a given year}}{\text{Mid-year population}} \times 1{,}000$$

2. Specific rates are for specific groups of population such as particular age, sex, marital status, occupation, etc.

$$\text{Specific rate} = \frac{\text{Number of events, which occurred among a specific group of population in a given geographical area during a given year}}{\text{Mid-year population of the specific group}} \times 1{,}000$$

Ratio

It is another measure of disease frequency. It is a comparison of two values relative to their size. It can be expressed as x:y or x to y or x/y. Example, nurse–patient ratio indicates the number of nurses available relative to the number of patients. Thus a 1:4 nurse–patient ratio indicates that one nurse is available for every four patients.

Proportion

Proportion is a ratio, which is defined as a part or a share in relation to the whole, generally expressed as a percentage. The numerator is always included in the denominator.

$$\text{Proportion}(\%) = \frac{\text{Number of patients from a village at certain time}}{\text{Total population of the village at the same time}} \times 100$$

The distinguishing characteristics of rate, ratio, and proportion are depicted in Flowchart 17.1.

BASIC MEASUREMENTS IN VITAL STATISTICS

Epidemiology focuses on measurement of fertility, morbidity, and mortality (Flowchart 17.2).

Measures of Fertility

Fertility is measured by a number of indicators: crude birth rate, general fertility rate, total fertility rate, gross reproductive rate, net reproductive rate, etc. Description of measures of fertility is provided in Table 17.1.

Measures of Morbidity

Morbidity is a state of being diseased. Morbidity rates describe the number and types of diseases present in the community and provide comprehensive and accurate information on patient characteristics. All these are needed for establishing priorities, for conducting basic research and for monitoring disease control activities. The following aspects of morbidity are generally measured using morbidity rates or ratios:

- *Frequency*: Measuring persons who are ill. The disease frequency is measured by incidence and prevalence rates.
- *Duration*: Number of days the person is exposed to disease. It is assessed by disability rate (disability/person).

Flowchart 17.1: Distinguishing characteristics of rate, ratio, and proportion

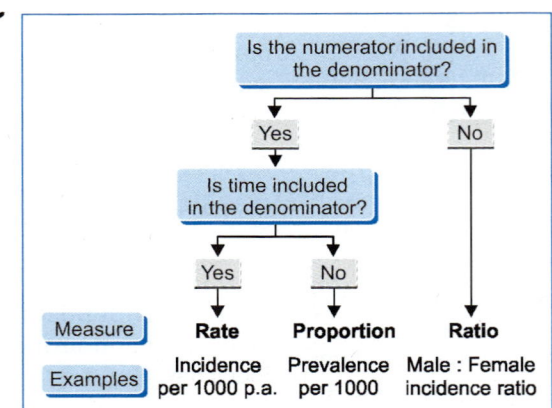

Flowchart 17.2: Basic measurements in vital statistics

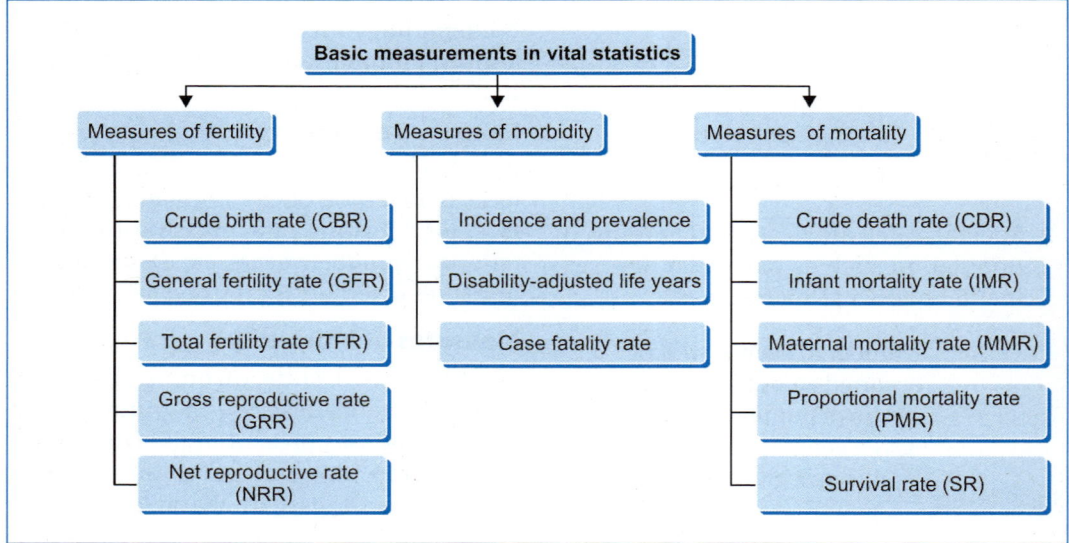

- ❖ *Severity*: Severity of illness they are experiencing. It is measured by case fatality rate.

Incidence and Prevalence

Incidence measures the rate (rapidity) at which new cases occur in a population. It is not influenced by the duration of the disease. The use of incidence is restricted to acute conditions. Information on rate of incidence is useful in taking preventive action so as to control disease and evaluate efficacy of preventive and therapeutic measures. For example, an increasing incidence rate might indicate ineffectiveness of current control programs and also suggest introduction of new preventive programs (Table 17.2).

Example:
If there had been 500 new tuberculosis cases in a population of 60,000 during a given year, the incidence rate can be calculated as under:

$$\text{Incidence rate} = \frac{500}{60,000} \times 1,000$$

$$= 8.33 \text{ per } 1,000 \text{ per year}$$

Table 17.1: Measures of fertility

Measure	Description	Equation
Crude birth rate (CBR)	Number of live births per 1,000 estimated mid-year population in a given year	$CBR = \dfrac{\text{Number of live births during the year}}{\text{Estimated mid-year population}} \times 1{,}000$
General fertility rate (GFR)	Number of live births per 1,000 women in the reproductive age group (15–49 years) in a given year	$GFR = \dfrac{\text{Number of live births in 1 year}}{\text{Mid-year female population aged 15-49 years}} \times 1{,}000$
Total fertility rate (TFR)	Average number of children that a woman would have over her childbearing years (i.e. age 15–49), based on current birth trends	It is calculated by adding up the average number of births per woman across 5-year age groups (i.e. age-specific fertility rates, or ASFR). The specific formula to calculate TFR is: $TFR = 5 \times \Sigma (ASFR)$ $= 5 \times \left(\dfrac{\text{number of births to women aged }15\text{-}19}{\text{number of women aged }15\text{-}19} + \ldots + \dfrac{\text{number of births to women aged }45\text{-}49}{\text{number of women aged }45\text{-}49} \right)$
Gross reproductive rate (GRR)	Average number of girls that would be born to a woman, if she experiences the current fertility pattern throughout her reproductive span assuming no mortality	$GRR = \dfrac{\text{Number of female births}}{\text{Total number of births}} \times TFR$
Net reproductive rate (NRR)	The number of daughters a newborn girl will bear during her life time assuming fixed age-specific fertility and mortality rates	$NRR = \dfrac{\text{Number of female infants born to mothers of specific age}}{\text{Number of women of specific age in the mid-year population}}$ • NRR = 1 means exact replacement • NRR > 1 means population is more than replacing itself • NRR < 1 means population is not replacing itself • NRR is always lower than GRR, as it takes into account that some women die before completing their childbearing years

Prevalence helps to estimate the magnitude (extent) of the disease problem in the community and identifies potential high-risk populations. Prevalence rates are utilized by the administration for planning purposes. For example, for estimation of manpower needs, rehabilitation facilities, hospital beds, etc. Prevalence is of two types: point and period (Table 17.3).

Disability-adjusted Life Years

It is a measure of overall disease burden, expressed as the number of years lost due to ill-health, disability or early death (Table 17.4).

Table 17.2: Incidence

Measure	Description	Equation
Incidence	Incidence refers to the number of new cases of a particular disease that are developed during the specific time period. Incidence rate lies between zero and infinity. The yearly incidence measures the number of new cases occurring during that particular year	$\text{Incidence rate} = \dfrac{\text{Number of new cases of specific disease during a given period}}{\text{Population at risk}} \times 1{,}000$

Table 17.3: Prevalence

Measure	Description	Equation
Prevalence	It refers to the total number of cases of disease that exist at a specific time point. It is the total number of all individuals who have disease at a particular time divided by the population at risk of having the disease at this point in time. Prevalence is often expressed as a percentage.	$\text{Prevalence (as \%)} = \dfrac{\text{Number of cases}}{\text{Number of people at risk}} \times 100$
Point prevalence	It is defined as the number of all current cases (old and new) of a disease at one point in time in relation to a defined population.	$\text{Point prevalence} = \dfrac{\text{Number of all old and new cases of a specific disease existing at a given point in time}}{\text{Estimated population at the same point in time}} \times 100$
Period prevalence	It measures the frequency of all current cases (old and new) existing during a defined period of time. It is expressed in relation to a defined population. It includes cases arising before but extending into the year as well as those cases arising during the year.	$\text{Period prevalence} = \dfrac{\text{Number of existing old and new cases of a specific disease during a given period of time interval}}{\text{Estimated mid-interval population of risk}} \times 100$

Table 17.4: Disability-adjusted life years (DALY)

Measure	Description	Equation
Disability-adjusted life years (DALY)	It is the sum of the years of life lost (YLL) due to premature mortality in the population and the years lost due to disability (YLD) for people living with the health condition	DALY = YLL + YLD (One DALY = One lost year of healthy life)

Case Fatality Rate

Also called case fatality ratio, it is used to measure disease severity, course, and outcome and evaluate the effect of new treatment (Table 17.5).

Measures of Mortality

Mortality is often monitored by public health authorities as the related measures are widely used for many purposes. They explain trends and differentials in overall mortality suggesting priorities for health action and the allocation of resources. Common mortality rates and ratios are crude death rate, specific death rate (infant mortality rate, maternal mortality rate), case fatality rate, proportional mortality rate, and survival rate (Table 17.6).

Table 17.5: Case fatality rate

Measure	Description	Equation
Case fatality rate (CFR)	It is the proportion of people who die from a specified disease among all individuals diagnosed with the disease over a certain period of time	$\text{Case fatality ratio} = \dfrac{\text{Total number of deaths due to a disease}}{\text{Total number of cases due to a disease}} \times 100$

Table 17.6: Measures of mortality

Measure	Description	Equation
Crude death rate (CDR)	The number of deaths from all causes in a given population during a year in a given place	$CDR = \dfrac{\text{Number of deaths during the year}}{\text{Mid-year population}} \times 1{,}000$
Infant mortality rate (IMR)	Number of deaths under 1 year of age among a given population in a particular area	$IMR = \dfrac{\text{Number of deaths under 1 year of age}}{\text{Number of live births}} \times 1{,}000$
Maternal mortality rate (MMR)	Number of deaths occurring due to puerperal cause (due to complications of pregnancy, childbirth, and puerperium) among a given population	$MMR = \dfrac{\text{Deaths from all puerperal causes in females}}{\text{Total live births}} \times 1{,}000$
Proportional mortality rate (PMR)	Number of deaths due to a particular cause per 100 total deaths	$PMR = \dfrac{\text{Number of deaths due to a specific disease in a year}}{\text{Total deaths from all causes in that year}} \times 100$
Survival rate (SR)	It is the proportion of survivors in a group of patients studied and followed over a period of time (e.g. 5-year period)	$\text{5 year SR} = \dfrac{\text{Total number of patients alive after 5 years}}{\text{Total number of patients diagnosed or treated}} \times 100$

STATISTICAL PACKAGES

Nurses are increasingly taking part in evidence-based practice to ensure better clinical decisions and improved patient outcomes. For this, the nurse must be able to read and evaluate research literature, familiarize with basic statistical procedures, choose appropriate statistical measures, and understand the author's interpretation of research results.

With quantitative research being carried out extensively, application of statistical software (SS) has come to play a very crucial role in data analysis. With the advent of digital age, the researchers have now moved to the more efficient and accurate form of statistical analysis, which use advanced statistical software (SS). The digital analysis has contributed immensely to the way demographic studies are being conducted, so also the social investigation among other professionals. The statistical packages are available both as proprietary (MS-Excel, SPSS, MINITAB, SAS) and free software (LibreOffice Calc, PSPP, Epi Info, R).

Statistical Methods Usable in the Software

- *Descriptive statistics*: Frequencies, cross-tabulation, and descriptive ratio statistics.
- *Bivariate statistics*: Analysis of variance (ANOVA), correlation, and nonparametric tests.
- *Numeral outcome prediction*: Linear regression.
- *Prediction for identifying groups*: Cluster analysis and factor analysis.

Uses of Statistical Packages

- All quantitative research studies rely upon statistical packages for analysis.
- Help in drawing conclusions and inference on which the decision is made.
- Present large data in understandable form, e.g. graphs and tables.
- Being a powerful tool, the statistical packages aid in advanced statistical analysis and data exploration.
- Extensively used in analyzing and presenting the research findings.
- Being compatible with a variety of file formats, they can be used with data in excel, plain text, or SQL data base.
- Help in drawing inferences and conclusions based on which the decisions are made.

Proprietary Software

- *MS-Excel*: It is a spreadsheet program included in Microsoft Office, which performs both basic and complex arithmetic operations. It is user-friendly and good for descriptive statistics. However, it is costly and more suitable for basic statistical analysis.
- *SPSS*: SPSS is the acronym of Statistical Package for the Social Science. It is one of the most powerful and widely used statistical packages by the academia that is easy to use. Designed for both interactive and noninteractive purposes, it can carry out data manipulation and perform highly complex analysis with simple instructions. It has a command line interface in addition to menu-driven user interface. However, it is very expensive.
- *MINITAB*: It is a software product used to analyze and manipulate the data, identify trends and patterns so as to arrive for answers to the current issues. It is easy to learn and often taught as a part of introductory statistics, also used in business. However, it is expensive and not ideal for complicated statistical analysis and thus not preferred for academic research.
- *SAS*: SAS stands for Statistical Analysis System that enables to perform data entry, retrieval, and management, and offers advanced analytics, multivariate

analysis, and numerous other tasks. It is very flexible and powerful. SAS is widely used by academia. However, the cost is exorbitant and not user-friendly. The graphic capabilities are relatively poor.

Free Software

- *LibreOffice Calc*: It is a *spreadsheet* application used to calculate, analyze, and manage data. The functionality is very similar to Microsoft Excel and user-friendly. It is good for basic descriptive statistics, charts, and plots and interoperable with Microsoft Office. Though it is a free software it is just sufficient to carry out most basic statistical analysis.
- *PSPP*: It is regarded as a free alternative of SPSS, which is user-friendly and good for statistical analysis. However, it is not widely used.
- *Epi Info*: It is developed by Centers for Disease Control and Prevention (CDC) for analyzing epidemiological studies. It consists of multiple modules to accomplish various tasks beyond just statistical analysis like the ability to rapidly develop and enter data into a questionnaire, customize the data entry process, and analyze the data. Though it is a free software, it is not a dedicated statistical package and not as powerful as commercial alternatives for performing advanced analysis.
- *R*: R is a language, which provides a variety of statistical and graphical techniques, including linear and nonlinear modeling, time–series analysis, classification, and clustering. It has a strong static graphics module with dynamic and interactive graphics available through additional packages. It is very powerful and flexible with a large user base. It is widely used and accepted by the academia. However, it is not user-friendly.

It can thus be concluded that statistical analysis is an integral part of any study and publication. While some free statistical software does not measure up, the commercial alternatives are very costly for the individual researchers.

USE OF COMPUTERS FOR DATA ANALYSIS

Data analysis is the process of checking, cleaning, organizing, feeding, and statistical testing of the data with the main aim of hypothesis testing, drawing generalizations, and interpretations. Computers play a key role in all these activities. They help in data analysis in the following ways:

- Data entry, data editing, data storage, and data management
- Analyzing statistical data using specially designed algorithms
- Monitoring the accuracy and completeness of the data as they are collected
- Examination of different dimension of variables or plot them in various charts using a statistical application
- Carry out calculations using various statistical software
- Calculation of sample size for a proposed study, hypothesis testing, and calculation of power of the study
- Display the results in graphical chart or graph form
- Store and access data from different sources via computer networks set up in research laboratories, which make collaboration simpler
- Contribute to scientific research across various disciplines by discovering new patterns and providing insights through various analytical software programs
- Provide an entirely new dimension to sharing of knowledge, access to latest research articles, and making international collaboration on scientific projects possible

BIBLIOGRAPHY

1. Sharma, K.S. (2014). *Nursing research and Statistics* (2nd ed.). Chennai: RR Donnelley Publishing India Pvt. Ltd.
2. Khanal B.A. (2016). *Mahajan's Methods in Biostatistics for medical students and research workers* (8th ed.). New Delhi: Jaypee Brothers Medical Publishers (P) Ltd.
3. Park K. (1995). *Preventive and Social Medicine* (14th ed.). Jabalpur: Banarsidas Bhanot Publishers.

REVIEW QUESTIONS

I. Long Essays

1. Explain various sources and uses of vital statistics.
2. Define and explain birth rate, maternal mortality rate, infant mortality rate, incidence rate, and prevalence rate.

II. Short Essays

1. Write short notes on infant mortality rate.
2. Explain measurement of fertility.
3. Explain uses of vital statistics.
4. Explain uses of statistical package.
5. Explain vital statistics.
6. Explain mid-year population.
7. Explain incidence and prevalence rate.

III. Multiple Choice Questions

1. Following are the sources of vital statistics, *except*:
    a. Civil registration system
    b. Sample registration system
    c. Health survey
    d. National survey
2. Data concerning birth, death, marriages, and fetal deaths are considered:
    a. Inferential statistics
    b. Descriptive statistics
    c. Vital statistics
    d. Nominal data
3. Vital health statistics is a:
    a. Record of birth, death and disease
    b. Record of vital signs
    c. Record of vital incidence of a region
    d. Record of vital history of a country
4. Who among the following cannot be considered as a beneficiary of vital health statistics:
    a. Researchers
    b. Public administrators
    c. Individuals
    d. Political leaders
5. Which of the following is not a method of obtaining vital statistics:
    a. Registration method
    b. Operational research method
    c. Census enumeration
    d. Analytical method
6. Which of the following stands true for the full form of SPSS:
    a. Statistical package for social system
    b. Statistical package for social science
    c. Statistical package for statistical science
    d. Statistical package for statistical system
7. Following are all morbidity measures, *except*:
    a. Period of stay in hospital
    b. Doctor population ratio
    c. Severity of illness
    d. Number of persons who are ill
8. Following all are mortality measures, *except*:
    a. Proportional mortality rate
    b. Crude birth rate
    c. Maternal mortality rate
    d. Survival rate
9. Incidence is defined as:
    a. Number of cases existing in a given population during a specific period
    b. Number of cases existing at a given time point

c. Number of new cases occurring during the specific time period
d. Number of old cases present
10. Prevalence is defined as:
    a. Total number of cases that exist at a specific time point
    b. Total number of new cases occurring during the specific time period
    c. Total number of old cases occurring during the specific time period
    d. Number of old cases present in that year

ANSWER KEY

| 1. d | 2. c | 3. a | 4. d | 5. b | 6. b |
| 7. b | 8. b | 9. c | 10. a | | |

Glossary

A

Abstract: An abstract is a brief overview of a research article, report, proposal, or review of a particular subject or discipline positioned at the beginning of a paper. It appears as a summary in searchable data bases and determines the paper's purpose.

Accessible population: Portion of the target population to which the researcher has a reasonable access.

Algorithm: A decision tree that provides a set of rules for solving particular practice problem. Its development usually is based on research evidence and theoretical knowledge.

Alpha: The risk of erroneous conclusions that the researcher is willing to accept the standard for statistical significance.

Analysis of covariance (ANCOVA): A statistical procedure used to test mean differences among groups on a dependent variable, while controlling for one or more extraneous variables (covariates).

Analysis of variance (ANOVA): A statistical procedure for testing mean differences among three or more groups by comparing variability between groups to variability within groups.

Analyzing research reports: Critical thinking skill that involves in determining the value of a study by breaking the contents of a study report into parts and examining the parts for accuracy, completeness, uniqueness of information, and organization.

Anonymity: Protection of participants in a study such that even the researcher cannot link individuals with the information provided.

Applicability and transferability: The ability of qualitative research findings to be applied to other samples and other settings.

Applied research: Scientific investigation conducted to find a solution to an immediate practical problem and generate knowledge that will in some way contribute to modification of practice.

Associative hypothesis: Hypothesis that identifies variables that occur or exist together in the real world, such that when one variable changes the other changes.

Assumption: A basic principle that is accepted as factual based on logic or reason, without proof or verification.

Attrition: Dropout of the subjects during the course of the research study, which can lead to bias by altering the composition of the initially drawn sample (particularly, if more participants are lost from one group than another) that can threaten the internal validity of the study.

Audit trail: Detailed documentation of sources of information, data, and design decisions related to qualitative research study.

B

Bar chart: A graphic presentation for nominal or ordinal data that represents the categories on the horizontal axis and frequency on the vertical axis.

Basic research: Scientific investigation for the pursuit of knowledge in a discipline for the sake of knowledge generation or theory construction.

Beneficence: An ethical principle that pursues to maximize benefits and above all prevent harm and exploitation of study participants.

Between group variance: A source of variation of the group means around the grand mean.

Bias: The distortion of true findings by factors other than those being studied.

Bibliography: A bibliography is a list of all the sources used during research process and background reading not just the ones cited in the writing. It includes books, articles, and papers. It is listed alphabetically by the author's surname.

Bivariate analysis: Analysis of two variables at a time, as in correlation studies.

Bivariate correlation: A measure of the extent of linear relationship between two variables.

Blind review: The review of a manuscript or proposal such that neither the author nor the reviewer is identified to the other party.

Blinded: The peer review is unaware of the author's identity, thus avoiding personal influence.

Borrowed theories: Theories taken from other disciplines and used as frameworks or models for nursing practice.

Box plot: A graphic presentation that marks the median of the values in the middle of the box and the 25th and 75th percentiles as the lower and upper edges of the box. It indicates the relative position of the data for each group and spread of the data for comparison.

Bracketing: The process of identifying and setting aside any preconceived beliefs and or opinions about the phenomena under study by a researcher in a qualitative study.

Breach of confidentiality: Accidental or direct action that allows an unauthorized person to have access to raw study data.

C

Calibration: The use of this procedure to minimize measurement error with physical instruments by objectively verifying that the instrument is measuring a characteristic accurately.

Case–control study: An intact group design that involves observation of subjects who exhibit a characteristic matched with subjects who do not. Differences between the subjects allow study of relationships between risk and disease without subjecting healthy individuals to illness.

Case study: The meticulous descriptive exploration of a single unit of study such as a person, family, group, community, or other entity.

Central limit theorem: A mathematical theorem that is the basis for the conclusion that larger samples will represent a population more accurately than smaller ones.

Chi-square test: A nonparametric test of statistical significance used to assess whether a relationship exists between two nominal-level variables; symbolized as χ^2.

Citation: It is a way of giving credit to the original author for his creative and intellectual work that have been used to support the research without plagiarizing.

Citation analysis: A way to measure quality and impact of research by noting how often researchers articles are referred to in another researchers works.

Closed questions: Questions that use a fixed number of alternative responses, wherein the respondents are forced to select answers or ratings on a scale provided by the researcher.

Cluster sampling: A sampling type in which large groups (clusters) are selected followed by successive subsampling of smaller units.

Cochran's Q test: Nonparametric test that is an extension of McNemar test for two related samples.

Coding: The process of converting raw data into standardized form for data analysis. While in quantitative research, it deals with the process of attaching numbers to categories; in qualitative research, it deals with the process of recognizing repetitive words, themes, or concepts within the data.

Coefficient of variation (CV): A calculation that produces a number that depicts the standard deviation relative to the mean.

Cohen's kappa: A measure of inter-rater or intercoder reliability between two raters or coders. The test yields the percentage of agreement and the probability of error.

Co-investigators: A co-investigator (CoI) assists the principal investigator in the management of the research project.

Comparison group: A subgroup of a quasi-experimental design sample from which the intervention is withheld. Subjects are similar to and compared with the experimental group, but are not randomly assigned.

Concept: An abstract idea that is used to describe or identify a phenomenon.

Conceptual definition: Clearly stated meanings of the abstract ideas or concepts used by a researcher in a study.

Conceptual model/conceptual framework: Inter-related concepts or phenomena put together in a rational manner for broader understanding by virtue of their relevance to a common theme.

Concurrent validity: It refers to the degree of correlation of two measures of the same concept administered at the same time.

Confidence interval: A range of values that includes, with a specified level of confidence, the actual population parameter.

Confidentiality: Protection of participants in a research study by not linking the individual identities to responses provided by them.

Confounding variables: Variables that cannot be controlled.

Consent form: A written form of subject's agreement signed both by the study participant and the researcher detailing the terms and conditions of voluntary participation in a study.

Construct: A broad or high level concept that is often complex and abstract.

Construct validity: An indication that a measurement captures the abstract concept that is the basis of the study.

Content analysis: A data analysis method that uses interpretations of the meaning in verbal responses or in documents.

Content validity: A subjective judgment about whether a measurement makes sense by assessing that items of the instrument are the attributes being measured (face validity) or by verifying items with a panel of experts.

Contingency table: A two-dimensional table that permits a cross-tabulation of the frequencies of two categorical variables.

Continuous variable: A variable that can take an infinite range of values along a continuum.

Control group: Randomly selected group of subjects in an experiment who are not exposed or receive the experimental intervention in a research study. The control group subject's performance provides a baseline against which the effects of the intervention can be measured.

Convenience sampling: A nonprobability method of selecting a sample that includes subjects who are available in a convenient way to the researcher.

Correlation analysis: A measure that depicts the strength and nature of the relationship between two variables.

Correlation coefficient: An index summarizing the degree of relationship between variables, typically ranging from +1 (for a perfect positive relationship) through 0 (for no relationship) to −1 (for a perfect negative relationship).

Correlation studies: A research design to quantify the strength and the direction of the relationship of two variables in a single subject or the relationship between a single variable in two samples without any active intervention by the researcher.

Cramer's V: An index describing the magnitude of relationship between nominal level data used when the contingency table to which it is applied is larger than 2 × 2.

Credibility: A qualitative data measure focused on ensuring that the results represent the underlying meaning of the data.

Criterion-related validity: Criterion validity (or criterion-related validity) determines how well one measure predicts an outcome for another measure. A test has this type of validity, if it is useful for predicting performance or behavior in another situation (past, present, or future).

Critique: Careful examination of all aspects of a study to judge its strengths, limitations, meaning, and significance.

Cross-sectional design: Cross-sectional studies involve observing a single phenomenon across multiple populations at a single point in time without any follow-up for determining the relationship between variables.

D

Data analysis: The systematic organization and synthesis of research data, and the testing of research hypotheses using those data.

Data collection: The process of gathering existing information or developing new information in a systematic manner so as to address a research problem.

Data source triangulation: A type of triangulation where multiple data sources are used in a study.

Data triangulation: The use of multiple data sources for the purpose of validating conclusions.

Data: Information collected during a study.

Database: An electronic index of information categorized by subject matter, authors, journals, and other relevant classification that can be searched using commands via computer technology.

Debriefing: Complete disclosure of the study purpose and results to study participants at the end of a study.

Deception: The deliberate withholding of information or providing false information to study participants with an intention to reduce potential biases.

Deductive reasoning: The process of developing specific predictions from general principles.

Degrees of freedom (df): A concept used in statistical testing, referring to the number of sample values free to vary given the values of other existing scores.

Delphi technique: A method of obtaining written judgments from a panel of experts about an issue of concern; experts are questioned individually in several rounds, with a summary of the panel's views circulated between rounds, to achieve some consensus.

Dependent variable: An outcome of interest in experimental studies that occurs after the introduction of an independent variable.

Descriptive statistics: Statistics used to describe and summarize data (e.g. mean, standard deviation).

Descriptive studies: Research designed to describe in detail some process, event, or outcome. The design is used when very little is known about the research question.

Descriptive variables: Characteristics that describe the sample and provide a composite picture of the subjects of the study; not manipulated or controlled by the researcher.

Diffusion: Process of communicating research findings (innovations) through various channels over time to the members of a discipline.

Directional hypothesis: A one-sided statement of the research question that is interested in only direction of change.

Discriminate validity: An approach to construct validity that involves assessing the degree to which a single method of measuring two constructs yields different results.

Dissertation: An extensive, usually original research project that is completed by a doctoral student as part of the requirements for a doctoral degree.

Double-blind experiment: An experiment in which neither the subjects nor those who administer the treatment know who is in the experimental or control group.

E

Effect size: The measure of the magnitude of impact an intervention is expected to have on an outcome.

Empirical literature: Published works that demonstrate how theories apply to individual behavior or observed events.

Epidemiology: The investigation of the distribution and determinants of disease within populations or cohorts.

Ethics: A type of philosophy that studies right and wrong.

Ethnography: A qualitative research method that investigates the features and interactions of a given culture.

Evidence-based practice: The use of best scientific evidence, integrated with clinical experience and incorporating patient values, and preferences in the practice of professional nursing care.

Ex post facto research: It is a type of research design that relies on observation of the relationship between naturally occurring differences in the intervention and outcome.

Exclusion criteria: Characteristics that eliminate a potential subject from the study.

Experimental design: A design that includes randomization, control group, and manipulation between or among variables to examine probability and causality among selected variables for the purpose of predicting and controlling phenomena.

Experimental group: The subjects in a group who receive the experimental treatment or intervention.

Experimental research: Highly structured studies of cause and effect, usually applied to determine the effectiveness of an intervention. Subjects are selected and randomly assigned to groups to represent the population of interest.

Exploratory study: Research approaches that are designed to explore and describe a given phenomenon and generate new knowledge.

External validity: The degree to which the study findings can be generalized beyond the sample used in the study.

Extraneous variable: Factors that exert an effect on the outcome but are not part of the planned experiment and may confuse the interpretation of the results.

F

Fabrication: A type of research misconduct where data or results are made-up.

Face validity: The extent to which a measuring instrument looks as though it is measuring what it purports to measure.

Factor analysis: A statistical procedure for reducing a large set of variables into a smaller set of variables with common characteristics or underlying dimensions.

Falsification: A type of research misconduct where the researcher manipulates results, changes procedures, omits data, or accepts subjects into the study who do not meet inclusion criteria.

Field notes: Detailed descriptions of the context, environment, and nonverbal communication observed during data collection and inserted by the researcher into the transcripts to enrich the data interpretation process.

Focus groups: Measurement strategy where groups are assembled to obtain the participants' perceptions in focused areas in settings that are permissive and non-threatening in a qualitative study.

Frequency: A count of the instances that an event occurs in a data set.

Friedman test: A nonparametric test analog of ANOVA used with paired groups or repeated measures situations.

Full disclosure: The communication of complete information to study participants about the nature of the study, potential risks, and benefits that would occur, and the right to refuse participation and withdrawal from the study.

G

Generalization: Extension of the implications of the findings from the sample to a larger population.

Grand theories: The most abstract and complex theories, broadest in scope, not amenable to testing, provide foundation for mid-range theories, and are central to the nursing profession.

Grounded theory: Aimed at discovering and developing a theory based on systematically collected data about a phenomenon. The intent is to discover a pattern of reactions, interactions, and relationships among people and their concerns.

Guttman scale: A scale with a set of items on a continuum or statements ranging from one extreme to another. Responses are progressive and cumulative.

H

Hawthorne effect: The effect on the dependent variable resulting from subjects' awareness that they are participants under study.

Heterogeneous sample: A sample in which subjects have a broad range of values being studied, which increases the representativeness of the sample and the ability to generalize from the accessible population to the target population.

Histograms: A visual display of information that organizes a group of data points using bars to show the frequency of a data item in successive intervals.

Historical research: Narrative description or analysis of events that occurred in the past.

Homogeneous sample: Sample in which subjects score on selected measurement methods in a study are similar, resulting in a limited distribution of scores.

Hypothesis: A tentative statement of the expected relationship between two or more variables under study.

I

Inclusion criteria: Guidelines for choosing subjects with a predetermined set of characteristics that include major factors important to the research question.

Independent variable: In experimental research, it is the manipulated variable; which is believed to cause the dependent variable.

Inductive reasoning: A process of reasoning from specific observations to broader generalizations and theories.

Inference: Generalization from a specific case to a general truth, from a part to the whole, from the concrete to the abstract, or from the known to the unknown.

Inferential statistics: Statistics to address research objectives and hypothesis in a study to allow inference from the study sample to the target population.

Informed consent: A process of information exchange in which participants are provided understandable information needed to make a participation decision, full disclosure of the risks and benefits, and the assurance that withdrawal is possible at any time without consequences. This process begins with recruitment and ends with a signed agreement document. Through informed consent patient's right to autonomy is protected.

Institutional Review Board (IRB): It is a committee having officially selected or nominated members to protect the rights, safety, and well-being of humans involved in a clinical trial by reviewing all aspects of the research study and approving its startup. This committee operates in accordance with national/local regulations as well as clinical practice guidelines.

Instrument: A tool or device used to collect the data, for example, a questionnaire, observational check list or a test, etc.

Internal validity: The extent to which the effects detected in the study are a true reflection of reality rather than the result of uncontrolled extraneous factors.

Interpretation of research outcomes: A process wherein the researcher makes sense of the study, examines its implications, explores the significance, and generalizes the findings.

Inter-rater reliability: The extent to which an instrument is consistent across raters, as measured with a percentage agreement or a kappa statistic.

Interval data: Data measured on a scale that has consistent intervals between measurement units and allows for broad selection of mathematical operations and analytic options.

Intervention: Intervention is a treatment that is manipulated while carrying out the experimental research study. It is an independent variable that produces an effect on the dependent variable.

Interview: It is a method of data collection in which an interviewer asks questions to another person either face-to-face or over telephone. It can be structured or unstructured.

Intuition: Insight or understanding of a situation or an event as a whole that usually cannot be logically explained.

Investigator triangulation: A type of triangulation where more than one person is used to collect, analyze, or interpret a set of data.

Item analysis: A type of analysis used to assess whether all the items on the scale are tapping the same construct and are sufficiently discriminating.

J

Journal club: A formally organized group that meets periodically to share and critique contemporary research in nursing with a goal of both learning about the research process and finding evidence for practice.

Journal impact factor: A way to measure quality and impact of research by calculating a ratio of current citations of the article to all the citations in the same time period.

Judgmental sampling (purposive sampling): It is a type of nonprobable sampling method in which the researcher selects study participants who will be most representative based on personal judgment.

Justice: A basic principle of ethics that incorporates a participant's right to fair treatment and fairness in distribution of benefit and burden.

K

Kendall's tau: Nonparametric test used to determine correlations among variables that have been measured at the ordinal level.

Key informant: Person in an ethnographic study with extensive knowledge and influence in a culture with whom a researcher may form a close bond. They are valuable sources of information to a researcher.

Key words: Important variables or concepts of a research topic used to search data base.

Kurtosis: Degree of peakedness of the curve that is related to the spread or variance of scores.

L

Landmark studies: Major projects generating knowledge that influence a discipline and sometimes a society in general.

Leptokurtic: Term used to describe an extremely peaked shape distribution of a curve, which means that the scores in the distribution are similar and have limited variance.

Level of significance: It is a probability level at which the results of statistical analysis are judged to indicate a statistically significant difference between groups. The level of significance for most nursing studies is 0.05. It is the risk of making type-I error in statistical analysis established by the researcher beforehand.

Levels of measurement: A system of classifying measurements according to a set of rules for assigning numbers to objects so that a hierarchy in measurement from low to high is established. The levels of measurement are nominal, ordinal, interval, and ratio.

Likert scale: It is a scale designed to determine the opinions or attitudes of subjects involving the summation of scores on a set of statements that respondents rate for their degree of agreement or disagreement. It contains a number of statements with a scale after each statement.

Limitations: They are the shortcomings, conditions, or influences that cannot be controlled by the researcher. These place restrictions on methodology and conclusions and decrease the generalizability of the findings.

Line graphs: A graphic presentation that plots means for a variable over a period of time.

Linear relationship: Relationship between two variables that remains consistent regardless of the values of each variable.

Literature review: A critical summary of research on a topic of interest, often prepared to generate a picture of what is known and not known about a particular problem.

Longitudinal design: Research design used to examine changes in the same subjects at different points of time over an extended time period. It might also be referred to as repeated measures.

Low-statistical power (Type-II error): Statistical issue that decreases the probability of concluding that there is no significant difference between samples when there actually is a difference.

M

Manipulation: A treatment or intervention introduced by the researcher in an experimental or quasi-experimental study to assess its impact on the dependent variable.

Mann–Whitney U test: A nonparametric statistic used to test the difference between two independent groups based on ranked scores.

MANOVA (Multivariate Analysis of Variance): A statistical procedure used to test the significance of differences between the means of two or more groups on two or more dependent variables considered simultaneously.

Matching: The pairing of subjects in one group with those in another group based on their similarity on one or more dimensions to enhance the overall comparability of groups.

Maturation: Threatens validity because the changes that occur in subjects do not occur as a result of the intervention, but because time has passed.

McNemar test: A statistical test for comparing differences in proportions when values are derived from paired groups.

Mean: The average; measure of central tendency.

Measurement: The process of assigning numbers to objects or situations or events according to some rules.

Measurement error: Difference between what exists in reality (true score) and what is measured by a research instrument (observed score).

Median test: A nonparametric statistical test involving the comparison of median values of two independent groups to determine if the groups are from populations with different medians.

Median: A measure of central tendency that is the exact mid-point of the numbers of the data set.

Member checking: Checking the accuracy of the observations and conclusions directly with subjects.

Meta-analysis: Meta-analysis is a statistical method of aggregating the results of quantitative studies so that an overall effect size can be evaluated.

Metasynthesis: The theories, grand narratives, generalizations, or interpretive translations produced from the integration or comparison of findings from qualitative studies.

Method triangulation: A type of triangulation where multiple data collection methods are used, such as interviews, observation, and document view.

Micro theories: Precise theories that are much narrower in scope and usually related to a particular situation or set of circumstances in nursing practice.

Middle-range theories: Nursing theories located midway between abstract and concrete theories that are more limited in scope and address-specific phenomena or concepts.

Mixed methods: A research approach that combines quantitative and qualitative elements; it involves the description of the measurable state of a phenomenon and the individuals subjective response to it.

Mode: A measure of central tendency that is the most frequently occurring value in the data set.

Multiple regression analysis: A statistical procedure for understanding the simultaneous effects of two or more independent variables on a dependent variable.

Multistage sampling: A sampling strategy that proceeds through a set of stages from larger to smaller sampling units. For example, from states to nursing institutions, to nursing students.

Multivariate analysis: Analysis of the effects of an independent variable on two or more dependent variables simultaneously.

N

n: The symbol designating the number of subjects in a subgroup or cell of a study.

N: The symbol designating the total number of subjects.

Network sampling: The sampling of participants based on referrals from others already in the sample, also called snowball sampling.

Nominal data: Data that can be named and placed into categories but cannot be ranked or measured on a scale.

Nondirectional hypothesis: It is a statement that indicates the existence of a relationship between two variables, without predicting the exact nature (direction) of the relationship.

Nonequivalent comparison group before/after design: The strongest type of quasi-experimental design in which subject responses in two or more groups are measured before and after an intervention.

Nonequivalent comparison group post-test only: A type of quasi-experimental design in which data are collected after the intervention is introduced. Lack of baseline data may introduce extraneous variables in the results.

Nonexperimental research: Studies in which the researcher collects data without introducing any intervention.

Nonparametric tests: Statistical tests that have no assumptions about the distribution of the data.

Nonprobability sampling: The selection of sampling units from a population using nonrandom procedures as in convenience and quota sampling.

Normal distribution: A theoretical distribution that is bell-shaped and symmetrical also called a normal curve.

Novelty effect: Threatens validity because subjects react to something because it is novel or new and not to the actual treatment or intervention itself.

Null hypothesis: A hypothesis stating no relationship between the variables under study.

Nursing research: Systematic inquiry designed to develop knowledge about issues of importance to the nursing profession.

O

Objectivity: The extent to which two independent researchers would arrive at similar judgments or conclusions.

Observational research: Studies in which data are collected by observing and recording behaviors or activities relating to a phenomenon of interest.

Odds ratio: A ratio of one odds to another odds; used in logistic regression as a measure of association and as an estimate of relative risk.

One-tailed test: A test of statistical significance in which only values at one extreme of a distribution are considered in determining significance; used when the researcher can predict the direction of a relationship.

Open access: Publication in a form that allows anyone to have access to the material without constraints.

Open-ended question: A question with no predetermined set of responses.

Operational definition: Description of how variables or concepts will be measured or manipulated in a study.

Ordinal data: Categorical data that can be put in rank order. The scales used contain intervals between entries that vary, limiting statistical analyses and comparison across the scales or between subjects.

Outcome research: Research designed to document the effectiveness of healthcare services and the end results of patient care.

Outliers: Values that lie outside the normal range of values for other cases in a data set.

P

p value: In statistical testing, the probability that the obtained results are due to chance alone; the probability of committing a type-I error.

Paradigm: An overall belief system or way of viewing the nature of reality and the basis of knowledge.

Parameter: A characteristic of a population.

Parametric tests: Statistical tests that are appropriate for data that are normally distributed (fall in a bell curve).

Pearson's r: A widely used correlation coefficient designing the magnitude of relationship between two variables measured on at least an interval scale; also called the product moment correlation.

Peer review: The process of subjecting research to the appraisal of a neutral third party. Common process of peer review includes evaluation of research manuscripts for publication and presentation in conferences.

Phenomenological research: A qualitative research design that uses inductive descriptive methodology for the purpose of describing lived experiences of the study participants.

Phenomenology: Investigations of the meaning of an experience among a group that has lived through it.

Phenomenon: The abstract concept under study, most often used by qualitative researchers as an alternate to the term variable.

Phi coefficient: A statistical index describing the magnitude of relationship between two dichotomous variables.

Pilot study: Smaller version of a proposed study conducted to develop and refine the methodology, such as intervention, instruments, or data collection processes to be used in the larger study.

Placebo: In a psychology experiment, a placebo is an inert treatment or substance that has no known effects. Researchers might utilize a placebo control group, who are exposed to the placebo or fake independent variable.

Plagiarism: A type of scientific misconduct with appropriation of another person's ideas, processes, results or words without giving appropriate credit, including those obtained through confidential review of others research proposals and manuscripts.

Point estimate: A statistic derived from a sample that is used to represent a population parameter.

Population: The entire set of subjects that are of interest to the researcher.

Post hoc test: A test for comparing all possible pair of groups following a significant test of overall group differences.

Poster presentation: A research report presented as a visual display, so it can be read and viewed by a large group of professionals in an informal setting.

Post-test only design: An experimental design in which data are collected from subjects only after the experimental intervention has been introduced also called an after only design.

Power: An analysis that indicates how large a sample is needed to adequately detect a difference in the outcome variable.

Power analysis: A procedure for estimating either the likelihood of committing a type-II error or sample size requirements.

Precision: The degree of reproducibility or the generation of consistent values every time an instrument is used.

Predictive validity: A measurement of criterion-related validity that is indicated when an instrument can predict future performance.

Pre-experimental design: A research design that does not include mechanisms to compensate for the absence of either randomization or a control group.

Pretest: Collection of data prior to the experimental intervention; sometimes called baseline data.

Pretest–post-test design: An experimental design in which data are collected from research subjects both before and after introducing the experimental intervention also called a before–after design.

Prevalence study: A study undertaken to determine the prevalence rate of some condition at a particular point in time.

Primary data: Data collected directly from the subject for the purpose of the research study. Examples include surveys, questionnaires, observations, or physiological measures.

Primary sources: Original, peer reviewed, and published research journal articles of studies conducted by the researcher.

Principal investigator: The individual who is primarily responsible for all elements of the study and is the first author listed on publications or presentations.

Probability or random sampling: A sampling process used in quantitative research in which every member of the available population has an equal probability of being selected for the sample.

Probing: Eliciting more useful or detailed information from a respondent in an interview.

Problem statement: A statement of disparity between what is known and what needs to be known and addressed by the research.

Projective technique: A method of measuring psychological attribute by providing respondents with unstructured stimuli to which to respond.

Prolonged engagement: Investment of sufficient time in the data collection process so that the researcher gains an in-depth understanding of the culture, language, or views of the group under study.

Prospective studies: Studies planned by the researcher for collection of primary data for the specific research and implemented in the future.

Psychometric instruments: Instruments used to collect subjective information directly from subjects, tested for reliability and validity.

Psychometrics: A theory underlying principles of measurement and the application of the theory in the development of measuring tools.

Purposive sampling: A nonprobability sampling method in which the researcher selects participants based on personal judgment.

Q

Q-sort: A data collection method in which participants sort statements into a number of piles (usually 9 or 11) according to some bipolar dimension.

Qualitative analysis: Organization and interpretation of non-numerical data for the purpose of discovering important underlying dimensions and patterns of relationships.

Qualitative research: A naturalistic approach to research where the focus is on systematic and subjective methodological approach to understand the meaning of life experiences.

Quantitative analysis: The manipulation of numeric data through statistical procedures for the purpose of describing the phenomenon or assessing the magnitude and reliability of relationships among them.

Quantitative research: A traditional approach to research where the focus is on formal, objective, and systematic process to identify variables and measure them in a reliable and valid way.

Quasi-experimental research: A type of quantitative research design that lacks one of the components (randomization or control group) of true experimental design.

Questionnaire: Printed self-report form designed to elicit information that can be obtained through written or verbal responses of the subject.

Quota sampling: A nonrandom selection of participants in which the researcher prespecifies characteristics of the sample to increase its representativeness.

R

***r*:** The symbol typically used to designate a bivariate correlation coefficient, summarizing the magnitude and direction of a relationship between two variables.

***R*:** The symbol used to designate the multiple correlation coefficients indicating the magnitude of the relationship between the dependent variables and multiple independent variables taken together.

Random assignment: Assignment of subjects to treatment or control groups in a random manner.

Random number table: A table displaying hundreds of numbers composed of digits (0 to 9) in a random order. The digits in each number have no predictable relationship to the other digits that precede or succeed it in the number. In short, the digits are arranged randomly.

Random sampling: Techniques in which every member of the population has an equal probability of being included in the study.

Random selection: A method of choosing a random sample using mathematical probability to ensure the selection of subjects is completely objective.

Randomization: It is the process of assigning subjects to treatment conditions in a random manner.

Randomized block design: An experimental design involving two or more factors, only one of which is experimentally manipulated.

Randomized controlled trial (RCT): A typical experiment in which subjects are randomly assigned to groups, one of which gets an experimental treatment while another is a control group. The experiment has high internal validity so that the researcher can draw conclusions after the effects of treatments.

Range: A measure of variability that is the distance between the two most extreme values in the data set.

Rate: A calculated count derived from dividing the frequency of an event in a given time period by all possible occurrences of the event during the same time period.

Rating scale: A scale that lists an ordered series of categories of a variable and is assumed to be based on an underlying continuum.

Ratio data: Data measured on interval scales that have a true zero.

Raw data: Data in the form in which they were collected without being coded or analyzed.

Reactivity: A measurement distortion arising from the study participants awareness of being observed are more generally from the effect of the measurement procedure itself.

Refereed journal: A journal in which decisions about the acceptance of manuscripts are made based on recommendations from peer reviewers.

Reflexivity: Sensitivity to the ways in which the researcher and the research process have shaped the data; based on introspection and acknowledgement of bias.

Regression analysis: A statistical procedure for predicting values of a dependent variable based on the values of one or more independent variables.

Reliability: The degree of consistency or dependability with which an instrument measures the attribute it is designed to measure.

Repeated measures design: An experimental design in which one group of subjects is exposed to more than one condition or treatment in a random order also called a crossover design.

Replicability: The likelihood that qualitative research outcomes or events will happen given the same circumstances.

Replication: Repeating a specific study in detail on a different sample. When a study has been replicated several times and similar results are found, the evidence can be used with more confidence.

Representativeness: Degree to which the sample, accessible population, and target population are alike.

Research: The systematic inquiry that uses orderly, disciplined methods to answer questions or solve problems.

Research design: The overall approach to or outline of the study that details all the major components of the research.

Research hypothesis: Alternative hypothesis to null hypothesis; states that a relationship exists between two or more variables.

Research objective: Clear, concise, declarative statement expressed to direct a study; focuses on identifying and describing variables and relationships among variables.

Research question: Concise interrogative statement developed to direct a study; focuses on describing variables, examines relationships among variables, and determines the differences between two or more groups.

Research report: A report that summarizes the major elements of a study and identifies the contributions of that study to nursing knowledge.

Research utilization: It is the process of synthesizing, disseminating, and using research-generated knowledge to make an impact on or change in the existing nursing practice.

Research variable: The qualities, properties, or characteristics identified in the research purposes and objectives that are observed or measured in a study.

Respect for persons: A basic principle of ethics stating that individuals should be treated autonomously, as capable of making their own decisions. Persons with limited autonomy or who are not capable of making their own decisions should be protected.

Response rate: The rate of participation in a study calculated by, dividing the number of persons participating by the number of persons sampled.

Retrospective design: A study design begins with the manifestation of the dependent variable in the present and then searches for the presumed cause occurring in the past.

Rigor: Excellence in research attained through the use of discipline, scrupulous adherence to detail, and strict accuracy.

Risk–benefit ratio: The relative costs and benefits to an individual subject and to society at large on account of participation in a study; also the relative costs and benefits of implementing an innovation.

Robust tests: Statistical tests that are able to yield reliable results even if underlying assumptions are violated.

S

Sample: A carefully selected subset of the population that represents the composition of that population.

Sample frame: List of every member of the population.

Sample size: Number of subjects, events, behaviors, or situations that are examined in a study.

Sampling: A process of selecting a portion of the population to represent the entire population.

Sampling bias: Distortions that arise when a sample is not representative of the population from which it was drawn.

Sampling error: A statistical value that indicates differences in results found in the same sample when compared to the population from which the sample was drawn.

Sampling frame: A list of all the elements in the population from which the sample is drawn.

Saturation: The point at which no new information is being generated and the sample size is determined to be adequate.

Scale: A type of closed question format where respondents put responses in rank order on a continuum.

Scatter plots: A graphic presentation that indicates the nature of the relationship between two variables.

Search strategy: The identification of search terms and search statements that will be used in the literature review.

Search terms: Words or phrases derived from elements in the problem statement, characteristics of the population of interest, and the theoretical framework that are used to conduct the literature search.

Secondary analysis: A form of research in which the data collected by one researcher are reanalyzed by another investigator to answer new research questions.

Secondary data collection: Data collected for other purposes but used in the current research study. Examples include patient medical records, employee or patient satisfaction surveys, organizational business reports, or governmental databases.

Secondary sources: Comments and summaries of multiple research studies on one topic such as systematic reviews, meta-analysis, and meta-syntheses, which are based on the secondary author's interpretation of the primary work.

Selection bias: A condition that occurs when subjects are selected for the study or assigned in groups in a way that is not impartial. This may pose a threat to validity of the study.

Self-report: A method of collecting data that involves a direct report of information by the person who is being studied.

Semistructured interview: An interview in which the researcher has listed topics to cover rather than specific questions to ask.

Sensitivity: A measure of discriminate validity in biomedical sciences, which indicates that an instrument has the capacity to detect a disease, if present.

Setting: The physical location and conditions in which data collection takes place in a study.

Sign test: A nonparametric test for comparing two paired groups based on the relative ranking of values between the pairs.

Significance level: The probability that an observed relationship could be caused by chance; significance at the 0.05 level indicates the probability that a relationship of the observed magnitude would be found by chance only 5 times out of 100.

Simple random sampling: A probability sampling technique, wherein sampling frame is created by listing all members of a population and then selecting a sample from it using random procedures.

Skewness: Absence of symmetry in the curve formed by the distribution of scores; distribution can be positively or negatively skewed.

Snowball sampling: A nonprobability sampling method that relies on referrals from the initial subjects to recruit additional subjects. This method is best used for studies involving subjects who possess sensitive characteristics.

Solomon four-group design: An experimental design that uses a before–after design for one pair of experimental and control groups and an after only design for a second pair.

Spearman's rank–order correlation (Spearman's rho): A correlation coefficient indicating the magnitude of a relationship between variables measured on the ordinal scale.

Specificity: A measure of discriminate validity in biomedical sciences, which indicates that an instrument has the capacity to differentiate when the disease is not present.

Split-half technique: A method to estimate the internal consistency of, the reliability of a test by correlating scores on half of the instrument with scores on the other half.

Stability: Type of measurement reliability that is concerned with the consistency of repeated measure; usually referred to as test–retest reliability.

Standard deviation: The most easily interpreted measure of variability of scores around the mean; represents the average amount of variation of data points about the mean.

Standard error: The error that arises from the sampling procedure; directly affected by variability and sample size.

Standard normal distribution: A bell-shaped distribution in which the mean is set at zero and a standard deviation at one.

Standardized scores: A measure of position that expresses the distance from the mean of single score in standard terms.

Statistical power: The ability of the research design to detect true relationships among variables.

Statistically significant: Differences between groups exceed standard error, the probability that differences are due to chance are less than 5%.

Stratified random sampling: It is a type of random sampling technique used when the researcher knows that some of the variables in the population are critical to achieving representativeness. In this technique, sample is divided into strata or groups and participants selected randomly from each strata.

Survey research: A nonexperimental research design in which information is obtained on activities, beliefs, preferences, and attitude of people through direct questioning of a sample of respondents.

Systematic bias: It is a phenomenon that occurs when the characteristics/measurement values of selected subjects vary in some way from those of the population.

Systematic error: A bias in measurement that is consistent but not accurate and that underestimates, overestimates, or misses data in a way that is not random.

Systematic review: A systematic review is a highly structured and controlled search of the available literature that minimizes the potential for bias and produces a practice recommendation as an outcome.

Systematic sampling: Selecting every K^{th} individual from an ordered list of all members of a population, using a randomly selected starting point.

T

Target population: Population determined by the sampling criteria.

Test blueprint: An outline for determining content validity that includes the analysis of basic content and the assessment objectives.

Test–retest reliability: Determination of the stability or consistency of a measurement technique by correlating the scores obtained from repeated measures.

Test statistic: A calculation of differences in group values compared to standard error.

Testing: Threatens validity due to the familiarity of the subjects with the testing, particularly when retesting is used in a study.

Themes: Implicit, recurring, and unifying ideas derived from the raw data in qualitative research.

Theoretical framework: Collection of interrelated concepts that depict a piece of theory that is to be examined as the basis for research study. These are the foundations that guide the research.

Theoretical sampling: Selecting additional members for the sample, often based on loosened inclusion criteria, to ensure divergent opinions are heard; a requirement for grounded theory development.

Theory triangulation: A type of triangulation where multiple perspectives from other researchers or published literature are obtained and used.

Theory: A method of perceiving reality and mapping the complex processes of human action and interaction that affect nursing care.

Therapeutic research: Studies in which the subject can be expected to receive a potentially beneficial treatment.

Thesis: Research project completed by a graduate student as a part of the requirements for a master's degree.

Time series design: A type of quasi-experimental design that involves one group that receives the intervention and outcome is measured overtime.

Transferability: Ability of qualitative research findings to apply in other settings or situations.

Triangulation: It refers to combining different methods to collect the data on the same concept by cross-checking information and conclusions using multiple data sources, research methods, theories, or researchers to improve the credibility and interpret the data.

Trustworthiness: Strength of a qualitative study determined by evaluating all study aspects.

t-test: A parametric statistical test for analyzing the difference between two means.

Two-tailed test: A statistical test in which both ends of the sampling distribution are used to determine improbable values.

Type-I error: It occurs when the researcher rejects the null hypothesis when it is true (incorrect rejection of a true null hypothesis). In reality, there is no relationship between variables or differences between group responses to the intervention but the researcher claims there is (false positive). Thus a type-I error occurs when the researcher concludes that a relationship exists while it actually does not.

Type-II error: It occurs when the intervention is effective or there is a relationship among the variables and the researcher concludes there is not, i.e. the intervention works but the researcher claims it does not. Here, null hypothesis is false but the researcher fails to reject it (false negative). In other words, it occurs when the researcher rejects the alternative hypothesis while it actually is true. Examples of type-II error would be—a laboratory investigation fails to detect a disease while the patient really has the disease; or a treatment or intervention failing to show that the treatment works when it really does.

U

Unimodal distribution: A distribution of values with one peak.

Univariate analysis: Analysis of a single variable in descriptive statistics or a single dependent variable in inferential analysis.

Unstructured interview: An oral self-report in which the researcher poses questions to a respondent without having a predetermined plan regarding the content or flow of information to be gathered.

Unstructured observation: Spontaneous observation and recording of what is seen. In this, the process of observation planning is minimal.

V

Validity: The degree to which an instrument measures what it is intended to measure.

Variable: Qualities, properties or characteristics of persons, things, or situations that change or vary and are manipulated or measured in research.

Variance: A measure of variability that gives information about the spread of scores around the mean.

Visual analog scale (VAS): A rating type scale where respondents mark location on the scale corresponding to their perception of a phenomenon on a continuum.

Vulnerable populations: Groups of people with diminished autonomy who cannot participate fully in the consent process. Such groups may include children, individuals with cognitive disorders, prisoners, and pregnant women.

W

Wilcoxon signed ranks test: A nonparametric statistical test for comparing two paired groups based on the relative ranking of values between the pairs.

Within subjects design: A research design in which a single group of subjects is compared under different conditions or at different points in time.

Z

Z-score: A standard score ranging from −3SD to +3SD that can be placed on a normal distribution curve, usually expressed as a number of standard deviations from the mean a data point is. Simply put, it is the measure of how many standard deviations below or above the population mean a raw score is. It can be arrived by knowing the mean μ and the population standard deviation σ.

Appendices

Appendix 1: Distribution of *t*-Probability

	Level of significance for one-tailed test					
	.10	.05	.025	.01	.005	.0005
	Level of significance for two-tailed test					
df	.20	.10	.05	.02	.01	.001
1	3.078	6.314	12.706	31.821	63.657	636.619
2	1.886	2.920	4.303	6.965	9.925	31.598
3	1.638	2.353	3.182	4.541	5.841	12.941
4	1.533	2.132	2.776	3.747	4.604	8.610
5	1.476	2.015	2.571	3.376	4.032	6.859
6	1.440	1.953	2.447	3.143	3.707	5.959
7	1.415	1.895	2.365	2.998	3.449	5.405
8	1.397	1.860	2.306	2.896	3.355	5.041
9	1.383	1.833	2.262	2.821	3.250	4.781
10	1.372	1.812	2.228	2.765	3.169	4.587
11	1.363	1.796	2.201	2.718	3.106	4.437
12	1.356	1.782	2.179	2.681	3.055	4.318
13	1.350	1.771	2.160	2.650	3.012	4.221
14	1.345	1.761	2.145	2.624	2.977	4.140
15	1.341	1.753	2.131	2.602	2.947	4.073
16	1.337	1.746	2.120	2.583	2.921	4.015
17	1.333	1.740	2.110	2.567	2.898	3.965
18	1.330	1.734	2.101	2.552	2.878	3.922
19	1.328	1.729	2.093	2.539	2.861	3.883
20	1.325	1.725	2.086	2.528	2.845	3.850
21	1.323	1.721	2.080	2.518	2.831	3.819
22	1.321	1.717	2.074	2.508	2.819	3.792
23	1.319	1.714	2.069	2.500	2.807	3.767
24	1.318	1.711	2.064	2.492	2.797	3.745
25	1.316	1.708	2.060	2.485	2.787	3.725
26	1.315	1.706	2.056	2.479	2.779	3.707
27	1.314	1.703	2.052	2.473	2.771	3.690
28	1.313	1.701	2.048	2.467	2.763	3.674
29	1.311	1.699	2.045	2.462	2.756	3.659
30	1.310	1.697	2.042	2.457	2.750	3.646
40	1.303	1.684	2.021	2.423	2.704	3.551
60	1.296	1.671	2.000	2.390	2.660	3.460
120	1.289	1.658	1.980	2.358	2.617	3.373
∞	1.282	1.645	1.960	2.326	2.576	3.291

Appendix 2: Significant Values of F

	$\alpha = .05$ (Two-tailed)								$\alpha = .025$ (One-tailed)	
$\dfrac{df_B}{df_W}$	1	2	3	4	5	6	8	12	24	∞
1	161.4	199.5	215.7	224.6	230.2	234.0	238.9	243.9	249.0	254.3
2	18.51	19.00	19.16	19.25	19.30	19.33	19.37	19.41	19.45	19.50
3	10.13	9.55	9.28	9.12	9.01	8.94	8.84	8.74	8.64	8.53
4	7.71	6.94	6.59	6.39	6.26	6.16	6.04	5.91	5.77	5.63
5	6.61	5.79	5.41	5.19	5.05	4.95	4.82	4.68	4.53	4.36
6	5.99	5.14	4.76	4.53	4.39	4.28	4.15	4.00	3.84	3.67
7	5.59	4.74	4.35	4.12	3.97	3.87	3.73	3.57	3.41	3.23
8	5.32	4.46	4.07	3.84	3.69	3.58	3.44	3.28	3.12	2.93
9	5.12	4.26	3.86	3.63	3.48	3.37	3.23	3.07	2.90	2.71
10	4.96	4.10	3.71	3.48	3.33	3.22	3.07	2.91	2.74	2.54
11	4.84	3.98	3.59	3.36	3.20	3.09	2.95	2.79	2.61	2.40
12	4.75	3.88	3.49	3.26	3.11	3.00	2.85	2.69	2.50	2.30
13	4.67	3.80	3.41	3.18	3.02	2.92	2.77	2.60	2.42	2.21
14	4.60	3.74	3.34	3.11	2.96	2.85	2.70	2.53	2.35	2.13
15	4.54	3.68	3.29	3.06	2.90	2.79	2.64	2.48	2.29	2.07
16	4.49	3.63	3.24	3.01	2.85	2.74	2.59	2.42	2.24	2.01
17	4.45	3.59	3.20	2.96	2.81	2.70	2.55	2.38	2.19	1.96
18	4.41	3.55	3.16	2.93	2.77	2.66	2.51	2.34	2.15	1.92
19	4.38	3.52	3.13	2.90	2.74	2.63	2.48	2.31	2.11	1.88
20	4.35	3.49	3.10	2.87	2.71	2.60	2.45	2.28	2.08	1.84
21	4.32	3.47	3.07	2.84	2.68	2.57	2.42	2.25	2.05	1.81
22	4.30	3.44	3.05	2.82	2.66	2.55	2.40	2.23	2.03	1.78
23	4.28	3.42	3.03	2.80	2.64	2.53	2.38	2.20	2.00	1.76
24	4.26	3.40	3.01	2.78	2.62	2.51	2.36	2.18	1.98	1.73
25	4.24	3.38	2.99	2.76	2.60	2.49	2.34	2.16	1.96	1.71
26	4.22	3.37	2.98	2.74	2.59	2.47	2.32	2.15	1.95	1.69
27	4.21	3.35	2.96	2.73	2.57	2.46	2.30	2.13	1.93	1.67
28	4.20	3.34	2.95	2.71	2.56	2.44	2.29	2.12	1.91	1.65
29	4.18	3.33	2.93	2.70	2.54	2.43	2.28	2.10	1.90	1.64
30	4.17	3.32	2.92	2.69	2.53	2.42	2.27	2.09	1.89	1.62
40	4.08	3.23	2.84	2.61	2.45	2.34	2.18	2.00	1.79	1.51
60	4.00	3.15	2.76	2.52	2.37	2.25	2.10	1.92	1.70	1.39
120	3.92	3.07	2.68	2.45	2.29	2.17	2.02	1.83	1.61	1.25
∞	3.84	2.99	2.60	2.37	2.21	2.09	1.94	1.75	1.52	1.00

Contd...

Appendix 2: Significant Values of F (contd...)

	α = .01 (Two-tailed)									α = .005 (One-tailed)	
$\frac{df_B}{df_W}$	1	2	3	4	5	6	8	12	24	∞
1	4052	4999	5403	5625	5764	5859	5981	6106	6234	6366
2	98.49	99.00	99.17	99.25	99.30	99.33	99.36	99.42	99.46	99.50
3	34.12	30.81	29.46	28.71	28.24	27.91	27.49	27.05	26.60	26.12
4	21.20	18.00	16.69	15.98	15.52	15.21	14.80	14.37	13.93	13.46
5	16.26	13.27	12.06	11.39	10.97	10.67	10.29	9.89	9.47	9.02
6	13.74	10.92	9.78	9.15	8.75	8.47	8.10	7.72	7.31	6.88
7	12.25	9.55	8.45	7.85	7.46	7.19	6.84	6.47	6.07	5.65
8	11.26	8.65	7.59	7.01	6.63	6.37	6.03	5.67	5.28	4.86
9	10.56	8.02	6.99	6.42	6.06	5.80	5.47	5.11	4.73	4.31
10	10.04	7.56	6.55	5.99	5.64	5.39	5.06	4.71	4.33	3.91
11	9.65	7.20	6.22	5.67	5.32	5.07	4.74	4.40	4.02	3.60
12	9.33	6.93	5.95	5.41	5.06	4.82	4.50	4.16	3.78	3.36
13	9.07	6.70	5.74	5.20	4.86	4.62	4.30	3.96	3.59	3.16
14	8.86	6.51	5.56	5.03	4.69	4.46	4.14	3.80	3.43	3.00
15	8.68	6.36	5.42	4.89	4.56	4.32	4.00	3.67	3.29	2.87
16	8.53	6.23	5.29	4.77	4.44	4.20	3.89	3.55	3.18	2.75
17	8.40	6.11	5.18	4.67	4.34	4.10	3.78	3.45	3.08	2.65
18	8.28	6.01	5.09	4.58	4.29	4.01	3.71	3.37	3.00	2.57
19	8.18	5.93	5.01	4.50	4.17	3.94	3.63	3.30	2.92	2.49
20	8.10	5.85	4.94	4.43	4.10	3.87	3.56	3.23	2.86	2.42
21	8.02	5.78	4.87	4.37	4.04	3.81	3.51	3.17	2.80	2.36
22	7.94	5.72	4.82	4.31	3.99	3.76	3.45	3.12	2.75	2.31
23	7.88	5.66	4.76	4.26	3.94	3.71	3.41	3.07	2.70	2.26
24	7.82	5.61	4.72	4.22	3.90	3.67	3.36	3.03	2.66	2.21
25	7.77	5.57	4.68	4.18	3.86	3.63	3.32	2.99	2.62	2.17
26	7.72	5.53	4.64	4.14	3.82	3.59	3.29	2.96	2.58	2.13
27	7.68	5.49	4.60	4.11	3.78	3.56	3.26	2.93	2.55	2.10
28	7.64	5.45	4.57	4.07	3.75	3.53	3.23	2.90	2.52	2.06
29	7.60	5.42	4.54	4.04	3.73	3.50	3.20	2.87	2.49	2.03
30	7.56	5.39	4.51	4.02	3.70	3.47	3.17	2.84	2.47	2.01
40	7.31	5.18	4.31	3.83	3.51	3.29	2.99	2.66	2.29	1.80
60	7.08	4.98	4.13	3.65	3.34	3.12	2.82	2.50	2.12	1.60
120	6.85	4.79	3.95	3.48	3.17	2.96	2.66	2.34	1.95	1.38
∞	6.64	4.60	3.78	3.32	3.02	2.80	2.61	2.18	1.79	1.00

Contd...

Appendix 2: **Significant Values of F** *(contd…)*

	α = .001 (Two-tailed)								α = .0005 (One-tailed)	
df_B / df_w	1	2	3	4	5	6	8	12	24	∞
1	405284	500000	540379	562500	576405	585937	598144	610667	623497	636619
2	998.5	999.0	999.2	999.2	999.3	999.3	999.4	999.4	999.5	999.5
3	167.5	148.5	141.1	137.1	134.6	132.8	130.6	128.3	125.9	123.5
4	74.14	61.25	56.18	53.44	51.71	50.53	49.00	47.41	45.77	44.05
5	47.04	36.61	33.20	31.09	29.75	28.84	27.64	26.42	25.14	23.78
6	35.51	27.00	23.70	21.09	20.81	20.03	19.03	17.99	16.89	15.75
7	29.22	21.69	18.77	17.19	16.21	15.52	14.63	13.71	12.73	11.69
8	25.42	18.49	15.83	14.39	13.49	12.86	17.04	11.19	10.30	9.34
9	22.86	16.39	13.90	12.56	11.71	11.13	10.37	9.57	8.72	7.81
10	21.04	14.91	12.55	11.28	10.48	9.92	9.20	8.45	7.64	6.76
11	19.69	13.81	11.56	10.35	9.58	9.05	8.35	7.63	6.85	6.00
12	18.64	12.97	10.80	9.63	8.89	8.38	7.71	7.00	6.25	5.42
13	17.81	12.31	10.21	9.07	8.35	7.86	7.21	6.52	5.78	4.97
14	17.14	11.78	9.73	8.62	7.92	7.43	6.80	6.13	5.41	4.60
15	16.59	11.34	9.34	8.25	7.57	7.09	6.47	5.81	5.10	4.31
16	16.12	10.97	9.00	7.94	7.27	6.81	6.19	5.55	4.85	4.06
17	15.72	10.66	8.73	7.68	7.02	6.56	5.96	5.32	4.63	3.85
18	15.38	10.39	8.49	7.46	6.81	6.35	5.76	5.13	4.45	3.67
19	15.08	10.16	8.28	7.26	6.61	6.18	5.59	4.97	4.29	3.52
20	14.82	9.95	8.10	7.10	6.46	6.02	5.44	4.82	4.15	3.38
21	14.59	9.77	7.94	6.95	6.32	5.88	5.31	4.70	4.03	3.26
22	14.38	9.61	7.80	6.81	6.19	5.76	5.19	4.58	3.92	3.15
23	14.19	9.47	7.67	6.69	6.08	5.65	5.09	4.48	3.82	3.05
24	14.03	9.34	7.55	6.59	5.98	5.55	4.99	4.39	3.74	2.97
25	13.88	9.22	7.45	6.49	5.88	5.46	4.91	4.31	3.66	2.89
26	13.74	9.12	7.36	6.41	5.80	5.38	4.83	4.24	3.59	2.82
27	13.61	9.02	7.27	6.33	5.73	5.31	4.76	4.17	3.52	2.75
28	13.50	8.93	7.19	6.25	5.66	5.24	4.69	4.11	3.46	2.70
29	13.39	8.85	7.12	6.19	5.59	5.18	4.64	4.05	3.41	2.64
30	13.29	8.77	7.05	6.12	5.53	5.12	4.58	4.00	3.36	2.59
40	12.61	8.25	6.60	5.70	5.13	4.73	4.21	3.64	3.01	2.23
60	11.97	7.76	6.17	5.31	4.76	4.37	3.87	3.31	2.69	1.90
120	11.38	7.31	5.79	4.95	4.42	4.04	3.55	3.02	2.40	1.56
∞	10.83	6.91	5.42	4.62	4.10	3.74	3.27	2.74	2.13	1.00

Appendix 3: Distribution of χ^2 Probability

df	Level of significance				
	.10	.05	.02	.01	.001
1	2.71	3.84	5.41	6.63	10.83
2	4.61	5.99	7.82	9.21	13.82
3	6.25	7.82	9.84	11.34	16.27
4	7.78	9.49	11.67	13.28	18.46
5	9.24	11.07	13.39	15.09	20.52
6	10.64	12.59	15.03	16.81	22.46
7	12.02	14.07	16.62	18.48	24.32
8	13.36	15.51	18.17	20.09	26.12
9	14.68	16.92	19.68	21.67	27.88
10	15.99	18.31	21.16	23.21	29.59
11	17.28	19.68	22.62	24.72	31.26
12	18.55	21.03	24.05	26.22	32.91
13	19.81	22.36	25.47	27.69	34.53
14	21.06	23.68	26.87	29.14	36.12
15	22.31	25.00	28.26	30.58	37.70
16	23.54	26.30	29.63	32.00	39.25
17	24.77	27.59	31.00	33.41	40.79
18	25.99	28.87	32.35	34.81	42.31
19	27.20	30.14	33.69	36.19	43.82
20	28.41	31.41	35.02	37.57	45.32
21	29.62	32.67	36.34	38.93	46.80
22	30.81	33.92	37.66	40.29	48.27
23	32.01	35.17	38.97	41.64	49.73
24	33.20	36.42	40.27	42.98	51.18
25	34.38	37.65	41.57	44.31	52.62
26	35.56	38.89	42.86	45.64	54.05
27	36.74	40.11	44.14	46.96	55.48
28	37.92	41.34	45.42	48.28	56.89
29	39.09	42.56	46.69	49.59	58.30
30	40.26	43.77	47.96	50.89	59.70

Appendix 4: Significant Values of the Correlation Coefficient

	Level of significance for one-tailed test				
	.05	.025	.01	.005	.0005
	Level of significance for two-tailed test				
df	.10	.05	.02	.01	.001
1	.98769	.99692	.999507	.999877	.9999988
2	.90000	.95000	.98000	.990000	.99900
3	.8054	.8783	.93433	.95873	.99116
4	.7293	.8114	.8822	.91720	.97406
5	.6694	.7545	.8329	.8745	.95074
6	.6215	.7067	.7887	.8343	.92493
7	.5822	.6664	.7498	.7977	.8982
8	.5494	.6319	.7155	.7646	.8721
9	.5214	.6021	.6851	.7348	.8471
10	.4973	.5760	.6581	.7079	.8233
11	.4762	.5529	.6339	.6835	.8010
12	.4575	.5324	.6120	.6614	.7800
13	.4409	.5139	.5923	.5411	.7603
14	.4259	.4973	.5742	.6226	.7420
15	.4124	.4821	.5577	.6055	.7246
16	.4000	.4683	.5425	.5897	.7084
17	.3887	.4555	.5285	.5751	.6932
18	.3783	.4438	.5155	.5614	.5687
19	.3687	.4329	.5034	.5487	.6652
20	.3598	.4227	.4921	.5368	.6524
25	.3233	.3809	.4451	.5869	.5974
30	.2960	.3494	.4093	.4487	.5541
35	.2746	.3246	.3810	.4182	.5189
40	.2573	.3044	.3578	.3932	.4896
45	.2428	.2875	.3384	.3721	.4648
50	.2306	.2732	.3218	.3541	.4433
60	.2108	.2500	.2948	.3248	.4078
70	.1954	.2319	.2737	.3017	.3799
80	.1829	.2172	.2565	.2830	.3568
90	.1726	.2050	.2422	.2673	.3375
100	.1638	.1946	.2301	.2540	.3211

Appendix 5: Mann-Whitney U Test Table

N_1 \ N_2	5	6	7	8	9	10	11	12	13	14	15	16	17	18	19	20
5	2	3	5	6	7	8	9	11	12	13	14	15	17	18	19	20
6	3	5	6	8	10	11	13	14	16	17	19	21	22	24	25	27
7	5	6	8	10	12	14	16	18	20	22	24	26	28	30	32	34
8	6	8	10	13	15	17	19	22	24	26	29	31	34	36	38	41
9	7	10	12	15	17	20	23	26	28	31	34	37	39	42	45	48
10	8	11	14	17	20	23	26	29	33	36	39	42	45	48	52	55
11	9	13	16	19	23	26	30	33	37	40	44	47	51	55	58	62
12	11	14	18	22	26	29	33	37	41	45	49	53	57	61	65	69
13	12	16	20	24	28	33	37	41	45	50	54	59	63	67	72	76
14	13	17	22	26	31	36	40	45	50	55	59	64	67	74	78	83
15	14	19	24	29	34	39	44	49	54	59	64	70	75	80	85	90
16	15	21	26	31	37	42	47	53	59	64	70	75	81	86	92	98
17	17	22	28	34	39	45	51	57	63	67	75	81	87	93	99	105
18	18	24	30	36	42	48	55	61	67	74	80	86	93	99	106	112
19	19	25	32	38	45	52	58	65	72	78	85	92	99	106	113	119
20	20	27	34	41	48	55	62	69	72'	83	90	98	105	112	119	127

Appendix 6: Table of Critical Values for the Wilcoxon Test

To use this table: Compare the obtained value of Wilcoxon's test statistic to the critical value in the table (taking into account N, the number of subjects). The obtained value is statistically significant if it is *equal* to or *smaller* than the value in the table.

Example: Suppose the obtained value is 22, and the number of participants is 15. The critical value in the table is 25: the obtained value is *smaller* than this, so one can conclude that the difference between the two conditions in the study was unlikely to occur by chance (p<.05 two-tailed test, or p<.025, one-tailed test).

n	Two-tailed test		One-tailed test	
	$\alpha = .05$	$\alpha = .01$	$\alpha = .05$	$\alpha = .01$
5	—	—	0	—
6	0	—	2	—
7	2	—	3	0
8	3	0	5	1
9	5	1	8	3
10	8	3	10	5
11	10	5	13	7
12	13	7	17	9
13	17	9	21	12
14	21	12	25	15
15	25	15	30	19
16	29	19	35	23
17	34	23	41	27
18	40	27	47	32
19	46	32	53	37
20	52	37	60	43
21	58	42	67	49
22	65	48	75	55
23	73	54	83	62
24	81	61	91	69
25	89	68	100	76
26	98	75	110	84
27	107	83	119	92
28	116	91	130	101
29	126	100	140	110
30	137	109	151	120

Appendix 7: Table of Random Numbers

36518	36777	89116	05542	29705	83775	21564	81639	27973	62413	85652	62817	57881
46132	81380	75635	19428	88048	08747	20092	12615	35046	67753	69630	10883	13683
31841	77367	40791	97402	27569	90184	02338	39318	54936	34641	95525	86316	87384
84180	93793	64953	51472	65358	23701	75230	47200	78176	85248	90589	74567	22633
78435	37586	07015	98729	76703	16224	97661	79907	06611	26501	93389	92725	68158
41859	94198	37182	61345	88857	53204	86721	59613	67494	17292	94457	89520	77771
13019	07274	51068	93129	40386	51731	44254	66685	72835	01270	42523	45323	63481
82448	72430	29041	59208	95266	33978	70958	60017	39723	00606	17956	19024	15819
25432	96593	83112	96997	55340	80312	78839	09815	16887	22228	06206	54272	83516
69226	38655	03811	08342	47863	02743	11547	38250	58140	98470	24364	99797	73498
25837	68821	66426	20496	84843	18360	91252	99134	48931	99538	21160	09411	44659
38914	82707	24769	72026	56813	49336	71767	04474	32909	74162	50404	68562	14088
04070	60681	64290	26905	65617	76039	91657	71362	32246	49595	50663	47459	57072
01674	14751	28637	86980	11951	10479	41454	48527	53868	37846	85912	15156	00865
70294	35450	39982	79503	34382	43186	69890	63222	30110	56004	04879	05138	57476
73903	98066	52136	89925	50000	96334	30773	80571	31178	52799	41050	76298	43995
87789	56408	77107	88452	80975	03406	36114	64549	79244	82044	00202	45727	35709
92320	95929	58545	70699	07679	23296	03002	63885	54677	55745	52540	62154	33314
46391	60276	92061	43591	42118	73094	53608	58949	42927	90993	46795	05947	01934
67090	45063	84584	66022	48268	74971	94861	61749	61085	81758	89640	39437	90044
11666	99916	35165	29420	73213	15275	62532	47319	39842	62273	94980	23415	64668
40910	59068	04594	94576	51187	54796	17411	56123	66545	82163	61868	22752	40101
41169	37965	47578	92180	05257	19143	77486	02457	00985	31960	39033	44374	28352

Appendix 8: Model Information Sheet for Research Participants and Consent Form

Investigator:

Contact details of the investigator: Address, phone number, e-mail ID.

The study aims to explore the wellbeing, quality of life, functional impairment of depressive patients and to develop and evaluate the effectiveness of a psychosocial group intervention based on the body-mind-spirit model approach. The findings from this study will be used to inform nursing practice and to ultimately improve quality of patient care.

What does participation in this study involve?

Participants will be asked to complete questionnaires that ask about their level of depression, wellbeing, quality of life, and functional impairment. These questionnaires will take approximately 30 minutes to complete. The investigator will assist you in completion of the questionnaire, if required. Participants in control group will receive routine care in the hospital and experimental group will receive group sessions for one month (one session per week), each session lasting for 150–180 minutes. Same questionnaires will be administered at 1-month, 2-month, 3-month and 6-month interval.

Consent to participate

I seek your consent to participate in this study. You are not under any obligation to consent to participate in this study. Taking part in this study is entirely voluntary. Non-participation will not affect any current or future care given.

Risk

There is no anticipated risk to your being involved in this study. The investigator is an experienced mental health nurse and will not place you under any pressure to complete the questionnaire or attend sessions.

Confidentiality

The data collected from this study will be reported in general terms and will not involve any identity names. All data will be kept confidential.

You can contact the investigator at any given time if you have any matter of concern regarding the research that you wish to discuss.

Contact details of the investigator:

Consent Form for Participation (Experimental Group Subjects)

I state that I am willing to participate in the study "Efficacy of Body-Mind-Spirit group intervention for depressive patients at a selected hospital" being conducted by ....

I have been explained that:
- This research is to investigate the efficacy of Body-mind-spirit intervention among depressive patients.
- I will undergo an assessment at the beginning of the study which will approximately take 30 minutes.
- The assessment questionnaire is anonymous and I do not have to provide my name.
- I will then be administered Body-Mind-Spirit Group Intervention over a period of 4-weeks (one session per week).
- I will undergo post-assessment at 1-month, 2-month, 3-month and 6-month interval.

I have been further explained that:
- Whatever information I provide will be used only for the study purpose and kept in strict confidence.
- I can approach the *investigator* for professional assistance at any point during the study; I also have the right to seek clarification about the study procedures at any point of time.
- I can withdraw my participation at any time during the study if I so desire.
- There will be no loss of benefit, treatment or penalty levied as a result of withdrawal.
- Any reports or publications resulting from this study will be reported in general terms and will not involve my being identified.

I have fully read the information sheet and understood the contents of the consent form. I agree to participate in this study and hereby give my free consent.

Date   Participant   Investigator

Consent Form for Participation (Control Group Subjects)

I state that I am willing to participate in the study "Efficacy of Body-Mind-Spirit group intervention for depressive patients at a selected hospital" being conducted by ....

I have been explained that:
- This research is to investigate the efficacy of Body-mind-spirit intervention among depressive patients.
- I will undergo an assessment at the beginning of the study which will approximately take 30 minutes.
- The assessment questionnaire is anonymous and I do not have to provide my name.
- I will then be administered routine care in the hospital.
- I will undergo post-assessment at 1-month, 2-month, 3-month and 6-month interval.

I have been further explained that:
- Whatever information I provide will be used only for the study purpose and kept in strict confidence.
- I can approach the investigator for professional assistance at any point during the study; I also have the right to seek clarification about the study procedures at any point of time.
- I can withdraw my participation at any time during the study if I so desire.
- There will be no loss of benefit, treatment or penalty levied as a result of withdrawal.
- Any reports or publications resulting from this study will be reported in general terms and will not involve my being identified.

I have fully read the information sheet and understood the contents of the consent form. I agree to participate in this study and hereby give my free consent.

Date   Participant   Investigator

Appendix 9: Model Letter to Institutional Ethics Committee

From
....
....

To
Chairperson/Member Secretary
Institutional Ethics Committee
....

Sir,
Sub: Ethical clearance for the research project entitled "..."

UNDERTAKING

With respect to the above said Research Project involving human subjects for which the ethical clearance is being sought, I am to state that I have gone through the "Institutional ethical guide lines ......" and am aware of rules governing the studies involving the human subjects. I am also aware that these guidelines are strictly to be followed while carrying out the above said research project involving human subjects.

Further, I also affirm that I will be responsible to keep the IEC informed of,
  i. Any serious and unexpected adverse events and remedial steps taken to tackle them.
  ii. Any new information that may influence the conduct of the study.
  iii. Any changes made in the consent form
  iv. In the event of need to amend the original protocol approved by the EC, the proposed amendment shall be brought to the notice of EC for its consideration and approval. Under no circumstances shall I/we deviate from the original approved protocol without prior consent to that effect from the IEC.

Date: Name and signature of the Principal Investigator

Appendix 10: Model Summary Sheet of the Research Project Submitted to the Institutional Ethics Committee

1.	Title of the project	
2.	Principal Investigators and their department(s)	
	Co-Investigators and their department(s)	
3.	Funded or non funded project? If yes, name of the funding agency (Government, private, foreign) Is the project being submitted for funding?	
4.	Are human subjects involved in the study?	
5.	Does the study involve healthy volunteers/vulnerable population	
6.	Type of study	
7.	Is the submission in IES format? (not the format of the funding agency)	
8.	Does the study involve any invasive procedures? If yes, list the procedures and the possible risk a. Greater than minimal b. Not more than minimal risk c. No risk d. Only part of the diagnostic test	
9.	Detail the measures taken for reducing the risk	
10.	Does the research/study involve:	
	a. Human exposure to infectious agents? b. Investigational new drug? c. New treatment regime? d. Use of new vaccines? e. Observation of public behavior? f. Pathological or diagnostic clinical specimen only? (Mention source...)	
11.	Is the informed consent form attached?	
12.	Does the informed consent form address the following: a. Provide adequate information in a layman language to the patient/surrogate? b. Are invasive procedures and possible risks adequately explained? c. Are financial implications explained to the patient/caregiver? d. If subject is minor, is there an appropriate assent form? e. Is the course of action, in case, any abnormalities are detected during the investigation, clearly spelt out? f. Is provision for the subject to opt out of the study made explicitly? g. Is confidentiality of the subjects' data assured?	
	h. If major risks are involved, is mechanism of compensation for any injury suffered? (e.g. insurance) clearly spelt out? i. Are the contact details of the investigator provided? j. Are translations of the information sheet and consent form in local languages provided?	

Contd...

Contd...

13.	In case of chart review/retrospective studies, please mention as to how the identity of the patient is delinked and how confidentiality is maintained?	
14.	Does the research deal with sensitive aspects of the subjects' behavior such as sexual behavior, alcohol use or illegal conduct such as drug use?	
15.	Are there any elements in the protocol that are likely to induce anxiety or distress to the subject (e.g. intrusive questionnaire, presentation of material that is unpleasant to the participant etc)	
16.	Are there any other ethical issues involved in the investigation? If yes, please give a brief description?	

Appendix 11: Model Research Proposal Format

TITLE OF THE PROJECT

....
....
....

Introduction:

Background of the problem:

Statement of the problem:

Short-term objectives:

Long-term objectives:

Study setting:

Sample and sampling procedure:

Measurements:

Methods of data collection:

Details of intervention any:

Timeline:

Date analysis:

Amount in grant-in-aid asked for:

Sl.	Particulars	1st year	2nd year	3rd year
1.	Staff			
2.	Contingencies			
3.	Recurring			
4.	Non-recurring			
5.	Travel			
6.	Institution overheads			

Total budget proposed:

References:

Appendix 12: CONSORT 2010 Checklist of Information to include When Reporting a Randomized Trial*

Section/Topic	Item No.	Checklist item	Reported on page No.
Title and abstract	1a	Identification as a randomized trial in the title	
	1b	Structured summary of trial design, methods, results, and conclusions (for specific guidance see CONSORT for abstracts)	
Introduction			
Background and objectives	2a	Scientific background and explanation of rationale	
	2b	Specific objectives or hypotheses	
Methods			
Trial design	3a	Description of trial design (such as parallel, factorial) including allocation ratio	
	3b	Important changes to methods after trial commencement (such as eligibility criteria), with reasons	
Participants	4a	Eligibility criteria for participants	
	4b	Settings and locations where the data were collected	
Interventions	5	The interventions for each group with sufficient details to allow replication, including how and when they were actually administered	
Outcomes	6a	Completely defined pre-specified primary and secondary outcome measures, including how and when they were assessed	
	6b	Any changes to trial outcomes after the trial commenced, with reasons	
Sample size	7a	How sample size was determined	
	7b	When applicable, explanation of any interim analyses and stopping guidelines	
Randomization			
Sequence generation	8a	Method used to generate the random allocation sequence	
	8b	Type of randomization; details of any restriction (such as blocking and block size)	
Allocation concealment mechanism	9	Mechanism used to implement the random allocation sequence (such as sequentially numbered containers), describing any steps taken to conceal the sequence until interventions were assigned	
Implementation	10	Who generated the random allocation sequence, who enrolled participants, and who assigned participants to interventions	
Blinding	11a	If done, who was blinded after assignment to interventions (for example, participants, care providers, those assessing outcomes) and how	
	11b	If relevant, description of the similarity of interventions	

Contd...

Contd...

Section/Topic	Item No.	Checklist item	Reported on page No.
Statistical methods	12a	Statistical methods used to compare groups for primary and secondary outcomes	
	12b	Methods for additional analyses, such as subgroup analyses and adjusted analyses	
Results			
Participant flow (a diagram is strongly recommended)	13a	For each group, the numbers of participants who were randomly assigned, received intended treatment, and were analyzed for the primary outcome	
	13b	For each group, losses and exclusions after randomization, together with reasons	
Recruitment	14a	Dates defining the periods of recruitment and follow-up	
	14b	Why the trial ended or was stopped	
Baseline data	15	A table showing baseline demographic and clinical characteristics for each group	
Numbers analyzed	16	For each group, number of participants (denominator) included in each analysis and whether the analysis was by original assigned groups	
Outcomes and estimation	17a	For each primary and secondary outcome, results for each group, and the estimated effect size and its precision (such as 95% confidence interval)	
	17b	For binary outcomes, presentation of both absolute and relative effect sizes is recommended	
Ancillary analyses	18	Results of any other analyses performed, including subgroup analyses and adjusted analyses, distinguishing pre-specified from exploratory	
Harms	19	All important harms or unintended effects in each group (for specific guidance see CONSORT for harms)	
Discussion			
Limitations	20	Trial limitations, addressing sources of potential bias, imprecision, and, if relevant, multiplicity of analyses	
Generalisability	21	Generalisability (external validity, applicability) of the trial findings	
Interpretation	22	Interpretation consistent with results, balancing benefits and harms, and considering other relevant evidence	
Other information			
Registration	23	Registration number and name of trial registry	
Protocol	24	Where the full trial protocol can be accessed, if available	
Funding	25	Sources of funding and other support (such as supply of drugs), role of funders	

*We strongly recommend reading this statement in conjunction with the CONSORT 2010 Explanation and Elaboration for important clarifications on all the items. If relevant, we also recommend reading CONSORT extensions for cluster randomized trials, non-inferiority and equivalence trials, non-pharmacological treatments, herbal interventions, and pragmatic trials.
Additional extensions are forthcoming: for those and for up to date references relevant to this checklist, see www.consort-statement.org.

Appendix 13: CONSORT Flow Diagram

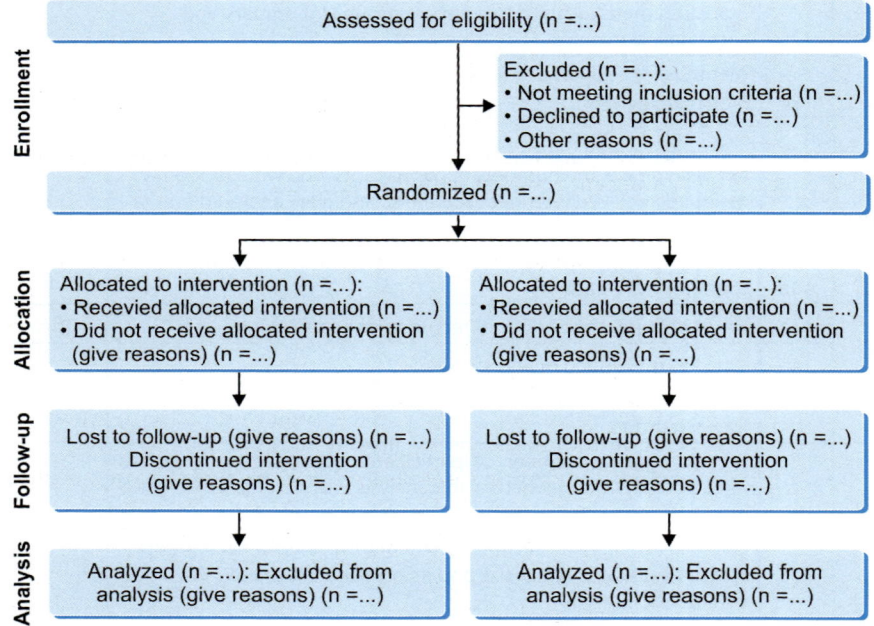

Appendix 14: The Strengthening the Reporting of Observational Studies in Epidemiology (STROBE) Statement: Checklist of Items that should be Addressed in Reports of Observational Studies

Item	Item number	Recommendation
Title and abstract	1	a. Indicate the study's design with a commonly used term in the title or the abstract. b. Provide in the abstract an informative and balanced summary of what was done and what was found.
Introduction		
Background/rationale	2	Explain the scientific background and rationale for the investigation being reported.
Objectives	3	State specific objectives, including any prespecified hypotheses.
Methods		
Study design	4	Present key elements of study design early in the paper
Setting	5	Describe the setting, locations, and relevant dates, including periods of recruitment, exposure, follow-up, and data collection.
Participants	6	a. Cohort study: Give the eligibility criteria, and the sources and methods of selection of participants. Describe methods of follow-up. Case-control study: Give the eligibility criteria, and the sources and methods of case ascertainment and control selection. Give the rationale for the choice of cases and controls. Cross-sectional study: Give the eligibility criteria, and the sources and methods of selection participants. b. Cohort study: For matched studies, give matching criteria and number of exposed and unexposed. Case-control study: For matched studies, give matching criteria and the number of controls per case.
Variables	7	Clearly define all outcomes, exposures, predictors, potential confounders, and effect modifiers. Give diagnostic if applicable.
Data sources/measurement	8*	For each variable of interest, give sources of data and details of methods of assessment (measurement). Describe comparability of assessment methods if there is more than one group.
Bias	9	Describe any efforts to address potential sources of bias.
Study size	10	Explain how the study size was arrived at.
Quantitative variables	11	Explain how quantitative variables were handled in the analyses. If applicable, describe which groupings were chosen, and why.
Statistical methods	12	a. Describe all statistical methods, including those used to control for confounding. b. Describe any methods used to examine subgroups and interactions. c. Explain how missing data were addressed. d. Cohort study: If applicable, explain how loss to follow-up was addressed. Case-control study: If applicable, explain how matching of cases and controls was addressed. Cross-sectional study: If applicable, describe analytical methods taking account of sampling strategy. e. Describe any sensitivity analyses.

Contd...

Contd...

Item	Item number	Recommendation
Results		
Participants	13*	a. Report the numbers of individual at each stage of the study—e.g. numbers potentially eligible, examined for eligibility, confirmed eligible, included in the study, completing follow-up, and analyzed. b. Give reasons for nonparticipation at each stage. c. Consider use of a flow diagram.
Descriptive data	14*	a. Give characteristics of study participants (e.g. demographic, clinical, social) and information on exposures and potential confounders. b. Indicate the number of participants with missing data for each variable of interest. c. Cohort study: Summarize follow-up time—e.g. average and total amount.
Outcome data	15*	Cohort study: Report numbers of outcome events or summary measures over time. Case-control study: Report numbers in each exposure category or summary measures of exposure. Cross-sectional study: Report numbers of outcome events or summary measures.
Main results	16	a. Give unadjusted estimates and, if applicable, confounder-adjusted estimates and their precision (e.g. 95% confidence intervals). Make clear which confounders were adjusted for and why they were included. b. Report category boundaries when continuous variables were categorized. c. If relevant, consider translating estimates of relative risk into absolute risk for a meaningful time period.
Other analyses	17	Report other analyses done—e.g. analyses of subgroups and interactions and sensitivity analyses.
Discussion		
Key results	18	Summarize key results with reference to study objectives.
Limitations	19	Discuss limitations of the study, taking into account sources of potential bias or imprecision. Discuss both direction and magnitude of any potential bias.
Interpretation	20	Give a cautious overall interpretation of results considering objectives, limitations, multiplicity of analyses, results from similar studies, and other relevant evidence.
Generalizability	21	Discuss the generalizability (external validity) of the study results.
Other information		
Funding	22	Give the source of funding and the role of the funders for the present study and, if applicable, for the original on which the present article is based.

* Give such information separately for cases and controls in case-control studies, and if applicable, for exposed and unexposed groups in cohort and cross-sectional studies.
An Explanation and Elaboration article (18–20) discusses each checklist item and gives methodological background and plublished examples of transparent reporting. The STROBE checklist is best used in conjunction with this article [freely available at www.annals.org and on the Websites of PLoS Medicine (www.plosmedicine.org) and Epidemiology (www.epidem.com)]. Separate versions of the checklist for cohort, case-control and cross-sectional studies are available on the STROBE website (www.strobe-statement.org).

Appendix 15: CARE Checklist (2013) of Information to Include When Writing a Case Report

Topic	Items	Checklist items description	Reported on page
Title	1	The words "case report" should be in the title along with what is of greatest interest in this case	
Key words	2	The key elements of this case in 2 to 5 key words	
Abstract	3a	Introduction—What is unique about this case? What does it add to the medical literature?	
	3b	The main symptoms of the patient and the important clinical findings	
	3c	The main diagnoses, therapeutics interventions and outcomes	
	3d	Conclusion—What are the main "take-away" lessons from this case?	
Introduction	4	Brief background summary of this case referencing the relevant medical literature	
Patient information	5a	Demographic information (such as age, gender, ethnicity, occupation)	
	5b	Main symptoms of the patient (his or her chief complaints)	
Clinical findings	6	Describe the relevant physical examination (PE) findings	
Timeline	7	Depict important milestones related to your diagnoses and interventions (Table or Figure)	
Diagnostic assessment	8a	Diagnostic methods (such as PE, laboratory testing, imaging, questionnaires)	
	8b	Diagnostic challenges (such as financial, language, or cultural)	
	8c	Diagnostic reasoning including other diagnoses considered	
	8d	Prognostic characteristics (such as staging in oncology) where applicable	
Therapautic intervention	9a	Types of intervention (such as pharmacologic, surgical, preventive, self-care)	
	9b	Administration of intervention (such as dosage, strength, duration)	
	9c	Changes in intervention (with rationale)	
Follow-up and outcomes	10a	Clinician-assessed outcomes and when appropriate patient-assessed outcomes	

Appendix 16: PRISMA 2009 Checklist for Reporting of Systematic Reviews and Meta-analyses

Section/topic	#	Checklist item	Reported on page #
Title			
Title	1	Identify the report as a systematic review, meta-analysis, or both.	See title, page 1
Abstract			
Structured summary	2	Provide a structured summary including, as applicable: background; objectives; data sources; study eligibility criteria, participants, and interventions; study appraisal and synthesis methods; results; limitations; conclusions and implications of key findings; systematic review registration number.	See abstract, page 2
Introduction			
Rationale	3	Describe the rationale for the review in the context of what is already known.	See introduction, page 3
Objectives	4	Provide an explicit statement of questions being addressed with reference to participants, interventions, comparisons, outcomes, and study design (PICOS).	See introduction, page 3
Methods			
Protocol and registration	5	Indicate if a review protocol exists, if and where it can be accessed (e.g. Web address), and, if available, provide registration information including registration number.	See methods, page 4
Eligibility criteria	6	Specify study characteristics (e.g. PICOS, length of follow-up) and report characteristics (e.g. years considered, language, publication status) used as criteria for eligibility, giving rationale.	See methods, page 3
Information sources	7	Describe all Information sources (e.g. databases with dates of coverage, contact with study authors to identify additional studies) in the search and date last searched.	See methods, page 4
Search	8	Present full electronic search strategy for at least on a database, including any limits used, such that it could be repeated.	See methods, page 3
Study selection	9	State the process for selecting studies (i.e. screening, eligibility, included in systematic review, and, if applicable, included in the meta-analysis).	See methods, page 4
Data collection process	10	Describe method of data extraction from reports (e.g. piloted forms, independently, in duplicate) and any processes for obtaining and confirming data from investigators.	See methods, page 4
Data items	11	List and define all variables for which data were sought (e.g. PICOS, funding sources) and any assumptions and simplifications made.	See methods, page 4

Contd...

Contd...

Section/topic	#	Checklist item	Reported on page #
Risk of bias in individual studies	12	Describe methods used for assessing risk of bias of individual studies (including specification of whether this was done at the study or outcome level), and how this information is to be used in any data synthesis.	See supplemental table 1
Summary measures	13	State the principal summary measures (e.g. risk ratio, difference in means).	See methods, page 4
Risk of bias across studies	15	Specify any assessment of risk of bias that may affect the cumulative evidence (e.g. publication bias, selective reporting within studies)	See supplemental table 1
Additional analyses	16	Describe methods of additional analyses (e.g. sensitivity or subgroup analyses, meta-regression), if done, indicating which were pre-specified.	See methods, page 4
Results			
Study selection	17	Give numbers of studies screened, assessed for eligibility, and included in the review, with reasons for exclusions at each stage, ideally with a flow diagram.	See figure 1
Study characteristics	18	For each study, present characteristics for which data were extracted (e.g. study size, PICOS, follow-up period) and provide the citations.	See table 1 and 2
Risk of bias within studies	19	Present data on risk of bias of each study and, if available, any outcome level assessment (see item 12).	See supplemental table 1
Results of individual studies	20	For all outcomes considered (benefits or harms), present, for each study: (a) simple summary data for each intervention group (b) effect estimates and confidence intervals, ideally with a forest plot.	See table 1 and 2
Synthesis of results	21	Present results of each meta-analysis done, including confidence intervals and measures of consistency.	See table 1 and 2
Risk of bias across studies	22	Present results of any assessment of risk of bias across studies (see item 15).	See results, page 8
Additional analysis	23	Give results of additional analyses, if done [e.g. sensitivity or subgroup analyses, meta-regression (see item 16)]	See results, pages 8-9
Discussion			
Summary of evidence	24	Summarize the main findings including the strength of evidence for each main outcome; consider their relevance to key groups (e.g. healthcare providers, users, and policy makers)	See discussion, pages 9-10
Limitations	25	Discuss limitations at study and outcome level (e.g. risk of bias), and at review-level (e.g. incomplete retrieval of identified research, reporting bias).	See discussion, pages 10-11
Conclusions	26	Provide a general interpretation of the results in the context of other evidence, and implications for future research.	See discussion, page 11
Funding			
Funding	27	Describe sources of funding for the systematic review and other support (e.g. supply of data); role of funders for the systematic review.	See discussion, page 11

Appendix 17: PRISMA (2009) Flow Diagram

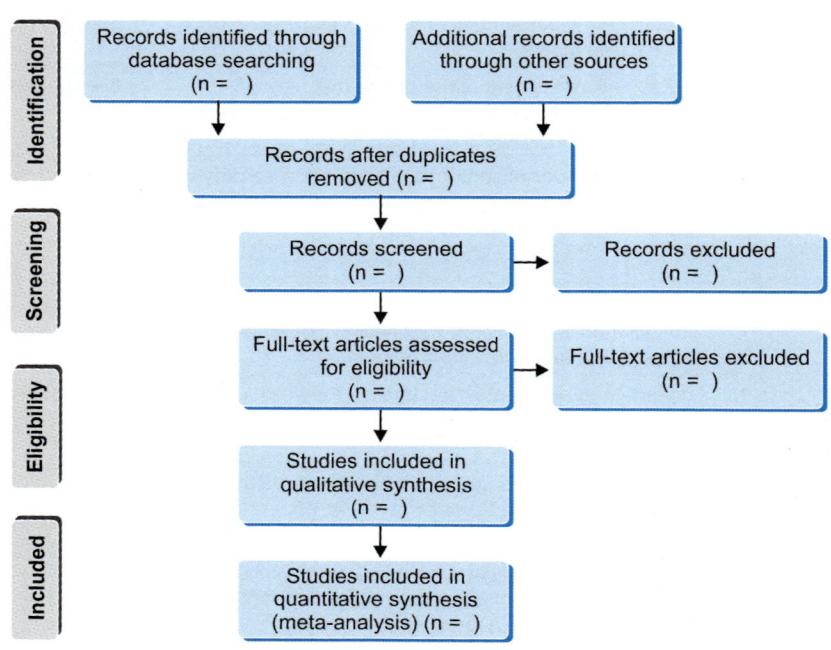

Source: Moher D, Liberati A, Tetziaff J, Altmon DG, The PRISMA Group. Preferred reporting items for systemic reviews and meta-analyses: The PRISMA statement. PLoS Med. 2009;6(6):e1000097. doi:10.1371/Journal.pmed1000097.
For more information, visit www.prisma-statement.org.

Appendix 18: TREND Statement Checklist

Paper Section/Topic	Item No	Descriptor	Reported? Page & line #	
Title and abstract				
Title and abstract	1	Information on how unit were allocated to interventions		
		Structured abstract recommended		
		Information on target population or study sample		
Introduction				
Background	2	Scientific background and explanation of rationale		
		Theories used in designing behavioral interventions		
Methods				
Participants	3	Eligibility criteria for participants, including criteria at different levels in recruitment/sampling plan (e.g. cities, clinics, subjects)		
		Method of recruitment (e.g. referral, self-selection), including the sampling method if a systematic sampling plan was implemented		
		Recruitment setting		
		Settings and locations where the data were collected		
Interventions	4	Details of the interventions intended for each study condition and how and when they were actually administered, specifically including: • Content: What was given? • Delivery method: How was the content given? • Unit of delivery: How were the subjects grouped during delivery? • Deliverer: Who delivered the intervention? • Setting: Where was the intervention delivered? • Exposure quantity and duration: How many sessions or episodes or events were intended to be delivered? How long were they intended to last? • Time span: How long was it intended to take to deliver the intervention to each unit? • Activities to increase compliance or adherence (e.g. incentives)		
Objectives	5	Specific objectives and hypotheses		
Outcomes	6	Clearly defined primary and secondary outcome measures		
		Methods used to collect data and any methods used to enhance the quality of measurements		
		Information on validated instruments such as psychometric and biometric properties		

Contd...

Contd…

Paper Section/Topic	Item No	Descriptor	Reported?	Page & line #
Sample size	7	How sample size was determined and, when applicable, explanation of any interim analyses and stopping rules		
Assignment method	8	Unit of assignment (the unit being assigned to study condition, e.g. individual, group, community)		
		Method used to assign units to study conditions, including details of any restriction (e.g. blocking, stratification, minimization)		
		Inclusion of aspects employed to help minimize potential bias induced due to non-randomization (e.g. matching)		
Blinding (masking)	9	Whether or not participants, those administering the interventions, and those assessing the outcomes were blinded to study condition assignment; if so, statement regarding how the blinding was accomplished and how it was assessed.		
Unit of analysis	10	Description of the smallest unit that is being analyzed to assess intervention effects (e.g. individual, group, or community)		
		If the unit of analysis differs from the unit of assignment, the analytical method used to account for this (e.g. adjusting the standard error estimates by the design effect or using multilevel analysis)		
Statistical methods	11	Statistical methods used to compare study groups for primary methods outcome(s), including complex methods of correlated data		
		Statistical methods used for additional analyses, such as a subgroup analyses and adjusted analysis		
		Methods for imputing missing data, if used		
		Statistical software or programs used		
Results				
Participant flow	12	Flow of participants through each stage of the study: enrollment, assignment, allocation, and intervention exposure, follow-up, analysis (a diagram is strongly recommended) • Enrollment: The numbers of participants screened for eligibility, found to be eligible or not eligible, declined to be enrolled, and enrolled in the study • Assignment: The numbers of participants assigned to a study condition • Allocation and intervention exposure: the number of participants assigned to each study condition and the number of participants who received each intervention • Follow-up: The number of participants who completed the follow-up or did not complete the follow-up (i.e. lost to follow-up), by study condition		

Contd…

Contd...

Paper Section/ Topic	Item No	Descriptor	Reported? Page & line #	
		• Analysis: The number of participants included in or excluded from the main analysis, by study condition		
		Description of protocol deviations from study as planned, along with reasons		
Recruitment	13	Dates defining the periods of recruitment and follow-up		
Baseline data	14	Baseline demographic and clinical characteristics of participants in each study condition		
		Baseline characteristics for each study condition relevant to specific disease prevention research		
		Baseline comparisons of those lost to follow-up and those retained, overall and by study condition		
		Comparison between study population at baseline and target population of interest		
Baseline equivalence	15	Data on study group equivalence at baseline and statistical methods used to control for baseline differences		
Numbers analyzed	16	Number of participants (denominator) included in each analysis for each study condition, particularly when the denominators change for different outcomes; statement of the results in absolute numbers when feasible		
		Indication of whether the analysis strategy was "intention to treat" or, if not, description of how non-compliers were treated in the analyses		
Outcomes and estimation	17	For each primary and secondary outcome, a summary of results for each estimation study condition, and the estimated effect size and a confidence interval to indicate the precision		
		Inclusion of null and negative findings		
		Inclusion of results from testing pre-specified causal pathways through which the intervention was intended to operate, if any		
Ancillary analyses	18	Summary of other analyses performed, including subgroup or restricted analyses, indicating which are pre-specified or exploratory		
Adverse events	19	Summary of all important adverse events or unintended effects in each study condition (including summary measures, effect size estimates, and confidence intervals)		
Discussion				
Interpretation	20	Interpretation of the results, taking into account study hypotheses, sources of potential bias, imprecision of measures, multiplicative analyses, and other limitations or weaknesses of the study		
		Discussion of results taking into account the mechanism by which the intervention was intended to work (causal pathways) or alternative mechanisms or explanations		

Contd...

Paper Section/ Topic	Item No	Descriptor	Reported?	
			Page & line #	
		Discussion of the success of and barriers to implementing the intervention, fidelity of implementation		
		Discussion of research, programmatic, or policy implications		
Generalizability	21	Generalizability (external validity) of the trial findings, taking into account the study population, the characteristics of the intervention, length of follow-up, incentives, compliance rates, specific sites/settings involved in the study, and other contextual issues		
Overall Evidence	22	General interpretation of the results in the context of current evidence and current theory		

Source: Des Jarlais, D.C., Lyles, C., Crepaz, N., & the Trend Group (2004). Improving the reporting quality of nonrandomized evaluations of behavioral and public health interventions: The TREND statement. *American Journal of Public Health*, 94, 361-366. For more information, visit: http://www.cdc.gov/trendstatement/

Appendix 19: TREND Flow Diagram

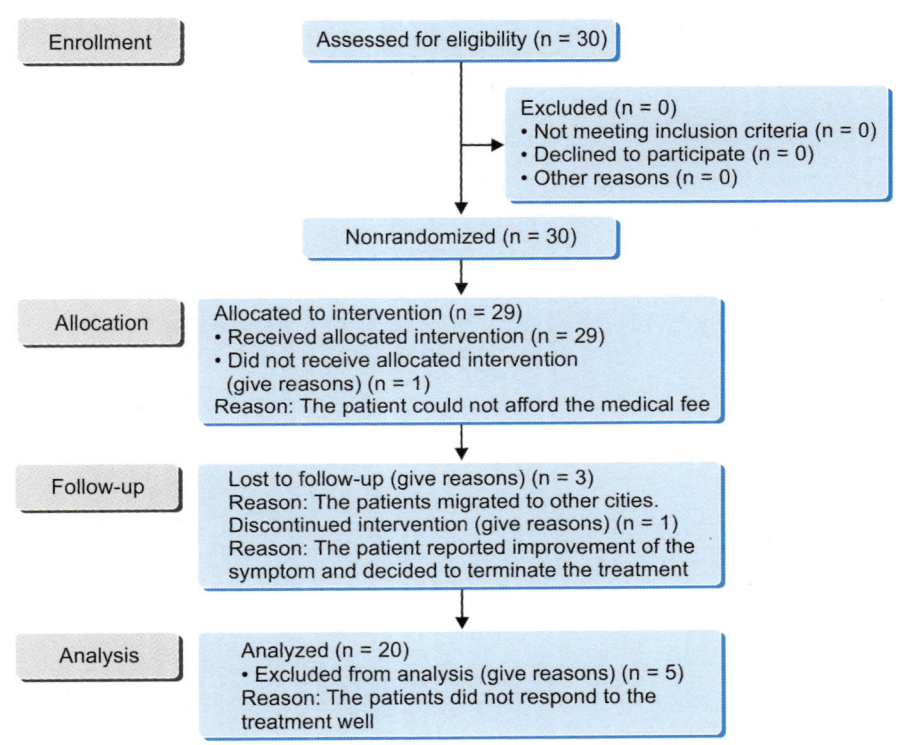

INDEX

Page numbers followed by *b* refer to box, *f* refer to figure, *fc* refer to flowchart, and *t* refer to table

A

Abbreviations 302, 303, 349
Absolute deviations, calculation of 385, 386
Abstract 302, 303, 313, 326, 471
Accessible population 174, 471
Accuracy 9, 329
Acknowledgments 296, 302
Action research 21
Active variables 69
Adaptation theory 110
Algorithm 471
Alpha 471
American Association of Colleges of Nursing 14
American Nurses Association 13
American Psychological Association 305, 308
    Style of Writing References 308, 309
Analysis of covariance 434, 471
Analysis of variance 196, 198, 343, 422, 427, 433, 466, 471
    test 422
    various forms of 434
Analysis, organize data for 45, 50
Analytic phase 45
    problems in 25
Analyze data 45, 50
Analyzing literature 97
Analyzing problem 6
Analyzing research reports 471
Analyzing solution 6
Anecdotes 94, 238
Annexure 302, 305
Annotated bibliography 306
Anonymity 471
Antiretroviral therapy 175
Appendices 302, 305, 329
    list of 303
Applied research 21, 471
Appropriateness 121, 255
Assembling and arranging subject-matter 292
Assessing internal consistency 251*f*
Assessing inter-rater reliability 250*f*
Associative hypothesis 78, 471
Assumptions 74, 75, 75*t*, 407, 433, 471
    of data, classification based on 272
    sources of 75
    theoretical based 75
    types of 75
    user of 74
Attitude
    questionnaire 224
    scale 224
        examples of 225*t*
Attribute variables 69
Attrition 139, 196, 471
Audit trail 471
Author date style 307
Authority 4
Authorship 297
Autobiographies 94
Autonomy 31
Average deviation 383

B

Background information 326
Bar chart 472
Bar graph 352, 354*f*, 355
    advantages of 354*t*
    disadvantages of 354*t*
    types of 352, 355, 355*t*
Basic research 21, 472
Beneficence 33, 472
Bias 472
    lack of 121
Bibliography 94, 305, 311, 311*t*, 316, 472
Biophysiological measures 240
    characteristics of 240, 240*f*
    types of 241
Biostatistics 337
    in field of nursing, significance of 338
    in medicine, user of 338
    scope of 338
Bivariate analysis 272, 472
Bivariate correlation 472
Bivariate statistics 466
Blind review 472
Body-mind-spirit 113
Borrowed theories 472
Borrowing 4
Box plot 472
Bracketing 472

Brainstorming 58
British Nursing Index 95
Budget
   estimation 328
   proposal 328*t*

C

Cafeteria questions 222
Calculate standard deviation 387, 389
Calculate variance 381
Calibration 472
Caption 348
CARE checklist 511
Carrying out interview 228
Case control studies 159, 159*t*, 472
Case fatality rate 465, 465*t*
Case report 295
Case study 90, 164, 472
Categorical variable 71*fc*
   types of 71, 71*t*
Causal hypothesis 78
Census 459
Central limit theorem 472
Central statistical organization 459
Central tendency 371*t*
   measures of 271, 364
Chain sampling 190
Checklist 236
Chi-square statistic 441
Chi-square test 198, 272, 422, 423, 440, 442, 472
   interpretation of 276
Choosing sampling approach 179
Citation 305, 472
   analysis 472
   within text 307, 308
Civil registration system 458
Class
   boundaries 347
   interval 339
      size of 347
   mid-point 339
   number of 347
   types of 347
Client advocate 20
Clinical research 23, 151
Clinical significance 277
Close-ended questions 221
Cluster analysis 466
Cluster sampling 188, 473
   technique 185, 185*f*, 186*fc*, 187*t*
   types of 186
Cochran's Q test 473
Coding 282, 473
   three stages of 283*b*

Coefficient of
   mean deviation, merits and demerits of 387*t*
   quartile deviation, merits and demerits of 379*t*
   variation, merits and demerits of 383*t*
Cognitive behavior therapy 432, 438
Cohen's kappa 473
Cohort study 158*f*
Collect data 45, 50, 211
Collecting reliable data 260
Commonly used true experimental designs, types of 145
Communicating
   research findings, importance of 288
   techniques 228
Comparative descriptive design 128, 129*f*
Comparative survey 137
Compensatory rivalry 140
Competency 32
Complete participant 238
Complex hypothesis 78
Complex table 350
Component bar graph 355
Comprehension 32
Computer
   assisted qualitative analysis software 50, 282
   for data analysis 467
   generated numbers 182
   in research process, role of 329
   in scientific research, importance of 329
Concepts, types of 107*fc*
Conceptual framework 43, 110, 473
   concepts and study variables 116*f*
   in quantitative and qualitative research 113*fc*
   theory, utilization of 117
Conceptual model 110, 111, 473
Conceptual papers 94
Conceptual phase 42
   problems in 24
Conceptual utilization 318
Conclusion 100, 296, 316
   meaning of 281*t*
Concurrent validity 254, 255, 473
Conduct pilot study 45
Conducting interview 228
Conducting pilot study 260
Conducting research 161
   critique 312, 313*t*
Conference proceedings 95
Confidence interval 416, 473
Confidentiality 473, 498
   breach of 472
Confirmation phase 322
Confounding variables 473
Consent form 473
   for participation 499, 500

Conservation model 110
Consort flow diagram 508
Construct 473
  validity 141, 253, 255, 473
Constructing graph 351
Consultation 58
Content analysis 473
Content validity 252, 255, 473
Contingency table 403, 404t, 473
Continuous data 339
Continuous frequency distribution 346t
Continuous variables 71fc, 473
Control group 473
  demoralization of 140
  subjects 500
Control sampling bias 200
Controlling external variables 25
Convenience sampling 187, 189f, 473
  technique
    advantages 189t
    disadvantages 189t
Convergent validity 254
Cooperation from sample, lack of 202
Correlation 399, 411
  analysis 474
  coefficient 399, 474
    features of 400
    significant values of 494
  measures of 403, 403f
  size of 405
  studies 474
  tests 466
  types of 400, 400fc
  values, interpretation of 405t
Correlational designs 128
  types of 130, 130fc
Correlational survey 137
Cramer's V 474
Criterion related validity 254, 474
Criterion sampling 202
Critique 474
Critiquing data collection methods 257
Critiquing ethical aspects of study, guidelines for 36
Critiquing hypothesis, guidelines for 81
Critiquing qualitative research design 167
Critiquing quantitative research design 160
Critiquing research report
  guidelines for 312
  importance of 311
  questions for 313-316
Critiquing sampling section of research report, guidelines for 203
Critiquing theoretical framework 118
Cross tabulation 403

Cross-over design 148, 148f
Cross-sectional design 131, 132f, 160, 160f, 474
Crude birth rate 463
Crude death rate 465
Cumulative frequency 339
  calculation of 379
  curve 359
  table 359t
Cumulative scale 243

D

Data 339, 474
  analysis 163, 164, 259, 316, 327, 474
    methods of 123
    plan for 265t
    techniques 196
  classification of 269, 344
  cleaning 268
  coding of 267
  collection
    method of 122, 212, 213f, 214, 214f, 215f, 327
    plan 210f
    procedure 210, 257, 259, 259b
    process 210f
    purposes of 208
    time points, number of 428
    tools and methods of 208
  editing of 266
  entry 267
  management 327
  organization of 268, 344
  presentation of 269, 344
  range of 339
  sets, dot plots of 374f
  source 209
    triangulation 474
  storage of 212
  tabulation of 345
  triangulation 165, 474
  types of 339, 341fc
  verification 268
Database 474
Decision phase 322
Declaration page 302
Deductive reasoning 5, 5f, 474
Defective measuring device 201
Delimitations 81, 83, 83t
  examples of 81t
  user of 82
Delphi technique 474
Demographic variables 69
Dependent variable 68, 69f, 70, 70f, 70t, 474
  measurement of 428
Descriptive correlational design 130, 130f

Descriptive design, types of 128, 128*fc*
Descriptive rating scale 237*f*
Descriptive statistics 270, 344, 466, 474
Descriptive studies 475
    sample size calculation for 199
Descriptive theories 109
Descriptive variables 475
Designing questionnaire 223*f*
Determining sample size 179
Develop sampling plan and select sample 44
Developing data collection plan 209
Developing research plan 167
Developing themes 283
Diagrammatic presentations 351
Difficulty index, estimation of 256
Diffusion 475
Direct observation 238
Directional hypothesis 79, 475
Disability-adjusted life years 463, 464, 464*t*
Disclosure, components of 32*b*
Discrete data 339, 381, 388
Discrete frequency distribution 345, 346*t*
Discrete variables 71*fc*
Discriminate validity 475
Discrimination index, estimation of 256
Discussion 296, 302, 304, 316
    meaning of 281*t*
Dispersion 375
Disproportionate stratified random sampling, 183
    example of 184*t*
Dissemination
    features of 288
    meaning of 288
    phase 46
    purposes of 288, 289*f*
Dissertation 94, 301, 475
    format of 302*t*
Distracters, evaluating effectiveness of 256
Distribution of χ^2 probability 493
Divergent validity 254
Documentary note style 306
Dotted diagrams 360
Double-blind experiment 475
Duplicate publication/submission 297

E

Educational programs in nursing, development of 11
Effective dissemination, criteria for 290*f*
Electronic literature searches 95
Electronic survey 137
Element 174
Eligible criteria 176, 177*t*
E-mail data collection 217, 218
Empirical based assumptions 75

Empirical evidence 9
Empirical literature 93, 475
Empirical phase 45
End report 305
Epidemiological research designs 157
    types of 158*fc*
Epidemiological survey 217
Epidemiology 475
Errors in hypothesis testing, types of 420*fc*
Establishing rapport 228
Estimating population parameters 414
Estimating sample size
    methods of 198, 198*f*
    thumb rules of 198
Ethical codes, history of 31
Ethical consideration 61, 124, 314, 327
Ethical issues 25, 99
Ethical neutrality 7
Ethical principles 34
    in research study, application of 34, 34*t*
Ethics 240, 475
    in nursing research, importance of 35
Ethnography 90, 161, 475
Evaluating data collection procedure, guidelines for 258
Evaluative research 22
Evidence hierarchy 29*f*
Evidence retrieval 28
Evidence-based nursing
    components of 27
    features of 27
Evidence-based practice 16, 26, 318, 475
    benefits of 29
    components of 27*f*
Ex post facto research 475
Exclusion criteria 176, 177, 475
Exclusive method 346
Executing sampling plan 180
Exhaustiveness 267
Experimental design 475
    validity of 138
Experimental group 475
    subjects 499
Experimental research 138, 475
    elements of 142
Experimental studies 212
    sample size calculation for 199
Experimenter effect 141
Explanatory theories 109
Exploratory design 128, 129*f*
Exploratory study 475
Exploratory survey 137
Expressive methods 245
    play techniques 245
    role playing 245

External criteria 60
External sources 58
External validity 141, 475
    threats to 138
Extraneous variable 69, 70, 70f, 70t, 475

F

Fabrication 35, 475
Face-to-face interviews 216, 218
Factor analysis 466, 476
Factorial design 149, 149f, 149t
Factors influencing sampling 191, 194f
Falsification 35, 476
Feasible, interesting, novel, ethical, and relevant criteria 61, 67
Fertility, measures of 461, 463t
Field notes 238, 476
Field trials 158
Fieldwork, activities in 161
Figures
    and figure captions 297
    list of 302, 303
Findings
    consider alternative explanations of 273
    considering significance of 276
    discussion of 273
    interpretation of 259
    meaning of 281t
Fisher exact test 443
    computation of 443
Florence Nightingale, work of 11
Focus, determine area of 235
Focused group interview 231
Footnote 305, 348
Framing review, methods of 99t
Free software 467
Freedom, degree of 421, 422, 422t, 474
Frequency 476
    curve 358f
    data 381, 388
    distribution 339, 345
    polygon 357, 357f
        advantages of 357t
        disadvantages of 357t
    table 345t
Friedman test 450, 476
F-test 272
Full disclosure 476
Funds, availability of 213

G

General fertility rate 463
Generalization 476
    meaning of 281t

Generates new questions 9
Getting representative sample 177
Goal attainment theory 110
Goals of analysis, classification based on 270
Good hypothesis, characteristics of 76, 76fc
Good measure of dispersion, properties of 375
Good question, qualities of 222
Good research
    characteristics of 8
    criteria for 9, 61b
Good researcher, qualities of 10, 10f
Good sample design, characteristics of 177, 177f
Good statistical
    average, characteristics of 364, 365f
    table, requirements of 348
Grand theories 108, 476
Graphic presentations 351
Graphic rating scale 237f
Graphical presentation 269
    types of 353f
Graphs 404
    types of 352
Greater accuracy and reliability 177
Gross reproductive rate 463
Grounded theory 90, 476
    approach 163
Group composition and size 232
Grouped data 384
Guttman scale 243, 476

H

Handling multiple variables 24
Harvard style 305
Hawthorne effect 141, 476
Head note 348
Health
    administration research 24
    and family planning programs 460
    care agency 319
    promotion model 110
    statistics 457
Healthcare organization 30
Helicobacter pylori infection 160
Heterogeneous sample 476
Histogram 354, 476
    advantages of 357t
    disadvantages of 357t
    important characteristics of 356
Historical notes 337
Historical research 90, 166, 476
Homogeneous sampling 202, 476
Hypothesis 43, 72, 73, 75, 75t, 79, 265, 327, 476
    alternative 418
        non-directional 80

example of 80*t*
formulation of 80
sources of 77, 77*f*
testing 417
    errors in 419
    interpretation of 276
    steps in 419
types of 78, 78*f*, 418, 418*fc*

I

Ideal study, rules of 313-316
Identify population 44
Identify study assumptions 43
Implementing research plan 257
Implementing solution 6
Implementing study intervention 212
Implications, meaning of 281*t*
Inappropriate sampling frame 200
Incidence 464*t*
Inclusion criteria 176, 177, 476
Inclusive method 347
Inconclusive trial 152
Independent samples T-test, interpretation of 275
Independent T-test 429, 430
    statistics 430
Independent variable 68, 69*f*, 70, 70*f*, 70*t*, 476
In-depth interviews 230
Indexes 95
Inductive reasoning 4, 5, 5*f*, 477
Infant mortality rate 465
Inference 477
    verification of 25
Inferential statistics 271, 344, 414, 477
    and hypothesis testing 414
    interpreting results of 274
    purposes of 414
    types of 414, 415*fc*
Information
    consort 2010 checklist of 506
    disclosure of 32
Informed consent 32, 33*b*, 477
    documentation for 33
Innovative approach 20
Institutional Ethics Committee 36, 502
Institutional Review Board 36, 477
Instrument 477
    assessing
        equivalence of 250*f*
        stability of 248*f*
Instrumental utilization 318
Integrative body-mind-spirit model
    application of 117*f*
    components of 117*f*
Intelligence quotient 74

Interdisciplinary collaboration 17
Internal consistency or scale homogeneity 251
Internal criteria 59
Internal validity 139, 477
    threats to 138
International Institute of Population Studies 459
Internet collection 217
Interpersonal theory 110
Interpret findings 46, 52
Interpretation, meaning of 281*t*
Interpretive phase 273
    components of 273*f*
Interquartile range 344, 376, 376*f*
    for continuous series, calculation of 378
    for discrete series, calculation of 378
    for raw data, calculation of 377
    merits and demerits of 377*t*
Inter-rater reliability 250, 477
Interval data 477
Interval estimation 415
Interval scale 342
Intervention 477
    implementation, low reliability of 142
Interventional studies 157
Interview 225, 477
    importance of 226
    process 226, 227*f*
    schedule 233, 233*t*
    types of 229, 229*f*
Intuition 4, 477
Investigator 498
    triangulation 477
Item analysis 255, 477
    calculation of 256
    purposes of 255
    steps in 256

J

Joint Commission on Accreditation of Healthcare Organization 14
Journal
    abstracts 94
    club 477
    impact factor 477
    publication in 293
Judgmental sampling 190, 477
Justice 478

K

Karl Pearson's correlation coefficient 408
Kendall's tau 478
Key words 478
Knowing target audience 290

Knowledge
  development of 20
  in sampling process, lack of 201
  sources of 3f
Kruskal-Wallis test 272, 423, 450
Kurtosis 478

L

Labeling missing values 268
Landmark studies 478
Legal use 460
Leptokurtic 478
Levine conservation model 114t
  application of 116f
Likert scale 478
Limitations 82, 83, 83t, 478
  examples of 82t
Line graph 358, 358f, 478
  advantages of 358t
  disadvantages of 358t
  important characteristics of 358
Linear correlation 402
Linear regression 466
  analysis, assumptions of 410
Linear relationship 478
Literature review 43, 48, 57, 62, 88, 94, 302, 313, 478
  elements of 89
  importance of 88
  in qualitative studies, purposes of 90t
  process 97f
    steps in 96
  purposes of 88
  types of 91
Logical reasoning 4
Logs 238
Longitudinal design 132, 478
Longitudinal study 133f
  types of 134, 134fc
Lottery method 181, 181f
Lower class limit 339
Low-statistical power 142, 478

M

Mail survey/self-completion data collection 216, 218
Main body 99, 303
Maintaining objectivity, problems in 25
Major organizations 459
Manifold table 350, 351t
Manipulation 478
Mann-Whitney U test 272, 423, 446, 478, 495
  statistic 447
Manpower resources, availability of 213
Maternal mortality rate 465

Mathematical functions 340
Maturation 479
McNemar test 443, 479
Mean
  absolute deviation 383
  calculation of 365
  characteristics of 365
  deviation 375, 383
    coefficient of 386
    formulae for 384t
    merits and demerits of 386t
  for frequency table data, calculation of 366
  for group frequency distribution, calculation of 366
  for ungrouped data, calculation of 365
  median, and mode 370, 371t
  merits and demerits of 365t
Measurability 9
Measurement 479
  error 479
  levels of 341, 344f, 478
  low reliability of 142
  sensitivity of 195
Mechanical devices 238
Median
  calculation of 367
  characteristics of 367
  for frequency table data, calculation of 367
  for grouped frequency distribution, calculation of 368
  for ungrouped data, calculation of 367
  merits and demerits of 367t
  test 479
Medical literature analysis and retrieval system online 96
Member, selection of 232
Meta-analysis 166, 479
Meta-synthesis 93, 479
Method triangulation 165, 479
Methodological studies 166
Methodological utilization 318
Methodology 302, 303, 327
Micro theories 479
Middle range theories 108, 479
Minimize measurement errors 122
Minnesota Multiphasic Personality Inventory 245
Missing values 268
Mixed method 479
  designs 165
Mixed research 23
Mobile short message services 137
Mode 369, 479
  calculation of 369
  characteristics of 369

for frequency table data, calculation of 369
for grouped frequency distribution, calculation of 370
for simple data, calculation of 369
merits and demerits of 369t
Model information sheet for research participants and consent form 498
Model registration scheme 458
Model research proposal format 504
Model table, components of 349t
Model testing correlational design 131, 131f
Mono-operation bias 141
Morbidity, measures of 461
Mortality, measures of 465, 465t
Multiple and confirmatory strategies, use of 16
Multiple bar graph 355
Multiple choice questions 221
Multiple correlation 402
Multiple linear regression 409
Multiple regression analysis 479
Multistage sampling 185, 186, 187f, 479
Multivariate analysis of variance 435, 479

N

Narrative reviews 91
Narrowing research topic, phase of 62b
National Center for Nursing Research 13
National Sample Survey Organization 459
Net reproductive rate 463
Network sampling 190, 480
Nominal data 480
Nominal scale 341
Nonconcealed observation 238
Nondirectional hypothesis 79, 480
Non-directive interview 230
Nonequivalent control group
  design 154, 155f
  interrupted time-series design 156, 156t
  pretest-post-test design 153, 154f
Nonexperimental designs 126
  types of 127, 127fc
Nonexperimental research 480
Noninferior trial 152
Nonlinear correlation 402
Nonparametric test 272, 339, 422-424, 425t, 426f, 440, 466, 480
Non-participant observation 238
Nonprobability sampling 193, 193f, 480
  methods 187
    summary of 192t
  techniques 187, 191, 193t
Non-randomized studies 295
Non-research reasons 89
Non-statistical factors 195b

Normal distribution 480
Novelty effect 480
Null hypotheses 79, 80, 418, 480
Number of variables in analyses, classification based on 272
Numbered style 307
Numeric pain rating scale 237f
Nurse
  administrators 324
  clinicians 324
  educators 324
  in ethical conduct of research, role of 36
  in research, role of 20
  researcher 325
Nursing
  associations, activities of 12
  education research 24
  evidence based 14
  health, and social research, problems in 24
  practice 57
    integrates, evidence-based 26b
  process, evidence-based 27b
  profession 319
  research 3, 10, 11b, 12, 14, 17, 26, 428, 480
    characteristics of 20
    development of 12
    funding organizations for 12
    importance of 19
    in India, evolution of 14, 15f
    purposes of 18, 19f
    registry of 96
    scope of 23, 23f
    Society of India, aims and objectives of 15b
    utilization of 323t
    visibility of 17
  theories 105
    basic elements of 105
    characteristics of 106
    elements of 106f

O

Objectives, types of 66
Observation 78, 234
  Method
    advantages of 239
    disadvantages of 239
    types of 236, 236f
  process, steps in 235
  sampling techniques 239
  scale, assessing stability of 249f
Observational data, validation of 239
Observational research 480
Observational studies 158, 295
  strengthening reporting of 509

Odds ratio 480
Ogive
    advantages of 360*t*
    disadvantages of 360*t*
One group pretest post-test design 155, 156*f*
One-sample T-test 421, 429
One-tailed test 418, 419, 480, 496
    significance for 489, 494
One-way analysis of variance 272, 435
    interpretation of 275
Open access 480
Open ended question 220, 480
Oral presentation 298
    advantage of 299*t*
    disadvantages of 299*t*
Oral survey 137
Ordinal data 480
    presence of 424
Ordinal scale 342
Organization 329
Organizational factors 323
Organize content 295
Orlando's theory of deliberative nursing process 109
Outcomes research 166, 480
Outliers 268, 480
    removal of 268

P

P value 481
Pain scores 446
Paired sample sign test 431, 445
Panel studies 134
Paradigm 481
Parameter 339, 481
Parametric test 272, 339, 422-424, 425*t*, 426*fc*, 428, 481
    assumptions of 423*f*
Parenthetical style 307
Partial correlation 400
Participant
    availability of 124
    observation 238
Pearson product-moment correlation, interpretation of 276
Peer review 481
Peplau's theory of interpersonal relations 109
Percentiles 379, 380*f*
Personality
    inventory 244
    measurement of 244, 244*f*
Persuasion phase 322
Persuasive utilization 318
Phenomena, control of 19
Phenomenological design 163

Phenomenological research 481
Phenomenology 481
Phenomenon 481
Phi coefficient 481
Pictogram 354
    advantages of 356*t*
    depicting population 356*f*
    disadvantages of 356*t*
Pictorial projective device 245
Pie diagram 352, 356
    advantages of 356*t*
    disadvantages of 356*t*
    important characteristics of 354
Pilot study 260, 481
Placebo 481
Plagiarism 35, 297, 481
Planning
    and empirical phase, problems in 24
    for data analysis, advantages of 265
Plot scatter diagram 404
Point estimation 414, 481
Point prevalence 464
Population 174, 327, 339, 481
    and sample 176*f*
    census 457
        main objectives of 459
    nature of 194, 195
    size 183, 184, 194
    standard deviation 388
    variance formula 381
Positive trial 152
Possible hypothesis test outcomes 420
Post hoc test 481
Poster layout 301*f*
Poster presentation 300, 481
    advantages of 301
    disadvantages of 301
Post-fieldwork, activities of 162
Post-test only control group design 145, 146*f*, 481
Power 122, 481
    analysis 481
Practice theories 108
Pre-analysis phase, steps in 267*fc*
Precision 122, 481
Prediction 19
Predictive correlational design 130
    example of 131*f*
Predictive theories 109
Predictive validity 254, 255, 481
Pre-experimental design 482
Pre-fieldwork, activities in 161
Preparing interview schedule 232
Preparing research report, guidelines for 292
Pretest-post-test control group design 146, 146*f*, 482

Prevalence 464, 464t
　study 482
Previous research findings 78
Primary data 482
　collection 215
Primary sources 93, 482
Principal investigator 20, 482
　responsibilities of 37
Prisma flow diagram 514
Probability 415, 482
　distribution curve 416f
　sampling 193f
　　methods 180, 188t
　　techniques 180, 191, 193t
Problem
　novelty of 60
　researchability of 60
　solving
　　and scientific method 6
　　approach 8
　　process 6f, 8, 8t
　statement, components of 63
Product moment correlation 408
Projective techniques 245, 482
Proportional mortality rate 465
Proportionate stratified random sampling 183
　example of 183t
Proprietary software 466
Prospective design 135, 136f
Prospective studies 482
Psychological measures 241
Psychometric instruments 482
Publication
　advantages of 298t
　decide type of 290
　disadvantages of 298t
　preparing manuscript for 294f
　select journal for 291
Published study, critiquing literature review in 101
Pubmed 96
Purpose of study, classification based on 127
Purposive sampling 190, 477, 482
　technique 190f
　　advantages 190t
　　disadvantages 190t
P-value and effect size, interpretation of 275

Q

Q-sort 482
　example of 246f
　procedures 246
Qualitative analysis 482
Qualitative data 339
　analysis 280, 281
　presentation 352
Qualitative information, ensuring validity of 52
Qualitative research 23, 52, 53t, 482
　advantages of 52, 52t
　designs 161
　　characteristics of 122
　　types of 162fc
　disadvantages of 52, 52t
　process 46
　　phases of 49fc, 51fc
　　steps in 48
　purposes of 48
　studies 281
　　sampling process in 202
Qualitative study
　sample size in 202
　types of 90
Quantitative analysis 482
　types of 270, 270fc
Quantitative data 339
　analysis, phases of 266, 266f
Quantitative research 22, 52, 53t, 90t, 482
　advantages of 46, 48t
　designs 124
　　characteristics of 121, 121f
　　types of 126
　disadvantages of 46, 48t
　process 41, 179f
　　phases of 42fc, 47fc
　　steps in 41
　purposes of 41
　sample size in 194
Quantitative study
　sampling process in 178
　types of 195
Quartile
　deviation, coefficient of 379
　user of 377
Quasi-experimental designs 153
　limitations of 157
　strengths of 157
　types of 153, 153fc
Quasi-experimental research 483
Questionnaire 217, 233t, 483
　administration, methods of 222, 222f
　types of 220
Questions
　plan sequence of 228
　types of 220, 220f, 226
Quota sampling 189, 483
　technique 189f
　　advantages 189t
　　disadvantages 189t

R

Random assignment 483
Random numbers, table of 181, 182b, 483, 497
Random sampling 482, 483
Randomization 143, 175, 483
Randomized block design 150, 150f, 150t, 483
Randomized control study 295
Randomized controlled trial 151, 483
Range for continuous series, calculation of 376
Range for discrete series, calculation of 375
Range for raw data, calculation of 375
Rank order questions 221
Rank sum test 272
Rate, ratio, and proportion, distinguishing characteristics of 462fc
Rating questions 222
Rating scale 236, 483
Ratio data 483
Ratio scale 342
Raw data 483
Reasonable sample size 198
Recommendations, meaning of 281t
Recording and reporting 9
Red blood cells 141
References 100, 297, 302, 305, 306, 311, 311t, 316, 328
    elements of 306
    errors in 306
    list 305
    purposes of 306
    style 306
    types of 306-310
Reflexivity 483
Regression 411
    analysis 409, 483
        types of 409
    equation 410, 411
    line 410, 410f
Relationship, measures of 399
Reliability 248, 483
Report, prepare outline of 291
Reporting findings of research study, guidelines for 295t
Reporting statistical significance 408
Representative sample, lack of 202
Representativeness 175, 177, 484
Research 8, 484
    approach 5
        and designs 120
    article, components of 313-316
    assumptions 75
    conduct and utilization of 320f
    critique 311
    design 126fc, 314, 327, 484
        factors influencing selection of 123f
        key elements of 122
        levels of 120fc
        purpose of 121
        selection of 123
        types of 124, 125fc, 165, 191
    ethical principles of 31, 34
    factors 324
    findings
        dissemination of 17, 288
        utilization of 288
    hypothesis 79, 484
    in nursing
        in nursing, historical evolution of 11
        project, conduct and utilization of 319
    methodology 314
    misconduct 35
    objectives 65, 484
        characteristics of 65f
        formulation of 66
        types of 66, 66t
    outcomes, interpretation of 477
    plan, components of 167
    problem 57, 80, 121, 122, 313
        and hypothesis 57
        and question 161, 163, 164
        formulating final statement of 62
        formulation of 61, 61f
        significance of 60
        sources of 57, 58f
        statement, examples of 72, 73
    process 41
    proposal 325
        format of 326
        functions of 325
        meaning of 325
    purpose 10, 313
    question 64, 88, 425, 484
    report 24, 291, 484
        characteristics of 292
        meaning of 292
        types of 293, 293f
    study
        example 113
        purposes of 64
        types of 213, 295
    team, member of 20
    title 313
    tool, characteristics of 247, 247f
    types of 21, 21f, 109
    utilization 312, 318, 484
        elements of 316
        importance of 318, 319

nursing model of 320f
process 317, 317f
studies 325
types of 317, 318, 318t
variable 484
Researcher's
competency 59
decision 420
interest 59
knowledge and experience of 123
own resources 59
triangulation 165
Resources 60
availability of 194, 196
lack of 201
Response error 201
Response rate 484
Results, interpretation of 274
Retrospective design 134, 484
Retrospective study 135f
Review 298
literature, purpose of 90
of literature
in qualitative research, purposes of 89
in quantitative research, purposes of 89
selected sources of 95f
sources of 93
organization of 98
selection of 98
Reviewing literature, general guidelines for 100
Revision 298
Rigor 484
Risk-benefit ratio 484
Robust tests 484
Roger's innovative diffusion model 322, 322f
Role modeling and mentorship 4
Rorschach Inkblot test 245
Rosenthal effect 141
Rules of thumb, sample size 198t

S

Safe guarding human rights 45
Sample 174, 339, 484
analyzed, number of 428
and sampling techniques 174
and statistical power 197
frame 484
registration system 458
size 183, 184, 194, 484
determining adequacy of 195
standard deviation 388
survey 459
variance formula 381

Sampling 188, 339, 484
advantages of 176
bias 176, 200, 485
potential sources of 200
disadvantages of 177
error 175, 201, 485
frame 174, 485
availability of 194
problems in 175
methods 180, 315
types of 180f
plan 176, 327
portion 183, 184
problems in 201
procedure 196
techniques 180
types of 180f
Saturation 485
Scales 241, 485
types of 242, 242f
Scatter diagram
benefits of 406
limitations of 406
Scatter plot 404, 485
interpretation of 404
types of 405, 405t, 406
Scattered diagram 360, 360f
advantages of 360t
disadvantages of 360t
Scientific approach 5
Scientific method 6, 8
characteristics of 7
steps of 7, 7t, 8t
Search strategy 485
Search terms 485
Searching literature 97
Secondary data collection 215, 485
Select data collection methods 49
Select effective communication channel 290
Select observers and provide training 235
Select research design 44, 49
Select sample 49
Selecting appropriate quantitative test 425
Selecting appropriate statistical test 428t
summary of 427fc
Selecting appropriate test 426f
Selecting research
criteria for 59fc
problem, criteria for 59
Selecting review topic 97
Selection bias 139, 176, 485
Selection of
research design, decision on 124
sources, criteria for 96

Index

Self-care deficit theory 110
Self-report 485
Semantic differential scale 243
Semi-structured interview 230, 485
Semi-structured questionnaire 220
Send query letter 294
Sensitivity 254, 485
Sentence completion techniques 245
Shared decision making 17
Sign test 444, 485
    types of 444
Significance
    criterion 197
    level of 80, 196, 421, 478, 485, 493
Significant values of F 490, 491, 492
Simple bar graph 355
Simple correlation 400
Simple hypothesis 78
Simple random sampling 188, 485
    technique 180, 181f
        advantages 181t
        disadvantages 181t
Simple table 350, 350t
Single-group interrupted time-series design 157, 157f
Skewness 485
Snowball sampling 190, 191f, 202, 485
    technique
        advantages 191t
        disadvantages 191t
Social issues 58
Solomon four-group design 147, 147f, 485
Spearman's rank
    coefficient 423
    correlation 407
Specify significance level 430, 432
Split-half technique 486
Stability 248, 486
Standard deviation 343, 344, 375, 387, 390, 486
    formula for 388t
    merits and demerits of 388t
Standard error 486
Standard normal distribution 486
Standardized scores 486
State null and alternative hypothesis 419, 430, 432
Stating limitations, importance of 83
Statistical analysis 269
Statistical conclusion validity 142
    threats to 138
Statistical packages 466
Statistical power 197, 486
Statistical significance 277, 486
    guidelines for 416t
Statistical test 265, 422t
    violated assumptions of 142
Statistics
    characteristics of 338
    limitations of 338
    types of 343, 344fc
Stetler model of research utilization 319, 321f
Stratified random sampling technique 182, 182f, 486
    advantages 183t
    disadvantages 183t
Student T-test 429, 430
Study
    and study objectives, determine purpose of 43
    design, control in 212
    nature of 213
    participants, recruitment of 210
    population 174
    protect integrity of 212
    purpose of 65, 191
    scope of 202, 213
    setting 327
    title of 259
    types of 72, 73
Subjects
    availability of 60
    nature of 214
Submit manuscript 297
Summary and conclusions 302, 305
Survey
    data collection
        advantages 218t
        disadvantages 218t
        methods 216f, 218t
    design
        advantages of 137
        disadvantages of 138
    method 216
    research 486
        designs 136
    types of 137, 137fc
Survival rate 465
Synthesizing literature 97
Systematic bias 200, 486
    factors responsible for 200f
Systematic error 486
Systematic review 16, 91, 92, 295, 486
    concept of 93f
Systematic sampling 188, 486
    technique 184, 184f
        advantages 184t
        disadvantages 184t
Systems model 110

T

Tables 348
   and table captions 297
   components of 348
   functions of 350
   list of 302, 303
   of contents 302
   title 348
   types of 350
Tabular presentation 269
Target population 174, 175, 486
Telephone interviews 216, 218, 231
Test
   assumptions of 428
   blueprint 486
   reliability, test of 248t
Testing hypothesis 417
Testing reliability, methods of 248, 252t
Test-retest method 248
Thematic apperception test 245
Themes 486
Theoretical framework 110, 314, 486
Theoretical literature 93
Theoretical papers 94
Theoretical sampling 487
Theory 57, 487
   classification of 107
   components of 106
   definitions of 105
   development of 107, 110fc
   overview of 105
   purposes of 106
   triangulation 165, 487
   types of 108, 109
Therapeutic research 487
Thesis 94, 301, 487
   format of 302t
Three-way table 350, 350t
Time
   and cost budgets 123
   and money 25
   and resources, availability of 124
   frame 60, 213
   of data collection, classification based on 131
   sampling 239
   series design 156, 487
Timeline 328
Title 326
   page 302
Tools used for
   structured observation 236b
   unstructured observation 238
Topic, nature of 202

Total fertility rate 463
T-probability, distribution of 489
Translation/application 321
Translational research 16
Trend flow diagram 519
Trend statement checklist 515
Triangulation 487
True experimental designs 143
   characteristics of 143f
   essential characteristics of 143
   limitations of 153
   strengths of 152
   types of 145fc
True experimental methods, use of 25
T-table value 430
T-test 196, 198, 272, 428, 487
   types of 429
Two data sets 374t
Two sample T-test 422, 430
Two-stage sampling 186
Two-tailed test 418, 419, 487, 496
Two-way table 350, 350t
Typical descriptive design 128, 128f

U

Unimodal distribution 487
Univariate analysis 272, 487
Univariate linear regression 409
Universal assumptions 75
Unstructured interview 230, 487
Unstructured observation 237, 487
Upper class limit 339
Use interviews 226
Use nonparametric test 424
Use observation method 234
Use parametric tests 423
Use quotation 306
Use relevant sources 96
Use surveys 216b
Using mathematical formulae 199
Using published tables 199
Utilization of research findings, barriers in 322

V

Validation 320
Validity 251, 488
   types of 253f, 255, 255t
Vancouver style 305
Variability
   degree of 197
   measures of 271, 374, 375, 375f
Variables 43, 68, 265, 327, 488

conceptual and operational definitions of 74
measuring 71
number of 196
types of 68, 68*f*
Variance 72, 73, 380, 488
across groups, homogeneity of 429
computing one-way analysis of 435
formulae for 381*t*
Variation, coefficient of 382, 473
Verbal projective techniques 245
Verifiability 7, 9
Verifying data 284
Vignettes 245
Visual analog scale 244, 244*f*, 488
Vital statistics 457
basic formulae in 460
basic measurements in 461
sources of 457, 458*f*
user of 459
Vulnerable populations 488

W

Watson's theory of human caring 109
Web surveys 217, 218
Wilcoxon signed-rank test 448, 488, 496

Wild code 268
removal of 268
Work plan 328
Wrap up interview 229
Writing
bibliography 293
case report 511
final draft 293
reference
different styles of 306
report 292, 293*f*
Vancouver style of 307, 307*t*
review 98, 99
style 313
Written survey 137

Y

Yates correction 442
criteria for 442
formula 442
Yearbooks 95

Z

Z-score 488
Z-test 272